Oculoplastic Surgery

*Educational grant very kindly provided by Altomed Limited
to support this publication*

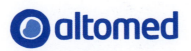

Oculoplastic Surgery

Second Edition

Brian Leatherbarrow BSc MBChB DO FRCS FRCOphth
Consultant Ophthalmologist and Ophthalmic Plastic Surgeon
Manchester Royal Eye Hospital
Oxford Road
Manchester, UK
www.eyelidsurgery.co.uk

Artwork by

Philip Ferguson Jones MMAA RMIP
Medical Illustrator
www.medicalartwork.co.uk

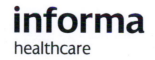

informa
healthcare

First edition published in 2002 by Martin Dunitz Ltd., The Livery House, 7-9 Pratt Street, London, UK.
This edition published in 2011 by Informa Healthcare, Telephone House, 69-77 Paul Street, London EC2A 4LQ, UK.

Simultaneously published in the USA by Informa Healthcare, 52 Vanderbilt Avenue, 7th Floor, New York, NY 10017, USA.

Informa Healthcare is a trading division of Informa UK Ltd. Registered Office: 37–41 Mortimer Street, London W1T 3JH, UK. Registered in England and Wales number 1072954.

A CIP record for this book is available from the British Library.

Library of Congress Cataloging-in-Publication Data available on application

ISBN-13: 9781841846859

Orders may be sent to: Informa Healthcare, Sheepen Place, Colchester, Essex CO3 3LP, UK
Telephone: +44 (0)20 7017 5540
Email: CSDhealthcarebooks@informa.com
Website: http://informahealthcarebooks.com/

For corporate sales please contact: CorporateBooksIHC@informa.com
For foreign rights please contact: RightsIHC@informa.com
For reprint permissions please contact: PermissionsIHC@informa.com

Typeset by Exeter Premedia Services Private Ltd., Chennai, India
Printed and bound in the United Kingdom

Dedication

This book is dedicated to my wife Angela, my son Michael and my daughter Erin.

Contents

Foreword   Keith D. Carter   *vii*
Preface   *viii*
Acknowledgments   *ix*

Basic Principles

1 Surgical principles   1

2 Applied anatomy   28

Eyelid Surgery

3 Lower eyelid entropion   75

4 Upper eyelid entropion   94

5 Abnormal eyelashes   106

6 Lower eyelid ectropion   110

7 Blepharoptosis   136

8 The management of thyroid-related
   eyelid retraction   177

9 Facial palsy   192

10 Eyelid/periocular tumors   205

11 Management of malignant eyelid/periocular tumors   227

12 Eyelid and periocular reconstruction   233

13 The use of autologous grafts in ophthalmic
    plastic surgery   279

Cosmetic Surgery

14 The evaluation and management of the
    cosmetic patient   300

15 Blepharoplasty   310

16 The management of brow ptosis   346

Orbital Surgery

17 Orbital disorders   362

18 Surgical approaches to the orbit   397

19 Thyroid eye disease   419

Lacrimal Surgery

20 The diagnosis and management of epiphora   445

Socket Surgery

21 Enucleation and evisceration   479

22 Secondary anophthalmic socket reconstruction   499

23 Orbital exenteration   520

Trauma

24 The management of eyelid and lacrimal trauma   531

25 Orbital wall blowout fractures   547

26 Zygomatic complex fractures   563

27 Other orbital fractures   569

28 Traumatic optic neuropathy   572

Index   *575*

Foreword

It is an honor to write the foreword to the second edition of Brian Leatherbarrow's *Oculoplastic Surgery*. There are many books in print addressing surgery in the periocular region, but this second edition of *Oculoplastic Surgery* is a must for all readers that want a refreshing and comprehensive approach to these surgical procedures. Brian Leatherbarrow brings a different perspective due to his combined training in England with Mr. Richard Collin and in the United States with Dr. Jeffrey Nerad and myself. During my time with Brian, I noted that he always approached patients in an organized manner based on facial and periorbital anatomical relationships. I have adopted some of his approaches, which have improved the surgical care of patients in my practice. Brian combines the best of his training and shares his 20 years of surgical practice in this book.

This second edition continues the practical approach to the diagnosis and management of a variety of oculoplastic, orbital, and lacrimal challenges. Brian shares his experience through the complete and anatomically-based descriptions of surgical procedures that have brought satisfactory results to his patients over the years. The chapters are comprehensive with regard to clinical presentations, patient selection, surgical indications, technical aspects of procedures, salient features for successful procedures, and potential complications. His narrative is exquisitely accented with both illustrations and numerous color photos of procedures and patients. Each chapter ends with suggested reading for further investigation. This approach provides an engaging presentation for the interested reader and a concise method of teaching that guides you to successful surgical procedures. This book adds to our understanding of the treatment of patients with oculoplastic conditions.

I congratulate Brian for undertaking the enormous task of a second edition to an already excellent textbook. There are ample improvements in this edition that will satisfy readers from any field with an interest in the area of oculoplastic and reconstructive surgery.

Keith D. Carter MD FACS
Lillian C & C.S. O'Brien Chair in Ophthalmology
Professor of Ophthalmology and Otolaryngology
University of Iowa
Iowa City, Iowa, USA

Preface

This book has been written with the intention of providing the reader with a pragmatic approach to the diagnosis and management of patients presenting with a broad range of oculoplastic, orbital, and lacrimal problems. Although aimed primarily at the ophthalmologist with a special interest in the subject, it should prove very useful to clinicians of all grades and experience in a number of other specialties that share an interest in the fields of ophthalmic plastic and reconstructive surgery, orbital and lacrimal surgery:

- Plastic surgeons
- Maxillofacial surgeons
- ENT surgeons
- Neurosurgeons
- Dermatologists and dermatological surgeons
- Radiologists

The reader should already have acquired a basic knowledge of eyelid, orbital, and facial anatomy and should seek to expand this knowledge as much as possible. As the eye, periocular area, and orbit represent a major crossroads of surgical anatomical dissection, the surgeon who wishes to contribute to this field should acquire a very detailed knowledge of the anatomy of this area and its adjacent structures. Applied anatomy relevant to each disorder and to each surgical procedure is presented in a dedicated chapter and the operative procedures described are based on anatomical principles as much as possible.

Important principles are highlighted in the text as key points in boxes. Pertinent clinical signs, investigations, surgical indications, important technical considerations, and complications receive appropriate emphasis in each chapter. The surgical techniques and procedures described are not exhaustive but represent those most commonly used in the author's own surgical practice. The text is accompanied by a considerable number of high-quality color photographs and complementary original illustrations. References have not been cited throughout the text; instead, further reading lists have been provided at the end of each chapter to serve as a starting point for those who may wish to pursue additional information.

Brian Leatherbarrow

Acknowledgments

I wish to convey my sincere gratitude to a number of people without whose assistance, time, influence, support, and encouragement I would not have been able to complete this work.

My wife, Angela, has shown enormous patience and forbearance in allowing me to write the second edition of this book in my "spare time" and during our holidays over a period of two years, 2008–2010.

My medical illustrator, Philip Jones, has devoted an enormous amount of time to this second edition. I am grateful not only for his skill and his patience but also for his enthusiasm, commitment, and great desire to achieve accuracy and effect in the many detailed drawings he has made. He has painstakingly observed my surgical procedures in order to achieve the best results.

My consultant anesthetic colleague and very close friend, Dr. Roger Slater, has taken most of the intraoperative photographs for me. I am grateful not only for the skill he has demonstrated in this task but for the dedication, patience, and forbearance he has displayed to me and my team over the last 17 years during our very lengthy operating sessions together. I am indebted to him. I, and my patients, have benefited enormously from his skills and experience in both general and local sedation anesthetic techniques that he has perfected for the safe delivery of anesthesia to patients undergoing the wide range of surgical procedures described in this book.

Lucy Clarke and Paul Cannon, my oculoplastic and orbital fellows at Manchester Royal Eye Hospital at the time of completion of this book, have given generously of their time in reviewing some of the manuscripts for this volume. I have appreciated their helpful suggestions, and constructive criticisms. I am also grateful to my consultant colleagues Austin McCormick and Bertie Fernando, and to Reshma Thampy and Konal Saha, specialist registrars, and to John Cooper, oculoplastic nurse practitioner, who have also very kindly reviewed manuscripts for me.

I am hugely indebted to my original preceptors Mr. JRO Collin, Dr. JA Nerad, and Dr. KD Carter from whose outstanding teaching and exemplary clinical and surgical skills I have benefited so much. They have greatly influenced the treatment philosophies and surgical approaches outlined in this text. I am also indebted to Mr. John Lendrum, consultant plastic surgeon, who very generously allowed me to assist at many operations and observe his head and neck plastic surgery practice for over a year before I embarked on my training fellowships in oculoplastic surgery at Moorfields Eye Hospital, London, UK, and in oculoplastic and orbital surgery at the University of Iowa, Iowa City, Iowa, USA.

I have been extremely privileged to have worked for many years in close cooperation with very skilled and excellent colleagues in other specialties who have been very generous in sharing their skills and knowledge with me. I am particularly indebted to Mr. Peter Richardson, consultant neurosurgeon, Dr. Roger Laitt, consultant neuro-radiologist, Dr. Nick Telfer, consultant dermatological and Mohs' micrographic surgeon, Mr. David Whitby, consultant plastic surgeon, Dr. Richard Bonshek, consultant ophthalmic histopathologist, and Mr. Elgan Davies, consultant ENT surgeon. In recent years I have also enjoyed the support of my close consultant oculoplastic colleagues and friends Mr. Saj Ataullah and Miss Anne Cook.

I am obliged to my colleagues in the Department of Medical Illustration at Manchester Royal Eye Hospital for their help with many of the photographs used in this book. I am particularly grateful to my friends and colleagues in the Department of Ocular Prosthetics at Manchester Royal Eye Hospital and to my dedicated oculoplastic nursing team, who have lent me such support with my work over many years.

I wish to acknowledge the multitude of patients who have so kindly and generously agreed to the use of their photographs for this book. I am also particularly grateful to so many colleagues throughout the United Kingdom and in many countries throughout the world who have referred so many challenging patients without whom this book would not have been possible.

Educational grant kindly provided to support this publication
by Karl Storz Endoscopy UK Ltd

1   Surgical principles

INTRODUCTION

The fundamental principles and techniques essential to success in ophthalmic plastic surgery are similar to those which underlie other branches of surgery. Careful attention to detail, meticulous surgical technique, and an utmost respect for the functional requirement of the eye are of paramount importance. The surgeon who is well versed in fundamental surgical principles and techniques will avoid unnecessary complications and the requirement for secondary procedures. In this chapter, the following basic principles will be discussed:

1. Preoperative patient evaluation
2. Documentation
3. Selection of the appropriate surgical procedure
4. Surgical planning and communication
5. Selection of the most appropriate type of anesthesia
6. Surgical instrumentation
7. Correct surgical site marking and allergy check
8. Preparation and draping of the patient
9. Surgical incision and exposure
10. Hemostasis
11. Wound closure
12. Postoperative pain management
13. Postoperative care

PREOPERATIVE PATIENT EVALUATION

The surgeon should develop a routine for questioning and examining patients in order not to omit important questions or crucial aspects of the examination. Obtaining a careful detailed history about the presenting problem from the patient is essential. Details should also be obtained about the past ophthalmic history, past medical and surgical history, current medications, allergies, family, and social history. Time spent in obtaining the history has additional benefits:

1. It provides the surgeon with information about the patient's potential expectations.
2. It provides an opportunity for the surgeon to establish a rapport with the patient.
3. It allows the surgeon to simply observe the patient and detect subtle physical signs, which may otherwise be overlooked, e.g., signs of aberrant re-innervation of the facial nerve, blepharospasm, hemifacial spasm, an abnormal head posture, frontalis overaction, and facial asymmetries.

The examination of the patient should be methodical. A record of the patient's corrected visual acuity and a basic ophthalmic examination should form part of the assessment of every patient presenting with an eyelid, orbital or lacrimal disorder. The detailed examination methods for various conditions are discussed in the ensuing chapters. Any ancillary laboratory or imaging investigations should be selected on the basis of the clinical evaluation of the patient and not simply performed as a blind "work-up."

It may be helpful to obtain copies of patient records from other institutions where the patient has previously been treated. The details of previous surgical procedures, the results of previous investigations and imaging, and original histology slides should be sought wherever this is relevant. A review of previous imaging and histology slides rather than a reliance on previous reports can prove to be invaluable.

DOCUMENTATION

The surgeon must ensure careful and accurate documentation of the history and examination findings as well as the diagnosis, management plan, and preoperative discussion with the patient.

Preoperative photographs are essential for the vast majority of patients who are to undergo ophthalmic plastic and reconstructive surgery. They serve a number of useful purposes:

1. A learning and teaching aid for the surgeon
2. A verification of the patient's disorder for health care insurance companies
3. An aid to defense in the event of a medicolegal claim
4. An aid to the patient in legal proceedings following accidents and assaults
5. To jolt the postoperative memory of the forgetful patient

> **KEY POINTS**
>
> Written patient consent should be obtained before the photographs are taken. It should be made clear to the patient how the photographs may be used.

The treatment options should be discussed with the patient. This should include the option of not being treated. The advantages, disadvantages, risks, and potential complications should be discussed with the patient and relatives if possible. The risks and the incidence of complications need to be outlined in an open and honest manner. Serious or frequently occurring risks must be discussed and documented. This should be undertaken in a manner which neither frightens nor offends. The consequences of complications and their management should also be outlined. If the patient expresses the wish not to be given this information, this must be clearly documented. The consultation should be followed by a detailed letter summarizing this information which should be sent to the patient's family practitioner and a copy should be sent to the patient or, in the case of children, to the parents.

Any surgical procedure can have serious complications. The surgeon should therefore avoid describing any periocular procedure as "basic," "straightforward," "simple," "minor," or "routine."

A surgeon who is fully conversant with the nature of the surgery, and who is qualified to take informed consent from a patient, should complete the surgical consent form. The consent form must be legible and must document the correct side and the precise details of the surgical procedure to be undertaken without the use of abbreviations. Serious or frequently occurring risks must be documented on the consent form and in the patient's records.

SELECTION OF THE APPROPRIATE SURGICAL PROCEDURE

The surgical procedure that is best suited to the individual requirements of the patient should be selected, e.g., a patient whose other eye is not functional should not be subjected to a Hughes tarsoconjunctival flap procedure for the reconstruction of a lower eyelid defect. An alternative surgical procedure should be selected.

An operation which is not indicated will not benefit a patient no matter how skillfully it is performed, e.g., a patient whose blepharoptosis is due to giant papillary conjunctivitis which has been overlooked by the failure to evert the upper eyelid will not benefit from any surgical procedure.

The patient's age and general health must be taken into consideration. It must also be borne in mind that under certain circumstances the patient's best interests may be served by advising against surgical intervention.

SURGICAL PLANNING AND COMMUNICATION

Each procedure should be planned carefully. Preoperative planning ensures that the surgical team is aware of the required instrumentation and materials. For elective operations, it is ideal to run a pre-assessment clinic in conjunction with a specialist oculoplastic nurse(s) who can coordinate preoperative investigations, ensure that investigation results are communicated to the anesthetist, communicate potential problems to the GP, e.g., previously undiagnosed hypertension, and liaise with the operating theatre nursing team, e.g., to ensure that the required range of orbital implant sizes and socket conformers is available. The operating list should be detailed and should not contain abbreviations.

The scrub nurse needs to be aware of the required preparation and draping of the patient, e.g., the proposed site for the harvesting of a skin graft or dermis fat graft. This ensures that the procedure can be performed efficiently, minimizing tissue exposure, operating and anesthetic time, and thereby minimizing risks to the patient. Preoperative planning is essential when operating as a team with other surgical disciplines.

The lead surgeon responsible for coordinating the preparations for surgery should be decided in advance.

The details of the planned surgical approach should be communicated to the anesthetist. The anesthetist is an essential member of the team and should know details about the following:

- The anticipated duration of the operation
- Special positioning of the patient, e.g., to harvest a dermis fat graft from the buttock
- The potential sites for harvesting autologous tissue, e.g., upper inner arm which may affect the siting of intravenous lines and a blood pressure cuff
- The requirement for hypotensive anesthesia
- The potential blood loss
- The potential risk of an oculocardiac reflex, e.g., during an enucleation or secondary orbital implant procedure
- Vasoactive agents to be used intraoperatively, including their concentration and volume, e.g., subcutaneous local anesthetic agent injections with adrenaline, topical intranasal cocaine solution
- The potential for postoperative pain, e.g., severe pain may be experienced following an enucleation with placement of an orbital implant requiring opiate analgesia, whereas severe pain following a lateral orbitotomy may indicate a retrobulbar hemorrhage which should be investigated and not merely suppressed with opiates
- The necessity to avoid anti-inflammatory agents for a patient following intraorbital surgery
- The requirement for a throat pack
- The requirement to position the endotracheal tube in a specific location, e.g., to one side of the mouth or intranasally when harvesting a mucous membrane graft or hard palate graft

The timing of surgical intervention may be crucial to the outcome, e.g., an orbital floor blowout fracture with signs of orbital tissue entrapment in a child should be managed without delay in contrast to the same clinical scenario in an adult where a delay of 10 to 14 days or more is usually advisable. Any significant delay in the management of the child could result in an ischemic contracture of the inferior rectus muscle with a poor prognosis for the restoration of a satisfactory field of binocular single vision.

SELECTION OF THE MOST APPROPRIATE TYPE OF ANESTHESIA

The types of anesthesia available are:

1. Topical anesthesia
2. Local anesthesia
3. Local anesthesia with intravenous sedation
4. Regional anesthesia
5. General anesthesia

The selection of the type of anesthesia for an individual patient depends on:

- The age of the patient
- The general health and emotional status of the patient

- The extent and anticipated duration of the surgery
- The requirement for intraoperative patient cooperation

The type of anaesthesia should allow the surgeon to complete the surgery in a safe and controlled manner while providing the best possible degree of comfort for the patient. This should be discussed with the patient in clinic.

Topical Anesthesia

Local anesthesia may be applied topically, e.g., proxymethocaine by pledget in the inferior fornix in order to perform a forced duction test. Proxymethocaine causes a minimal degree of discomfort and acts very rapidly. For this reason it is preferred to other topical anesthetic agents for surface anesthesia of the cornea and the conjunctiva. It should be borne in mind that topical anesthetic agents last for a short period of time and should be instilled at regular intervals during surgery on the conscious patient. Care should also be taken to ensure that the anesthetized cornea is protected during the course of surgery, e.g., Lacrilube ointment should be instilled into both eyes of a patient following the application of the topical anesthetic agent if a traction suture has not been used to close the eye.

Topical agents applied to the skin are very useful to reduce the pain of injections, e.g., EMLA cream, which contains lidocaine and prilocaine, applied to the eyelids prior to the injection of a local anesthetic agent. A minimum period of 10 to 15 min should be allowed and great care should be taken to ensure that the cream does not enter the eye. The same topical agent can be very effective for other procedures, e.g., the injection of a soft tissue filler for the cosmetic improvement of nasolabial folds associated with a mid-face ptosis. It should be borne in mind, however, that a minimum period of 30 to 45 min is required for the topical agent to take effect in an area of the face where the skin has a much greater thickness.

Topical cocaine 5% is a very effective topical anesthetic agent for use in intranasal surgery, e.g., a dacryocystorhinostomy (DCR). Co-phenylcaine (phenylephrine–lidocaine mixture) nasal spray is a very effective topical anesthetic agent for use in intranasal examinations and minor intranasal procedures in clinic.

Local Anesthesia

Local anesthesia is most commonly achieved by local infiltration with either lidocaine 2% containing 1:80,000 units of adrenaline for relatively short procedures or bupivacaine (0.5% for adults and 0.25% for children) containing 1:200,000 units of adrenaline for longer procedures. For some procedures, it is preferable to use a 50:50 mixture of lidocaine and bupivacaine. A period of 5 to 10 min should be allowed for the local anesthetic agent and the adrenaline to take effect. The duration of action of lidocaine is approximately 45 to 60 min while that of bupivacaine is approximately 2 to 3 hours. The amount of local anesthetic agent used in relation to the age and body weight of the patient should be noted and care taken not to exceed safe levels, particularly in children. The anesthetic agent should be warmed prior to use to reduce the pain associated with its injection.

Subcutaneous injections in the eyelid should be placed just beneath the skin, avoiding injections into the orbicularis muscle. This reduces the risk of causing a hematoma, which can distort the tissue planes and cause a mechanical ptosis in the upper eyelid, making ptosis surgery more difficult to perform. The volume used in the eyelids should rarely exceed 2 ml per eyelid for most procedures. A 25-gauge, 24-mm needle is used to avoid the need for multiple injections, which further predispose to bleeding and hematoma. Injections into the eyelid should be performed from the temporal side of the patient, with the needle parallel to the eyelid. This reduces the risk of perforation of the globe in the event of sudden inadvertent movement of the patient. Immediate pressure and massage should be applied over the injection site for 5 mins.

Additional local anesthetic agent should be kept available in a sterile syringe on the scrub nurse's trolley if required during the surgical procedure.

Local Aanesthesia with Sedation

Many oculoplastic procedures can be safely and satisfactorily performed with the use of a combination of local anesthesia and neuroleptic sedation. An anaesthetist can provide safe conscious sedation, and monitoring and management if required of a variety of medical conditions, e.g., hypertension, arrhythmias, while providing safe intravenous sedation, which can be titrated to the individual patient's requirements and rapidly reversed. The agents most commonly used for this purpose are a combination of Midazolam and Propofol. This is ideal for the anxious patient who requires a levator aponeurosis advancement procedure. The patient is sedated during the administration of the injections but is fully cooperative during the intraoperative assessment and adjustment of the eyelid height and contour. For a more invasive, potentially painful procedure, e.g., an enucleation, an opiate can be used in addition, e.g., Remifentanil, a potent ultra short-acting synthetic opioid analgesic drug. The agents to be used by the anaesthetist should be selected taking into consideration whether or not the patient is undergoing the procedure on a day case or an in-patient basis.

Great care must be taken when administering periocular local anesthetic injections to a sedated patient. Such a patient may lose all inhibitions and become aggressive during a painful injection. This should be anticipated and assistance sought to prevent the patient from moving or raising his/her hands toward the face. This is particularly important in younger strong patients. In addition, the operating team and the anesthetist should be fully aware of the risk posed by the sternutatory reflex (from the Latin: sternuere, to sneeze). This reflex affects a large proportion of patients sedated with Midazolam and Propofol. The reflex is suppressed by deep sedation and by the additional administration of an opiate, e.g., Remifentanil. The reflex may occur without warning and poses a risk during the administration of local anesthesia around the eye.

KEY POINTS

Safe conscious sedation for oculoplastic procedures requires skill and experience on the part of the anesthetist, a good understanding of the procedure to be performed and the surgeon's requirements. Intravenous sedation should be used with great caution during lacrimal drainage surgery, as the airway may not be adequately protected from the effects of bleeding or use of irrigation fluid.

Regional Anesthesia

Regional nerve blocks are useful to supplement the effects of subcutaneous injections for a limited number of surgical procedures under local anesthesia. An infratrochlear block can be combined with local tissue infiltration and intranasal cocaine for an external DCR. A peribulbar injection of 0.5% bupivacaine with 1:200,000 units of adrenaline mixed with hyaluronidase is ideal for an enucleation or an evisceration procedure. Regional nerve blocks targeting the supraorbital, supratrochlear, infratrochlear, infraorbital, zygomatico-facial, zygomatico-temporal, and lacrimal nerves in addition to such a peribulbar injection, in combination with safe intravenous sedation, can permit an orbital exenteration to be performed on a conscious patient who is unfit for general anesthesia.

General Anesthesia

General anesthesia is required for children and uncooperative patients and is indicated for longer and more extensive surgical procedures, e.g., a lateral orbitotomy. It is also required for patients undergoing procedures that are likely to result in bleeding from the nose or mouth in order to protect the airway. The patient's general health will determine the suitability of the patient for general anesthesia. The patient with a history of general medical disorders who is to undergo elective surgery should be identified to the anesthetist at the pre-assessment clinic.

Bupivacaine injections containing adrenaline (1:200,000 units) are used in combination with general anesthesia to assist hemostasis and to provide immediate postoperative pain relief. The use of such injections in combination with hyaluronidase prior to enucleation or evisceration surgery can be very effective in blocking the effects of the oculocardiac reflex. The anesthetist should be made aware of the potential for such a reflex, which can cause severe bradycardia and, rarely, asystole.

SURGICAL INSTRUMENTATION

The variety of delicate surgical instruments used in ophthalmic plastic surgery attests to the special demands of surgery in this region.

A basic ophthalmic plastic surgery instrument set should be available for oculoplastic cases (Fig. 1.1). Separate instrument sets should be available for enucleation/evisceration (Fig. 1.2), external DCR (Fig. 1.3), endoscopic DCR and endoscopic brow lift surgery (Fig. 1.4), and orbital surgery (Fig. 1.5). A variety of accessory instruments should be readily available (Fig. 1.6). These instruments must be kept in good repair and should be respected and used appropriately. Alternatively, consideration can be given to the use of disposable instruments which are now of very good quality. Inappropriate use of instruments can result in damage to delicate instruments and damage to tissues. The nurse assistant should ensure that dried blood, tissue, and char are carefully removed from the instruments as these are handed back during the course of surgery. The surgeon should ensure that the instruments are carefully handed to the nurse assistant, avoiding injury from sharp blades and needles.

KEY POINT

The surgeon should ensure that instruments are never passed across the patient's face.

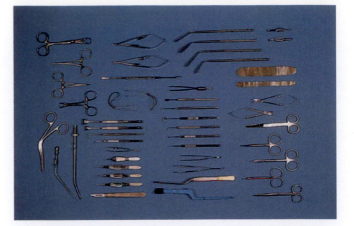

Figure 1.1 A basic oculoplastic instrument set (non-disposable).

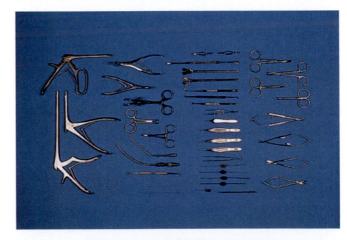

Figure 1.2 An enucleation/evisceration instrument set used in conjunction with a basic oculoplastic set.

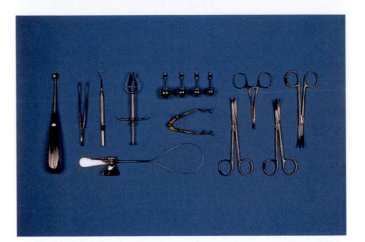

Figure 1.3 An external DCR instrument set.

A number of basic principles apply to the use of ophthalmic instruments. Toothed forceps or skin hooks should be used to avoid crushing and damaging tissue. A variety of forceps of varying size are available and should be selected according to the type of tissue to be handled. The most commonly used toothed forceps to assist with dissection of the eyelids are Paufique forceps. The 0.12 Castroviejo forceps are ideal for the handling of delicate eyelid skin when suturing. Skin hooks

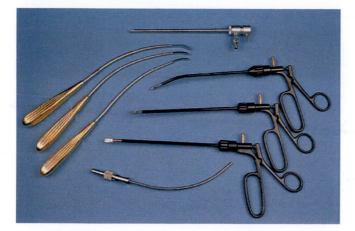

Figure 1.4 Endoscopic brow lift instruments.

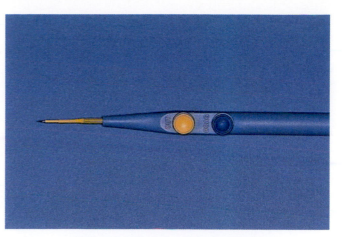

Figure 1.7 A Colorado needle and hand piece.

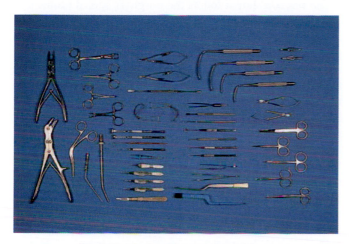

Figure 1.5 A basic orbitotomy instrument set.

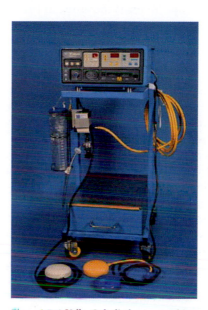

Figure 1.8 A Valley Lab diathermy machine.

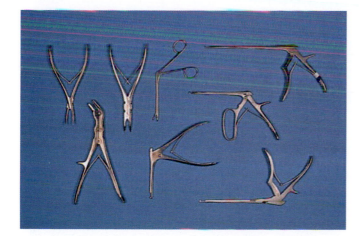

Figure 1.6 A variety of accessory bone rongeurs and forceps for orbital surgery.

must be handled with great care to avoid inadvertent injury to the globe. The eyelid skin is very delicate and it is preferable to hold and lift the underlying orbicularis muscle, and not the skin, to dissect underlying tissue planes. Adson forceps are more robust and are used for handling the cheek, lower face, and scalp tissues.

A variety of scissors may be used during surgery. These are curved, straight, sharp, or blunt-tipped. Curved, blunt-tipped

Westcott scissors are used for the dissection of tissue planes in eyelid surgery and conjunctival surgery. They should not be used to blunt dissect tissue planes. Steven's tenotomy scissors are more appropriate for this purpose and for the dissection of thicker tissue, e.g., a glabellar flap. Westcott scissors should not be used for cutting sutures. Sharp-tipped Westcott scissors are used for punctal surgery, e.g., a three-snip procedure, and for the removal of the posterior eyelid margin in a lateral tarsorrhaphy.

The more gross separation of tissue planes should be accomplished with blunt-tipped Stevens tenotomy scissors which minimize the risk of bleeding, e.g., they are used to blunt dissect Tenon's fascia from the globe in an enucleation, and the orbicularis muscle in an external DCR. Sharp-tipped iris scissors are used for performing eyelid wedge resections. Small suture scissors should be used for cutting sutures.

A Colorado needle is an efficient instrument for the precise, delicate and bloodless dissection of tissue planes in the eyelids. An earthing plate must first be attached to the patient and care must be taken to ensure that the patient has removed all metallic objects from their clothing. The needle has both cutting and monopolar coagulation modes (Fig. 1.7). It is used in conjunction with a Valley Lab diathermy machine (Fig. 1.8). The author uses this instrument ubiquitously in his practice for making skin crease incisions, subciliary incisions, and transconjunctival incisions in addition to general eyelid dissections, e.g., to perform blepharoplasties, to expose the levator aponeurosis, and the inferior orbital margin. Alternatively, it can be used for soft tissue dissection in the eyelids after making the initial skin incision with a no. 15 Bard Parker blade. Its use requires a dry surgical field. The tissues to be dissected should be held under some tension. The tip of the needle should be moved constantly across the tissue to be dissected when the instrument is activated to avoid burning the tissues and should be used with a delicate stroking motion without applying pressure to the tissues.

Artery clips are used routinely to fixate traction sutures and Jaffe retractor bands to the surgical drapes. It is preferable to use curved clips that lie flat against the surface of the drapes unlike straight clips. To fixate the suture or bands, one limb of the clips should lie beneath a fold of the drapes before the clips are closed.

Enucleation scissors in a variety of curvatures and sizes should be available and used whenever the use of a snare is inappropriate, e.g., where a long piece of optic nerve is required, the presence of a soft globe, a previous corneal section, or a penetrating keratoplasty. A snare may transect the posterior aspect of a soft globe and can cause a globe weakened by previous surgery to rupture causing intraocular fluid to spray out under pressure. A snare is otherwise very useful for enucleation surgery and its use is associated with minimal bleeding (Fig. 1.9).

Spring handle needle holders are available in a variety of sizes and may be curved or straight. These are excellent for use in oculoplastic surgery. These are selected according to the size of needle to be used. Needle holders designed to hold small needles, e.g., 7/0 Vicryl, will be damaged if used inappropriately to hold larger needles. The Castroviejo needle holders are preferred as these have a simple locking mechanism that permits the needle to be loaded securely and held between suture passes. Ring handle needle holders (e.g., the Webster needle holder) are used to hold suture needles larger than 4/0 in size.

A variety of bone punches are available for bone removal, e.g., for an external DCR (Fig. 1.6). It is important that these are used appropriately. The delicate bone of the lacrimal fossa floor can be removed using a fine punch, e.g., a Hardy sella

punch. This should then be replaced by progressively larger Kerrison rongeurs for the removal of the anterior lacrimal crest and nasal bone. The continued use of the delicate Hardy sella punch for the thicker bone will result in damage to this instrument.

CORRECT SURGICAL SITE MARKING AND ALLERGY CHECK

It is the responsibility of the surgeon to ensure that he/she has seen the patient prior to surgery and has clearly marked the correct surgical site after carefully checking the patient's consent form and the patient's identification bracelet. When the patient arrives in the anesthetic room the surgeon should pause. The pause before anesthesia and surgery begin is known as "time out" and is intended to make everyone slow down for a few moments and double check what they are about to do.

The surgeon should follow the hospital's agreed protocol to ensure that the correct patient has arrived, that every member of the surgical team agrees that the correct operation is to be performed on the correct side, that the appropriate scans are available, and that all required surgical equipment, implants, and disposables are available. In addition, where appropriate, the availability of cross-matched blood should be checked and the availability of a pathologist confirmed whenever a frozen section is required. A checklist should be completed and signed.

The surgeon should check the patient's allergy history prior to giving any injections and prior to prepping the patient. The surgeon should also inform the anesthetist prior to the administration of any injections. The surgeon should always prep and drape the patient himself/herself, and should not allow himself/herself to be distracted during this very important process.

The surgeon should also ensure that all members of the surgical team are wearing eye protection prior to the commencement of surgery and that suction is available for the evacuation of surgical smoke.

KEY POINT

Ensure that "time out" is called prior to the commencement of anesthesia and surgery.

PREPARATION AND DRAPING OF THE PATIENT

If the patient is under local anesthesia, with or without sedation, the whole of the patient's face should be cleaned with Betadine diluted 50:50 with sterile water, commencing with the eyelids and moving outward. The face should then be dried. If the patient is under general anesthesia, the area to be operated on should be cleaned but both eyes should be left exposed whenever there is a need to check the symmetry of the globe positions. Additional areas may need to be cleaned, e.g., the postauricular area or the upper inner arm if a skin graft is required. The eyes should be instilled with Lacrilube ointment. The drapes should be applied by the surgeon so that there is no restriction on the movement of a local tissue flap or pressure on the eyebrow when undertaking a ptosis procedure.

SURGICAL INCISION AND EXPOSURE

Incisions should be planned preoperatively to provide adequate surgical access and yet result in a minimally conspicuous scar. Wherever possible, skin incisions should be planned to

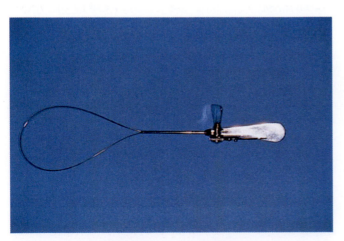

Figure 1.9 An enucleation snare.

follow the relaxed skin tension lines (RSTL). These lines lie within normal skin creases or folds, enabling incisions to be hidden or disguised (Fig. 1.10). The lines correspond to the directional pull existing in relaxed skin; this is determined by the underlying structures and the depth of subcutaneous tissue and fat. Incisions that run parallel to the RSTL tend to remain narrow after wound closure in contrast to those running perpendicular to them, which are more likely to gape.

Incisions which interrupt lymphatic drainage should be avoided, as these can lead to persistent postoperative lymphedema, e.g., incisions directly over the infraorbital margin.

Skin incisions should be marked prior to the injection of the local anesthetic agent as this may obscure anatomic landmarks, e.g., the upper eyelid skin crease. Marking is best achieved with the use of a cocktail stick inserted into a gentian violet marker block (Fig. 1.11). This results in a fine line (Fig. 1.12). Grease on the skin surface should first be removed with a small alcohol wipe.

In very young patients or in patients who are prone to hypertrophic or keloid scar formation (Fig. 1.13), skin incisions may be avoided for certain procedures, e.g., a DCR may be performed endoscopically, an orbital floor blow-out fracture may be approached via a conjunctival incision.

Skin incisions which are commonly used in ophthalmic plastic surgery are shown in Figure 1.14. The Stallard Wright lateral orbitotomy incision is used for older patients, but for younger patients an upper lid skin crease incision is used instead, and the incision carried into a "laughter" line at the lateral canthus.

Skin incisions should be made perpendicular to the skin surface, except in the eyebrow region or scalp where the incision should be beveled. For eyelid skin incisions, the Colorado needle is a very effective alternative to the use of a no. 15 Bard Parker blade. It results in less bleeding and permits a layer-by-layer dissection of the tissues, allowing identification of blood vessels which can be cauterized before they are cut.

When making a skin incision with either a blade or the Colorado needle, the incision should be made with a continuous motion to avoid jagged wound edges. The skin should be held taut. Skin incisions in the eyelids are aided by the use of 4/0 silk traction sutures placed through the gray line. A 4/0 black silk suture on a reverse-cutting needle is passed into the gray line of the eyelid and the curvature of the needle followed until the needle emerges from the gray line again. The delicate eyelid skin should be held with fine-toothed forceps, e.g., Bishop Harmon forceps. Skin hooks should be used with great care in the periocular region because of the risk of inadvertent injury to the globe.

Incisions along the gray line of the eyelids, e.g., a gray line split into the upper eyelid as part of an upper eyelid entropion procedure or in both eyelids as part of a tarsorrhaphy procedure, should be made with a Beaver micro-sharp blade (7530) on a Beaver blade handle (Fig. 1.15).

Surgical exposure is aided by the use of a variety of retractors or by the use of traction sutures. In upper eyelid levator surgery or an orbital floor fracture repair, the use of self-retaining Jaffe retractors enables the surgeon to operate without the requirement for a surgical assistant in contrast to Desmarres retractors (Figs. 1.16 and 1.17). Desmarres retractors are very useful and are available in different sizes. They are also used to evert the upper and lower eyelids in conjunction with a gray line traction suture to undertake posterior

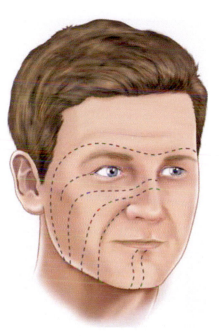

Figure 1.10 Relaxed skin tension lines.

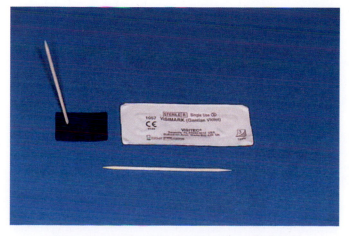

Figure 1.11 A gentian violet pad used with a cocktail stick.

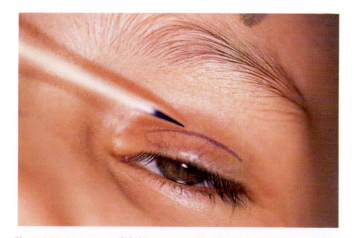

Figure 1.12 An upper eyelid skin crease incision being marked with a cocktail stick which has been inserted into a gentian violet marker pad.

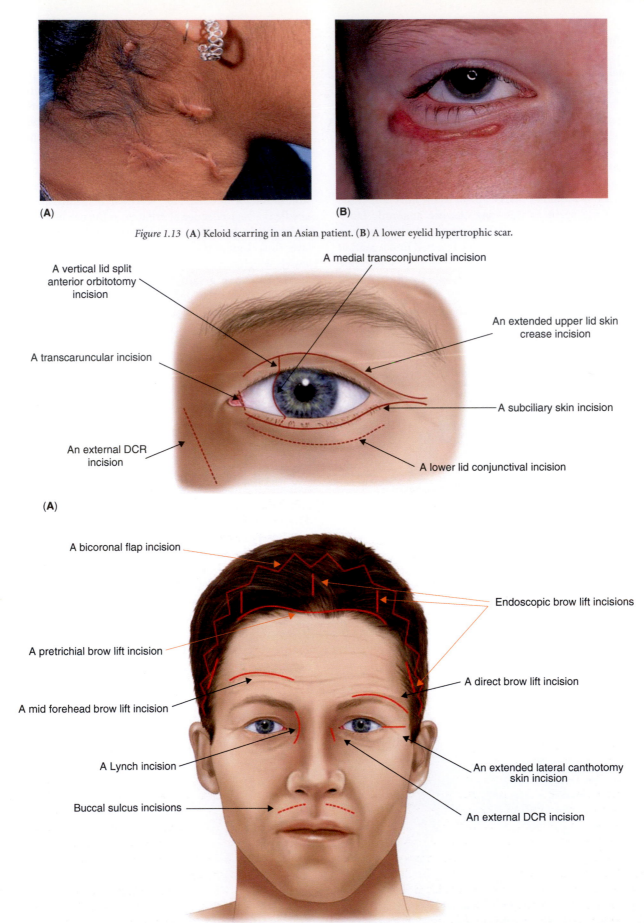

Figure 1.13 (**A**) Keloid scarring in an Asian patient. (**B**) A lower eyelid hypertrophic scar.

Figure 1.14 (**A**) Periocular incisions commonly used in ophthalmic plastic surgery. (**B**) Periocular and facial incisions commonly used in ophthalmic plastic surgery. (*Continued*)

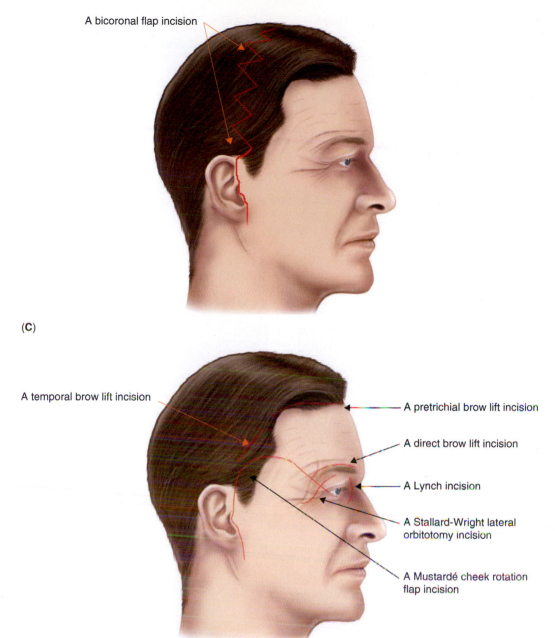

A bicoronal flap incision

(C)

A temporal brow lift incision

A pretrichial brow lift incision

A direct brow lift incision

A Lynch incision

A Stallard-Wright lateral orbitotomy incision

A Mustardé cheek rotation flap incision

(D)

Figure 1.14 (Continued) (**C**) A bi-coronal flap incision extended as a face lift incision as seen from the side. (**D**) Some examples of periocular and facial incisions commonly used in ophthalmic plastic surgery seen from the side.

approach surgery, e.g., a posterior approach Müller's muscle resection. It is important to use the appropriate size of Desmarres retractor to evert the eyelid.

Sewall retractors (Fig. 18.18) are used to retract the orbital contents during an orbital fracture repair, an orbital decompression, or during an orbital exenteration. The blades are available in different sizes and should be selected appropriately. They can be used in conjunction with a piece of Supramid to improve the retraction of orbital fat during these procedures. Typically, these retractors are placed into the subperiosteal space. Great care, however, must be taken by the assistant when using these retractors as great force can be applied to the globe. In addition, it is easy to "toe-in" the tip of the retractor and tear the periorbita. This can also lead to direct trauma to the optic nerve.

Wright's retractors (Fig. 18.19) are more delicate retractors, which are used to retract tissues in the orbit during the course of the exploration of an orbital mass or during the course of an optic nerve sheath fenestration. Malleable retractors are mainly used to protect the orbital contents from the use of drills and saws. The use of retractors in orbital surgery is discussed in more detail in chapters 17 to 19.

Traction sutures not only improve surgical exposure but also assist in hemostasis, e.g., in an external DCR (Fig. 1.18).

Safe surgical dissection is greatly facilitated by adequate magnification and illumination of the surgical field. The surgeon should wear surgical loupes, which do not unduly restrict the visual field. The loupes should be comfortable and should not require adjustment; typically, they provide 2.5 to 3.5 times magnification, and should be fitted with protective side shields (Fig. 1.19).

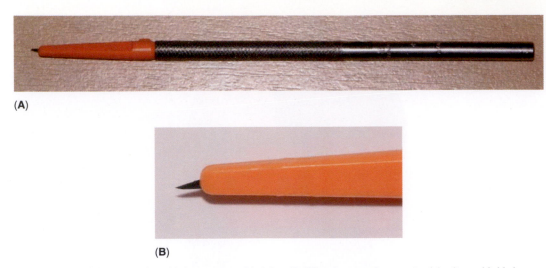

(A)

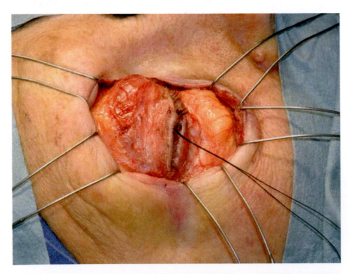

(B)

Figure 1.15 (**A**) A micro-sharp blade on a Beaver blade handle. (**B**) A close-up photograph of the disposable blade.

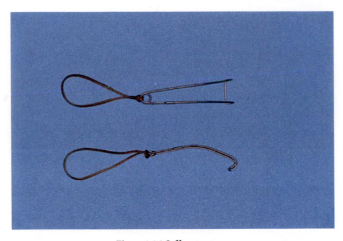

Figure 1.16 Jaffe retractors.

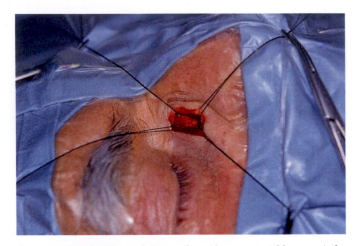

Figure 1.18 Traction sutures being used to aid exposure and hemostasis for an external dacryocystorhinostomy.

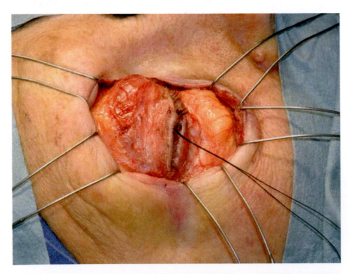

Figure 1.17 Jaffe retractors being used during the course of an orbital exenteration.

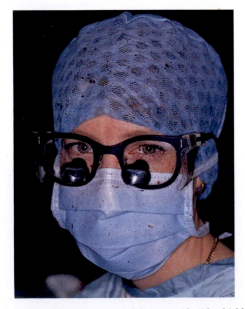

Figure 1.19 Designs for Vision surgical loupes with side shields, offering ocular protection from sudden unexpected bleeding.

The use of a headlight offers a number of advantages over an overhead operating lamp. The light is always focused on the surgical field, which is not placed in shadow by the surgeon's or assistant's hands. The use of a headlight is essential in surgery within cavities, e.g., an external DCR, an orbital decompression.

HEMOSTASIS

Meticulous attention to hemostasis is essential in ophthalmic plastic surgery. The process of hemostasis begins preoperatively and continues postoperatively. Intraoperative bleeding can obscure and distort tissue planes, making surgical dissection difficult and prolonging the operative procedure. Eyelid hematoma formation can prevent accurate intraoperative assessment of eyelid height and contour in levator surgery. Hematomas retard healing, promote scarring, and act as a nidus for the growth of microorganisms. Postoperative bleeding in the orbit can result in compressive optic neuropathy and blindness.

Preoperative Evaluation

A careful medical history should be taken to identify medical conditions which predispose the patient to intraoperative and postoperative bleeding, e.g., systemic hypertension. Steps should be taken to ensure that this is adequately controlled before surgery is undertaken, particularly for elective procedures. The patient should be questioned about any history of a bleeding disorder, a tendency to bruise easily or a prior history of intraoperative bleeding.

It is important to identify patients who have a cardiac pacemaker, as the use of a radio-frequency device is contraindicated in such patients. The use of sympathomimetic agents, e.g., adrenaline and cocaine, may be contraindicated in patients with a history of cardiac arrhythmias, myocardial infarction, cerebrovascular accident, or hypertension.

A careful drug history should be taken. The use of aspirin, nonsteroidal anti-inflammatory agents (NSAIAs), and other antiplatelet agents should be discontinued for at least 10 days prior to surgery *unless this is contraindicated*, e.g., a patient with cardiac stents or a previous history of transient ischemic attacks should not discontinue the use of prescribed aspirin. Patients should be specifically asked about the use of aspirin, as this information is rarely volunteered. It is preferable to liaise with a hematologist for the management of patients who are taking anticoagulants. Patients taking warfarin who have undergone heart valve surgery should be admitted and converted to heparin preoperatively.

Preoperative Injection

The subcutaneous/submucosal injection of local anesthetic agents containing adrenaline (1:80,000 or 1:200,000 units) is very helpful in minimizing intraoperative bleeding. Five minutes should be spent by the surgeon scrubbing, and a further 5 min should be spent prepping and draping the patient. This allows 10 min for the adrenaline to work. The anesthetist must be informed prior to the use of any adrenaline.

Nasal Packing

For operations involving the nose, e.g., external or endoscopic DCR, the nose should be packed prior to surgery with small patties or a nasal epistaxis tampon, which are moistened with 5% cocaine solution. This is very effective in decongesting the nasal mucosa. Its use may be contraindicated, e.g., in children, patients with cardiovascular disease. For these patients, oxymetazoline should be substituted. Small patties moistened in 1:1,000 units of adrenaline may be placed directly over bleeding nasal mucosa in patients without a contraindication to the use of topical adrenalin.

Positioning of the Patient

Correct positioning of the patient can aid in achieving hemostasis. A gentle head-down position allows identification of the external angular vessels prior to marking the proposed skin incision in an external DCR procedure. The patient should then be placed into a reverse Trendelenburg position as soon as this is permitted by the anesthetist. This reduces venous pressure within the head and face and can significantly reduce bleeding.

Surgical Technique

A meticulous gentle surgical technique is essential to avoid bleeding. The surgeon must be familiar with vascular anatomy of the periocular and orbital region (Fig. 1.20). The vessels which are commonly encountered in ophthalmic plastic surgery are:

1. The marginal and peripheral eyelid arcades in eyelid surgery
2. The angular vessels in an external DCR
3. Branches of the infraorbital vessels and orbital floor blowout fracture surgery/orbital decompression
4. The anterior and posterior ethmoidal vessels in an orbital exenteration, a medial orbital wall decompression/fracture repair
5. The zygomaticofacial and zygomaticotemporal vessels in a lateral orbitotomy/lateral orbital wall decompression
6. The supraorbital/supratrochlear vessels in brow lift surgery

The use of the Colorado needle aids meticulous surgical dissection with ready identification of tissue planes. The tissue must be handled with great care to avoid tearing and maceration. It is essential to avoid traction on orbital fat, which can risk rupture of deeper orbital vessels. The surgical dissection should be restricted to that required to expose the area of interest.

Blunt dissection can avoid unnecessary intraoperative bleeding; e.g., in secondary orbital implant surgery, blunt dissection of deep orbital fibrous bands with blunt-tipped Steven's tenotomy scissors, also aided by digital dissection, is preferred.

The Application of External Pressure

Intraoperative pressure tamponade is useful to assist hemostasis prior to the application of cautery. It is particularly useful following enucleation. Postoperatively, capillary oozing may be limited by the application of a pressure dressing. This is particularly useful following anophthalmic socket surgery. It must be used with great caution, however, in situations where postoperative bleeding may lead to compressive optic neuropathy, e.g., following an anterior orbitotomy for an incisional orbital biopsy.

Suction

Suction is an important aid to hemostasis and must be used appropriately. There are a number of different suction tips available which should be selected according to the surgery to

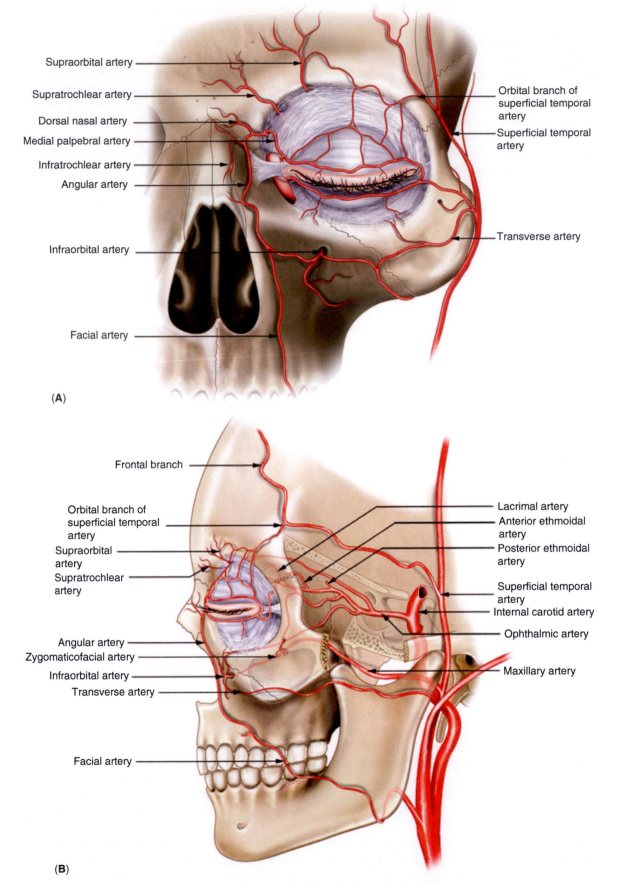

Supraorbital artery

Supratrochlear artery

Dorsal nasal artery

Medial palpebral artery

Infratrochlear artery

Angular artery

Infraorbital artery

Facial artery

Orbital branch of superficial temporal artery

Superficial temporal artery

Transverse artery

(A)

Frontal branch

Orbital branch of superficial temporal artery

Supraorbital artery

Supratrochlear artery

Angular artery

Zygomaticofacial artery

Infraorbital artery

Transverse artery

Facial artery

Lacrimal artery

Anterior ethmoidal artery

Posterior ethmoidal artery

Superficial temporal artery

Internal carotid artery

Ophthalmic artery

Maxillary artery

(B)

Figure 1.20 Vascular anatomy of the periocular and orbital region.

be undertaken. A small Frazier suction tube is appropriate to use in the non-dominant hand when performing dissection with a Freer periosteal elevator held in the dominant hand during an external DCR procedure. A Baron suction tube is smaller and very useful to use in more delicate situations, e.g., in the course of delicate orbital surgery. It is helpful to apply a

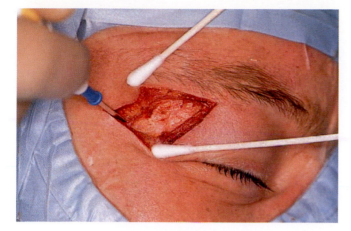

Figure 1.21 A cutting diathermy blade.

moistened swab or neurosurgical cottonoid over orbital fat to prevent this from being drawn into the sucker. Suction can then be applied to the swab or cottonoid. The suction can be increased, if necessary, by occluding a port on the suction tube with the surgeon's forefinger.

The Yankauer tonsil suction catheter is used for suctioning the oropharynx following lacrimal surgery, and intraoral surgery, e.g., following the removal of a hard palate graft.

Instrumentation

Hemostasis can be greatly influenced by the choice of instrumentation. For example, hemostasis is aided in enucleation surgery by the use of a snare. Contraindications to the use of a snare must, however, be observed, e.g., a soft globe, a previous corneal section or penetrating keratoplasty.

Cautery

A Colorado needle has both a cutting mode and a monopolar cautery facility. This is very useful for cauterizing fine vessels in the eyelids. For larger vessels, bipolar cautery is used. Fine-tipped jeweler's forceps limit tissue destruction to the zone between the tips of the instrument. A bayonet style of forceps is used for cautery of vessels at deeper levels within the orbit or socket. The forceps should be gently approximated until cauterization of tissue is seen to occur. A common error is to grasp tissue too firmly with the opposing tips of the forceps forced against each other. The surgeon should ensure that he/she is familiar with the required settings on the machine before using bipolar or monopolar cautery. Charred tissue should not be allowed to accumulate on the tips of the forceps.

Cautery should be used with great care. Overuse of cautery may compromise the blood supply to periorbital flaps. The underuse of cautery may place a skin graft at jeopardy. If bleeding occurs beneath a skin graft, or mucosal graft, the graft may fail.

A larger cutting diathermy blade (Fig. 1.21) can be used for fast bloodless incisions in the periorbital area, e.g., to aid in exenteration surgery. The blade can also be used in a fulgurate mode to prevent or stop bleeding from bone.

Great care should be taken with the use of disposable thermal hot-wire cautery close to the eye or within the orbit. It is useful in the treatment of simple periocular skin lesions, particularly in a clinic setting. It is essential that non-inflammable moistened swabs be used in conjunction with such cautery devices.

Bleeding should first be stopped by the application of pressure. Small bleeding vessels are rolled with a cotton-tipped applicator until the vessel can be identified and cauterized. The applicators should not be wiped across the tissue, which removes clot and provokes more bleeding. For more profuse bleeding, a gauze swab should be applied and gently removed until the vessels can be identified.

There is little justification for the use of a CO_2 laser to aid in hemostasis in ophthalmic plastic surgery. Most of the advantages of the CO_2 laser are also gained by the use of the Colorado needle without the numerous disadvantages of the CO_2 laser: significant expense, the requirement for nonflammable drapes, the risks of inadvertent injury to adjacent structures, the requirement for non-reflective instrumentation, the need to avoid supplemental oxygen, and the need for the operating room personnel to use protective eyewear.

Topical Hemostatic Agents

The topical hemostatic agents commonly used during ophthalmic plastic surgery are:

- Adrenaline
- Thrombin
- Surgicel
- Bone wax
- Tisseel®
- Fibrin sealant

The application of 1:1000 units of adrenaline to the donor site of a mucous membrane or hard palate graft on a cottonoid is particularly useful prior to the use of cautery. This prevents mucosal capillary oozing and allows a more conservative use of bipolar cautery with less tissue destruction.

Thrombin is a protease that facilitates the clotting cascade by converting fibrinogen to fibrin. It is applied to tissue with gelfoam, an absorbable sponge, as a carrier. This is particularly useful to stop oozing from a tumor bed in the orbit following an incisional biopsy. It is preferable to remove the gelfoam from the orbit once hemostasis has been achieved.

Surgicel is oxidized cellulose that is applied dry to produce a local reaction with blood, promoting the formation of an artificial clot. It is non-toxic and creates very little local tissue reaction. Although it can be left in situ, it is preferable to remove Surgicel at the completion of surgery as it can promote local swelling and a compartment syndrome in the orbit.

Bone wax is used to arrest bleeding from small perforating vessels in bone. The wax is applied on a cotton-tipped applicator or on the blunt end of a Freer periosteal elevator to plug the bleeding sites. It is important to dry the surrounding bone first to enable the wax to adhere.

Tisseel is a topically applied fibrin sealant which contains human fibrinogen, bovine aprotinin, calcium chloride, human thrombin, fibronectin, and factor XIII. It is both a tissue adhesive as well as a topical hemostatic agent. It is available in a ready-to-use prefilled double chamber syringe. It is very effective. It has many potential applications in oculoplastic surgery, e.g., its use has been advocated to assist the placement of full thickness skin grafts, saving surgical time devoted to suturing,

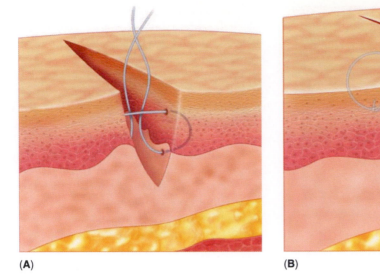

Figure 1.22 (**A**) Buried subcutaneous suture. (**B**) Technique of suture placement ensures that the knots are buried deep in the wound.

and to assist hemostasis and fixation of the forehead in brow lift surgery. Its potential advantages must be weighed against the cost, and the very small potential risks of transmissible disease and anaphylactic reactions.

Postoperative Hemostasis

The maintenance of a head-up position overnight following surgery can help to prevent postoperative bleeding. Restriction of activity postoperatively can also be important. The patient should be instructed to avoid blowing the nose following a DCR or orbital decompression procedure. The use of a surgical drain may be indicated following certain procedures, e.g., it can help to prevent the occurrence of a hematoma following a Mustardé cheek rotation procedure. It should be noted, however, that a drain is not a substitute for good intraoperative hemostasis.

WOUND CLOSURE

Although some periocular wounds can be left to heal by secondary intention with good functional and cosmetic results, avoiding the additional scars associated with skin flap reconstructions, most periocular, scalp and facial wounds, and tissue graft donor sites require a formal closure.

Suture Closure of Wounds

Meticulous wound closure is essential to obtain good cosmetic and functional results. Although the skill and technique of the surgeon are important, the selection of wound closure materials is also important. The purpose of these materials is to maintain wound closure until the wound is secure enough to withstand daily tensile forces and to enhance wound healing when the wound is most vulnerable.

A number of factors are important in successful wound closure:

- The proper anatomical realignment of tissues
- The avoidance of undue wound tension
- Atraumatic tissue handling
- The elimination of "dead space"
- The appropriate selection of needles
- The appropriate selection of suture materials

"Dead space" within a wound must be eliminated as this may act as a reservoir for hematoma and microorganisms; it may prevent anatomical realignment of the tissues and may delay or impair wound healing. The appropriate deep closure of wounds reduces tension on the cutaneous wound, reducing the risk of wound breakdown or widening of the scar.

Deep wounds should be closed with 5/0 or 4/0 Vicryl (polyglactin 910) sutures, e.g., in the lateral thigh following the harvesting of autogenous fascia lata the subcutaneous tissues are realigned with interrupted 4/0 Vicryl sutures. The suture should be placed while everting the wound edge. The needle is inserted into the subcutaneous tissue so that the needle reaches 2 to 3 mm back from the wound edge. The sutures' knots are buried to prevent interference with skin closure or postoperative erosion of the sutures through the skin wound. To bury the knot, the needle is first passed from deep to superficial in the wound and then from superficial to deep. Both ends of the suture should lie on the same side of the loop and the suture should be tied by pulling its ends along the line of the wound (Fig. 1.22).

Wound strength gradually increases during the process of healing. After 2 weeks, a wound has less than 10% of its final healed strength. By this time, most skin sutures are removed, and the resulting wound has little to rely on for strength unless additional support is provided. Wound strength increases to approximately 20% by 3 weeks and 50% by 4 weeks. At 3 to 6 months, a skin wound achieves its maximum strength, which is 70 to 80% that of normal skin.

Selection of Suture Needles

Suture needles are selected according to their size, curvature and cutting characteristics, and the characteristics and location of the tissues to be sutured. The needles commonly used in ophthalmic plastic surgery are:

- Cutting (Fig. 1.23)
- Reverse cutting (Fig. 1.24)
- Spatula (or side-cutting) (Fig. 1.25)
- Taper (Fig. 1.26)

The needles are most commonly 3/8, 1/4, or 1/2 circle: 3/8 circle needles are more commonly used, e.g., 5/0 Vicryl, for the

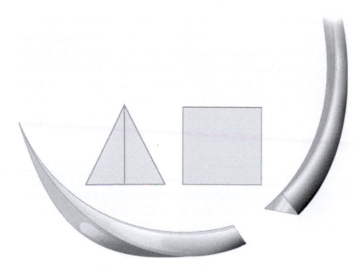

Figure 1.23 Conventional cutting needle.

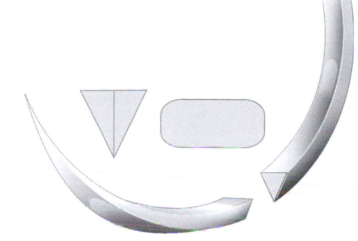

Figure 1.24 Reverse cutting needle.

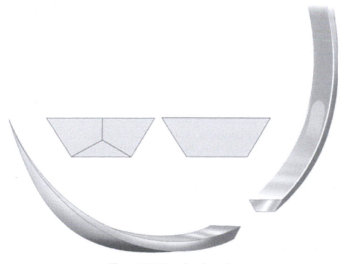

Figure 1.25 Spatulated needle.

reattachment of the levator aponeurosis to the tarsus; a 1/2 circle needle is used in a more confined space, e.g., 5/0 Vicryl, for the closure of mucosal flaps in external DCR surgery, or for the fixation of a lateral tarsal strip to the periosteum of the

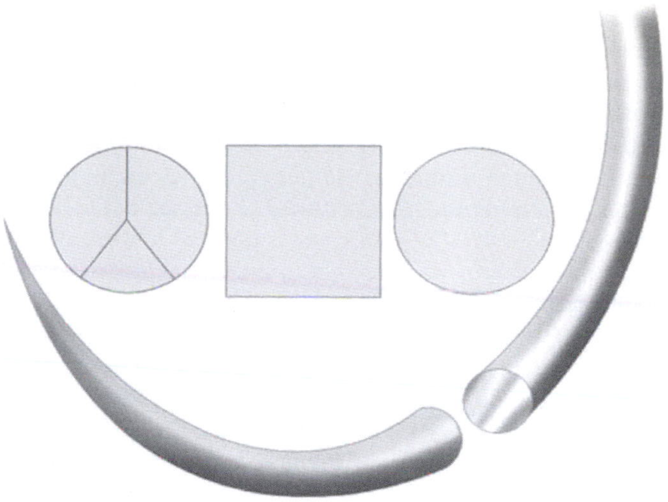

Figure 1.26 Taper needle.

lateral orbital margin. Cutting and reverse cutting needles pass through tissue very easily and are particularly suited to skin closure and general purpose use.

Reverse cutting needles are the most frequently used needles in ophthalmic plastic surgery. The reverse cutting needle has a third cutting edge located on the outer convex curvature of the needle. This offers several advantages:

- Reverse cutting needles have more strength than similar-sized conventional cutting needles
- The danger of tissue cut out is greatly reduced
- The hole left by the needle leaves a wide wall of tissue against which the suture is to be tied

The side-cutting edges of spatulated needles are designed for ophthalmic surgery. They permit the needle to separate or split through the thin layers of tissue, e.g., sclera. They are suited to partial-thickness passage through tarsus.

Taper needles are designed to limit the cutting surface to the tip, making them more suitable for passage through more vascular tissues, e.g., extraocular muscles. They cause the smallest possible hole in the tissue and the minimum cutting of tissue. This needle is therefore most suited for use as a superior rectus bridle suture.

The actual placement of the needle in the patient's tissue can cause unnecessary trauma if performed incorrectly. The following principles should be borne in mind:

1. Force should be applied in the same direction as the curve of the needle.
2. Excessively large bites of tissue should not be taken with a small needle.
3. A blunt needle should not be forced through tissue. It should be replaced.
4. The needle should not be forced or twisted in an effort to bring the point through the tissue.
5. The needle should not be used to bridge or approximate tissues for suturing.
6. If the tissue is tougher than anticipated, a heavier gauge needle should be used.
7. If a deep confined area prevents ideal placement of the needle, then it should be exchanged for a heavier gauge needle or a different curvature.

Selection of Suture Materials

Suture materials are selected according to the type of tissue to be sutured, its physical location, the degree of wound tension, and the suitability of the patient for suture removal. The size denotes the diameter of the suture material. In general, the smallest diameter suture that will adequately support the wound is chosen to minimize trauma caused by passage of the suture through the tissue. The suture size is denoted numerically: as the number of 0s in the suture size increases, the diameter of the suture decreases, e.g., size 7/0 is smaller than size 6/0.

Understanding the various characteristics of available suture materials is important to enable a surgeon to make an educated selection of a suture. No single suture possesses all the desirable characteristics. The optimal suture should be easy to handle and have high tensile strength and knot security. Any tissue reaction should be minimal, and the material should resist infection and have good elasticity and plasticity to accommodate wound swelling. A low cost is obviously preferred. Although some of the newer materials available have many of these properties, no one material is ideal and compromises have to be made.

The physical characteristics of a suture material determine its utility; these characteristics include configuration, diameter, capillarity and fluid absorption, tensile strength, knot strength, elasticity, plasticity, and memory.

The configuration of a suture is based on the number of strands of material used to fabricate it. *Monofilament* sutures are made of a single strand of material. They encounter less resistance than *multifilament* sutures as they pass through tissue. They also resist harboring microorganisms which may cause suture line infection, and cause little tissue reaction. The sutures tie easily but crushing or crimping of this suture type can create a weak spot, predisposing to breakage. Multifilament sutures consist of several filaments braided together. This provides greater tensile strength, pliability, and flexibility. They may be coated to assist in passage through tissues.

Plasticity refers to the ability of the suture to retain its new form and length after stretching. Plasticity allows a suture to accommodate wound swelling, thereby decreasing the risk of strangulating tissues. However, as swelling subsides, the suture retains its new size and may not continue to support the wound edges adequately.

Elasticity refers to the ability of a suture to regain its original form and length after stretching. After the swelling of a wound subsides, the suture returns to its original length and keeps the wound well supported. Most sutures provide elasticity. Few are "plastic."

Memory refers to the ability of a suture to return to its original shape after being tied. Memory is also related to plasticity and elasticity. Sutures with a high degree of memory, particularly monofilament sutures, are stiff and difficult to handle. As a consequence, the knots are less secure and may require extra throws to prevent loosening, e.g., polypropylene.

Pliability refers to the ease with which a suture can be bent. The more pliable a suture, the easier it is to tie.

Sutures may be *absorbable* or *nonabsorbable*. Absorbable sutures are defined by the loss of most of their tensile strength within 60 days after placement. Synthetic absorbable sutures are hydrolyzed. They are used primarily as buried sutures to close the dermis and subcutaneous tissues, and to reduce tension on the wound. The only natural absorbable suture available is surgical gut or catgut but these are no longer used in the United Kingdom. Synthetic multifilamentous materials include polyglycolic acid (Dexon; Syneture) and Polyglactin 910 (Vicryl; Ethicon). Monofilamentous forms include polydioxanone (PDS; Ethicon), polytrimethylene carbonate (Maxon; Syneture), poliglecaprone (Monocryl; Ethicon), Glycomer 631 (Biosyn; Syneture), and Polyglytone 6211 (Caprosyn; Syneture).

Nonabsorbable sutures are defined by their resistance to enzymatic digestion or hydrolysis by the body. They are most useful in percutaneous closures. Surgical silk is a natural material. Synthetic nonabsorbable monofilament sutures are most commonly used in cutaneous procedures and include nylon and polypropylene. Synthetic nonabsorbable multifilament sutures composed of nylon and polyester are used occasionally in oculoplastic surgery. The most recently developed monofilament nonabsorbable synthetic suture is polybutester (Novafil; Syneture).

The suture materials commonly used in ophthalmic plastic surgery are listed in Table 1.1

Polyglactin 910 (Vicryl)

Polyglactin 910 has good tensile strength and is absorbed relatively quickly after subcutaneous placement. It retains approximately 60% of its tensile strength 14 days postoperatively and only 8% of its original strength at day 28. It is completely hydrolyzed by 60 to 90 days. Tissue reactivity with polyglactin is low. It has easy tissue passage, precise knot placement, and a smooth tie down. It is usually dyed violet. Although used primarily as a buried suture, it can also be used for skin closure without adverse outcomes.

Vicryl Rapide is Polyglactin 910 that has been ionized with gamma rays to speed its absorption. This suture is useful as a buried suture in a wound requiring limited dermal support. It is completely absorbed in 35 days. It is very useful for skin wound closure in the periocular area in children.

Coated Vicryl Plus Antibacterial is coated with triclosan. This suture inhibits bacterial colonization with both methicillin-sensitive and methicillin-resistant *Staphylococcus aureus* and *Staphylococcus epidermidis*. This suture may be useful in wounds at increased risk of infection.

4/0 Vicryl is used for subcutaneous wound closure in the thigh, e.g., following fascia lata removal, in the abdominal wall, e.g., following dermis fat graft removal, or in the brow, e.g., following a direct brow lift.

5/0 Vicryl is used for subcutaneous wound closure in the periocular region and for the attachment of the levator aponeurosis to the tarsus, for the advancement of the lower lid retractors to

Table 1.1 Sutures Most Commonly Used in Ophthalmic Plastic Surgery
Polyglactin (Vicryl)
Silk
Polyester (Ethibond)
Nylon
Polybutester (Novafil)
Polydioxanone (PDS)
Polypropylene

the tarsus, for a lateral tarsal strip and medial spindle procedures, and for lower lid everting sutures. It is also used to reapproximate the mucosal flaps in external DCR surgery and for the attachment of the extraocular muscles to an orbital implant.

7/0 Vicryl is typically used for eyelid skin wound closure. It may be removed in adults, but in uncooperative patients or children it can be left to disintegrate spontaneously aided by the application of warm saline compresses and the application of antibiotic ointment. They do not cause an inflammatory reaction or leave visible suture tracks. Although more expensive, Vicryl Rapide is preferable for use in children.

8/0 Vicryl is typically used for conjunctival wound closure.

Silk

Silk is a braided material formed from the protein fibers produced by silkworm larvae. Although silk is considered a nonabsorbable material, it is gradually degraded by the body over a period of 2 years. Silk has excellent handling and knot-tying properties and is the standard to which all other suture materials are compared. Its knot security is high, tensile strength low, and tissue reactivity high. Silk sutures are usually dyed black for easy visibility in tissue.

6/0 silk is typically used to close an eyelid margin defect.

4/0 silk sutures are used for eyelid traction sutures or to assist in wound exposure, e.g., during an external DCR or a lateral orbitotomy.

2/0 silk sutures are passed through the eyelid margins and used for traction in an exenteration procedure.

Nylon

Nylon is available in both monofilamentous and multifilamentous forms. It has a high tensile strength, and, although it is classified as nonabsorbable, it loses tensile strength when implanted in the body. Multifilamentous forms retain no tensile strength after being in tissue for 6 months, whereas monofilamentous forms retain as much as two-thirds of their original strength after more than 10 years. Monofilament nylon is stiff; therefore, handling and tying are difficult and knot security is low. The suture also may cut easily through thin tissue. Multifilamentous forms have better handling properties but greater tissue reactivity and cost. They are not used very frequently in oculoplastic surgery. Monofilament nylon (Ethilon) is relatively inexpensive.

Ethilon sutures are particularly suited to skin closure because of their elasticity. Monofilament nylon sutures also have good memory. More throws are therefore required to securely hold monofilament nylon sutures.

4/0 Ethilon is used as a Frost suture and for temporary suture tarsorrhaphies. It is used for wound closure under tension, e.g., a thigh skin wound following the removal of a fascia lata graft, upper inner arm skin graft donor wound site closure.

6/0 Ethilon is used for facial skin wound closure.

Polyester (Ethibond)

Ethibond sutures comprise untreated fibers of polyester closely braided into a multifilament strand. The suture does not weaken when wetted prior to use, causes minimal tissue reaction, retains its strength for extended periods, and gradually becomes encapsulated in fibrous connective tissue. The coating of the suture allows easy passage through tissue and provides pliability, good handling qualities, and a smooth tie down. The suture is available in white or dyed green. Ethibond is no longer used very frequently in ophthalmic plastic surgery as it is associated with an increased risk of granuloma formation.

5/0 Ethibond is typically used to reattach the tarsus to the posterior lacrimal crest.

2/0 Ethibond is typically used for the fixation of the scalp tissues to a bone tunnel in endoscopic brow lift procedures.

Polybutester (Novafil)

This suture combines many of the desirable characteristics of polypropylene and polyester. Polybutester has a high tensile strength with good handling qualities. Its memory is lower than that of polypropylene, and therefore, its knots are more secure. Polybutester is not a plastic suture, but it has unique elastic properties that allow it to optimally respond to wound edema. Like polypropylene, polybutester has a low coefficient of friction and is an excellent choice for a running subcuticular closure. Polybutester is available as a clear or a blue suture. Its cost is comparable to that of polypropylene.

6/0 Novafil is typically used for the subcuticular closure of skin wounds which are not under tension, e.g., a lateral orbitotomy wound. It is also used for the percutaneous closure of a variety of facial skin wounds.

Polypropylene (Prolene)

Polypropylene is a monofilament synthetic suture which, unlike nylon, does not degrade over a number of years and can be considered permanent. It has extremely low tissue reactivity. Its handling, tying, and knot security are poor as a result of its stiff nature and high memory. An additional throw is needed for adequate knot security. Polypropylene is more expensive than nylon and is available as a clear or a blue suture.

4/0 Prolene is the ideal material to be used in brow suspension surgery for patients at risk of exposure keratopathy as it can be cut easily and the eyelid position instantly reversed. It can also be used as a running subcuticular suture.

Staples

Staples are formed from high-quality stainless steel. They are relatively easy to place and can save surgical time. The staplers are disposable. Most regular staples are 4 to 6 mm wide and 3.5 to 4 mm high. Their use results in a less precise wound approximation. The cost is usually more than that of suture material.

In order to place the staples, the stapler is held on the surface of the skin, perpendicular to the wound, and the handle squeezed, injecting the staple into the skin to form an incomplete rectangle. The depth of penetration depends on the pressure exerted on the stapler against the skin. To disengage the staple, the handle is released. If the stapler has an ejector-spring release, it is lifted vertically off the skin.

The correct placement of staples is important to avoid tissue strangulation. Staples should be inserted at 45° or 60° angles. As the wound swells, a staple placed at an acute angle rotates into a vertical position, leaving a space between the cross-member and the skin surface to accommodate swelling. If placed at a 90° angle, however, the staple is unable to move, having no plasticity or elasticity, and is likely to strangulate the tissues as they swell. Staples are removed painlessly by using a specialized set of extractors.

The primary utility of staples is in the closure of wounds under high tension on the trunk, extremities, and scalp. In oculoplastic surgery, the main use is the closure of a temple wound following the removal of a temporalis fascial graft, and for the closure of the central and paramedian scalp wounds following an endoscopic brow lift.

Tissue Adhesives
Cyanoacrylate adhesive (Dermabond® Ethicon) is useful for the closure of simple facial laceration in children but it has a small role to play in the closure of most periocular wounds. It can be applied to external DCR wounds to save surgical time.

Surgical Tapes (Steri-Strip Skin Closures 3M)
Tapes are strips of microporous nonocclusive material backed by a thin film of acrylic polymer adhesive. They are useful as an adjunct to other wound closure materials, and in oculoplastic surgery are most often used to reinforce a wound after placement of sutures, e.g., to support the wound following a direct brow lift.

It is essential to maximize adhesion of the tapes to the skin using a tincture of benzoin.

Skin Suturing Techniques
Most skin wounds should be closed with a slight eversion of the skin edges to prevent an inverted wound. The exception to this is where skin wounds are to be hidden within a natural skin crease, in which case a slight inversion of the wound is desirable, e.g., in a direct brow lift.

The skin wound edges should not be under undue tension. If this cannot be achieved, undermining of the tissues may be required. Overly tight sutures should be avoided, as these will cheese wire through the tissues or impair the vascular supply of the tissues, resulting in wound breakdown.

The surgeon should use a needle holder that is appropriate to the size of the needle. The self-locking Castroviejo needle holders are the most appropriate for use. The needle holder should be loaded properly. The needle should be grasped at the junction of the proximal two thirds with the distal one third, with approximately 1 mm of the needle holders overlapping the needle (Fig. 1.27). This will prevent rotation of the needle or the inadvertent springing of the needle from the jaws of the needle holder.

The curvature of the needle should be followed as it is passed through the tissue. The tip of the needle should be avoided when grasping the needle to remove it from the tissues. For speed, the needle can be re-grasped with the needle holders so that the surgeon is ready for the next pass of the needle when using a continuous suture technique.

Interrupted percutaneous standard sutures are useful to approximate skin edges in small wounds that are not under tension. The needle should be inserted at a slight outward angle to achieve a slight eversion of the wound edges (Fig. 1.28).

In the upper eyelid, these sutures should incorporate a bite of the levator aponeurosis to recreate a skin crease.

A running percutaneous suture is useful to close a longer wound that is not under tension, e.g., a lower eyelid subciliary incision (Fig. 1.29).

An interlocking running percutaneous suture is useful for efficient fast wound closure, e.g., for a postauricular wound under moderate tension following the removal of a skin graft (Fig. 1.30).

A running subcuticular suture, e.g., 6/0 Ethilon, is useful for wounds under minimal tension where the dermis is relatively thick, e.g., the forehead, brow. Such a suture is used in conjunction with buried subcutaneous sutures for deep closure. The suture can be supplemented with the use of sterile

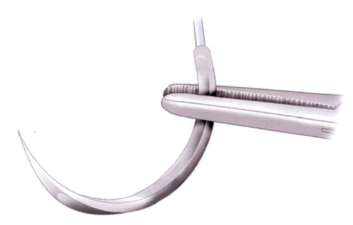

Figure 1.27 Correct arming of needle holder.

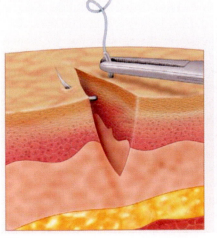

(A)

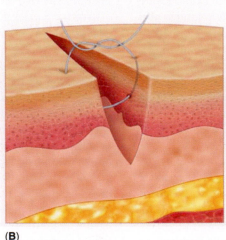

(B)

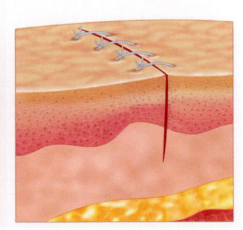

(C)

Figure 1.28 Technique of simple interrupted suture placement.

adhesive tape. The needle should be inserted through the skin approximately 1 cm beyond one end of the incision. It is brought into the wound and an artery clip attached to the free end of the suture to prevent the suture from being inadvertently pulled through the wound. The needle is then passed into the edge of the skin while everting the wound edges slightly with toothed forceps. The needle is curved through the skin for an arc of approximately 1 cm. The entire course of the suture is within the skin. The skin is then entered on the opposite side at the same point it exited the first side. The sides are alternated in this fashion until the end of the wound is reached. The wound is exited as it was entered (Fig. 1.31). The suture ends are attached to the skin with sterile adhesive tape.

Vertical mattress sutures provide both superficial and deep support to the wound and assist in everting the skin edges.

This technique is good for closing an external DCR wound with 7/0 Vicryl sutures, but elsewhere on the face, may leave unnecessary suture marks. Such a closure is very useful in the upper inner arm following the removal of a skin graft after undermining the skin edges, or for the closure of an abdominal dermis fat graft donor site wound (Fig. 1.32).

The sutures should be tied correctly. The desired tension should be obtained with an initial double throw of the suture. It is important to avoid tying sutures for tissue approximation too tightly, as this may contribute to tissue strangulation. Additional single throws are used to maintain this tension. The tension should not be adjusted by the additional throws. The suture should be pulled through leaving a short end to grasp. This avoids unnecessary wastage of suture material and avoids an annoying loop of suture when attempting to tie the knots. Extra throws do not add to the strength of a properly tied knot, only to its bulk.

> **KEY POINT**
>
> Avoid tying sutures too tightly. "Approximate—do not strangulate." Extra throws do not add to the strength of a properly tied knot, only to its bulk.

The timing of suture removal depends on the suturing technique, which has been used, the type of sutures used, and the tension of the wound, e.g., eyelid margin sutures should not be removed prior to 14 days following surgery. A subcuticular suture can usually be removed after 5 to 7 days with the wound further supported by the use of sterile adhesive tape.

Flap Techniques

Flap techniques mobilize local tissue to close tissue defects and, where necessary, to add tissue bulk. Flap techniques can be faster than the use of a skin graft, require a shorter period of time for the application of a compressive dressing postoperatively and are preferred in a situation where the recipient bed is unlikely to allow the survival of a graft.

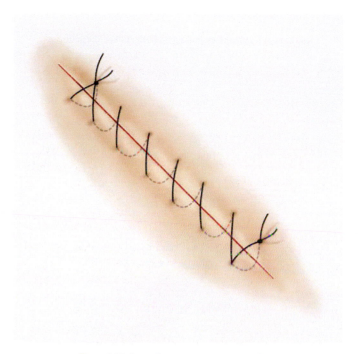

Figure 1.29 A continuous percutaneous suture.

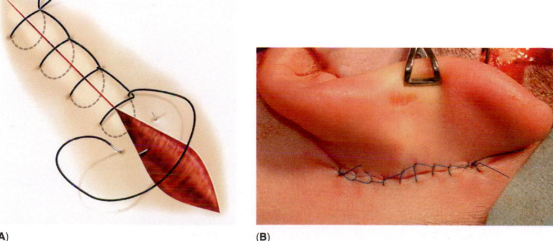

(A)   **(B)**

Figure 1.30 (**A**) A continuous interlocking percutaneous suture. (**B**) A continuous interlocking percutaneous suture used to close a postauricular skin graft donor site wound.

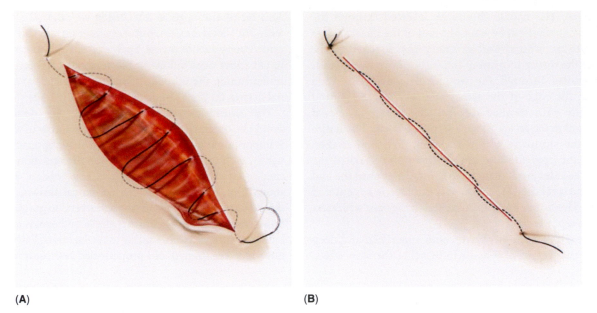

(A)   **(B)**

Figure 1.31 (**A**) Placement of a continuous subcuticular suture. (**B**) The wound edges are approximated by pulling on both ends of the suture.

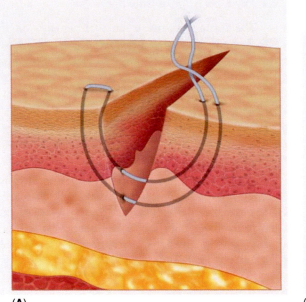

(A)

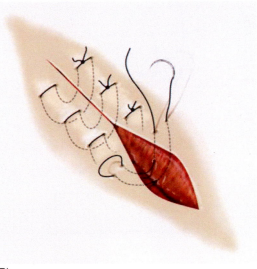

(B)

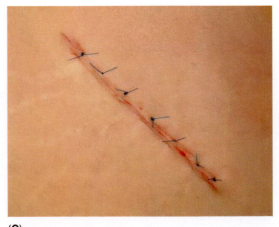

(C)

Figure 1.32 (**A**) Placement of a vertical mattress suture. (**B**) Wound closed with series of interrupted vertical mattress sutures. (**C**) Vertical mattress sutures (4/0 Nylon) used to close an abdominal dermis fat graft donor site.

Flaps used in ophthalmic plastic surgery are either "random" or "axial." The random flap receives its blood supply from the underlying dermal plexus, whereas the axial flap is based upon a direct cutaneous artery. The midline forehead flap is an example of an axial flap, based upon the frontal branch of the ophthalmic artery.

Local flaps may also be classified as:

- Advancement flaps
- Rotation flaps
- Transpositional flaps

An advancement flap is usually rectangular in shape and is advanced directly into a defect. An example is the lower eyelid advancement flap, which is used in conjunction with an upper eyelid tarsoconjunctival flap for the reconstruction of a lower eyelid defect. This is usually combined with the excision of Burow's triangles (Fig. 1.33).

A rotation flap rotates about a pivot point and is rotated into an adjacent tissue defect. An example is the Mustardé cheek rotation flap (Fig. 1.34).

A transposition flap is mobilized into a nonadjacent tissue defect. Examples are the Limberg rhomboid flap and the bilobed flap. The rhomboid flap is a very versatile flap, which is particularly useful in the closure of defects lateral to the lateral canthus and of medial canthal defects (Fig. 1.35). Care should be taken in designing the flap, taking into consideration the configuration of the resultant scars. The bilobed flap is also a very versatile flap (Fig. 1.36).

The Z-plasty very rarely finds practical application in ophthalmic plastic surgery. This technique is based upon the transposition of two triangular flaps (Fig. 1.37). Its aims are to lengthen skin in the direction of a linear scar, to achieve a cosmetic improvement in the scar by redirecting it within the RSTL and to reduce the effects of traction by the scar, e.g., a "bow string" DCR scar. The angles of each limb of the Z to the central scar are usually 60° (Fig. 1.38).

Free flaps, used for the reconstruction of large defects, e.g., the radically exenterated socket, are removed from one site and transplanted into the defect where the feeding artery and draining vein are attached to local blood vessels, e.g., the superficial temporal vessels. Examples are the rectus abdominis and radial forearm free flaps.

Flaps should be handled with great care as they have a delicate blood supply. Care should be taken in the use of cautery, in placing sutures without undue tension at appropriate intervals and in ensuring that there is no kinking of the pedicle of the flap. Excessive pressure from dressings should also be avoided.

The Dog-Ear Deformity

A dog-ear deformity typically occurs when a circular or elliptical defect is closed directly or when one side of an elliptical defect is longer than the other. The deformity is managed by

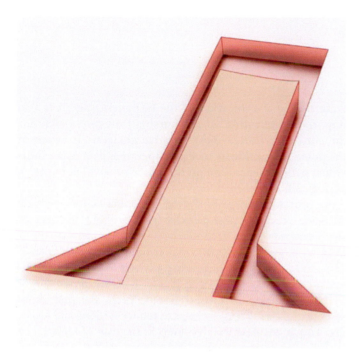

Figure 1.33 An advancement flap with the excision of Burow's triangles.

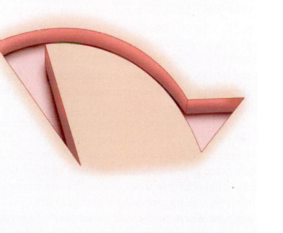

(A)

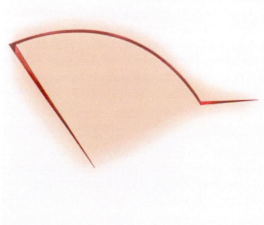

(B)

Figure 1.34 (A) A rotation flap being mobilized. (B) The rotation flap completed.

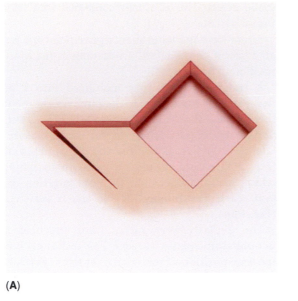
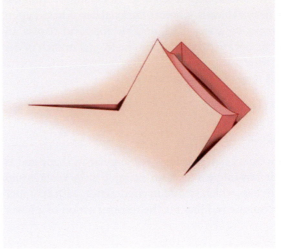

(A)   (B)

Figure 1.35 (**A**) A rhomboid flap dissected. (**B**) The flaps transposed.

elevating the dog ear, incising along one side of the dog ear with straight sharp scissors following the line of the original incision, and elevating the resulting flat triangle of skin, which is then incised along its base with the same scissors (Fig. 1.39).

Dog-ear deformities can be avoided in a number of situations by incorporating small triangular excisions into the wound closure, e.g., Burow's triangles (Fig. 1.33). This is typically required in the use of a skin-muscle advancement flap used as part of a Hughes flap reconstruction of a lower eyelid defect.

The principle of halving can be employed in closing an elliptical wound where one edge is longer than the other, e.g., an upper eyelid blepharoplasty wound. The wound is bisected with sutures until it is closed. Traction applied to both ends of the ellipse aids this closure.

An alternative method is to attempt to equalize the length of the wound edges by excising a triangle, e.g., the lower skin edge of a subciliary incision following a lower eyelid wedge resection procedure (Fig. 1.40).

POSTOPERATIVE PAIN MANAGEMENT

The majority of procedures undertaken by the ophthalmic plastic surgeon rank low on the pain scale. There are a few notable exceptions, e.g., enucleation with an orbital implant, or secondary orbital implant surgery. Careful surgery with the minimal degree of iatrogenic tissue trauma reduces postoperative pain.

KEY POINT

Pain following eyelid and orbital surgery should be investigated immediately and not merely suppressed with analgesic agents as such pain may indicate a sight-threatening orbital hemorrhage.

It is important to communicate the anticipated level of postoperative pain to the anesthetist who is normally responsible for the prescription of postoperative analgesia

regimens for the duration of the in-patient stay. It is also important to ensure that the nursing staff responsible for the administration of postoperative analgesia is aware of the potential significance of postoperative pain in an individual patient depending on the procedure which has been performed.

Postoperative analgesia should be prescribed to provide adequate relief for postoperative pain without the risk of significant side effects. It should be noted that older patients or those with systemic disorders may require lower doses of analgesia. In general, patients who are anxious require more postoperative analgesia.

The application of crushed ice packs in the first 24 to 48 hours following surgery helps to reduce swelling and bleeding. This is not practical, however, in the case of children or where compressive dressings have been applied. Great care should be taken to avoid excessive application of ice packs, however, as these can cause cryogenic burns, especially when the effects of local anesthesia have not yet worn off. The packs should not be applied directly to the eyelids but should be applied over sterile swabs.

For procedures undertaken under general anesthesia, the use of a further injection of a longer-acting local anesthetic agent, e.g., bupivacaine, as a local infiltration or a regional block is very helpful. Following an enucleation with an orbital implant or a secondary orbital implant procedure, a deep orbital injection of bupivacaine is recommended at the completion of surgery.

Moderate to severe pain is normally controlled postoperatively with narcotic agents, e.g., morphine, or NSAIAs such as ketorolac. NSAIAs avoid the side effects of opiate agents but may cause gastrointestinal irritation and decreased renal function. Intramuscular ketorolac or intravenous paracetamol are very effective for immediate postoperative pain relief for day case procedures performed under general anesthesia. This can be continued orally on discharge for 4 to 5 days. For mild postoperative pain, codeine and paracetamol (Kapake) are usually adequate.

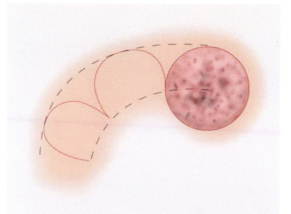

(A)

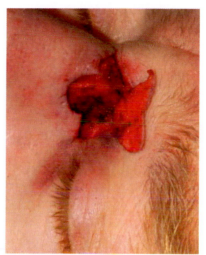

(B)

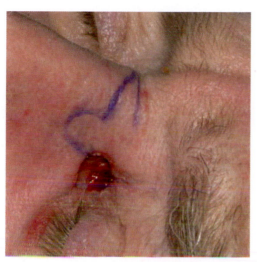

(C)

(D)

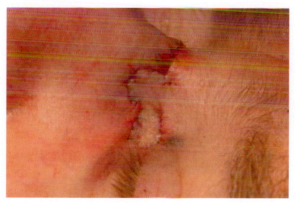

(E)

Figure 1.36 (**A**) A drawing of a bilobed flap outlined. (**B**) A drawing depicting the flaps transposed. (**C**) A bilobed flap outlined with gentian violet. (**D**) The bilobed flap dissected. (**E**) The appearance of the reconstructed defect.

KEY POINT

Any drug allergies, interactions, contraindications and systemic disorders should always be considered before prescribing any analgesic agents.

POSTOPERATIVE CARE

Clear effective communication is essential. An operation record should be detailed and clearly legible. Ideally, this should be type written immediately following surgery and a signed copy entered into the patient's records. Postoperative instructions should also be clearly specified in the patient's records. A GP discharge letter should also be dictated following the completion of surgery and a copy given to the patient.

The nursing staff responsible for the immediate postoperative aftercare of the patient should be carefully instructed about:

- Topical and systemic antibiotic treatment
- Dressings

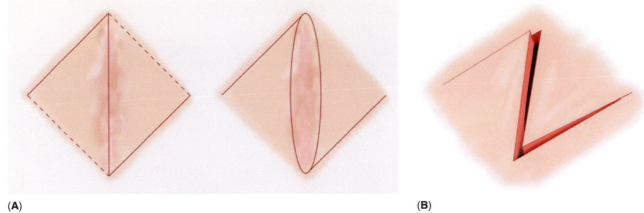

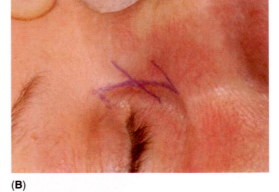

(A)   **(B)**

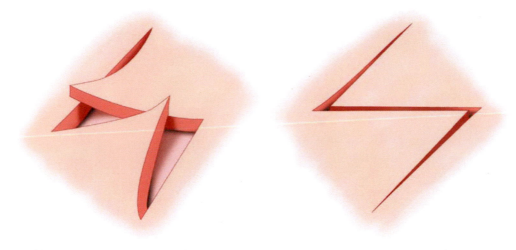

(C)

Figure 1.37 (**A**) The Z-plasty is marked out based on the vertical scar and the scar is excised. (**B**) The flaps are dissected. (**C**) The flaps are transposed.

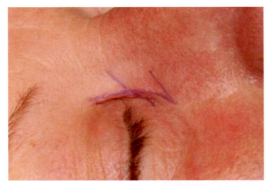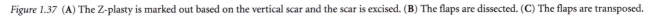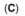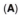

(A)   **(B)**

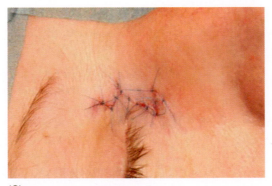

(C)

Figure 1.38 (**A**) A 'bow stringed' external DCR scar marked with double Z-plasty incisions. (**B**) The skin of the bridge of the nose stretched to demonstrate the positions of the incision marks. (**C**) The Z-plasty flaps have been transposed and sutured.

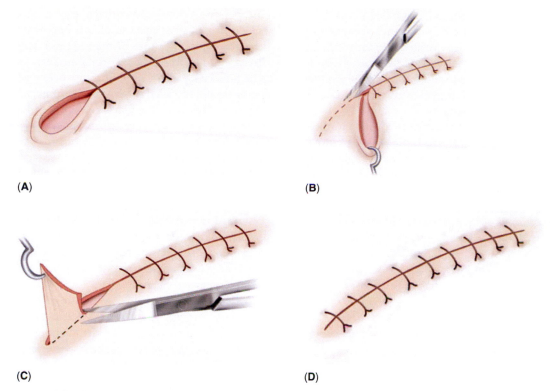

Figure 1.39 (**A**) A dog-ear deformity. (**B**) The apex of the dog ear is drawn away from the line of the wound with a skin hook and an incision is made along the line of the wound. (**C**) The triangle of skin and subcutaneous tissue is laid across the wound and the excess tissue is trimmed away. (**D**) The wound is closed.

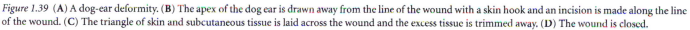

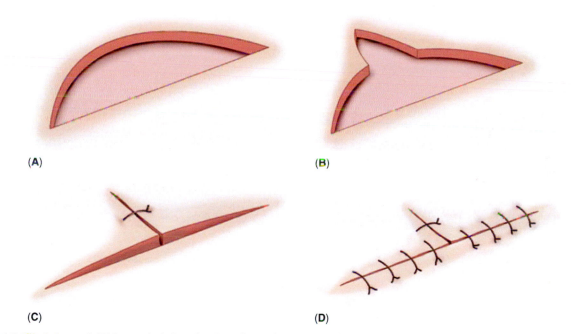

Figure 1.40 (**A**) Elliptical wound. (**B**) Removal of triangular piece of tissue from apex of ellipse. (**C**) Closure of triangular skin wound. (**D**) Closure of remaining wound.

- Drains
- Head positioning
- Visual monitoring
- Management of bleeding, e.g., postoperative epistaxis
- Activity restrictions
- Postoperative wound care
- Timing of suture removal
- Dietary restrictions
- Use of ice packs
- Postoperative analgesia

Patients should also be given clear written instructions about their aftercare on discharge from hospital. They should also be given emergency contact numbers. Postoperative instruction sheets for specific operations are particularly useful. A successful outcome without complications depends on good quality aftercare.

Topical antibiotic ointment should be applied to wounds at the end of surgery after rechecking the patient's allergy history with the nursing staff. This is also instilled into the conjunctival sac where ocular protection is required. The use of systemic antibiotics should be restricted to those cases for which there are specific indications, e.g., immuno-compromised patients undergoing lacrimal drainage surgery.

A Frost suture may be used in children following ptosis surgery: 4/0 nylon should be used, as this is more easily removed. If eyelid traction sutures are to be left in place for longer than 48 hours, they should be placed over small rubber bolsters. The suture is taped to the forehead with sterile adhesive tape.

Dressings may be left in place for a variable period of time depending on the operative procedure. Where firm compression is required, e.g., following an enucleation, it is preferable to apply tincture of benzoin to the forehead and cheek. Vaseline gauze should be placed over the wounds before eye pads are applied. Micropore tape is applied followed by a bandage.

Drains are rarely used in ophthalmic plastic surgery. They are mainly used following the drainage of subperiosteal abscesses or following a Mustardé cheek rotation flap. They are removed once the drainage from them has ceased.

It is preferable to advise patients to keep the head elevated following ophthalmic plastic surgery: this helps to reduce postoperative edema.

It is important to perform regular postoperative visual checks following certain procedures where there is a risk of a postoperative orbital hemorrhage, e.g., a lateral orbitotomy and excision of an orbital tumor. It is important to ensure that the nursing staff is aware of the required frequency of these checks, e.g., hourly following orbital surgery; and the protocol to be followed, e.g., the level of acuity below which an on-call doctor should be called to see the patient immediately.

Postoperative bleeding may be anticipated following certain procedures, e.g., following an endoscopic DCR. Restricting activity for the first few hours following this operation reduces the risk of bleeding.

Dietary restrictions are required following the removal of mucous membrane or hard palate grafts. The patient should be restricted to a bland soft diet for a few days and should be prescribed an antiseptic oral mouth wash such as Difflam to be used for a few days.

Careful instructions on the use of ice packs postoperatively should be given to ensure that these are not overused with the risk of a cryogenic burn.

Postoperative wound care can greatly influence the outcome of surgery. Patients must be instructed on the necessity for thorough hand washing prior to touching any wounds. All debris should be gently soaked away with cotton wool moistened with boiled water or sterile saline. The patient should be instructed on the use of postoperative wound massage with Lacrilube ointment. This reduces wound edema, softens scars, and prevents wound contracture (Figs. 1.41 and 1.42). This can very successfully obviate the need for further surgery, e.g., postoperative massage commenced within 48 to

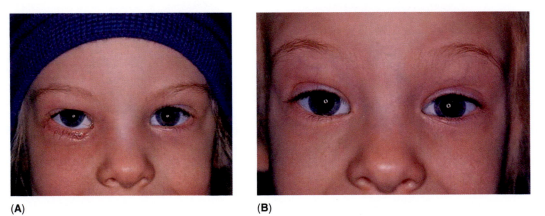

(A)   **(B)**

Figure 1.41 (**A**) Right lower eyelid retraction following wound repair in a child. (**B**) Satisfactory position of lower eyelid after 3 months of regular massage.

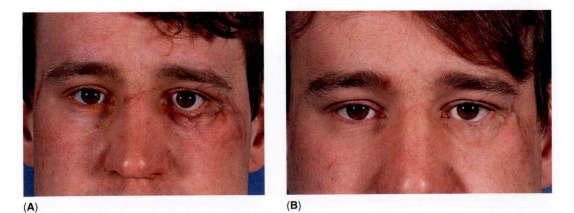

(A)   **(B)**

Figure 1.42 (**A**) Periocular scarring and a left lower eyelid retraction following a poor repair of irregular lacerations in a young adult. (**B**) Appearances after 3 months of regular wound massage.

72 hours of a lower lid dissection for the management of a blowout fracture can prevent eyelid retraction.

CONCLUSION

Although the fundamental principles and techniques essential to success in ophthalmic plastic surgery are similar to those which underlie other branches of surgery, the functional requirements of the globe and the ocular adnexal tissues and their delicate anatomical structure demand precise attention to detail, and a meticulous surgical technique. The surgeon who is well versed in fundamental surgical principles as well as specific surgical techniques will achieve successful results, avoiding unnecessary complications and the requirement for secondary procedures.

FURTHER READING

1. Albert D, Lucarelli M, eds. Ophthalmic plastic techniques: basic considerations. In: Clinical Atlas of Procedures in Ophthalmic Surgery. Chicago, IL: AMA Press, 2004: 241–7.
2. Backster A. Teo A. Swift M. Polk HC Jr. Harken AH. Transforming the surgical "time-out" into a comprehensive "preparatory pause". J Cardiac Surg 2007; 22(5): 410–16.
3. Bloom LH, Sheie HG, Yanoff M. The warming of local anaesthetic agents to prevent discomfort. Ophthal Surg 1984; 15(7): 603.
4. Borges AF. Relaxed skin tension lines (RSTL) versus other lines. Plast Reconstr Surg 1984; 73: 144.
5. Christie DB, Woog JJ. Basic surgical techniques, technology, and wound repair. In: Bosniak S, ed. Principles and Practice of Ophthalmic Plastic and Reconstructive Surgery. Philadelphia, PA: WB Saunders, 1996: 281–93.
6. Dortzbach RK, ed. Ophthalmic Plastic Surgery: Prevention and Management of Complications. Philadelphia, PA: Lippincott, Williams & Wilkins, 1993.
7. Egerton MT. The Art of Surgical Technique. Baltimore, MD: Williams and Wilkins, 1988.
8. Nerad JA. Techniques in Ophthalmic Plastic Surgery—A Personal Tutorial. London, UK: Elsevier Inc., 2010: 1–24 (ISBN: 978-1-4377-0008-4).
9. Linberg JV, Mangano LM, Odoni JV. Comparison of nonabsorbable and absorbable sutures for use in oculoplastic surgery. Ophthal Plast Reconstr Surg 1991; 7: 1–7.
10. McCord C Jr, Codner MA. Basic principles of wound closure. In: McCord C, ed. Eyelid Surgery: Principles and Techniques, 3rd edn. Philadelphia, PA: Lippincott-Raven, 1995: 23–8.
11. McGregor IA. Fundamental Techniques of Plastic Surgery, 8th edn., Edinburgh: Churchill Livingstone, 1989.
12. Parkin B, Manners R. Aspirin and warfarin therapy in oculoplastic surgery. Br J Ophthalmol 2000; 84: 1426–7.
13. Sherman DD, Dortzbach RK. Monopolar electrocautery dissection in ophthalmic plastic surgery. Ophthal Plast Reconstr Surg 1993; 9: 143–7.
14. Sierra CA, Nesi FA, Levine MR: Basic wound repair: surgical techniques, flaps and grafts. In: Levine MR, ed. Manual of Oculoplastic Surgery. Boston, MA: Butterworth- Heinemann, 2003: 23–9.
15. Tandara AA, Mustoe TA. The role of the epidermis in the control of scarring: evidence for mechanism of action for silicone gel. J Plast Reconstr Aesthetic Surg 2008; 61: 1219–25.
16. Tanenbaum M. Skin and tissue techniques. In: McCord CD, Tanenbaum M, Nunery WR, eds. Oculoplastic Surgery, 3rd edn. New York, NY: Raven Press, 1995: 1–49.
17. Younis I, Bhutiani RP. Taking the "ouch" out—effect of buffering commercial Xylocaine on infiltration and procedure pain—a prospective, randomised, double-blind controlled trial. Ann R Coll Surg Engl 2004; 86(3): 213–17.

2 Applied anatomy

INTRODUCTION
A sound working knowledge of eyelid, orbital, nasal, and facial anatomy is essential before embarking upon oculoplastic, oculofacial, orbital, and lacrimal surgery. The surgical procedures, which are described throughout this book, are much easier to understand and to undertake when a good working knowledge of this anatomy has been acquired. This chapter aims to present detailed and practical anatomical descriptions as they apply directly to these surgical procedures, and to a variety of clinical problems. The order in which the anatomy is presented has been selected to make the chapter easier to read, and more relevant to the order in which the subsequent chapters appear.

THE EYELIDS
In the adult the normal interpalpebral fissure varies in vertical height from 8 to 11 mm. The peak of the upper eyelid usually lies just nasal to the midline of the pupil. The horizontal length of the interpalpebral fissure measures approximately 30 to 32 mm. The angle between the upper and lower eyelids medially and laterally measures approximately 60°. Laterally the eyelids should be in contact with the globe but medially the eyelids are displaced away from the globe creating a space, the lacus lacrimalis. Within the lacus lacrimalis lies the caruncle and immediately lateral to the caruncle lies the plica semilunaris (Fig. 2.1A). The plane between the caruncle and the plica semilunaris is commonly used to gain access to the medial orbital wall, e.g., to drain a subperiosteal abscess. This is referred to as a "transcaruncular" approach.

The lateral canthal angle usually lies approximately 2 to 3 mm higher than the medial canthal angle (Fig. 2.1B). This angle and its location should be borne in mind when surgery is undertaken on the lateral canthus, e.g., a lateral eyelid tightening procedure undertaken during the course of a lower eyelid blepharoplasty.

The eyelid margin is covered by conjunctival epithelium along the posterior half and meets the anterior margin, which is covered with cutaneous epidermis at the gray line. The meibomian gland orifices lie within the conjunctival epithelium while the eyelashes emerge within the cutaneous epidermis.

The eyelid can be divided into five structural planes:

1. The eyelid skin and subcutaneous fascia
2. The orbicularis oculi muscle
3. The orbital septum
4. The eyelid retractors
5. The tarsal plates and conjunctiva

The upper eyelid skin crease is created by attachments from the superficial aspect of the levator aponeurosis into the orbicularis muscle and the subcutaneous tissue (Fig. 2.2). The skin crease varies in height and tends to lie 5 to 6 mm above the eyelid margin centrally in males and 7 to 8 mm above the eyelid margin centrally in females. Medially the crease extends to within 3 to 4 mm of the eyelid margin while laterally it lies approximately 5 to 6 mm above the eyelid margin (Fig. 2.3A). This should be borne in mind when marking the desired position of the upper lid skin crease in patients undergoing ptosis repair or an upper lid blepharoplasty. In oriental patients, the upper lid skin crease is typically poorly developed or absent because the orbital septum inserts onto the levator aponeurosis in a lower position. This anatomical arrangement allows the pre-aponeurotic fat to extend further into the eyelid.

The Eyelid Skin
The eyelid skin is the thinnest in the body and unique in having no subcutaneous fat. This, along with the color match, makes the upper eyelid an ideal donor site for a small full thickness skin graft to be used for lower eyelid reconstruction. The skin can be removed easily and quickly and does not need to be thinned in contrast to skin harvested from other donor sites.

The Orbicularis Oculi Muscle
The orbicularis oculi muscle is divided anatomically into three parts (Fig. 2.4)

- Orbital
- Pre-septal
- Pre-tarsal

The orbital portion of the orbicularis muscle lies over the bony orbital margins. It arises from the frontal process of the maxillary bone in front of the anterior lacrimal crest, from the orbital process of the frontal bone, and from the medial canthal tendon. The fibers of the orbicularis pass around the orbital margins without interruption at the lateral canthus and the bony insertions lie just below the points of origin.

The palpebral part of the orbicularis muscle extends from the orbital margins to the margins of the eyelids. The muscle fibers pass circumferentially around the eyelids and are fixed medially and laterally at the medial and lateral canthal tendons. The palpebral part of the orbicularis muscle is further subdivided into the pre-septal and pre-tarsal orbicularis muscles.

The pre-septal part of the orbicularis muscle lies over the orbital septum in the upper and lower eyelids. Its muscle fibers arise in a perpendicular fashion from the upper and lower borders of the medial canthal tendon. In the upper lid, the muscle arises by anterior and posterior heads. The anterior head arises as a broad extension from the superior surface of the common part of the medial canthal tendon. The posterior head arises from the superior arm and also from the posterior arm of the medial canthal tendon. The inferior pre-septal muscle arises as a single head from the whole length of the common medial canthal tendon.

The superior limb of the medial canthal tendon fuses to the fundus of the lacrimal sac by a layer of fibrovascular fascia. When the deep head of the pre-septal muscle pulls on the lacrimal sac via this fascia, it contributes to the lacrimal pump

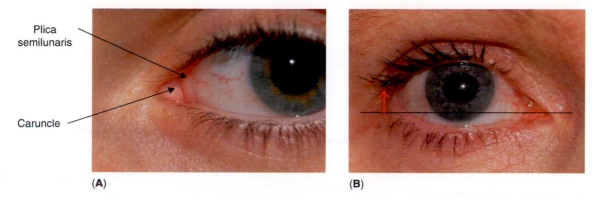

Plica semilunaris

Caruncle

(A)

(B)

Figure 2.1 The canthal angles.

mechanism. The pre-septal muscles extend in an arc around the eyelids and insert along the lateral horizontal raphé.

The pre-tarsal orbicularis muscle lies over the tarsal plates. The fibers of the muscle in both the upper and lower eyelids arise from the medial canthal tendon by means of superficial and deep heads. The superficial heads extend from the eyelid and continue anterior to the upper and lower limbs of the medial canthal tendons. The muscles thicken and surround the limbs of the medial canthal tendon and the canaliculi superiorly, anteriorly, and inferiorly. Contraction of these muscle fibers also contributes to the lacrimal pump mechanism.

Close to the common canaliculus, the deep heads of the pretarsal orbicularis muscle fuse together to form a prominent bundle of muscle fibers referred to as Horner's muscle which extends just behind the posterior limb of the medial canthal tendon. Horner's muscle continues posteriorly to insert onto the posterior lacrimal crest immediately behind the posterior limb of the medial canthal tendon. A few fibers continue more posteriorly 3 to 5 mm along the medial orbital wall. As Horner's muscle passes to the posterior lacrimal crest, it is joined by the medial horn of the levator aponeurosis, the posterior layer of the orbital septum, and the medial rectus check ligament (Fig. 2.5). The function of Horner's muscle is to maintain the posterior position of the medial canthal angle and to tighten the eyelids against the globe during eyelid closure. It is thought that it also contributes to the lacrimal pump mechanism.

The pre-tarsal orbicularis muscle fibers join together along the surface of the lateral canthal tendon and the lateral horizontal raphé. Additional bundles of thin muscle fibers run along the upper and lower eyelid margins. These are referred to as muscles of Riolan. These are firmly fixated to the tarsus. Medially these muscles insert into the puncta and ampullae of the lacrimal drainage system. Some deeper fibers past posterior to the canaliculi and merge into the deep heads of the pretarsal orbicularis muscle. These muscle fibers run in various directions in contrast to the rest of the orbicularis muscle.

KEY POINT

A detailed working knowledge of the anatomical arrangements of the orbicularis muscle is the key to success in undertaking a conservative or radical orbicularis myectomy in the surgical management of a patient with essential blepharospasm.

Lying between the orbicularis muscle and the orbital septum/ levator aponeurosis fascial complex is an avascular fascial plane composed of loose areolar tissue. This fascial plane extends to the margin of the eyelid as the gray line. The gray line itself marks the anatomical separation of the anterior skin muscle lamella from the posterior tarso-conjunctival lamella. The post-orbicularis fascial plane is surgically important as it allows a bloodless dissection permitting careful identification of the underlying orbital septum during the initial phase of ptosis surgery. It also permits a bloodless approach to the superior and inferior orbital margins (Fig. 2.6).

The post-orbicularis fascial plane allows slight movement between the orbicularis muscle and the underlying orbital septum while maintaining an integrated lamellar structure. Undue disruption of the fibrous connections within the post-orbicularis fascial plane during upper lid surgery results in an inferior slippage of the anterior lamella after anterior approach levator advancement surgery or upper lid blepharoplasty surgery. This inferior slippage of the anterior lamella can be prevented by fixating the orbicularis muscle and skin edges to the levator aponeurosis with interrupted 7/0 Vicryl sutures during the skin closure.

A deep plane of fat lies posterior to the orbital part of the orbicularis muscle superiorly and inferiorly. The sub-orbicularis oculi fat (SOOF) lies over the inferior orbital margin. The retro-orbicularis oculi fat (ROOF) lies over the superior orbital margin (Figs. 2.2 and 2.6).

The Orbital Septum

The orbital septum is a fibrous multi-layered membrane of variable thickness, which arises from the arcus marginalis, a line of periosteal condensation, along the superior and inferior orbital margins. In young patients, the orbital septum is usually relatively thick and quite easily identified at surgery. In contrast the orbital septum may be very thin and dehiscent in older patients. The orbital septum is continuous with the inner layers of the periorbita. Within the orbit the periorbita lines the bony orbital walls and is composed of an outer layer of periosteum and an inner layer continuous with the orbital fascia. These layers separate at the arcus marginalis with the outer periosteum continuing over the orbital margins as the periosteum of the forehead and facial bones. In the upper eyelid the inner fascial layer separates into two further layers at the arcus marginalis. The superficial layer continues over the brow where it is continuous with the deep fascia over the frontalis muscle and the galea aponeurotica above the eyebrow. The deep layer becomes the orbital septum in the upper eyelid. In the lower eyelid the inner fascial layer extends into the eyelid as the orbital septum (Fig. 2.7).

Laterally the orbital septum inserts into the lateral canthal tendon and also passes behind the tendon inserting onto the lateral retinaculum together with the lateral horn of the levator aponeurosis. In the superomedial aspect of the orbit the orbital septum extends inferiorly and posteriorly along the posterior

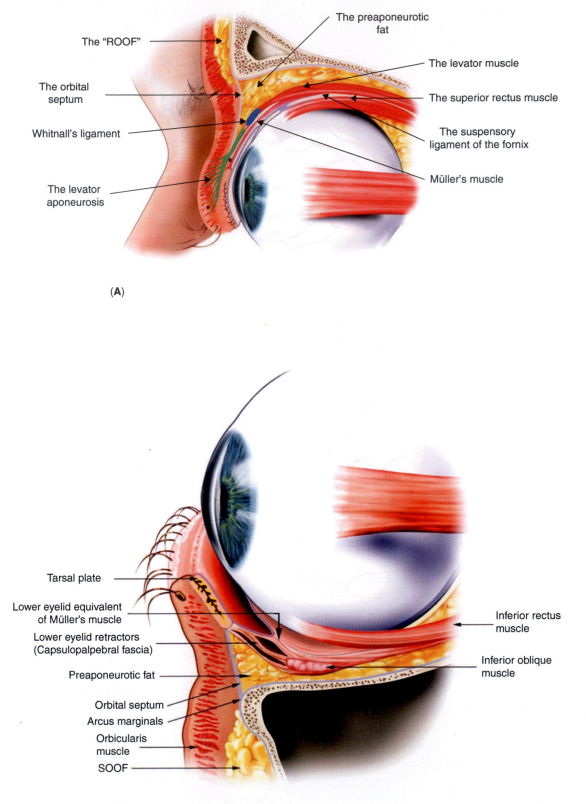

(A)

(B)

Figure 2.2 (**A**) The anatomy of the upper eyelid and adjacent structures. (**B**) The anatomy of the lower eyelid and adjacent structures.

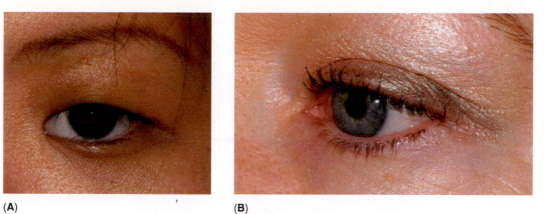

(A)   **(B)**

Figure 2.3 (**A**) An oriental female upper eyelid with an apparent lack of any skin crease. (**B**) A normal female upper eyelid skin crease.

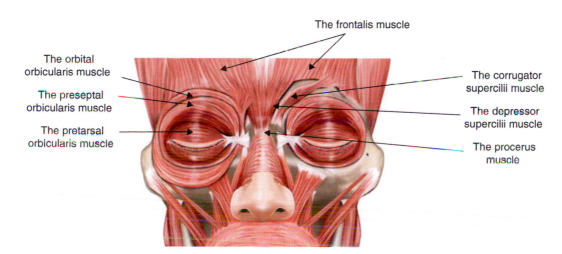

The frontalis muscle

The orbital orbicularis muscle

The corrugator supercilii muscle

The preseptal orbicularis muscle

The depressor supercilii muscle

The pretarsal orbicularis muscle

The procerus muscle

Figure 2.4 The brow depressor muscles.

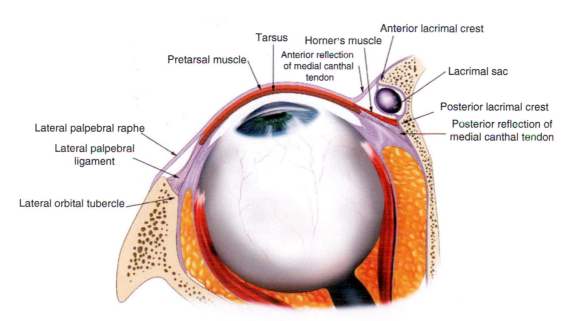

Anterior lacrimal crest

Tarsus   Horner's muscle

Pretarsal muscle   Anterior reflection of medial canthal tendon

Lacrimal sac

Lateral palpebral raphe

Posterior lacrimal crest

Lateral palpebral ligament

Posterior reflection of medial canthal tendon

Lateral orbital tubercle

Figure 2.5 Horner's muscle.

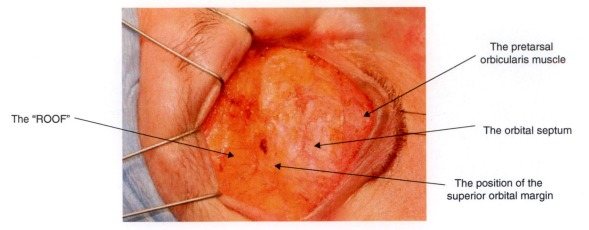

The "ROOF"

The pretarsal
orbicularis muscle

The orbital septum

The position of the
superior orbital margin

Figure 2.6 The orbital septum has been exposed in a patient who is undergoing an orbicularis oculi myectomy procedure for the control of essential blepharospasm.

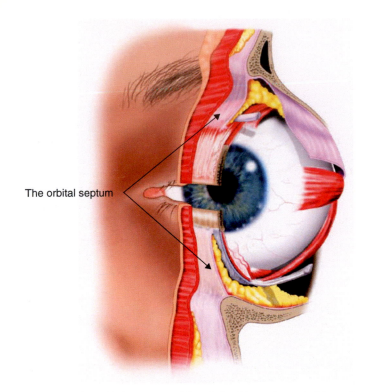

The orbital septum

Figure 2.7 The orbital septum and its relationship to the periorbita and periosteum.

lacrimal crest. Here it inserts just posterior to Horner's muscle and the posterior limb of the medial canthal tendon. The orbital septum passes around the lip of the lacrimal foramen where it fuses to the lacrimal sac fascia (Fig. 2.8). The inferior orbital septum joins the superior orbital septum medially at the anterior lacrimal crest.

Superomedially at the orbital margin the orbital septum thins and becomes dehiscent allowing for the passage of the infratrochlear neurovascular bundle and branches of the superior ophthalmic vein. In the central aspect of the upper lid, the inferior aspect of the orbital septum fuses with the anterior surface of the levator aponeurosis (Fig. 2.2). The point at which the orbital septum fuses with the levator aponeurosis varies from a position approximately 3 to 5 mm above the superior aspect of the tarsal plate to as far as 10 to 15 mm

above the tarsal plate. In the lower eyelid, the orbital septum fuses with the capsulopalpebral fascia a few millimeters below the inferior aspect of the tarsal plate (Fig. 2.2). This common fascial sheet then inserts into the lower edge of the inferior tarsal plate.

The orbital septum can be readily identified during surgery by noting the firm resistance to traction applied to it because of its attachment to the arcus marginalis. The pre-aponeurotic fat pads lie immediately posterior to the orbital septum in the upper and lower eyelids (Fig. 2.2). It is extremely important not to confuse an extension of the brow fat pad into the post-orbicularis fascial plane of the upper eyelid with the pre-aponeurotic fat pads. The orbital septum may be incorrectly identified as the levator aponeurosis in such patients and an inadvertent advancement of this septal layer will result in marked lagophthalmos. Likewise it is important not to advance the capsulopalpebral fascia in the lower eyelid without first separating the orbital septum to avoid a resultant lower eyelid retraction. It is also important that the orbital septum is not sutured following eyelid surgery to avoid inadvertent shortening resulting in lagophthalmos or eyelid retraction.

KEY POINTS

It is extremely important not to confuse an extension of the brow fat pad into the post-orbicularis fascial plane of the upper eyelid with the pre-aponeurotic fat pads. It is important not to advance the capsulopalpebral fascia in the lower eyelid without first separating the orbital septum to avoid a resultant lower eyelid retraction.

The Tarsal Plates

The tarsal plates are made up of dense fibrous tissue which provides the main structural integrity to the eyelids. The upper and lower tarsal plates are approximately 25 mm in length horizontally and are gently curved. They are approximately 1 to 1.5 mm in thickness and centrally the vertical height of the tarsal plate varies from 8 to 12 mm in the upper lid and 3.5 to 4 mm in the lower eyelid. The medial and lateral aspects of the tarsal plates taper to 2 mm in height as they pass into the medial and lateral canthal tendons. A row of approximately 25 meibomian glands lie within the upper lid tarsus and

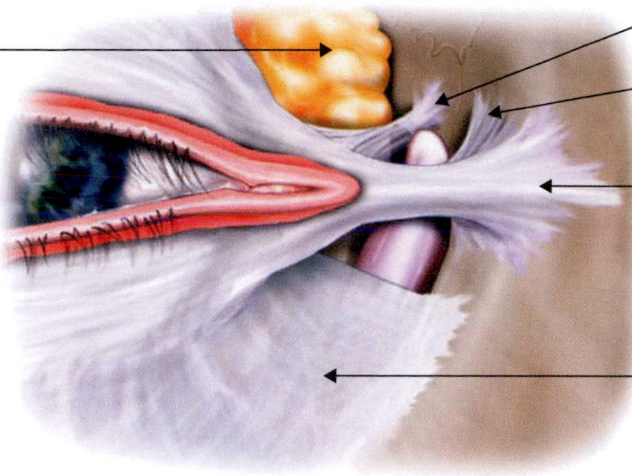

The medial
orbital fat pad

The posterior limb of
the medial canthal
tendon

The superior limb of the
medial canthal tendon

The anterior limb of
the medial canthal
tendon

The orbital septum

Figure 2.8 A diagram demonstrating the anatomy of the medial canthal tendon.

approximately 20 in the lower tarsus. The meibomian glands are holocrine sebaceous glands which are multi-lobulated and empty into a tiny central duct. The duct opens onto the posterior eyelid margin behind the gray line. These glands produce the lipid layer of the pre-corneal tear film.

The Canthal Tendons

The tarsal plates continue into fibrous bands medially which form the crura of the medial canthal tendon. These crura lie between the orbicularis muscle anteriorly and the conjunctiva posteriorly. The superior and inferior crura fuse together to form a common medial canthal tendon. This tendon inserts onto the adjacent bones by means of three arms: the anterior, posterior, and superior arms. The anterior arm inserts onto the orbital process of the maxillary bone anterior and above the anterior lacrimal crest (Fig. 2.8).

The width of the tendon on insertion is approximately 4 to 5 mm. The anterior arm provides the main support for the medial canthal angle. The posterior arm arises from the common tendon close to the junction of the superior and inferior crura and passes posteriorly between the superior and inferior canaliculi. The posterior arm continues along the postero-lateral aspect of the lacrimal sac. It continues posteriorly fanning out to form a broad sheet between 6 and 9 mm in vertical height. The posterior arm inserts onto the posterior lacrimal crest just anterior to Horner's muscle. The posterior arm serves to direct the vector forces of the canthal angle posteriorly to maintain a close apposition of the lids to the globe.

KEY POINT

It is the posterior arm of the medial canthal tendon inserting into the posterior lacrimal crest that must be repaired meticulously when a lower eyelid has been avulsed to avoid an anterior malposition of the lower eyelid.

The superior arm of the medial canthal tendon takes origin from the anterior and posterior arms and passes superiorly 7 to 10 mm inserting onto the orbital process of the frontal bone (Fig. 2.8). The superior arm may serve to provide vertical support to the canthal angle and may also play a role in the lacrimal pump mechanism.

Laterally the tarsal plates extend into less well-defined fibrous strands that become the superior and inferior crura of the lateral canthal tendon. The lateral canthal tendon measures approximately 5 to 7 mm in length. It is approximately 3 mm in width at the point where the superior and inferior crura unite but it broadens to a width of approximately 6 to 7 mm as it inserts into the lateral orbital tubercle 1.5 mm inside the lateral orbital margin. The lateral horn of the levator aponeurosis blends with the superior border of the lateral canthal tendon. The lateral canthal tendon and the lateral horn of the levator aponeurosis extend superiorly to a position 4 to 5 mm below the fronto-zygomatic suture line forming a broad tendon-like insertion (Fig. 2.9).

The inferior crus of the lateral canthal tendon is divided during the course of a lateral tarsal strip procedure and to effect a rapid orbital decompression for the management of an acute retrobulbar hemorrhage. It can be seen from Figure 2.9 why the division of the superior crus of the lateral canthal tendon can be associated with significant morbidity due to the proximity of important adjacent structures, i.e., the lateral horn of the levator, Whitnall's ligament, and the lacrimal gland.

These fibers continue posteriorly along the lateral orbital wall fusing with fibers of the lateral check ligament. Along with the lateral canthal tendon complex the infero-lateral fibers of Whitnall's superior suspensory ligament and the lateral portion of Lockwood's inferior suspensory ligament insert onto the lateral tubercle forming the lateral retinaculum (Fig. 2.10).

A small lobule from the pre-capsulopalpebral fat pad extends superiorly between the orbital septum and the lateral canthal tendon. This is referred to as Eisler's pocket. This is thought to act like a bursa allowing some independent movement of the lateral canthal tendon during eyelid movement particularly on lateral gaze.

The Pre-aponeurotic Fat Pads

The pre-aponeurotic fat pads in the upper eyelid and the pre-capsulopalpebral fat pads in the lower eyelid are anterior extensions of the extraconal orbital fat. The fat pads are enveloped by thin fibrous sheaths that represent forward continuations of the anterior orbital septal system. The individual lobules of fat within the fat pockets are surrounded by fine interlobular septa. The fibrous sheaths surrounding the fat pads are connected to the overlying orbital septum and the underlying levator aponeurosis by very fine fibrous bands. The eyelid fat pads are very important surgical landmarks

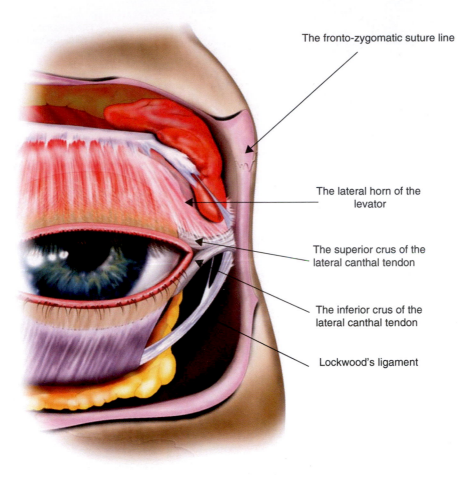

The fronto-zygomatic suture line

The lateral horn of the levator

The superior crus of the lateral canthal tendon

The inferior crus of the lateral canthal tendon

Lockwood's ligament

Figure 2.9 The lateral canthal tendon and its adjacent structures.

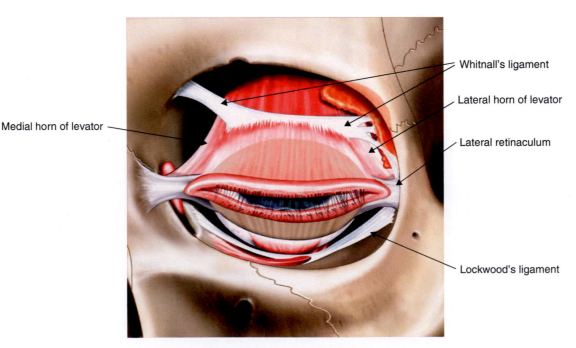

Whitnall's ligament

Lateral horn of levator

Lateral retinaculum

Medial horn of levator

Lockwood's ligament

Figure 2.10 The lateral retinaculum.

which assist in the identification of the eyelid retractors which lie immediately posterior to the fat pads (Fig. 2.2).

In the upper eyelid, there are two fat pads: one medially and one centrally (Fig. 2.11).

These are separated by fine fascial bands, which are continuous with the trochlea. The medial fat pad is paler than the central fat pad and contains thicker and more abundant interlobular septa. In the lateral aspect of the upper eyelid, the lacrimal gland is located in the lacrimal gland fossa just posterior to the orbital margin (Fig. 2.9).

The lacrimal gland is isolated within its own fascial compartment. If this fascial support system of the lacrimal gland becomes loose the gland may prolapse into the lateral aspect of the eyelid where it must not be mistaken for pre-aponeurotic fat (Fig. 2.12).

The appearance of the lacrimal gland is quite distinctive appearing pink in color (Fig. 2.13).

It is also firm in contrast to pre-aponeurotic fat.

There are three fat pads in the lower eyelid each of which is separated by fibrous septa, which are continuous with the orbital connective tissue system (Fig. 2.14).

The central and lateral fat pads are separated by a connective tissue band referred to as the arcuate expansion which extends from Lockwood's ligament to the inferolateral orbital margin. The inferior oblique muscle runs between the medial and central fat pockets (Fig. 2.15).

The Eyelid Retractors

The levator palpebrae superioris muscle arises from the lesser wing of the sphenoid bone just above the annulus of Zinn and superolateral to the optic canal (Fig. 2.16).

The muscle is approximately 35 mm in length. At its origin it is approximately 4 mm in width widening to approximately 8 mm in the mid-section of the orbit. As the muscle passes forward, it lies in intimate contact with the superior rectus muscle (Fig. 2.2). The levator and the superior rectus muscles are connected by fine fibrous strands of the superior orbital fascial system. Extensive fibrous tissue strands connect the sheath of the levator muscle with the superior rectus muscle below and with the superior conjunctival fornix and Tenon's capsule just behind Whitnall's ligament.

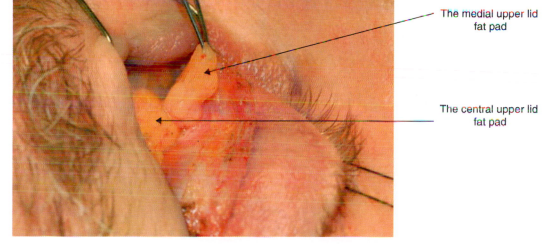

The medial upper lid fat pad

The central upper lid fat pad

Figure 2.11 The medial and central upper lid fat pads. The medial fat pad is paler than the central fat pad.

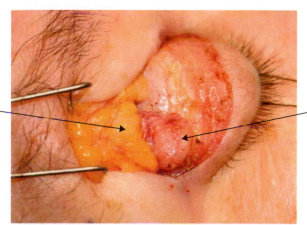

The central upper eyelid preaponeurotic fat

A prolapsed lacrimal gland

Figure 2.12 A prolapsed lacrimal gland contrasted against central upper eyelid pre-aponeurotic fat.

These fibrous tissue strands function as check ligaments but permit coordinated movement of the upper eyelid with alterations in the vertical ocular gaze position. The levator muscle widens to approximately 18 mm just posterior to the superior orbital margin. In this location, a condensation of variable thickness and density is seen running along the muscle sheath in a horizontal direction. This is Whitnall's superior transverse ligament (Fig. 2.17).

Whitnall's ligament attaches to the fascia adjacent to the trochlea medially and laterally inserts into the lacrimal gland capsule and the periorbita of the lower aspect of the frontal bone (Fig. 2.10).

The ligament is firmly attached to the levator muscle sheath medially and laterally but only very loosely attached to the levator muscle centrally. A very thin sheet of fascia passes from Whitnall's ligament to insert into the superior orbital margin.

Whitnall's ligament appears to function as a check ligament against posterior movement of the levator and superior rectus muscles. Whitnall's ligament forms a circum-orbital fascial ring in conjunction with Lockwood's ligament. During ptosis surgery Whitnall's ligament should be maintained intact wherever possible. If Whitnall's ligament is severed, the levator muscle prolapses. This loss of support results in the need for a greater

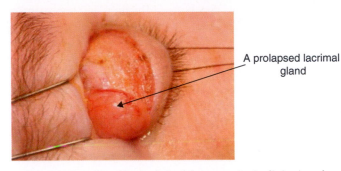

Figure 2.13 A prolapsed lacrimal gland demonstrating its distinctive color.

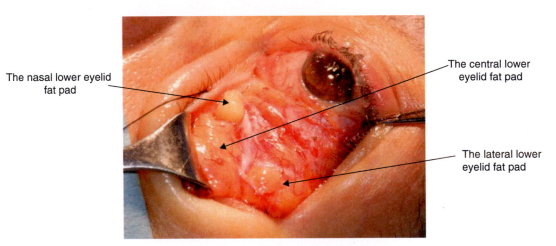

Figure 2.14 The lower eyelid fat pads as seen during a lower eyelid transconjunctival blepharoplasty.

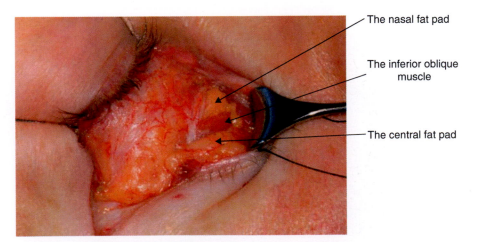

Figure 2.15 The inferior oblique muscle lying between the nasal and the central lower eyelid fat pads.

resection than would otherwise be required. The ligament can also be used as an internal sling during ptosis surgery.

The levator muscle attaches to the fibrous levator aponeurosis in close proximity to Whitnall's ligament (Fig. 2.2). The levator aponeurosis continues inferiorly approximately 15 to 20 mm to insert onto the superior two thirds of the anterior tarsal surface (Fig. 2.2). Delicate fibers also continue forward from the levator aponeurosis to insert onto the septum of the pre-tarsal orbicularis muscle and the skin (Fig. 2.2). The delicate fibers from the levator aponeurosis retract the pre-tarsal skin and muscle and orbicularis muscle preventing an overhang of these structures on elevation of the eyelid. The superior limits of the attachment of these layers are marked by the upper lid skin crease. This relationship is disturbed by a dehiscence of the levator aponeurosis, which results in an apparent superior displacement of the upper lid skin crease (Fig. 2.18).

The levator aponeurosis widens to form the medial and lateral levator horns as it passes inferiorly from Whitnall's ligament (Fig. 2.19).

The medial horn is more tenuous accounting for a lateral shift of the superior tarsus in older patients. Great care should be taken to avoid further intraoperative damage to the medial horn as this will result in a further lateral shift of the superior tarsus, and an unsatisfactory temporal displacement of the peak of the eyelid. The lateral horn, which is a better defined structure, separates the lacrimal gland into orbital and palpebral lobes (Fig. 2.20).

The lateral levator horn inserts onto the lateral orbital tubercle of the zygomatic bone at the level of the lateral retinaculum (Fig. 2.20). It also joins with fibers of the capsulopalpebral fascia of the lower eyelid.

The medial horn of the levator aponeurosis inserts onto the posterior limb of the medial canthal tendon and the posterior lacrimal crest (Fig. 2.19). The medial and lateral levator horns help to distribute the forces generated by the levator muscle

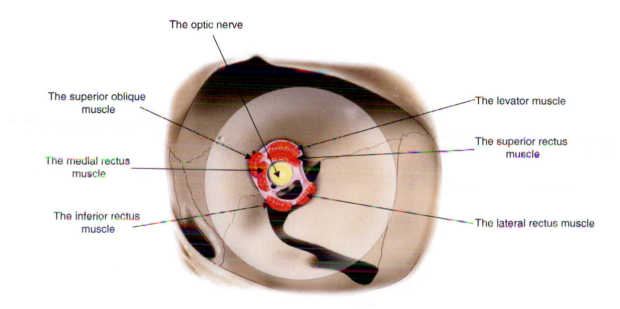

Figure 2.16 The origin of the levator palpebrae superioris muscle.

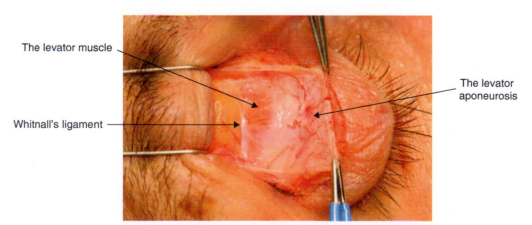

Figure 2.17 Whitnall's ligament.

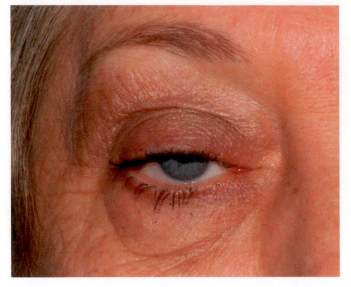

Figure 2.18 A patient with a ptosis due to dehiscence of the levator aponeurosis. Note the very high skin crease typically seen in such a ptosis.

along the levator aponeurosis allowing the central aspect of the eyelid to elevate to the greatest extent. The lateral levator aponeurosis horn is severed during levator aponeurosis recession procedures undertaken for the management of thyroid-related eyelid retraction. In contrast, however, during surgery to advance to the levator aponeurosis for the management of a blepharoptosis, the levator horns should be preserved wherever possible.

KEY POINT

During a levator aponeurosis advancement procedure the medial and lateral horns of the levator muscle should be preserved.

Müller's muscle is joined to the overlying levator aponeurosis by a very loose connective tissue layer. This avascular plane can usually be dissected easily during ptosis surgery procedures (Fig. 2.21).

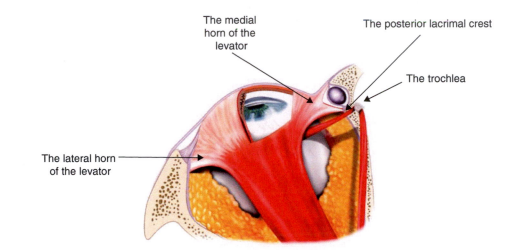

Figure 2.19 The medial and lateral horns of the levator.

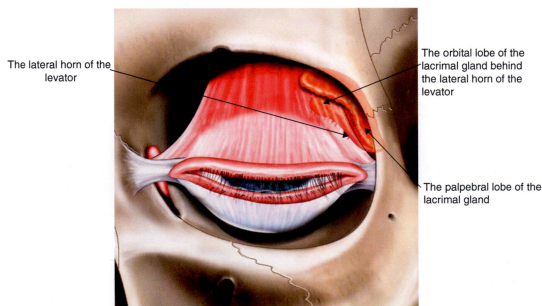

Figure 2.20 The lateral horn of the levator divides the lacrimal gland into orbital and palpebral lobes.

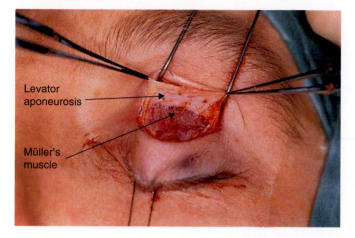

Figure 2.21 The levator aponeurosis elevated to demonstrate the avascular plane between the levator aponeurosis and the underlying Müller's muscle.

Müller's muscle takes origin from the under surface of the levator muscle at a point just distal to Whitnall's ligament (Fig. 2.2). Müller's muscle runs inferiorly posterior to the levator aponeurosis. It measures approximately 8 to 12 mm in length and has a variable thickness of 0.1 to 0.5 mm. Müller's muscle inserts onto the anterior edge of the superior border of the tarsus (Fig. 2.2). Müller's muscle is innervated by sympathetic nerve fibers, which pass to the orbit via the internal carotid plexus. These sympathetic nerve fibers originate in the hypothalamus. Disruption of the sympathetic innervation of Müller's muscle results in the ptosis seen in a Horner's syndrome.

In the lower eyelid, the capsulo-palpebral fascia is a fibrous sheet, which arises from Lockwood's ligament and the inferior rectus and inferior oblique muscle sheaths (Fig. 2.2). As it passes superiorly the fascia fuses with the orbital septum approximately 4 to 5 mm below the inferior border of the tarsal plate (Fig. 2.2). From this position, a common fascial sheet passes superiorly and inserts onto the inferior border of the tarsus (Fig. 2.2). Fine fibers pass anteriorly from this fascial sheet to the orbital septum and the skin creating the lower eyelid crease in a manner analogous to that of the upper eyelid.

Smooth muscle fibers analogous to Müller's muscle in the upper eyelid lie posterior to the capsulo-palpebral fascia forming a very thin muscular layer (Fig. 2.2). These fibers are also innervated by the sympathetic nervous system. Disruption of the sympathetic innervation of these muscle fibers results in a slight rise in the lower eyelid seen in a Horner's syndrome.

The Conjunctiva

The conjunctiva is a mucous membrane, which can be arbitrarily divided into palpebral, forniceal, and bulbar portions. The palpebral portion is very closely applied to the posterior surface of the tarsus in the upper and lower eyelids from which it cannot be separated. This portion is also closely applied to Müller's muscle in the upper lid and the equivalent smooth muscle fibers in the lower lid (Fig. 2.22).

The palpebral portion continues into the forniceal portion. The superior fornix is situated approximately 10 mm above the superior corneal limbus. The superior fornix is supported by a fine fibrous suspensory ligament, which

arises from the fascia of the levator muscle and the superior rectus muscle. The inferior fornix is situated approximately 8 mm below the inferior corneal limbus and is supported by a fine suspensory ligament which arises from Lockwood's ligament. This is situated just posterior to the capsulo-palpebral fascia and functions to retract the fornix inferiorly during down gaze.

The conjunctiva contains a series of small accessory lacrimal glands. Lymphatic blood vessels and sensory nerves run in the conjunctival submucosa. A small, elevated structure consisting of sebaceous glands, sweat glands, and fine hairs lies within the medial canthal angle. This is the caruncle. A vertical fold of conjunctiva the plica semilunaris lies just lateral to the caruncle. The medial wall of the orbit can be accessed via an incision made between these two structures, e.g., a transcaruncular approach to the drainage of a medial subperiosteal orbital abscess complicating orbital cellulitis.

Sensory Nerve Supply of the Eyelids

The sensory innervation of the eyelids is provided by branches of the ophthalmic and maxillary divisions of the trigeminal nerve. The upper eyelid is innervated by the supraorbital, supratrochlear, and lacrimal nerves (Fig. 2.23).

The medial aspect of the upper and lower eyelids is supplied by the infratrochlear nerve. Branches of the infratrochlear nerve also supply parts of the adjacent eyebrow, forehead, and nose (Fig. 2.23). The lateral aspect of the upper eyelid and temple is supplied by the zygomatico-temporal branch of the maxillary nerve (Fig. 2.23). The central aspect of the lower eyelid is supplied by infraorbital nerve, a branch of the maxillary nerve and the lateral aspect of the lower eyelid is supplied by the zygomaticofacial branch of the maxillary nerve. (A more detailed description of the periorbital sensory nerve supply is outlined later in this chapter.)

Vascular Supply to the Eyelids

The eyelids have a very rich blood supply with multiple anastomoses (Fig. 2.24).

The anterior lamellae of the eyelids are supplied by branches of the external carotid artery namely the transverse facial, superficial temporal, and angular arteries in conjunction with multiple anastomoses with vessels passing through the orbit (Fig. 2.24). The posterior lamellae of the eyelids are supplied by vascular arcades. In the upper eyelid, a marginal arcade runs horizontally about 2 mm above the eyelid margin (Fig. 2.24). A more peripheral arcade runs along the superior border of the tarsus between the levator aponeurosis and Muller's muscle (Fig. 2.25).

These arcades are supplied medially by the superior medial palpebral artery, a terminal branch of the ophthalmic artery, while laterally the arcades are fed by the superior lateral palpebral artery, a branch of the lacrimal artery (Fig. 2.24).

The lymphatic drainage channels are extensive and well developed and lie anterior to the orbital septum. Lymph from the lateral two thirds of the upper eyelid and the lateral one third of the lower eyelid drains laterally and inferiorly into the deep and superficial parotid and submandibular lymph nodes. Lymph from the medial one third of the upper eyelid and the medial two thirds of the lower eyelid drains medially and inferiorly into the anterior cervical lymph nodes (Fig. 2.26).

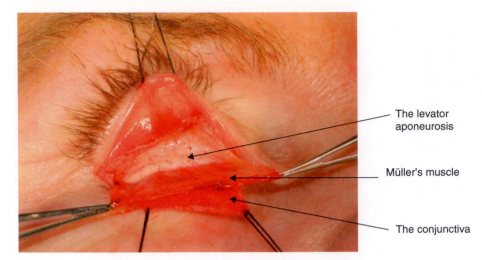

The levator
aponeurosis

Müller's muscle

The conjunctiva

Figure 2.22 Müller's muscle as seen during a posterior approach Müller's muscle resection.

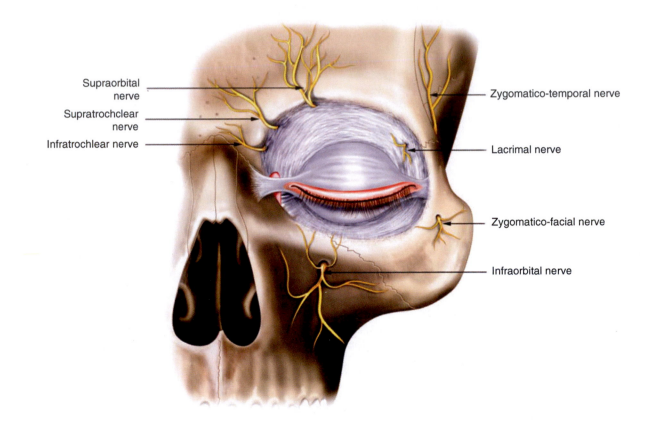

Supraorbital
nerve

Supratrochlear
nerve

Infratrochlear nerve

Zygomatico-temporal nerve

Lacrimal nerve

Zygomatico-facial nerve

Infraorbital nerve

Figure 2.23 The sensory innervation of the eyelids and periorbital area.

Extensive disruption of these lymphatic channels results in lymphoedema.Figure 2.1 The canthal angles.

THE EYEBROWS

The eyebrows consist of thickened skin overlying the supra-orbital prominences from which the eyebrows are separated by the brow fat pads (Fig. 2.2). The eyebrows contain coarse hairs, which emerge from the skin surface at an oblique angle. The eyebrows are raised by the frontalis muscle and are depressed by the actions of the procerus, corrugator and depressor supercilii muscles, and the orbicularis oculi muscles (Figs. 2.4 and 2.27).

The brow elevators and the brow depressors are all inner-vated by branches of the facial nerve.

The eyebrows tend to be heavier and flatter in males and higher and more arched in females although there are great inter-individual variations. The brows tend to become pro-gressively ptotic with age.

The muscle fibers of the frontalis muscle lie vertically on the forehead and form the anterior belly of the occipitofrontalis muscular fascial complex. The occipital and frontalis muscles are separated by the galea aponeurotica (Fig. 2.28).

The frontalis muscle connects to the galea aponeurotica in the region of the coronal suture line and runs inferiorly to the

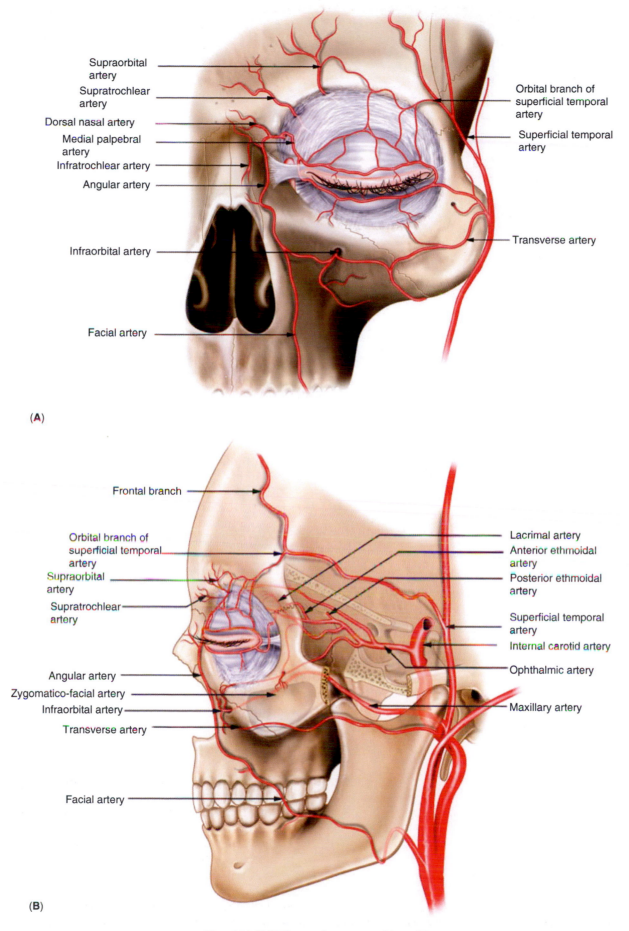

Supraorbital artery

Supratrochlear artery

Dorsal nasal artery

Medial palpebral artery

Infratrochlear artery

Angular artery

Infraorbital artery

Facial artery

Orbital branch of superficial temporal artery

Superficial temporal artery

Transverse artery

(A)

Frontal branch

Orbital branch of superficial temporal artery

Supraorbital artery

Supratrochlear artery

Angular artery

Zygomatico-facial artery

Infraorbital artery

Transverse artery

Facial artery

Lacrimal artery

Anterior ethmoidal artery

Posterior ethmoidal artery

Superficial temporal artery

Internal carotid artery

Ophthalmic artery

Maxillary artery

(B)

Figure 2.24 (**A,B**) The vascular anatomy of the eyelids.

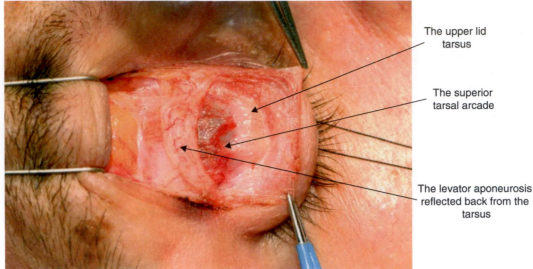

Figure 2.25 The peripheral vascular arcade in the upper eyelid.

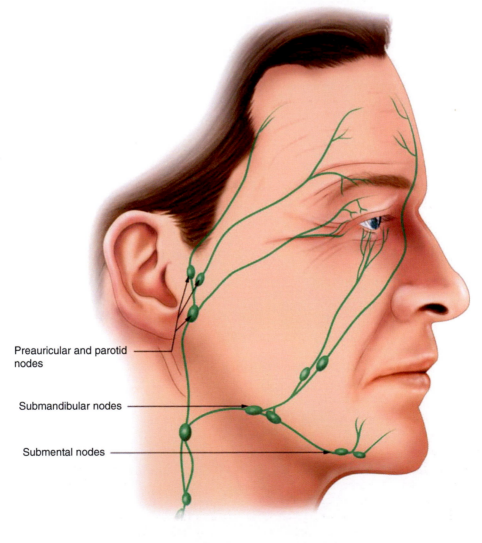

Figure 2.26 The lymphatic drainage of the eyelids.

superior orbital margin. The galea aponeurotica forms a narrow extension that runs between the bellies of the frontalis muscle onto the bridge of the nose. The frontalis muscle has no bony attachments at all. Medially the muscle fibers interdigitate with those of the procerus muscle and laterally the frontalis muscle fibers interdigitate with the corrugator

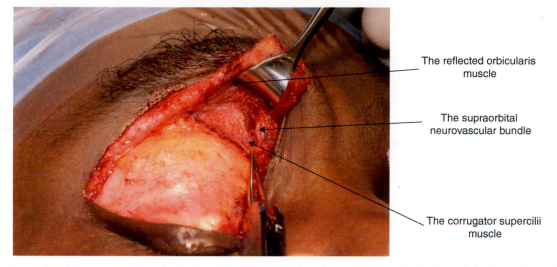

Figure 2.27 A patient undergoing an upper eyelid orbicularis myectomy for essential blepharospasm. The orbicularis muscle had been dissected away from the tarsus and the orbital septum.

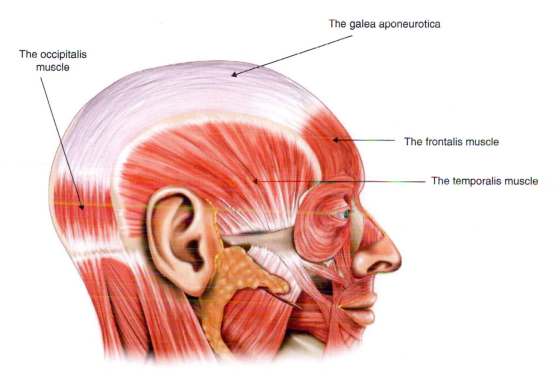

Figure 2.28 The frontalis and occipitalis muscles joined by the galea aponeurotica.

supercilii muscles and the orbital portion of the orbicularis oculi muscles. In the region of the superior orbital margin, a deep fat pad separates the frontalis muscle from the underlying deep fascia. This brow fat pad continues into the upper eyelid where it fuses with the layer of fascia lying posterior to the orbicularis oculi muscle. In some patients particularly those over the age of 50, globules of fat may descend into the eyelid and these should not be confused with the central pre-aponeurotic fat pads.

The frontalis muscle acts as an elevator of the brow and also serves as an accessory retractor of the upper eyelid. Over action of the frontalis muscle is seen in patients with a blepharoptosis.

It is for this reason that the frontalis muscle should be firmly immobilized when measuring a patient's levator function.

The corrugator supercilii muscle has a pyramidal shape and lies medially beneath the frontalis muscle and the orbital portion of the orbicularis oculi muscle (Fig. 2.4). It arises from the medial end of the frontal bone at the superior orbital margin. It extends obliquely superiorly and laterally. The muscle inserts into the deep fascia of the frontalis muscle along the lateral third of the eyebrow by means of a series of slips. In this area, the deep fascia comprises several distinct layers, and fibers of the corrugator supercilii muscle interdigitate among these. Contraction of the corrugator supercilii muscles causes the brow to move in a medial and downward direction and creates vertical folds in the glabella.

The depressor supercilii muscle is distinct from the corrugator supercilii muscle and the medial head of the orbital portion of the orbicularis oculi muscle. It arises from most individuals as two distinct heads from the frontal process of the maxilla approximately 1 cm above the medial canthal tendon, with the angular vessels passing between the two muscle heads. The muscle inserts into the dermis approximately 13 to 14 mm above the medial canthal tendon (Fig. 2.4).

The procerus muscle has a pyramidal shape. It arises from the fascia covering the lower part of the nasal bone and upper lateral nasal cartilage. It extends vertically between the eyebrows and inserts into the skin lying over the lower aspect of the forehead (Fig. 2.4). The fibers of the procerus muscle merge with those of the medial aspect of the frontalis muscle. Contraction of the procerus muscle pulls the medial aspect of the brows in a downward direction and produces transverse lines over the bridge of the nose.

The orbital portion of the orbicularis muscle runs in a circular direction and overlies the bony orbital margins (Fig. 2.4). Within the eyebrow the orbicularis muscle fibers interdigitate with those of the frontalis muscle and subcutaneous fascia. Contraction of the orbital portion of the orbicularis oculi muscle draws the brows downward and produces the lateral rhytids of the lateral canthi.

The frontalis muscle is responsible for the appearance of horizontal creases in the forehead skin. These creases can be reduced for aesthetic reasons with the use of botulinum toxin injections, but great care should be taken in administering such injections as weakening the action of the frontalis muscle can result in an unsatisfactory brow ptosis. The corrugator and depressor supercilii muscles are responsible for the appearance of frown lines in the glabellar region. The injection of botulinum toxin into these muscles can remove or soften the appearance of such lines, which can be responsible for facial miscues, giving the unwanted impression of anger. This is particularly noticeable in patients with thyroid eye disease (Fig. 2.29).

The superolateral part of the orbicularis oculi muscle is responsible for the appearance of lateral canthal rhytids and for depression of the temporal aspect of the eyebrow. The injection of botulinum toxin into this part of the muscle can remove or soften the appearance of these lines and can also result in a temporal brow lift due to the unopposed action of the frontalis muscle. In some individuals, this action can, however, result in an unwanted peaking of the temporal brow.

THE FACIAL NERVE

A very good understanding of the relationship of the facial nerve and its branches to the fascial planes of the face is essential. The facial nerve exits the stylomastoid foramen and gives off the postauricular nerve and the branch to the posterior belly of the diagastric and stylo-hyoid muscles. The main trunk then usually bifurcates into the upper (temporo-zygomatic) and lower (cervico-facial) branches

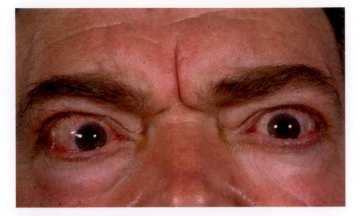

Figure 2.29 Marked glabellar frown lines in a patient with thyroid eye disease.

as it approaches the postero-medial border of the parotid gland. As it passes forward within the substance of the parotid gland, it lies between the superficial and deep lobes. The nerve divides in a variable pattern into the main distal branches (the temporal or frontal, zygomatic, buccal, mandibular, and cervical branches) (Fig. 2.30).

At the anterior border of the parotid gland, these branches lie on the surface of the masseter muscle deep to the parotido-masseteric fascia. The temporal nerve is the smallest of the branches and has the least number of interconnections. In the majority of individuals, the temporal branch is a terminal branch. It is the branch which frequently shows the least degree of recovery following a facial palsy.

The temporal branch becomes superficial once it crosses the zygomatic arch where the nerve is most vulnerable to injury. The approximate position of this branch (branches) is indicated in Figure 2.31.

Three to five branches cross the zygomatic arch. The most posterior branch is always anterior to the superficial temporal vessels. The anterior hairline at the level of the lateral canthus represents the junction of the posterior and middle branches of the nerve. The most anterior branch crosses the zygomatic arch approximately 2 cm posterior to the posterior aspect of the lateral orbital margin (Fig. 2.30). In the brow region, the frontal branch runs approximately 2 cm above the brow. In the temple the nerve runs within the superficial temporoparietal fascia and supplies the frontalis muscle, the superior fibers of the orbicularis muscle, the procerus and corrugator supercilii muscles. It is important to stay on the glistening fibers of the deep temporal fascia deep to the temporoparietal fascia to avoid injury to the nerve during surgical dissections in this area, e.g., when undertaking an endoscopic brow lift.

The zygomatic and buccal branches of the facial nerve pass medially across the surface of the masseter muscle under the parotidomasseteric fascia where they are relatively well protected. At the anterior border of the masseter muscle, the branches pass over the buccal fat pad and course forward to supply the inferior fibers of the orbicularis oculi muscle, the zygomaticus major and minor muscles, and the levator labii muscle by accessing the muscles from their deep surface.

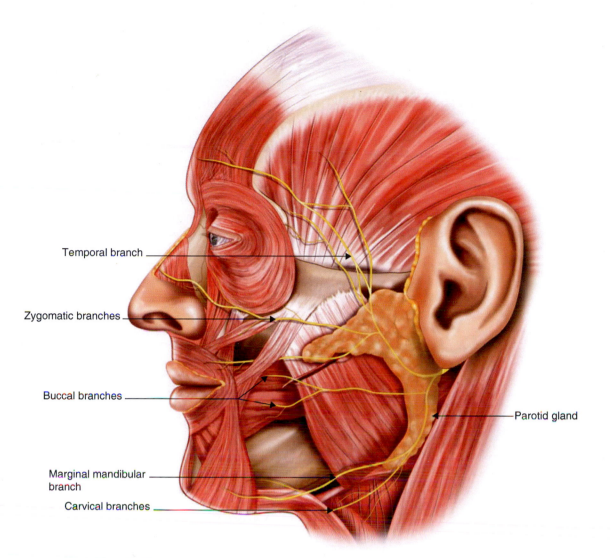

Figure 2.30 Branches of the facial nerve.

Temporal branch

Zygomatic branches

Buccal branches

Parotid gland

Marginal mandibular branch

Carvical branches

KEY POINT

It is extremely important to understand the different anatomical planes which are traversed by branches of the facial nerve in order to avoid intraoperative damage to these. The safe planes of dissection:

- Pre-auricular area: superficial to the parotid gland
- Over the zygomatic arch: in the subcutaneous fat
- 1 cm above the zygomatic arch: in the subcutaneous fat or deep to the superficial layer of the deep temporal fascia
- In the temple: just superficial to the deep layer of the temporal fascia
- Over the frontalis muscle: in the subcutaneous fat or deep to the galea aponeurotica
- In the mid-face: in the subcutaneous fat
- In the lower face: in the subcutaneous fat

The marginal mandibular nerve passes from the lower pole of the parotid gland and descends below the mandible in the area posterior to the facial artery lying 1 to 2 cm inferior to its lower border (Fig. 2.30). In older individuals and with extension of the neck, it can lie even lower. Like the frontal branch of the facial nerve, the marginal mandibular branch is a terminal branch and is most liable to injury. Its injury causes an obvious clinical deficit due to paralysis of the depressor labii inferioris muscle. It enters the platysma muscle along its deep surface and is liable to injury in operations requiring elevation and division of platysma in the upper neck. In 10 to 15% of patients, there are connections between this nerve and the buccal branches. In these patients, considerable recovery of function will take place even if this nerve is transected

The cervical branch is the most inferior of the facial nerve branches. Below the parotid gland, it passes deep to the platysma muscle which it innervates.

THE BONY ORBIT

In the adult, the bony orbit is pyramidal in shape. The volume of the orbit in the average adult is approximately 30 cm^3. The globe contributes approximately 7.5 cm^3. The anterior entry to the orbit forms an approximate rectangle 4 cm in width, by 3.5 cm in height. The widest dimension of the orbit is attained approximately 1 cm posterior to the anterior orbital margin. The anterior–posterior axes of the orbits form a 45° angle between them. The lateral orbital walls form a 90° angle between them (Fig. 2.32).

The dimensions of the orbit vary from patient to patient. For this reason, a surgeon cannot rely on any specific measurements as a guide to the precise location of the optic canal or of the superior orbital fissure. Great care should therefore be taken when injecting fat for example into the posterior orbit of an anophthalmic patient as the cannula could penetrate the intracranial cavity. The precise location of the anterior and posterior ethmoidal foramina cannot be determined accurately prior to surgical dissection. For this reason, great care must be taken in undertaking dissections in the medial and posterior orbit during an orbital decompression procedure or during the exploration of a medial orbital wall blowout fracture. The inferior orbital fissure may lie within 10 to 15 mm of the anterior orbital margin. It should be noted that the floor of the orbit ends at the posterior wall of the maxillary sinus and does not extend to the apex of the orbit (Fig. 2.33).

KEY POINT

The dimensions of the orbit vary from patient to patient. For this reason, a surgeon cannot rely on any specific measurements as a guide to the precise location of the optic canal or of the superior orbital fissure.

The Orbital Margin

The anterior orbital margin is rounded and thickened. The superior orbital margin is the most prominent due to expansion of the underlying frontal sinus. The supraorbital neurovascular bundle forms a notch or a foramen in the medial third of the superior orbital margin (Fig. 2.34).

A notch is present in approximately two thirds of all orbits whereas a foramen is seen in the remaining third. An awareness of the location of the supraorbital notch or foramen is important in order to avoid injury to the nerve during brow lifting surgery, during coronal flap approaches to the superomedial orbit, during superomedial anterior orbitotomy procedures, and orbicularis myectomy procedures. Between the supraorbital notch or foramen and the medial canthal tendon, the supratrochlear and infratrochlear neurovascular bundles and the dorsal nasal artery emerge (Fig. 2.24). The cartilaginous trochlea of the superior oblique tendon lies just within the orbital rim in this location (Fig. 2.35).

The superior orbital margin passes downward medially to the posterior lacrimal crest where this ends at the entrance to the lacrimal canal (Fig. 2.36).

The inferior orbital margin medially passes upward as the anterior lacrimal crest to a position just above the medial canthal tendon insertion. The lacrimal sac fossa therefore represents a discontinuity in the medial orbital margin. The sutura notha containing a branch of the infero-orbital artery lies just in front of the anterior lacrimal crest and is seen as a vertical groove in the bone (Fig. 2.37).

This is an important and constant landmark during an external dacryocystorhinostomy (DCR) and should not be mistaken for the medial edge of the anterior lacrimal crest.

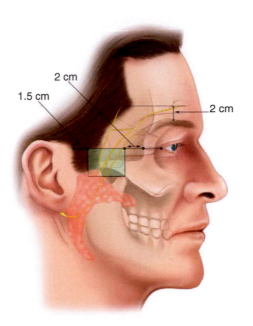

Figure 2.31 The course of the temporal branch of the facial nerve.

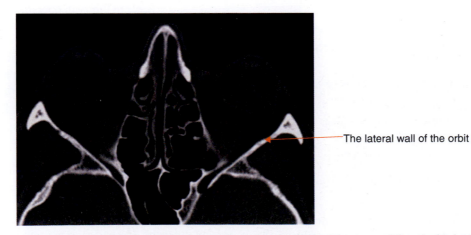

Figure 2.32 Axial CT scan of the orbits demonstrating the 90° angle between the lateral orbital walls. (The apparent bilateral orbital apical masses are the enlarged inferior recti of a patient with thyroid eye disease.)

The maxillary bone medially and the zygomatic bone laterally form the inferior orbital margin (Fig. 2.38).

The inferior orbital foramen, through which passes the inferior orbital neurovascular bundle, is located approximately 4 to 8 mm below the central portion of the inferior orbital margin (Fig. 2.38). Great care must be taken to avoid damage to the inferior orbital neurovascular bundle in elevating the periosteum anterior to the inferior orbital rim during orbital decompression surgery, orbital floor blowout fracture repair surgery and mid face lift procedures.

The lateral orbital margin is formed by the zygomatic process of the frontal bone superiorly and the frontal process of the zygomatic bone inferiorly (Fig. 2.39).

These meet at the fronto-zygomatic suture line of the supra-temporal aspect of the orbit. This represents an important surgical landmark as the anterior cranial fossa lies approximately 5 to 15 mm above this suture. The suture is relatively weak and is frequently seen as a point of separation in zygomatico-maxillary complex (ZMC) fractures. The lateral orbital tubercle, a smooth raised area of bone lying just on the inside edge

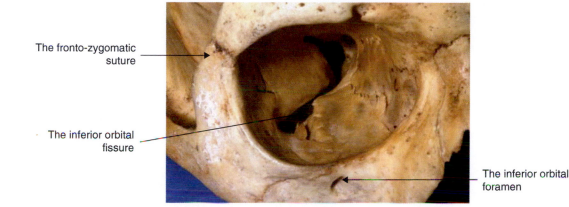

The fronto-zygomatic suture

The inferior orbital fissure

The inferior orbital foramen

Figure 2.33 The floor of the orbit.

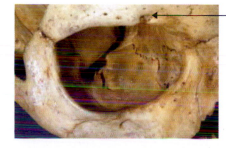

The supraorbital notch

Figure 2.34 The supraorbital notch.

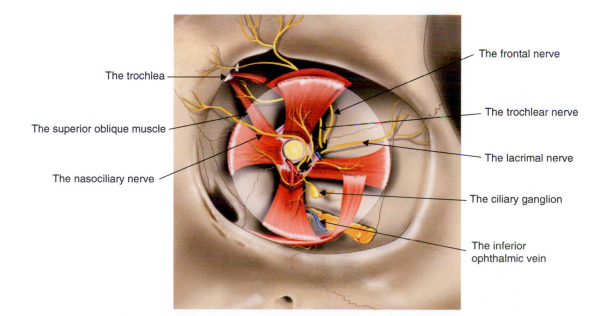

The trochlea

The superior oblique muscle

The nasociliary nerve

The frontal nerve

The trochlear nerve

The lacrimal nerve

The ciliary ganglion

The inferior ophthalmic vein

Figure 2.35 The position of the trochlea and the structures at the apex of the orbit.

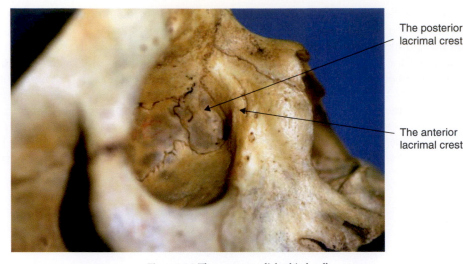

Figure 2.36 The antero-medial orbital wall.

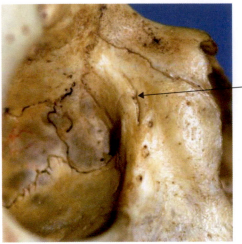

Figure 2.37 The sutura notha.

of the lateral orbital margin, serves as the site of insertion of the posterior crus of the lateral canthal tendon, Lockwood's inferior suspensory ligament, the lateral horn of the aponeurosis of the levator palpebrae superioris, the lateral check ligament of the lateral rectus muscle, and the deepest layer of the orbital septum (Fig. 2.40).

Failure to re-align these structures during a repair of ZMC fractures results in a typical cosmetic deformity (Fig. 2.41).

The Medial Orbital Wall

The medial wall of the orbit is formed by four bones: the maxillary, lacrimal, ethmoid, and sphenoid bones (Fig. 2.42).

The medial orbital wall measures approximately 45 to 50 mm in length from the medial orbital margin to the apex of the orbit. The frontal process of the maxillary bone contains the anterior lacrimal crest and forms the anterior part of the lacrimal sac fossa. The posterior part of the lacrimal sac fossa is formed by the lacrimal bone, which is a very small thin and fragile bone (Fig. 2.37). The posterior lacrimal crest runs vertically along the mid-point of the lacrimal bone. The lacrimo-maxillary suture lies vertically in the center of the lacrimal sac fossa in the majority of patients but in a small proportion of patients this suture lies more posteriorly. In such patients

creating a bony osteotomy during an external DCR will be more difficult, and a coarse diamond burr may be required to thin the bone prior to its removal with a Rongeur.

The lamina papyracea lies behind the posterior lacrimal crest. This forms the lateral wall of the ethmoid sinuses. This bone is very thin and offers little resistance to blunt trauma. It also offers little resistance to the spread of infection from the ethmoid sinuses to the orbit.

Superiorly the medial orbital wall is formed by the frontal bone, which joins the lamina papyracea at the fronto-ethmoidal suture line (Fig. 2.42). This is an important surgical landmark lying on a level with the roof of the ethmoid sinuses and the floor, and the anterior cranial fossa. The cribriform plate lies just medial to the roof of the ethmoid sinuses (the fovea ethmoidalis) and may extend 5 to 10 mm below the level of the fronto-ethmoidal suture line (Fig. 2.43).

This relationship must be borne in mind during surgery along the medial orbital wall particularly during orbital decompression surgery. The position of the cribriform plate should be ascertained on coronal CT scans prior to the performance of an orbital decompression procedure and before the use of a transnasal wire in medial canthal reconstructive surgery.

> **KEY POINT**
>
> The cribriform plate lies just medial to the roof of the ethmoid sinuses (the fovea ethmoidalis) and may extend 5 to 10 mm below the level of the fronto-ethmoidal suture line.

It should also be noted that the anterior cranial fossa may be as little as 1 to 2 mm above the superior border of the medial canthal tendon at the mid-portion of the lacrimal fossa. It is for this reason that it is unwise to detach the medial canthal tendon during external lacrimal drainage surgery. It is preferable to leave the medial canthal tendon attached and to use this position as a guide for the upper-most limit of the osteotomy to avoid the risk of a cerebrospinal fluid (CSF) leak.

The anterior and posterior ethmoidal foramina are very variable in their position. They tend to lie within the

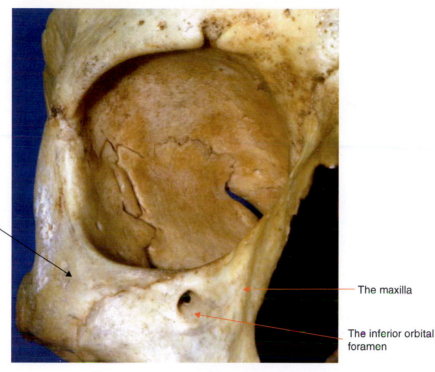

The zygoma

The maxilla

The inferior orbital foramen

Figure 2.38 The inferior orbital margin.

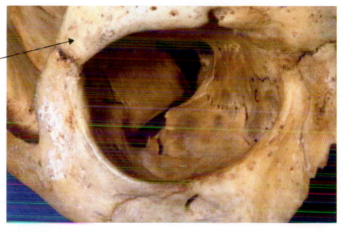

The zygomatic process of the frontal bone

Figure 2.39 Lateral orbital margin.

fronto-ethmoidal suture line but may lie above this line (Fig. 2.42). The posterior foramen may be absent or both foramina may be multiple. The foramina transmit branches of the ophthalmic artery and nasociliary nerve. In the majority of patients, the anterior ethmoidal foramen lies approximately from 20 to 25 mm behind the anterior lacrimal crest but may lie as close as 16 mm and as far as 42 mm behind the anterior lacrimal crest. The posterior ethmoidal foramen lies approximately 5 to 10 mm anterior to the optic canal. Damage to the ethmoid arteries can result in severe bleeding and the formation of a sub-periosteal hematoma. These neurovascular bundles should be carefully identified and cauterized during orbital exenteration surgery. The neurovascular bundles should be avoided completely during medial orbital wall decompression surgery.

The most posterior portion of the medial wall is formed by the body of the sphenoid bone. The optic canal is situated in the superomedial aspect of the orbital apex and is enclosed by the body of the sphenoid bone medially, the lesser wing of the sphenoid superiorly, and the optic strut infero-laterally (Fig. 2.44).

The Orbital Floor

The orbital floor is composed of three bones: the maxillary, zygomatic, and palatine bones (Fig. 2.33). The orbital plate of the maxillary bone makes the greatest contribution to the orbital floor. This also forms the roof of the maxillary sinus. The zygomatic bone contributes a small portion of the orbital floor anterolaterally while the palatine bone lies at the extreme posterior end of the orbital floor, in the orbital apex. The floor extends medially to the maxillo-ethmoid suture line and anterolaterally to the zygomatico-maxillary suture line. In the mid- and posterior aspects of the orbit, the orbital floor finishes at the inferior orbital fissure and

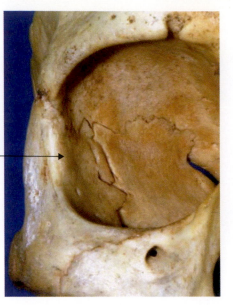

The lateral orbital
tubercle

Figure 2.40 The lateral orbital tubercle.

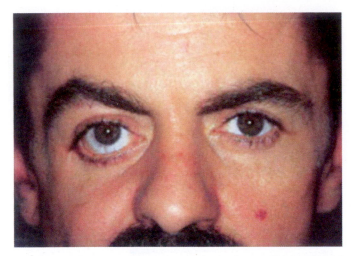

Figure 2.41 Patient with a right zygomatic complex fracture with lower eyelid retraction, malar flattening, and inferior displacement of the lateral canthus.

the posterior extent of the maxillary sinus. It should be noted that the orbital floor does not extend to the apex of the orbit but ends at the pterygo-palatine fossa. The orbital floor is the shortest of the orbital walls and extends approximately 35 to 40 mm from the inferior orbital margin. Surgical dissection in the management of orbital floor blowout fracture should not be continued further than the posterior wall of the maxillary sinus.

> **KEY POINT**
>
> Surgical dissection in the management of orbital floor blowout fracture should not be continued further than the posterior wall of the maxillary sinus.

The thinnest part of the orbital floor lies medial to the inferior orbital canal. This is the part of the orbital floor, which is usually affected by blowout fractures. The infraorbital sulcus containing the infraorbital nerve, a branch of the maxillary division of the trigeminal nerve, and the associated infraorbital artery and vein from the pterygopalatine fossa, runs from the posterior aspect of the orbital floor centrally in a postero-anterior direction. In the majority of patients, the maxillary bone covers the sulcus to form the infraorbital canal. This bone is pierced by one or more small foramina, which transmits an anastomotic branch from the infraorbital artery to the inferior muscular branch of the ophthalmic artery. This constant vessel(s) is seen 5 to 10 mm behind the inferior orbital margin during a surgical exploration of the orbital floor. Failure to identify and cauterize this vessel can lead to sudden brisk hemorrhage.

The infraorbital canal continues forward to the inferior orbital margin where it appears as the infraorbital foramen. It is important to recognize the position of the infraorbital canal and its very thin bony roof in order to avoid damage to the infraorbital nerve during orbital floor explorations. The infraorbital neurovascular bundle is quite large. Trauma to the infraorbital

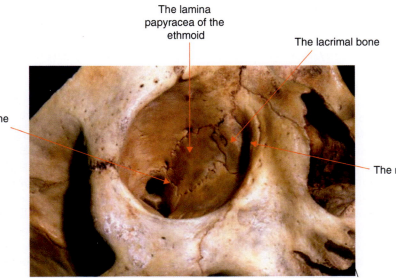

The lamina
papyracea of the
ethmoid

The lacrimal bone

The body of the
sphenoid

The maxillary bone

Figure 2.42 The medial orbital wall.

nerve results in anesthesia of the cheek, the lower eyelid, the lateral aspect of the nose, the upper lip, and the anterior teeth. Such anesthesia is commonly seen in patients who have suffered an orbital floor blowout fracture. Inadvertent trauma to the infraorbital vessels can result in severe hemorrhage.

The orbital floor is separated from the lateral orbital wall by the inferior orbital fissure. The fissure runs in an antero-lateral to postero-medial direction and measures approximately 20 mm. The inferior orbital fissure joins the superior orbital fissure at the orbital apex below the optic canal (Fig. 2.33). The inferior orbital fissure transmits vessels and nerves from the pterygo-palatine fossa posteriorly, and from the infra-temporal fossa anteriorly. Branches of the inferior ophthalmic vein pass through the inferior orbital fissure to the pterygoid venous plexus (Fig. 2.45).

The maxillary division of the trigeminal nerve passes from the foramen rotundum through the inferior orbital fissure to the infraorbital sulcus, and becomes the infraorbital nerve. Postganglionic parasympathetic secretory and vasomotor neural branches from the pterygo-palatine ganglion pass to the orbit through the inferior orbital fissure. Here they join with the maxillary nerve before passing to the lacrimal gland.

The Lateral Orbital Wall

The lateral orbital wall is composed of the zygomatic bone anteriorly and the greater wing of the sphenoid bone posteriorly (Fig. 2.46).

The inferior orbital fissure separates the lateral wall from the orbital floor. The superior orbital fissure partly separates the lateral orbital wall from the roof of the orbit. The lateral wall of the orbit is the thickest orbital wall, the thinnest part of which lies at the zygomatico-sphenoid suture approximately 10 mm behind the lateral orbital margin. The sphenoid bone begins to thicken approximately 10 mm posterior to the zygomatico-sphenoid suture. This represents the anterior aspect of the middle cranial fossa. In this location, the cranio-orbital foramen may be seen transmitting an anastomotic branch between the middle meningeal artery and branches of the ophthalmic artery.

Two or more foramina perforate the lateral orbital wall just behind the lateral orbital margin laterally and inferiorly and transmit the zygomatico-temporal and zygomatico-facial neurovascular bundles (Fig. 2.24). The zygomatico-temporal and zygomatico-facial nerves are branches of the maxillary division of the trigeminal nerve. The nerves are severed during surgery on the lateral orbital wall, e.g., a lateral orbitotomy. This results in a small area of hypoesthesia postoperatively over the zygoma and temple but this is usually insignificant in contrast to the sensory loss that follows damage to the infraorbital nerve. The zygomatico-temporal and zygomatico-facial arteries are branches of the lacrimal artery, which itself is a branch of the ophthalmic artery. These vessels are encountered when the periorbita is raised from the lateral orbital wall. These vessels should be cauterized before they are severed.

The superior orbital fissure is situated between the roof and lateral wall of the orbit and between the greater and lesser wings of the sphenoid bone. This fissure is divided into superior and inferior parts by the fibrous annulus of Zinn, from which the recti muscles take origin. The superior part of the fissure transmits the lacrimal, frontal and trochlear nerves, the superior ophthalmic vein and the anastomosis of the recurrent lacrimal, and middle meningeal arteries, while the inferior part transmits the superior and inferior divisions of the oculomotor nerve, the

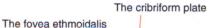

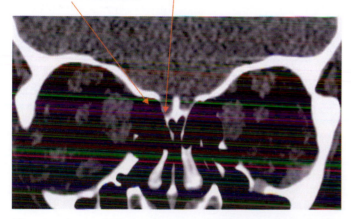

Figure 2.43 A coronal CT scan of a patient with thyroid eye disease showing the fovea ethmoidalis and the position of the cribriform plate.

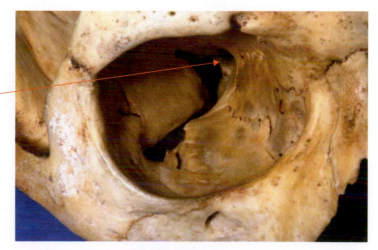

Figure 2.44 The orbital apex.

nasociliary nerve, the abducens nerve, and sympathetic nerves (Fig. 2.35).

The Orbital Roof

The orbital roof is triangular in shape and mainly formed by the orbital plate of the frontal bone with a small portion being made by the lesser wing of the sphenoid bone posteriorly (Fig. 2.44). The anterior superolateral aspect of the orbital roof is a shallow concavity within which lies the lacrimal gland. In the superomedial aspect of the orbital roof, approximately 3 to 5 mm behind the superomedial orbital margin lies the trochlea. Great care

should be exercised when operating in this area as the trochlea is susceptible to iatrogenic trauma, which can result in an acquired Brown's syndrome (superior oblique tendon sheath syndrome). The bone of the orbital roof is very thin and, particularly in older patients, may have areas of bony dehiscence (Fig. 2.47).

For this reason, great care must be taken when elevating the periorbita from the roof of the orbit as a periosteal elevator may encounter exposed dura and perforate it leading to a CSF leak. Surgery performed along the orbital roof should be undertaken under direct vision and should not be performed "blind."

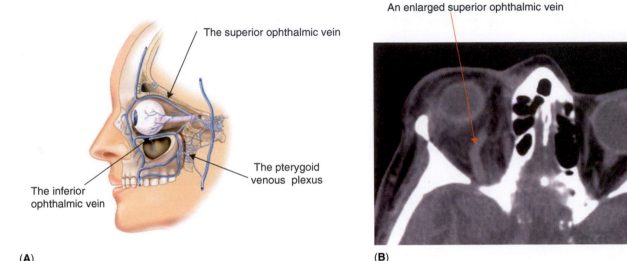

Figure 2.45 The venous drainage of the orbit. (**A**) A diagram depicting the venous drainage of the orbit. (**B**) A contrast-enhanced axial CT scan of a patient with a carotico-cavernous fistula demonstrating a markedly enlarged superior ophthalmic vein.

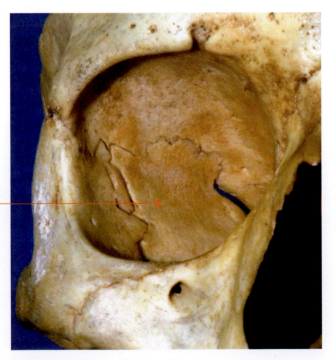

Figure 2.46 The lateral wall of the orbit.

The frontal sinus is situated within the frontal bone in the antero-medial part of the orbital roof. The frontal sinus is very variable in size and may extend as far laterally as the lacrimal gland fossa and as far posteriorly as the optic canal.

The Optic Canal

The optic canal is housed within the roof of the orbital apex. The optic canal changes shape as it extends from the orbit to the intracranial cavity. The canal is vertically oval at the orbital end and measures approximately 5 to 6 mm in diameter. Centrally the optic canal is circular. The intracranial end has an oval shape in the horizontal plane. The optic canal measures approximately 8 to 12 mm in length; it transmits the ophthalmic artery from the intracranial cavity to the orbit.

Along its entire intracanalicular length the optic nerve is strongly tethered to the very rigid adjacent structures. The annulus of Zinn forms a tight stricture around the optic nerve as it enters the canal from the orbit. Within the optic canal, the dural sheath is tightly adherent to the periosteum. As the optic nerve exits intracranially, it is restrained superiorly by a dural fold. The intracranial optic nerve continues its superomedial course to the optic chiasm. To expose the intracranial portion of the optic nerve, the dura must be opened.

For purposes of surgical anatomy, the optic canal may be considered as a triangle:

- The medial wall of the canal abuts the posterior ethmoid sinus and the sphenoid sinus
- The lateral wall of the canal is formed by the bone of the optic strut, which separates it from the superior orbital fissure
- The roof lies adjacent to the cranial vault

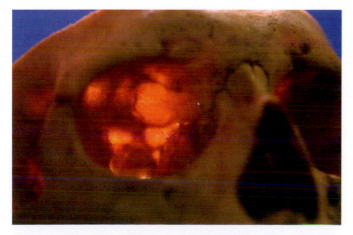

Figure 2.47 The orbital roof has been transilluminated to demonstrate how thin the bone can be, particularly in an elderly patient.

When assessing a computed tomography (CT) scan, it is helpful to recall that the anterior clinoid process lies just lateral to the optic canal, a constant feature on axial and coronal images. The superior orbital fissure can be confused with the optic canal on CT scans. A number of findings assist in distinguishing these:

- The superior orbital fissure lies at a different level to the optic canal on axial images
- The superior orbital fissure lies on the same level as the cavernous sinus—the lateral wall of the cavernous sinus is usually visible on CT
- The optic canal typically lies at the same level as the superior rectus muscle

The Periorbita

The periorbita covers all the bones of the internal orbit. Unlike the periosteum covering bones elsewhere, the periorbita is loosely adherent over the orbital walls and can be very easily elevated from the underlying bone, except at the orbital suture lines and along the orbital margins, where it is tightly adherent to the bone.

Surgical Spaces of the Orbit

Anatomically, the orbital spaces are divided into:

- Sub-Tenon's space
- Intraconal space
- Extraconal space
- Subperiosteal space

A good understanding of the surgical spaces of the orbit is essential in order to select the most appropriate surgical approach and to assist in navigation within the orbit during surgery (Fig. 2.48).

Sub-Tenon's Space

The sub-Tenon's space is a potential space situated between the globe and Tenon's capsule. It is not commonly involved in pathological processes. The space may be enlarged with fluid visible on echography in posterior scleritis, air following trauma (Fig. 2.48B), or by infiltration by extraocular extension of intraocular tumors, e.g., choroidal melanoma.

Intraconal Space

The intraconal space lies within the recti and their intermuscular septa. The intraconal space contains the following:

- The optic nerve
- Intraconal orbital fat
- Nerves
- Blood vessels

Tumors of the optic nerve lie within this space. The intraconal space may be accessed via a number of surgical approaches: e.g., in order to perform an optic nerve sheath fenestration, the optic nerve may be approached superomedially via an upper eyelid skin crease incision, medially via a conjunctival incision with disinsertion of the medial rectus muscle or laterally via a lateral orbitotomy, with or without bone removal.

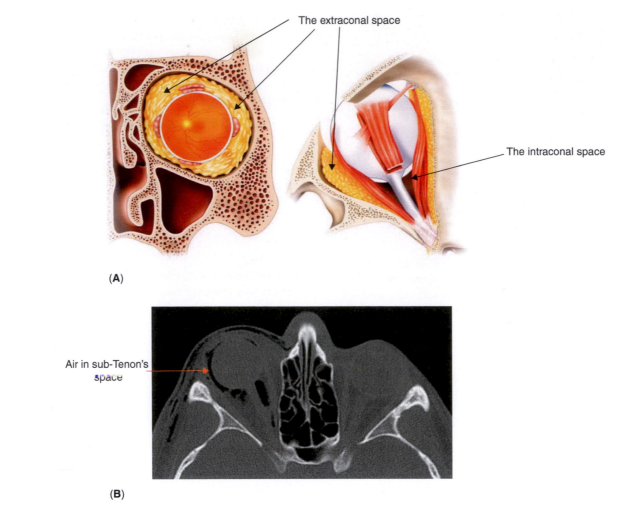

Figure 2.48 (**A**) The intraconal and extraconal spaces of the orbit. (**B**) An axial CT scan showing air within the sub-Tenon's space following trauma.

During a lateral orbitotomy approach with bone removal, the intraconal space is usually accessed by dissecting between the lacrimal gland and the lateral rectus muscle.

Extraconal Space
The extraconal space lies outside the recti and their intermuscular septa and contains the following:

- The lacrimal gland
- The oblique muscles
- The trochlea
- Extraconal orbital fat
- The superior and inferior ophthalmic veins
- Nerves and other vessels

The extraconal fat includes the pre-aponeurotic fat that is important in the identification of the underlying eyelid retractors. Extraconal fat can be removed superiorly via an upper eyelid skin crease incision. Medial, lateral, and inferior extraconal fat can be removed via transconjunctival incisions.

The anterior portion of the superior ophthalmic vein lies in the extraconal space. This can be accessed via an upper eyelid skin crease incision. In patients with arteriovenous shunts, the vein is dilated and can provide alternative access for the insertion of platinum coils in conjunction with an interventional radiologist in selected cases.

Subperiosteal Space
The subperiosteal space is a potential space that lies between the periorbita and the bony orbital walls. The periorbita has a loose attachment to the bone and can be easily separated from the bone except at the orbital suture lines and along the orbital margins. The subperiosteal space can be filled with blood (a subperiosteal hematoma) or pus (a subperiosteal abscess). In such cases, the periorbita is lifted from the walls of the orbit in a characteristic dome-shaped fashion that is limited by the orbital suture lines (Fig. 2.49).

This space is accessed surgically for the repair of orbital wall blowout fractures, for the drainage of subperiosteal abscesses or hematomas, for bony orbital decompression surgery or for the insertion of subperiosteal orbital implants in anophthalmic patients. This space can be accessed via a variety of transcutaneous or transconjunctival incisions.

The Optic Nerve
The optic nerve runs from the optic chiasm to the globe (Fig. 2.50A). The length of the optic nerve is approximately 45 to 50 mm. It is divided into four parts:

- Intraocular (1 mm)
- Intraorbital (30 mm)
- Intracanalicular (5 mm)
- Intracranial (10 mm)

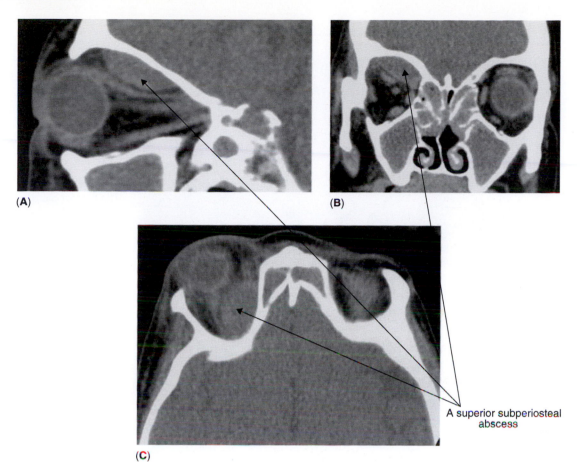

(A)

(B)

(C)

A superior subperiosteal abscess

Figure 2.49 Sagittal, coronal, and axial CT scans demonstrating a superomedial subperiosteal orbital abscess. The inferomedial extension of the abscess is limited by the attachment of the periorbita at the fronto-ethmoidal suture line.

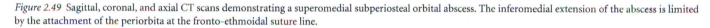

The nerve normally has an S-shaped configuration in the orbit. In contrast, the nerve is straightened in patients with proptosis. Dura, arachnoid, and pia mater surround the nerve from the optic canal to the globe. The subarachnoid space is continued to the globe and is filled with cerebrospinal fluid. The space is enlarged just posterior to the globe in a bulbous part of the nerve. This is the site where an optic nerve sheath fenestration is performed for patients with benign intracranial hypertension. The central retinal artery enters the optic nerve in a variable position, usually on the inferomedial aspect approximately 10 mm posterior to the globe.

The intracanalicular part of the optic nerve is immobile as the dural sheath is fused to the periosteum of the optic canal. The anatomical arrangement of the nerve in this location leaves the nerve vulnerable to damage from blunt head trauma, which can lead to shearing of the pial vessels supplying the nerve. The intracanalicular nerve is also vulnerable to edema.

The intracranial part of the nerve extends from the chiasm to the optic canal. The dura of the anterior cranial fossa has to be opened to gain access to the nerve in this location. This part of the nerve is closely related to the frontal lobe, the anterior cerebral, anterior communicating, middle cerebral and internal carotid arteries, and the cavernous sinus (Fig. 2.50B).

The Periorbital Sensory Innervation
The ophthalmic and maxillary divisions of the trigeminal nerve provide sensation to the periorbital area with considerable overlap of the branches of the sensory nerves (Fig. 2.51).

The ophthalmic and maxillary divisions of the trigeminal nerve arise from the semilunar (trigeminal) ganglion, which lies in Meckel's cave over the apex of the petrous temporal bone, in the floor of the middle cranial fossa. They pass anteriorly in the lateral wall of the cavernous sinus (Fig. 2.50).

The Ophthalmic Division of the Trigeminal Nerve
The ophthalmic nerve divides into three main branches as it leaves the cavernous sinus:

- The lacrimal nerve
- The frontal nerve
- The nasociliary nerve

The arrangement of these nerves in the superior orbital fissure is illustrated in Figure 2.35.

The largest branch is the frontal nerve. This travels forward from the orbital apex lying between the levator muscle and the periorbita (Fig. 2.52).

It is clearly visible when the periorbita is opened from above. It divides midway in the orbit into two branches:

- The supratrochlear nerve
- The supraorbital nerve (Fig. 2.52C)

The supratrochlear nerve passes above the trochlea and supplies the lower part of the forehead and the medial aspect of the upper eyelid. The supraorbital nerve passes through the supraorbital foramen or notch and supplies the forehead to the vertex of the scalp, the upper eyelid, and superior conjunctiva.

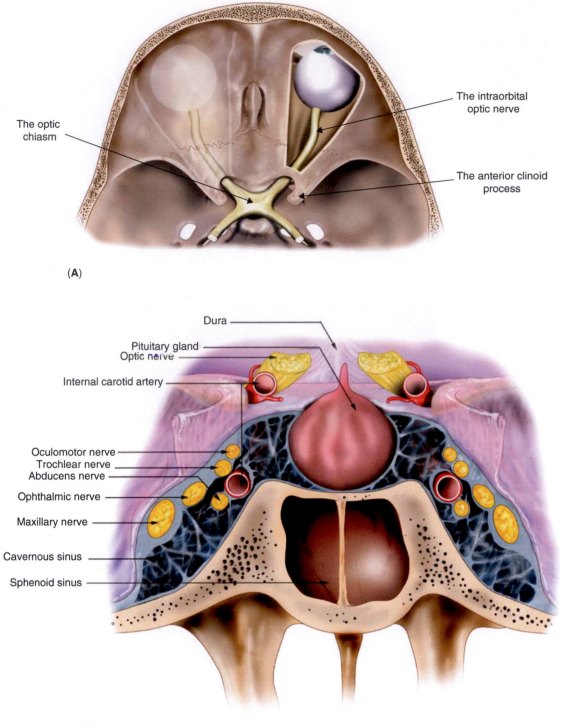

Figure 2.50 (**A**) The course of the optic nerve. (**B**) The anatomy of the cavernous sinus.

The nasociliary nerve innervates the globe. It crosses over the optic nerve from a lateral position after entering the orbit (Fig. 2.52). It gives rise to a number of branches:

- The short ciliary nerves
- The long ciliary nerves
- The anterior ethmoidal nerve
- The posterior ethmoidal nerve

A small branch, the sensory root, runs along the lateral aspect of the optic nerve and enters the ciliary ganglion. The ciliary ganglion lies close to the apex of the orbit between the optic nerve and the lateral rectus muscle. The short ciliary nerves (5–20) then arise from the ciliary ganglion, and run with short ciliary arteries to the posterior aspect of the globe. They penetrate the sclera and provide sensory innervation to the cornea, the iris and the ciliary body. They also carry

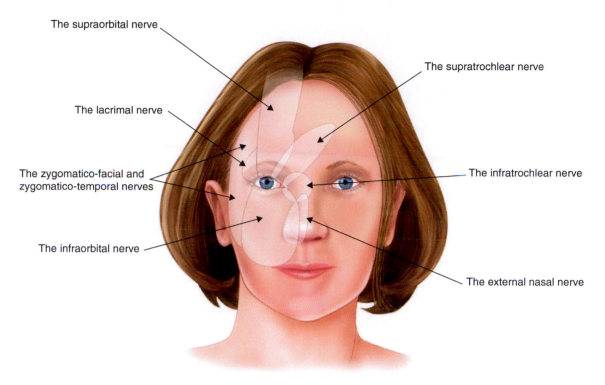

The supraorbital nerve

The supratrochlear nerve

The lacrimal nerve

The zygomatico-facial and zygomatico-temporal nerves

The infratrochlear nerve

The infraorbital nerve

The external nasal nerve

Figure 2.51 A diagram demonstrating the overlap of the periorbital sensory innervation.

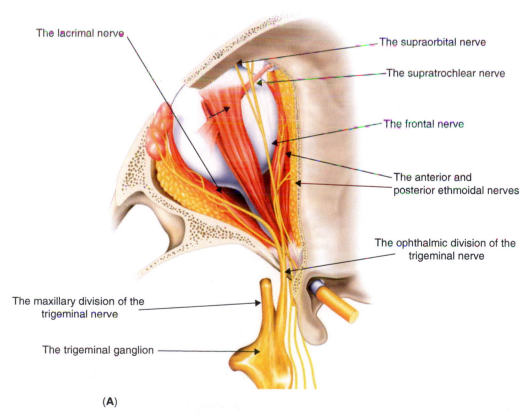

The lacrimal nerve

The supraorbital nerve

The supratrochlear nerve

The frontal nerve

The anterior and posterior ethmoidal nerves

The ophthalmic division of the trigeminal nerve

The maxillary division of the trigeminal nerve

The trigeminal ganglion

(A)

Figure 2.52 (**A**) A diagram demonstrating the course of the frontal nerve. (*Continued*)

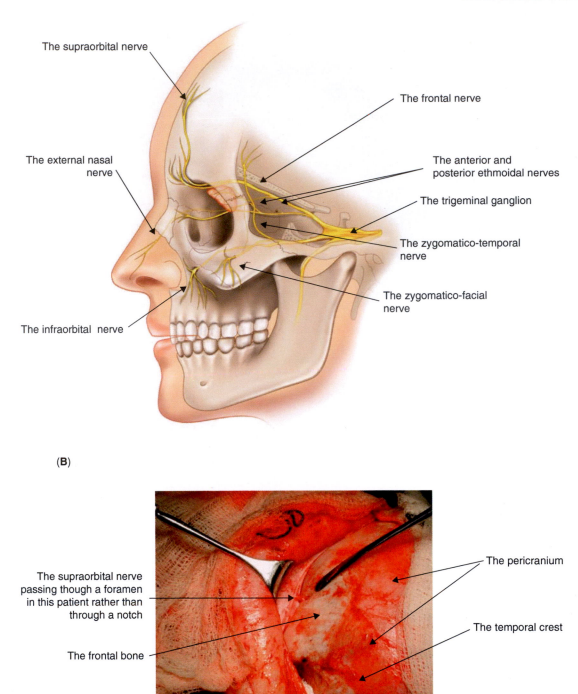

The supraorbital nerve

The frontal nerve

The external nasal nerve

The anterior and posterior ethmoidal nerves

The trigeminal ganglion

The zygomatico-temporal nerve

The zygomatico-facial nerve

The infraorbital nerve

(B)

The supraorbital nerve passing though a foramen in this patient rather than through a notch

The pericranium

The frontal bone

The temporal crest

(C)

Figure 2.52 (Continued) (**B**) A diagram showing the main orbital branches of the trigeminal nerve from a sagittal perspective. (**C**) The supraorbital nerve seen at the superior orbital margin during a bicoronal flap approach to the antero-superior orbit.

parasympathetic nerve fibers to the ciliary body, and the sphincter pupillae muscle.

The nasociliary nerve gives rise to the long ciliary nerves (2–3), which enter the sclera posteriorly and extend anteriorly along the medial and lateral aspects of the globe to provide sensory innervation to the cornea, iris, and ciliary body. These nerves also carry sympathetic nerve fibers from the superior cervical ganglion to the dilator pupillae muscle. After crossing the optic nerve, the posterior ethmoidal nerve is given off followed by the anterior ethmoidal nerve more anteriorly (Fig. 2.52). This branch in turn gives rise to medial and lateral nasal branches and to the external nasal nerve. These branches provide sensory innervation to the nasal cavity and dorsum of the nose. After the anterior ethmoidal

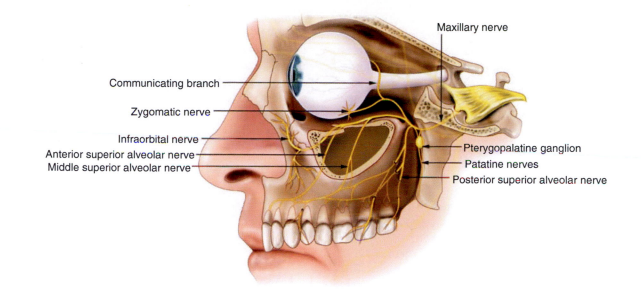

Figure 2.53 The branches of the maxillary division of the trigeminal nerve.

nerve has branched away, the nasociliary nerve continues as the infratrochlear nerve (Fig. 2.52). This runs along the superior aspect of the medial rectus muscle and perforates through the orbital septum below the trochlea. It provides sensory innervation to the medial aspect of the skin of the eyelids, the lateral aspect of the nose, the lacrimal sac, and the caruncular area. A regional block of this nerve permits good anesthesia for an external DCR.

The lacrimal nerve runs along the lateral orbital wall above the lateral rectus muscle (Fig. 2.52). As it runs to the lacrimal gland, it is joined by parasympathetic nerve fibers branching from the zygomatico-temporal nerve.

The Maxillary Division of the Trigeminal Nerve

The maxillary division of the trigeminal nerve leaves the middle cranial fossa through the foramen rotundum and enters the pterygopalatine fossa. A number of branches arise in the pterygopalatine fossa (Fig. 2.53):

- The zygomatic nerve
- The sphenopalatine nerves
- The posterior, superior alveolar nerves

The zygomatic nerve enters the orbit through the inferior orbital fissure, runs along the lateral aspect of the orbit, and divides into the zygomaticofacial and zygomatico-temporal nerves. The posterior, superior alveolar nerves provide sensation to the upper molar teeth, the gingiva, and the mucous membrane of the maxillary sinus.

The maxillary division enters the orbit through the central aspect of the inferior orbital fissure and continues forward as the infraorbital nerve through the infraorbital groove and infraorbital canal. In the canal it gives rise to:

- The middle superior alveolar nerve
- The anterior, superior alveolar nerve
- The superior labial nerve

The middle superior alveolar nerve provides sensation to the upper premolar teeth. The anterior, superior alveolar nerve supplies the upper incisor teeth and canines, and the mucous membrane of the maxillary sinus, and of the inferior meatus of the nose. The superior labial nerve supplies the skin of the cheek and the skin and mucous membrane of the upper lip. These areas are affected by trauma to the infraorbital nerve following an orbital floor blowout fracture.

The Motor Nerves to the Extraocular Muscles

The Oculomotor Nerve

The oculomotor nerve provides motor innervation for:

- The levator muscle
- The superior rectus muscle
- The medial rectus muscle
- The inferior rectus muscle
- The inferior oblique muscle

It provides the pathway for parasympathetic nerve fibers to the ciliary muscle and the sphincter pupillae muscle.

The nerve leaves the lateral wall of the cavernous sinus and enters the orbit, where it divides into superior and inferior branches. It enters the orbit through the superior orbital fissure within the annulus of Zinn (Fig. 2.35). The superior branch rises over the lateral aspect of the optic nerve and enters the under surface of the superior rectus muscle at the junction of the posterior third with the anterior two-thirds. A branch of this nerve passes through or around the medial aspect of the superior rectus muscle to reach the levator muscle. The inferior branch gives rise to three further branches supplying the medial rectus, the inferior rectus, and the inferior oblique muscles. The latter gives off a short root to the ciliary ganglion.

The Trochlear Nerve

The trochlear nerve supplies the superior oblique muscle. The nerve enters the orbit through the superior orbital fissure outside the annulus of Zinn (Fig. 2.35). It passes anteriorly and medially over the levator muscle and enters the superior oblique muscle on its outer aspect as three or four branches at the junction of the posterior third with the anterior two-thirds. The trochlear nerve is the only nerve that enters an extraocular muscle from the outer aspect. The other nerves enter the muscles from the conal surface.

The Abducens Nerve

The abducens nerve supplies the lateral rectus muscle. The nerve enters the orbit within the annulus of Zinn. It enters the lateral rectus muscle on its conal surface at the junction of the posterior third with the anterior two-thirds.

The Orbital and Periocular Arterial System

The internal carotid artery provides the main arterial blood supply to the brain, the orbit, and the globe. The external carotid artery mainly supplies the face, the scalp and parts of the neck (Fig. 2.24). The main orbital arteries arise from the ophthalmic artery. The terminal branches of the ophthalmic artery anastomose with terminal branches of the external carotid artery to form a rich arterial network of collateral circulation in the periocular region, making the tissues resistant to the effects of ischemia and infection.

The External Carotid Artery

The external carotid artery branches from the common carotid artery at the level of the upper border of the thyroid cartilage and, taking a slightly curved course, passes upward and forward, and then inclines backward to the space behind the neck of the mandible, where it divides into two main branches, the superficial temporal and maxillary arteries, within the parotid gland. There are numerous branches within the neck but the most important of these is the facial artery. The facial artery crosses the mandible just anterior to the masseter muscle and courses toward the side of the nose where it becomes the angular artery. This artery is commonly encountered during the course of an external dacryocystorhinostomy procedure.

The maxillary artery supplies the mandibles, the palate, and the internal aspect of the nose. It gives rise to the infraorbital artery in the pterygopalatine fossa. This courses forward in conjunction with the infraorbital nerve, entering the orbit through the inferior orbital fissure, the inferior orbital groove, and the infraorbital canal to emerge onto the cheek through the infraorbital foramen.

The superficial temporary artery is the terminal branch of the external carotid artery. The artery crosses the zygomatic arch just in front of the ear and lies in the temporo-parietal fascia, the same plane as the temporal branch of the facial nerve. It gives rise to the frontal, zygomatic, and transverse facial arteries.

The Internal Carotid Artery

The internal carotid artery runs perpendicularly upward in the carotid sheath, enters the skull through the carotid canal, traverses the cavernous sinus, and pierces the dura close to the intracranial opening of the optic canal where it gives rise to the ophthalmic artery.

Ophthalmic Artery

The ophthalmic artery is the first main branch of the internal carotid artery (Fig. 2.24). It is divided into intracranial, intracanalicular, and intraorbital parts. The intracranial part lies below the optic nerve. The intracanalicular part lies below the optic nerve within its dural sheath. It enters the orbit inferolateral to the optic nerve and crosses either above or below the nerve, running toward the medial orbital wall.

The ophthalmic artery gives off a number of branches:

- Central retinal artery
- Medial and lateral posterior ciliary arteries
- Collateral branches to the optic nerve
- Multiple muscular arteries
- Lacrimal artery
- Supraorbital artery
- Supratrochlear artery
- Anterior and posterior ethmoidal arteries
- Infratrochlear artery
- Medial palpebral arteries

Lacrimal Artery

The lacrimal artery passes along the lateral orbital wall above the lateral rectus muscle. The branches from the lacrimal artery are:

- Recurrent meningeal artery
- Zygomatic artery
- Artery to the lacrimal gland
- Lateral palpebral artery

The zygomatic branches, the zygomatico-temporal and zygomatico-facial arteries, pass through foramina within the zygomatic bone and anastomose with anterior deep temporal and transverse facial arteries (Fig. 2.24).

Supraorbital Artery

The supraorbital artery branches from the ophthalmic artery as it crosses over the optic nerve. It runs along the medial border of the superior rectus and levator muscles. The artery exits the orbit through the supraorbital notch or foramen, supplying the forehead, brows, and upper eyelid regions.

Supratrochlear Artery

The supratrochlear artery is one of the terminal branches of the ophthalmic artery. It supplies the medial aspect of the forehead and scalp and the superior medial canthal area.

Infratrochlear Artery

The infratrochlear artery is another of the terminal branches of the ophthalmic artery. It runs above the medial canthal tendon and anatomoses with the angular artery. It supplies the nasal bridge, scalp, medial forehead, and medial canthal areas.

Medial Palpebral Arteries

The medial palpebral arteries are also terminal branches of the ophthalmic artery and arise from the arteries lying just below the trochlea. They pass into the eyelids and anastomose with the lateral palpebral arterial branches.

Ethmoidal Arteries

The anterior and posterior ethmoidal arteries form important surgical landmarks. They exit the orbit via their respective ethmoidal foramina sheathed by periorbita. Inadvertent damage to these arteries can lead to brisk bleeding and the rapid development of a subperiosteal orbital hematoma.

The Orbital Venous System

Venous blood is drained from the orbit through three main systems:

- The cavernous sinus
- The pterygoid plexus
- The anterior venous system

The superior ophthalmic vein drains to the cavernous sinus. The inferior ophthalmic vein drains both to the superior ophthalmic vein and also to the pterygoid plexus (Fig. 2.54).

The venous system communicates anteriorly via the angular vein and its tributaries from the face and forehead.

The Superior Ophthalmic Vein

The superior ophthalmic vein is formed by the confluence of the supraorbital vein and the angular vein. It extends posteriorly from the medial aspect of the orbit to the medial border of the superior rectus muscle. It then runs below the superior rectus muscle and along its lateral margin to the superior orbital fissure and the cavernous sinus.

A supraorbital vein can be cannulated in order to pass a radio-opaque dye to perform an orbital venogram. The superior ophthalmic vein itself can be dissected and cannulated via an upper eyelid skin crease incision in order to embolize a dural vascular shunt if an alternative endovascular route cannot be accessed by an interventional neuroradiologist (Fig. 2.55).

The Inferior Ophthalmic Vein

The inferior ophthalmic vein forms from a plexus of veins on the floor of the orbit. The vein runs posteriorly to communicate by a branch with the superior ophthalmic vein and by another smaller branch with the pterygoid plexus via the inferior orbital fissure.

The Central Retinal Vein

The central retinal vein exits from the optic nerve at a variable distance from the globe. It usually passes directly to the cavernous sinus.

The Lacrimal System

The lacrimal system comprises the tear-producing glands, the lacrimal gland and accessory lacrimal glands of the conjunctiva and eyelids, the tear film, and the lacrimal drainage system. The eyelids distribute the tears across the eye by the act of blinking and also contribute to tear drainage by means of the "lacrimal pump" mechanism. Any abnormality of these components of the lacrimal system can give rise to the complaint of a " watery" eye.

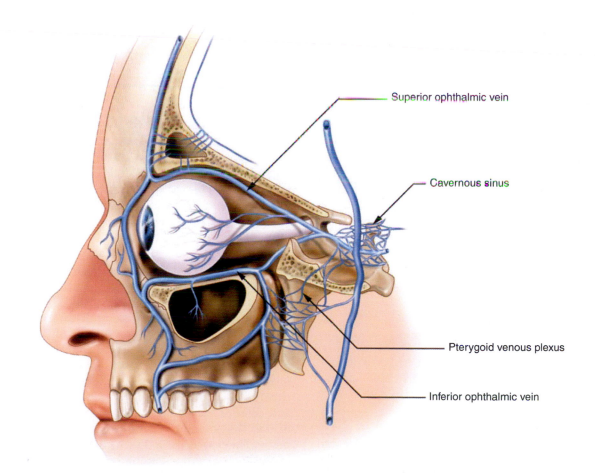

Figure 2.54 The venous drainage of the orbit.

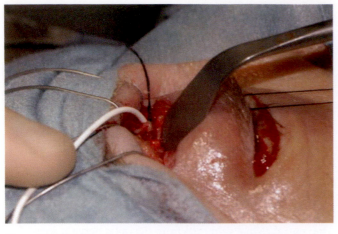

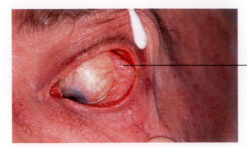

→ Palpebral lobe of lacrimal gland

Figure 2.56 The palpebral lobe of the lacrimal gland visible in the patient on raising the upper eyelid.

Figure 2.55 The dilated superior ophthalmic vein in this patient has been exposed via an upper eyelid skin crease incision and has been cannulated.

The Tear Film

The tear film consists of three layers:

- The mucinous layer
- The aqueous layer
- The lipid layer

The mucinous layer is produced by the many goblet cells throughout the conjunctiva. The aqueous layer is produced by the lacrimal gland and by the many accessory lacrimal glands. The lipid layer serves to retard the evaporation of the aqueous layer and is produced by the sebaceous glands of the eyelids and caruncle. The tear film can be stained with a fluorescein strip, and its stability observed between blinks. The tear film should remain stable for approximately 10 to 12 s under normal conditions.

The Lacrimal Gland

The lacrimal gland lies in the concavity of the lacrimal gland fossa in the superolateral aspect of the orbit. Its two lobes, the orbital and palpebral lobes, are separated by the lateral expansion (the lateral horn) of the levator aponeurosis. The orbital lobe lies within the orbit above the palpebral lobe. The palpebral lobe lies against the conjunctiva in the superolateral aspect of the superior fornix. This lobe is visible in many patients on everting the upper eyelid (Fig. 2.56).

The lacrimal ductules pass through the palpebral lobe from the orbital lobe into the superolateral fornix (Fig. 2.57). The ductules can be seen on slit lamp examination with the use of high magnification after applying a fluorescein strip to the conjunctiva of the superolateral fornix.

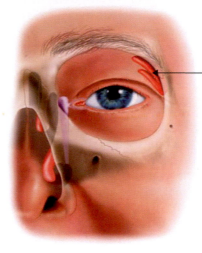

→ The lacrimal gland and the lacrimal gland ductules

Figure 2.57 The location of the lacrimal gland and the lacrimal ductules.

The Puncta

The lacrimal drainage system commences with the puncta, which are situated approximately 5 mm from the medial commissure. Each punctum lies on the lacrimal papilla, a slight elevation of the eyelid margin. The inferior punctum lies in apposition to the tear meniscus and should not be visible on slit lamp examination without manual eversion of the eyelid. There are no eyelashes medial to the punctum.

The Canaliculi

The puncta lead to the canaliculi, which are initially vertical for approximately 2 mm and which then turn to lie horizontally for approximately 8 mm (Fig. 2.58A). They are approximately 1 to 1.5 mm in diameter. The junction of the vertical and horizontal portions of the canaliculi is referred to as the ampulla and is slightly dilated. In the majority of patients, the superior and inferior canaliculi join to form a common canaliculus before entering the lacrimal sac. In a small proportion of patients, the superior and inferior canaliculi enter the lacrimal sac independently. This should be borne in mind when using a pigtail probe. The canaliculi lie directly beneath the anterior limb of the medial canthal tendon before entering the lacrimal sac (Fig. 2.58B). This relationship is important to recall when performing a canaliculo-dacryocystorhinostomy.

KEY POINT

Any surgery performed in the superolateral conjunctival fornix, e.g., surgery to remove a congenital dermolipoma, risks damage to the lacrimal ductules and a dry eye.

The Lacrimal Drainage System

The lacrimal drainage system comprises the superior and inferior puncta, the superior and inferior canaliculi, the common canaliculus, the lacrimal sac, and the nasolacrimal duct (Fig. 2.58).

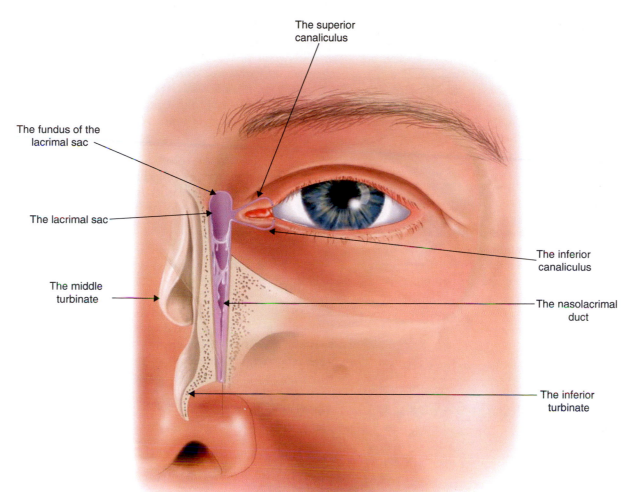

The superior
canaliculus

The fundus of the
lacrimal sac

The lacrimal sac

The middle
turbinate

The inferior
canaliculus

The nasolacrimal
duct

The inferior
turbinate

(A)

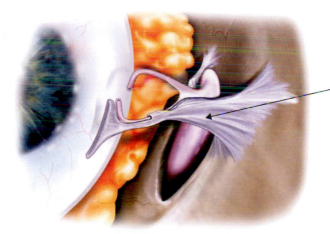

The anterior limb of the medial
canthal tendon which has been
partially removed to show the
relationship of this to the
lacrimal sac and to the
canaliculi

(B)

Figure 2.58 (**A**) The lacrimal drainage system. (**B**) A drawing depicting the relationship of the canaliculi and lacrimal sac to the medial canthal tendon.

The Lacrimal Sac

The lacrimal sac lies within the lacrimal sac fossa. The fossa is bounded anteriorly by the anterior lacrimal crest and posteriorly by the posterior lacrimal crest. The floor of the fossa comprises part of the maxillary bone, which usually forms the anterior two-thirds, and the lacrimal bone. A vertical suture lies between these bones. This represents a weak area, which is broken at the commencement of the creation of the bony osteotomy during a dacryocystorhinostomy procedure. Occasionally, anterior ethmoid air cells may be situated very anteriorly and even extend into the anterior lacrimal crest. It is important to recognize this and differentiate friable ethmoid sinus mucosa from normal nasal mucosa.

The lacrimal sac measures approximately 12 to 15 mm in vertical height and is approximately 2 to 3 mm wide in its resting semi-collapsed state. The fundus of the sac rises above the level of the anterior limb of the medial canthal tendon. The body of the sac gives rise to a narrowed neck, which joins the nasolacrimal duct. The anterior limb of the medial canthal tendon marks the superior limit of the osteotomy in an external dacryocystorhinostomy procedure. The cribriform plate can lie within 2 to 3 mm of this tendon in some patients. The anterior limb of the medial canthal tendon is a firm structure and prevents distension of the fundus of the sac by fluid or mucus in the presence of a nasolacrimal duct obstruction. For this reason, a mucocele or amniocoele distends the lacrimal sac below the level of the medial canthal tendon (Fig. 2.59).

The tendon offers no such resistance to a lacrimal sac tumor. Any enlargement of the lacrimal sac above the tendon should therefore suggest a tumor process until proven otherwise. In infants, other medial canthal lesions should be considered, e.g., a meningoencephalocoele, a dermoid cyst (Fig. 2.60), a capillary hemangioma or a rhabdomyosarcoma.

KEY POINT

Any enlargement of the lacrimal sac extending above the medial canthal tendon should suggest a neoplastic lesion until proven otherwise.

The Nasolacrimal Duct
The membranous portion of the nasolacrimal duct extends from the inferior aspect of the lacrimal sac and travels within the bony nasolacrimal duct to open beneath the inferior turbinate in the inferior meatus of the nose (Fig. 2.58). The nasolacrimal duct ostium is located at the junction of the anterior and middle thirds of the inferior meatus (Fig. 2.61).

In an adult, the ostium is approximately 1.5 cm above the floor of the nose. The nasolacrimal duct is approximately 15 mm in length. A common misconception is that the duct is much longer, with the result that probes are often passed too far through the system, abutting the floor of the nose or passing into the nasopharynx.

A number of valves are present within the lacrimal drainage system, which prevent the retrograde passage of tears or air. The most important are:

- The valve of Rosenmüller
- The valve of Hasner

The valve of Rosenmüller is situated at the junction of the common canaliculus and the lacrimal sac. Although not a true valve, it functions to prevent retrograde flow of tears from the lacrimal sac to the conjunctival sac. If the valve is competent in the presence of a nasolacrimal duct obstruction, a tense mucocele or acute dacryocystitis will occur.

External pressure applied to the lacrimal sac will cause pain. In contrast, if the valve is incompetent a mucocele can be decompressed by external pressure applied to the lacrimal sac with a regurgitation of mucus through the canaliculi and puncta into the conjunctival sac.

The valve of Hasner is situated at the inferior aspect of the nasolacrimal duct. This area represents the last portion of the lacrimal drainage system to develop embryologically. It is not uncommon for a thin membranous obstruction to occur in this region in the newborn. The vast majority of such obstructions spontaneously resolve by the age of 2 years. Failure to do so by this age warrants surgical intervention by simple probing of the nasolacrimal duct.

The nasolacrimal duct ostium is very variable in its anatomy. Two distinct variations are recognized:

1. Apical: The ostium is located at the most superior point of the inferior meatus of the nose and is open without any valve of Hasner evident.
2. Lateral: The ostium is located in an oblique groove on the lateral wall of the inferior meatus of the nose and has a mucosal valve of Hasner.

Other named valves are present but these have no clinical significance.

THE NOSE
It is important to have a good knowledge of nasal anatomy to be able to examine the nose as part of the clinical evaluation of a patient presenting with epiphora and to be able to undertake endonasal lacrimal drainage procedures.

The Nasal Septum
The nasal cavity is divided into two halves by the nasal septum. It comprises an anterior membranous and cartilaginous

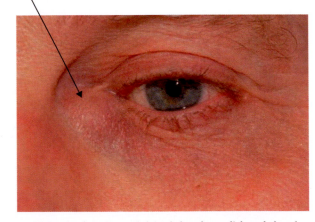

A lacrimal sac mucocele

Figure 2.59 Lacrimal sac mucocele lying below the medial canthal tendon.

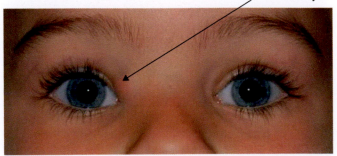

A dermoid cyst

Figure 2.60 A right medial canthal dermoid cyst lying above the medial canthal tendon.

portion and a posterior bony part. The anterior most part or the columella is formed by the medial crurae of the two alar cartilages and are connected to the free caudal border of the septal cartilage by the membranous septum. The quadrilateral or the septal cartilage articulates postero-superiorly with the perpendicular plate of the ethmoid and postero-inferiorly with the vomer. The latter two form the bony part of the nasal septum. The perpendicular plate of the ethmoid articulates anteriorly with the nasal bone and the nasal spine of the frontal bone, superiorly with the cribriform plate of the ethmoid, and posteriorly with the crest of the sphenoid. The vomer articulates inferiorly with the nasal crest of the maxilla and the palatine bone (Fig. 2.62).

The nasal cavity derives its blood supply from branches of both the external, as well as the internal carotid arteries. The antero-superior quadrant of the nose is supplied by the anterior and posterior ethmoidal arteries, which are branches of the ophthalmic artery. The facial artery and the superior labial artery supply the vestibular area. The sphenopalatine artery supplies, the posterior and inferior quadrants. It is a branch of the internal maxillary artery, which in turn is a branch of the external carotid artery. An area of anastomosis between all these arteries is present on the antero-inferior part of the nasal

septum, which is termed the Little's area or the Kiesselbach's plexus and is the commonest site of epistaxis.

It is common for the nasal septum to show some minor degrees of deviation. A significant degree of deviation, e.g., following a previous nasal fracture, can prevent intranasal access (Fig. 2.63). Surgery to correct such a deviation (a submucosal resection or SMR) may be required to permit some lacrimal drainage surgery procedures to be performed, e.g., placement of a Lester Jones tube. Such a procedure can also be performed endoscopically at the time of lacrimal drainage system surgery.

The Turbinates

The middle and inferior turbinates are important landmarks in lacrimal drainage procedures (Fig. 2.64).

The superior turbinate plays no role in lacrimal drainage surgery. The turbinates are seen as projections from the lateral wall of the nose. Their purpose is to warm and moisten air drawn through the nose. A space, the meatus, lies beneath each turbinate. The nasolacrimal duct opens beneath the inferior turbinate into the inferior meatus. The inferior meatus can be particularly narrow in some infants, necessitating an in-fracture of the inferior turbinate to gain access

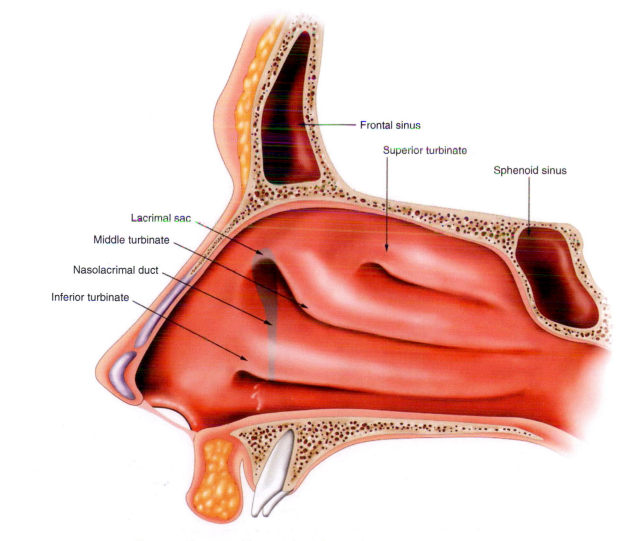

Figure 2.61 The course of the nasolacrimal duct and its opening beneath the inferior turbinate.

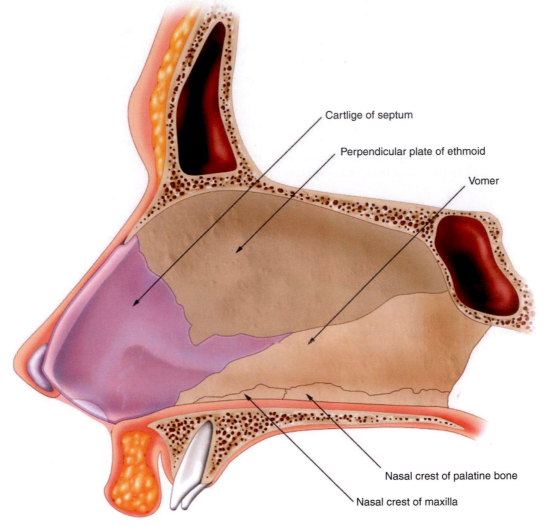

Cartlige of septum

Perpendicular plate of ethmoid

Vomer

Nasal crest of palatine bone

Nasal crest of maxilla

Figure 2.62 The nasal septum seen in sagittal section.

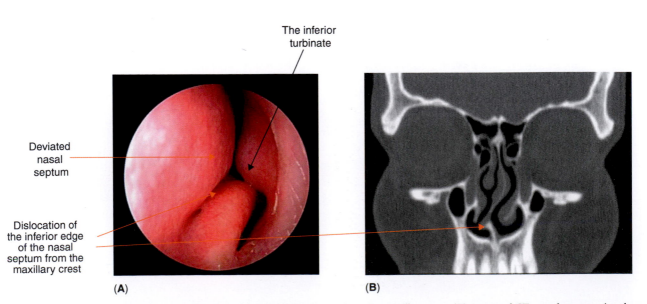

The inferior
turbinate

Deviated
nasal
septum

Dislocation of
the inferior edge
of the nasal
septum from the
maxillary crest

(A)   **(B)**

Figure 2.63 (**A**) A deviated nasal septum with an inferior dislocation of the septum from the maxillary crest. (**B**) A coronal CT scan demonstrating the septal deviation to the left and the inferior septal dislocation.

to the inferior meatus. The area can be directly visualized with a pediatric (2.7 mm) endoscope after decongesting the mucosa.

The middle turbinate is seen at a higher level within the nose. The anterior tip of the middle turbinate lies adjacent to the lacrimal sac. Sometimes ethmoid air cells invade the middle turbinate, a condition referred to as concha bullosa. It is very occasionally necessary to resect a small portion of the middle turbinate if it obstructs a dacryocystorhinostomy osteum. As the root of the middle turbinate joins the cribriform plate, great care should be taken if surgery is performed on the middle turbinate to avoid creating a CSF leak. The middle turbinate's function should be respected and it should never be routinely resected, e.g., during endoscopic orbital decompression surgery. The frontonasal duct from the frontal sinus drains into the middle meatus. The anterior and middle ethmoid sinuses and the maxillary sinus drain into the middle meatus.

The Paranasal Sinuses

- Frontal sinuses
- Ethmoidal sinuses
- Sphenoidal sinuses
- Maxillary sinuses

The frontal, ethmoidal, sphenoidal, and maxillary paranasal sinuses vary in size and shape in different individuals. Most are rudimentary, or even absent, at birth. They enlarge considerably during the time of eruption of the permanent teeth and after puberty, and this growth is a factor in the alteration in the size and shape of the face at these times. They are lined with mucous membrane continuous with that of the nasal cavity, an important fact in connection with the spread of infections. The mucous membrane resembles that of the respiratory region of the nasal cavity, but is thinner, less vascular and more loosely adherent to the bony walls of the sinuses. The mucus secreted by the glands in the mucous membrane is swept into the nose through the apertures of the sinuses by the movement of the cilia covering the surface.

The Frontal Sinuses

Two frontal sinuses are posterior to the superciliary arches, between the outer and inner tables of the frontal bone. They are rarely symmetrical as the septum between them frequently deviates from the median plane (Fig. 2.65).

The frontal sinus is sometimes divided into a number of communicating recesses by incomplete bony partitions. Rarely, one or both sinuses may be absent, and the degree of prominence of the superciliary arches is no indication of the presence or size of the frontal sinuses. The part of the sinus extending upward in the frontal bone may be small and the orbital part large, or vice versa. Sometimes one sinus may overlap in front of the other. The sinus may extend posteriorly as far as the lesser wing of the sphenoid but does not invade it. Each opens into the anterior part of the corresponding middle meatus of the nose, either through the ethmoidal infundibulum or the frontonasal duct, which traverses the anterior part of labyrinth of the ethmoid. Rudimentary or absent at birth, they are generally fairly well developed between seventh and eighth years, but reach their full size only after puberty.

The frontal sinuses are usually larger in males, giving the profile of the head an obliquity that contrasts with the vertical or convex outline usually seen in children and females. The arterial blood supply of the sinus is from the supraorbital and anterior ethmoidal arteries, and the venous drainage is into the anastomotic vein in the supraorbital notch connecting the supraorbital and superior ophthalmic veins. The lymphatic drainage is to the submandibular nodes. The nerve supply is derived from the supraorbital nerve.

The Ethmoidal Sinuses

The ethmoidal sinuses consist of thin-walled cavities in the ethmoidal labyrinth. They vary in number and size from three large to eighteen small sinuses on each side, and their openings into the nasal cavity are very variable. They lie between the upper part of the nasal cavity and the orbits, and are separated from the latter by the extremely thin orbital plates of the ethmoid, the lamina papyracea (Fig. 2.66).

Infection can spread readily from the sinuses into the orbit and produce orbital cellulitis.

On each side, they are arranged in three groups—anterior, middle, and posterior. The three groups are not sharply delineated from each other and one group may encroach on the territory generally occupied by another. The groups are really only distinguishable on the basis of their sites of

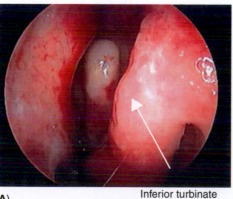
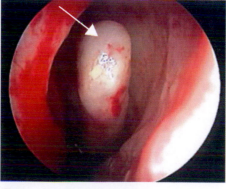

Figure 2.64 (**A**) An endoscopic view of the nose following the use of a nasal decongestant. The inferior turbinate is indicated by the arrow. The inferior meatus and the opening of the nasolacrimal duct lie under the inferior turbinate. (**B**) The middle turbinate is indicated by the arrow. The middle meatus lies beneath this.

communication with the nasal cavity. In each group the sinuses are partially separated by incomplete bony septa. The anterior group varies up to 11 in number and opens into the ethmoidal infundibulum or the frontonasal duct by one or more orifices; one sinus frequently lies in the agger nasi and the most anterior sinuses may encroach upon the frontal sinus. The middle group generally comprises three cavities that open into the middle meatus by one or more orifices on or above the ethmoidal bulla. The posterior group varies from one to seven in number and usually opens by one orifice into the superior meatus inferior to the superior turbinate, though one may open into the highest meatus (when present), and one or more sometimes opens into the sphenoidal sinus. The posterior group is very closely related to the optic canal and optic nerve.

The ethmoidal sinuses are small at birth growing rapidly between the sixth and eighth years and after puberty. They derive their arterial blood supply from the sphenopalatine and the anterior ethmoidal and posterior ethmoidal arteries and are drained by the corresponding veins. The lymphatics of the anterior and middle groups drain into the submandibular nodes and those of the posterior group into the retropharyngeal nodes. The ethmoidal sinuses are supplied by the anterior and posterior ethmoidal nerves, and the orbital branches of the pterygo-palatine ganglion.

The Sphenoidal Sinuses

The two sphenoidal sinuses lie posterior to the upper part of the nasal cavity. Contained within the body of the sphenoid bone, they are related to the optic chiasm superiorly, and the pituitary, and, on each side, to the internal carotid arteries and the cavernous sinuses (Fig. 2.50B). If the sinuses are small, they lie in front of the pituitary. They vary in size and shape, and, because of the lateral displacement of the intervening septum, are frequently asymmetrical. One sinus is often larger than the other and extends across the median plane behind the sinus of the opposite side. One sinus may overlap above the other, and rarely there is a communication between the two sinuses. Occasionally one or both sinuses may extend close to and even partially encircle the optic canal on its own side. For this reason sphenoid sinusitis may be responsible for an optic neuropathy. When exceptionally large they may extend into the roots of the pterygoid processes or greater wings of the sphenoid, and may invade the basilar part of the occipital bone. Occasionally there are gaps in the bony walls and the mucous membrane may lie directly against the dura.

Bony ridges, produced by the internal carotid artery and the pterygoid canal, may project into the sinuses from the lateral wall and floor, respectively. The proximity of the carotid artery must be borne in mind when attempting to decompress the optic canal through the sphenoid sinus following a fracture with a compressive optic neuropathy. A posterior ethmoidal sinus may extend into the body of the sphenoid and largely replace a sphenoidal sinus. Each sinus communicates with the spheno-ethmoidal recess by an aperture in the upper part of its anterior wall. They are present as minute cavities at birth, but their main development occurs after puberty. Their blood supply is by one of the posterior ethmoidal vessels and the lymph drain is to the retropharyngeal nodes. Their nerve supply is from the posterior ethmoidal nerves and the orbital branches of the pterygopalatine ganglion.

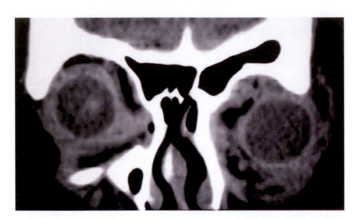

Figure 2.65 Asymmetric frontal sinuses seen in a coronal CT scan. (This patient had a left carotico-cavernous fistula.)

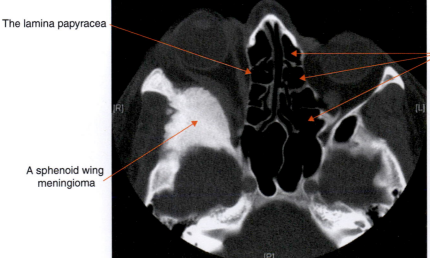

The lamina papyracea

The ethmoid sinuses

A sphenoid wing meningioma

Figure 2.66 An axial CT scan of a patient with a right sphenoid wing meningioma. The ethmoid sinuses are well demonstrated on this CT scan.

The Maxillary Sinuses

The two maxillary sinuses, which are the largest accessory air sinuses of the nose, are pyramidal cavities in the bodies of the maxillae (Fig. 2.67).

The base of each is formed by the lateral wall of the nasal cavity; the apex extends into the zygomatic process of the maxilla. The roof, which forms the orbital floor, is frequently ridged by the infraorbital canal. The size of the maxillary sinus varies in different skulls, and even between the two sides of the same skull. In some patients, a large maxillary sinus may extend into the zygomatic bone. The sinus communicates with the lower part of the hiatus semilunaris through an opening in the antero-superior part of its base. A second orifice is frequently seen in, or immediately below, the hiatus. Both are nearer the roof than the floor of the sinus. The maxillary sinus does not reach its full size until after the eruption of all the permanent teeth. The blood supply of the sinus is by means of the facial, infraorbital and greater palatine vessels; the lymph drainage is to the submandibular nodes. The nerve supply is derived from the infraorbital and the anterior, middle and posterior, superior alveolar nerves.

THE FACE

It is important to understand the various layers of the face and the tissue planes, which can be safely accessed for a variety of reconstructive and aesthetic procedures.

The Scalp

The central scalp consists of five layers (Fig. 2.68):

- Skin
- Subcutaneous fibrofatty tissue
- Galea aponeurotica
- Loose areolar tissue
- Pericranium

The galea aponeurotica links the frontalis and occipitalis muscles. The sub-galeal plane is relatively avascular and the forehead can be peeled forward in this plane after making a bicoronal scalp incision. The pericranium is very vascular and a pericranial flap can be used to reconstruct deep medial canthal defects in conjunction with a full thickness skin graft. The pericranium can be lifted from the underlying bone very easily, and the space thus created is avascular. This space is accessed for endoscopic brow lift surgery.

The Temple

The anatomy of the temple can be confusing because of the different nomenclature often used to describe the fascial layers in the temple. The temple consists of the following layers:

- Skin
- Subcutaneous tissue
- Superficial temporal fascia (temporo-parietal fascia)
- The deep temporal fascia
- Temporalis muscle

The superficial temporal fascia is continuous with the galea aponeurotica. It contains the frontal branch of the facial nerve and the superficial temporal artery. The deep temporal fascia is easily recognized by its thick white glistening surface. A nick can be made in the deep temporal fascia to expose the underlying temporalis muscle and to confirm the nature of the anatomical

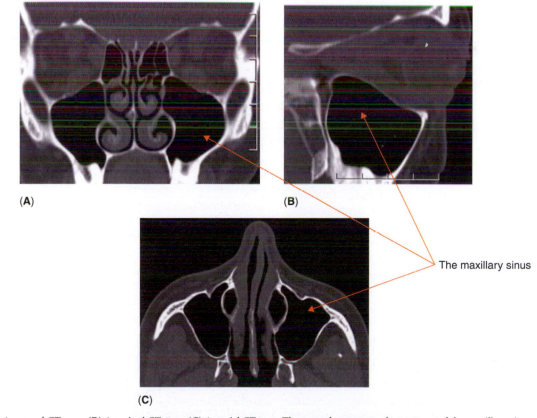

(A)

(B)

The maxillary sinus

(C)

Figure 2.67 (**A**) A coronal CT scan. (**B**) A sagittal CT scan. (**C**) An axial CT scan. The scans demonstrate the anatomy of the maxillary sinuses. Note the normal configuration and shape of the orbital floor.

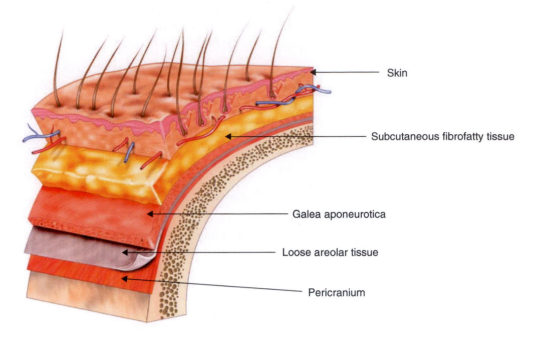

Figure 2.68 The layers of the central scalp.

layer. A dissection undertaken from the temple to the orbital margin in the course of an endoscopic brow lift should be made along this layer, with the frontal branch of the facial nerve lying protected in the superficial temporal fascia above this.

A few centimeters above the zygomatic arch the deep temporal fascia splits into two layers: *the superficial and the deep layers of the deep temporal fascia.* These insert onto the antero-superior and postero-superior aspects of the zygomatic arch, respectively. Between these two layers lies the temporal fat pad (Figs. 68 and 69).

The Superficial Musculoaponeurotic System (SMAS)

The SMAS is a superficial continuous fibromuscular layer of the face and neck, which invests and interlinks all the superficial muscles of facial expression (Fig. 2.70). It extends from the malar region superiorly to become continuous with the galea aponeurotica, inferiorly to join the platysma, and laterally to invest in the parotid fascia overlying the parotid gland. In the temporal region, the SMAS blends into the superficial temporoparietal fascia.

The SMAS invests the superficial mimetic muscles, including the platysma muscle, orbicularis oculi muscle, occipitofrontalis muscle, zygomaticus muscles, and the levator labii superioris muscle. The SMAS attaches to the skin via ligamentous extensions. The SMAS, although a true anatomical structure, is not a very distinct layer. It varies in thickness from patient to patient. It becomes much thinner and less distinct as it extends toward the nasolabial fold. The malar fat pad is a collection of fat overlying the malar eminence, which lies on and within the anterior surface of the SMAS.

In the lower part of the face, the facial nerve branches are deep to the SMAS, and innervate the facial muscles on their undersurface. The deep facial muscles are an exception to this rule: the levator anguli oris, the buccinator, and the mentalis are all innervated on their superficial surface. These facial

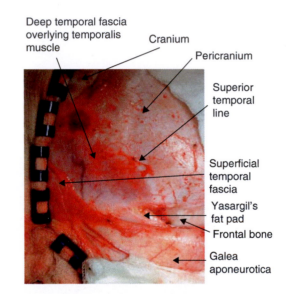

Figure 2.69 An intraoperative photograph during a bicoronal flap dissection demonstrating layers of fascia in the right temple.

nerve branches are protected if a dissection is kept superficial to the SMAS in this location.

The SMAS can be divided and repositioned, partially excised and sutured, or plicated as required to augment or contour the elevation of the malar fat pad. Tightening the SMAS plays a major role in the surgical rejuvenation of the lower third of the face. Tightening the SMAS also provides a suitable support framework for platysmal plication.

The Retaining Ligaments

These are condensations of fibrous tissue that run from deeper structures to the overlying dermis, and help to anchor the skin and mobile soft tissues to the underlying skeleton (Fig. 2.71). There are two types of retaining ligaments: true and false. True retaining ligaments are short and stout fibrous bands that run

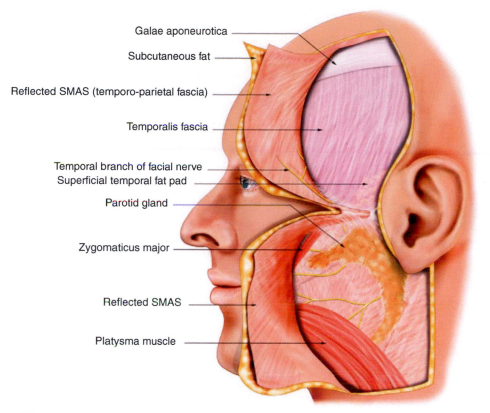

Galae aponeurotica

Subcutaneous fat

Reflected SMAS (temporo-parietal fascia)

Temporalis fascia

Temporal branch of facial nerve
Superficial temporal fat pad

Parotid gland

Zygomaticus major

Reflected SMAS

Platysma muscle

(A)

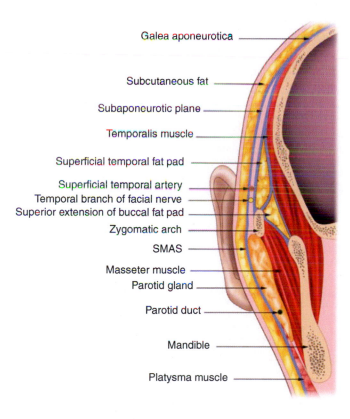

Galea aponeurotica

Subcutaneous fat

Subaponeurotic plane

Temporalis muscle

Superficial temporal fat pad

Superficial temporal artery
Temporal branch of facial nerve
Superior extension of buccal fat pad

Zygomatic arch

SMAS

Masseter muscle

Parotid gland

Parotid duct

Mandible

Platysma muscle

(B)

Figure 2.70 (**A**) The reflected SMAS depicted in a sagittal drawing of the face. (**B**) The SMAS layer and its relationship to surrounding structures depicted in a coronal drawing of one half of the face.

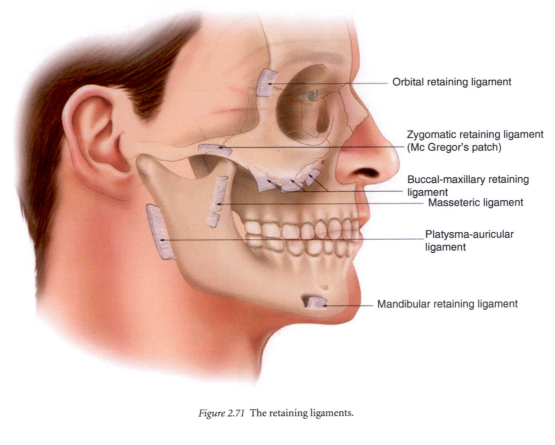

Figure 2.71 The retaining ligaments.

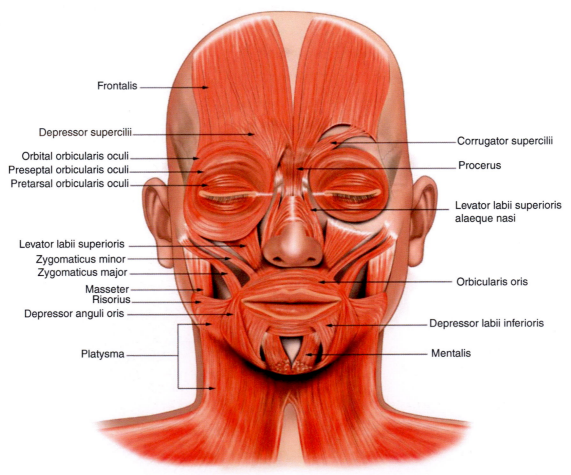

Figure 2.72 The muscles of the facial expression.

from then periosteum to the dermis. They are found in four locations in the mid- and lower face:

- Orbital
- Zygomatic
- Buccomaxillary
- Mandibular

The orbital ligaments are located over the zygomatico-frontal suture and over the malar eminence. The zygomatic ligaments attach the fat to the underlying zygomatic eminence (McGregor's patch). The buccomaxillary ligaments have both true and false components. The true components attach the skin to zygomatico-maxillary suture. The mandibular ligaments attach the parasymphyseal dermis to the underlying bone and help support the chin pad to the underlying bone.

The false retaining ligaments fix the SMAS to the deep fascia and function to prevent gravitational descent. They are located in three regions and are accordingly named platysma auricular ligaments, masseteric ligaments, and buccomaxillary ligaments.

The malar soft tissues are suspended from the malar eminence and maxilla by the zygomatic ligaments laterally and bucco-maxillary ligaments medially. With aging, as these ligaments become lax, there is a descent of the malar tissues and a characteristic submalar hollow. This soft tissue ptosis occurs adjacent to the line of fixation along the nasolabial fold. This leads to the prominence of the nasolabial fold with aging. The attenuation of the masseteric ligaments leads to a descent of the soft tissues of the cheek below the mandibular border and the formation of jowls.

The platysma-auricular ligaments form a thick fascial aponeurosis that attaches the postero-superior border of the platysma to the lobule of the ear. They provide a dissection plane in the subcutaneous preauricular region that leads directly to the external surface of the platysma.

In the young person, the retaining ligaments are taut, keeping the mobile superficial facial tissues firmly anchored to the underlying skeleton or deep fascia. Years of muscle action and gravity result in fascial and ligamentous laxity which, in combination with dermal elastosis, result in a descent of all soft tissues of the face.

The Muscles of the Mid-face and Lower Face

The perioral muscles are responsible for the movement of the upper and lower lips and of the angles of mouth (Fig. 2.72). They are situated in two planes—superficial and deep. The SMAS splits to invest the superficial muscles:

- Zygomatic major
- Zygomatic minor
- Risorius
- Depressor anguli oris
- Orbicularis oris—superficial portion
- Platysma

The facial nerve branches innervate these along their deep surface. The zygomatic major and minor muscles are the predominant smile muscles.

The deep perioral muscles are:

- Levator labii superioris
- Levator anguli oris

- Buccinator
- Mentalis
- Depressor labii inferioris
- Orbicularis oris—deep portion

The facial nerve branches innervate these muscles along their superficial surface. The buccal fat pad is situated deep to buccinator. The lip elevators are responsible for the nasolabial crease and lip depressors (depressor anguli oris) for labiomandibular crease.

The platysma blends into the inferior extent of the SMAS. This superficial muscle consists of two flat muscles, which join together in the central neck. Fat lies superficial to the platysma and can be removed with liposuction or directly excised in the central neck area. Fat also lies just deep to the muscle. The platysma can be plicated, suspended with sutures, or even partially excised as needed to further define a good cervicomental angle.

A knowledge of the anatomy of the greater auricular nerve is important as it is liable to injury during face lift surgery. It is located approximately 6.5 cm inferior to the external auditory meatus crossing the sternocleidomastoid muscle (Fig. 2.73). It is located deep to the superficial cervical fascia, which is a continuation of the SMAS in the neck. As long as the subcutaneous undermining of the lateral neck flap does not violate this fascia, this nerve is safe. Damage to this nerve can result in sensory loss to the external ear.

SUMMARY

It cannot be over-emphasized that a sound working knowledge of eyelid, orbital, nasal, and facial anatomy is essential before embarking upon oculoplastic, oculofacial, orbital, and lacrimal surgery. The surgeon in training and the

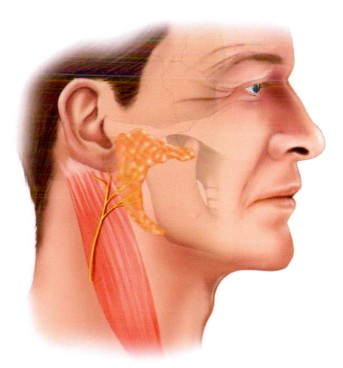

Figure 2.73 The greater auricular nerve.

inexperienced surgeon should take the time to carefully review the relevant aspects of this chapter in preparation for any operative procedure. The recognition of anatomical structures altered and distorted by pathological processes comes with experience.

FURTHER READING

1. Anderson RL, Beard C. The levator aponeurosis. Arch Ophthalmol 1977; 95:1437–41.
2. Codère F, Tucker NA, Renaldi B. The anatomy of Whitnall ligament. Ophthalmology 1995; 102:2016–19.
3. Cook BE Jr. Lucarelli MJ. Lemke BN. Depressor supercilii muscle: anatomy, histology, and cosmetic implications. Ophthal Plast Reconstr Surg 2001; 17(6):404–11.
4. Doxanas MT, Anderson RL, eds. Clinical Orbital Anatomy. Baltimore: Williams & Wilkins, 1984.
5. Doxanas MT, Anderson RL. Oriental eyelids: an anatomic study. Arch Ophthalmol 1984; 102:1232.
6. Dutton J. Clinical anatomy of the orbit. In Yanoff M, Duker J, eds. Ophthalmology. London: Mosby, 2004: 744–51.
7. Dutton J.J. Atlas of Clinical and Surgical Orbital Anatomy. Philadelphia, PA: WB Saunders Company. 1994 (ISBN: 0-7216-5427-4).
8. Ettl A, Priglinger S, Kramer J, Koornneef L. Functional anatomy of the levator palpebrae superioris muscle and its connective tissue system. Br J Ophthal 1996; 80(8):702–7.
9. Horner WE. Description of a small muscle at the Internal Commissure of the Eyelid. J Med Phys 1823; 8:70–80.
10. Kanize DM, ed. The Forehead and Temporal Fossa: Anatomy and Technique. Philadelphia, PA: Williams & Wilkins, 2001.
11. Koornneef L. Orbital septa: anatomy and function. Ophthalmology 1979; 86(5):876–80.
12. Larrabee WF, Jr, Makielski KH. Surgical Anatomy of the Face. 1993, New York, NY: Raven Press (ISBN: 0-88167-945-3).
13. Lucarelli MJ, Khwarg SI, Lemke BN, Kozel JS, Dortzbach RK. The anatomy of midfacial ptosis. Ophthal Plast Reconstr Surg 2000; 16(1):7–22.
14. Mendelson BC, Jacobson SR. Surgical anatomy of the midcheek: facial layers, spaces, and the midcheek segments. [Review] [34 refs] Clin Plast Surg 2008; 35(3):395–404; discussion 393.
15. Mendelson BC, Muzaffar AR, Adams WP, Jr. Surgical anatomy of the midcheek and malar mounds. Plast Reconstr Surg 2002; 110(3):885–96; discussion 897–911.
16. Meyer DR, Linberg JV, Wobig JL, McCormick SA. Anatomy of the orbital septum and associated eyelid connective tissues. Implications for ptosis surgery. Ophthal Plast Reconstr Surg (1991) 7:104–13.
17. Muzaffar AR, Mendelson BC, Adams WP, Jr. Surgical anatomy of the ligamentous attachments of the lower lid and lateral canthus. Plast Reconstr Surg 12002; 10(3):873–84; discussion 897–911.
18. Seery GE. Surgical anatomy of the scalp. Dermatol Surg 2002; 28(7): 581–7.
19. Shorr N, Hoenig JA, Cook T: Brow lift. In: Levine MR, ed. Manual of Oculoplastic Surgery, 3rd edn, Boston: Butterworth-Heinemann, 2003: 61–75.
20. Tucker NA, Tucker SM, Linberg JV. The anatomy of the common canaliculus. Arch Ophthal 1996; 114(10):1231–4.
21. Tucker SM, Linberg JV. Vascular anatomy of the eyelids. Ophthalmology 1994; 101(6):1118–21.
22. Wobig JL, Dailey RA. Surgery of the mid face, lower face and neck. In: Wobig JL, Dailey RA, eds. Oculofacial Plastic Surgery, Face, Lacrimal System and Orbit. New York: Thieme, 2004: 103–25.
23. Wobig JL, Dailey RA. Surgery of the upper eyelid and brow. In: Wobig JL, Dailey RA, eds. Oculofacial Plastic Surgery, Face, Lacrimal System and Orbit. New York, NY: Thieme, 2004: 34–53.
24. Zide BM, Jelks GW. Surgical Anatomy of the Orbit. New York, NY: Raven Press, 1985. ISBN: 0-88167-054-5.

3   Lower eyelid entropion

INTRODUCTION

Lower eyelid entropion is an eyelid malposition in which the lower eyelid margin is turned inward against the globe. The keratinized skin of the eyelid margin and the eyelashes rub against the inferior cornea and bulbar conjunctiva, causing irritation. Patients with a lower lid entropion tend to seek medical attention early because of the troublesome symptoms. Lower lid entropion can be classified into four types.

CLASSIFICATION

1. Involutional entropion
2. Cicatricial entropion
3. Acute spastic entropion
4. Congenital entropion

Involutional Entropion

The majority of entropia are involutional and therefore seen in older patients. In the lower eyelid, involutional changes typically result in either a lower lid entropion or ectropion, whereas in the upper eyelid the same changes result in ptosis. A combination of factors has been proposed to account for the eyelid malposition. These are:

1. Laxity, dehiscence, or disinsertion of the lower eyelid retractors (Fig. 3.1A)
2. Over-riding of the preseptal orbicularis oculi muscle over the pretarsal orbicularis oculi muscle
3. Horizontal eyelid laxity
4. Enophthalmos

Any surgical treatment should aim to address these factors with the exception of enophthalmos. Enophthalmos has not been shown to be a significant factor in the aetiology of involutional lower eyelid entropion. Laxity, dehiscence, or disinsertion of the lower eyelid retractors is the primary cause of involutional entropion. This lower eyelid retractor problem allows the inferior edge of the tarsus to rotate away from the globe. Horizontal eyelid laxity leads to instability of the eyelid. The preseptal orbicularis appears to force the lower eyelid margin inwards.

> **KEY POINT**
>
> Laxity of the eyelid retractors is the primary cause of involutional lower eyelid entropion

Cicatricial Entropion

Any condition that causes contracture of the conjunctiva can result in a cicatricial entropion (Fig. 3.2). Such conditions include chemical burns, surgical or accidental trauma, topical glaucoma medications, ocular cicatricial pemphigoid, trachoma, and Stevens–Johnson syndrome. It may also be seen with the extrusion of an orbital floor implant through the inferior fornix.

Acute Spastic Entropion

This form of entropion is seen in susceptible individuals with blepharospasm that has been induced by ocular irritation. Although treatment of the underlying cause of ocular irritation may reverse the eyelid malposition, a permanent entropion may ensue which will require surgical intervention.

Congenital Entropion

Congenital lower eyelid entropion is a rare condition. It differs from congenital epiblepharon, a much more common condition, by the fact that the tarsus is inverted (Fig. 3.3). This eyelid malposition does not resolve spontaneously and requires surgical intervention to prevent corneal morbidity. It has been postulated that an abnormal insertion of the lower lid retractors is the underlying cause.

APPLIED SURGICAL ANATOMY

A thorough understanding of lower eyelid anatomy is essential to the surgical management of lower eyelid entropion (Fig. 3.4). For a more detailed description of the anatomy of the lower eyelid, refer to chapter 2.

The lower eyelid can be considered to consist of three lamellae:

- Anterior—skin and orbicularis oculi muscle
- Middle—orbital septum and inferior eyelid retractors
- Posterior—tarsus and conjunctiva

The lower eyelid tarsus is approximately 3 to 4 mm in height and 1 mm in thickness. The normal lower eyelid margin is flat, ending at right angles anteriorly and posteriorly. The most posterior aspect of the normal eyelid margin is the mucocutaneous junction where the mucosa of the palpebral conjunctiva ends and the keratinized skin of the eyelid margin begins. The meibomian gland orifices lie just anterior to the mucocutaneous junction. Anterior to the meibomian gland orifices lies the gray line. The gray line is used as a surgical landmark to separate the anterior and posterior lamellae of the eyelid. The eyelashes lie anterior to the gray line. These lie in one or two irregular rows in the lower eyelid and three or four irregular rows in the upper eyelid.

The tarsal conjunctiva is firmly adherent to the tarsus and cannot be dissected freely. The forniceal conjunctiva, in contrast, is very loosely attached to the underlying retractors. The lower eyelid skin crease is variable but usually situated approximately 4 to 5 mm below the eyelid margin. The lateral canthal angle normally sits approximately 2 mm higher than the medial canthal angle.

The lower eyelid retractor complex consists of an aponeurotic expansion from the inferior rectus muscle. This aponeurotic expansion, known as the capsulopalpebral fascia, extends anteriorly to envelop the inferior oblique muscle, where it

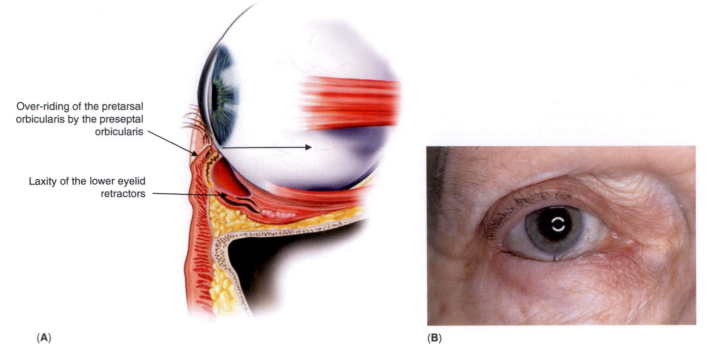

Over-riding of the pretarsal orbicularis by the preseptal orbicularis

Laxity of the lower eyelid retractors

(A)   **(B)**

Figure 3.1 (**A**) Laxity of the lower eyelid retractors and overriding of the preseptal orbicularis muscle over the pretarsal orbicularis, causing lower eyelid entropion. (**B**) A typical lower eyelid involutional entropion.

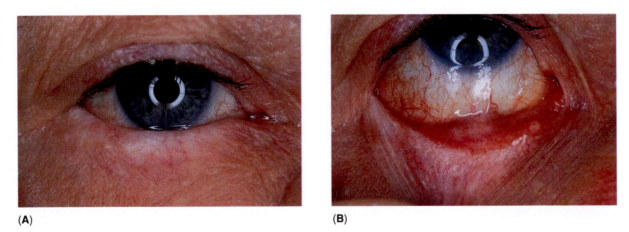

(A)   **(B)**

Figure 3.2 (**A**) A lower eyelid cicatricial entropion. The lower eyelid lashes have been removed by previous cryotherapy. (**B**) Eversion of the lower eyelid reveals conjunctival scarring.

fuses with the inferior suspensory ligament (Lockwood's ligament). The fascia also contains fibers which insert into the inferior margin of the tarsus, the preseptal orbicularis muscle at the level of the lower lid skin crease, and the inferior fornix. The fascia is also accompanied by some smooth muscle fibers. The retractors pull the lower eyelid inferiorly on down gaze acting synchronously with the inferior rectus muscle. Normal tension on the lower eyelid retractors is essential in the maintenance of a stable lower eyelid.

The orbital septum fuses with the fascia approximately 4 to 5 mm below the tarsus. The orbital septum extends from the arcus marginalis of the inferior orbital margin to the inferior border of the tarsus. Posterior to this lie the three lower lid fat pockets.

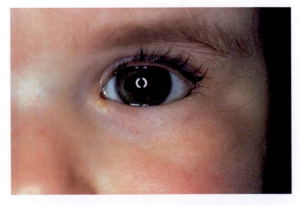

Figure 3.3 Congenital lower eyelid entropion.

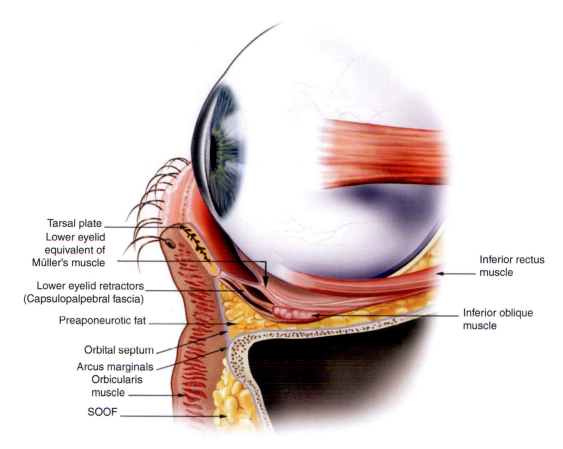

Figure 3.4 A diagram illustrating the anatomy of the lower eyelid and adjacent structures.

The anatomy of the lower eyelid resembles that of the upper eyelid. Although the tarsus is much smaller, the capsulopalpebral fascia is analogous to the levator aponeurosis. The smooth muscle fibers accompanying this fascia are analogous to Müller's muscle. Lockwood's ligament is analogous to Whitnall's ligament. The fat in the lower eyelid lies posterior to the septum but anterior to the capsulopalpebral fascia and is analogous to the upper lid preaponeurotic fat. There are three fat pads in the lower eyelid: medial, central, and lateral. These lie between the capsulopalpebral fascia and the orbital septum. The inferior oblique muscle lies between the medial and central fat pads. The central and lateral fat pads are separated by the arcuate expansion.

In the lower eyelid, an anastomotic arterial arcade runs in the orbicularis oculi muscle plane approximately 4 to 5 mm below the eyelid margin.

It is very helpful to consider the individual layers of the lower eyelid that are encountered during a surgical dissection. A full thickness horizontal incision made through the eyelid at a point 4 to 5 mm below the tarsus would pass through the following structures:

- Skin
- Orbicularis oculi muscle
- Orbital septum
- "Preaponeurotic" fat
- Lower eyelid retractors
- Conjunctiva

"Preaponeurotic" fat is often encountered a few millimeters inferior to this position, particularly in an elderly patient. The orbital septum is very attenuated in this age group and should be opened more inferiorly to expose the fat. This ensures that the septum has been opened and released and the inferior retractors (the capsulopalpebral fascia) are correctly identified. This lies beneath the fat and above the conjunctiva.

The involutional entropion presents the trainee oculoplastic surgeon with the ideal opportunity to appreciate eyelid anatomy, to improve surgical skill in eyelid dissection, to perfect the use of the Colorado needle and bipolar cautery in achieving good hemostasis, to practice suturing, and to perfect patient communication during surgery under local anesthesia.

PATIENT ASSESSMENT
History
Patients who present with a lower eyelid entropion complain of irritation, photophobia, and a red eye. Occasionally they will complain of discharge. The patient may experience only intermittent symptoms and may show no physical abnormalities when they present. Such a history in an older patient should lead to the suspicion that an intermittent involutional entropion is the cause of the patient's complaints. Some patients discover that the eyelid can be manually repositioned offering temporary relief from the symptoms. Others present with tape placed at the eyelid–cheek junction to prevent the re-occurrence of the entropion.

Patients with involutional entropion are frequently elderly with multiple medical problems. The patient's age and medical and drug history must be taken into account when determining the appropriate management. Most elderly, infirm patients are better suited to the placement of simple lower lid everting sutures in clinic. These are quick and simple to place, very effective, and easy to repeat in the event of a recurrence of the entropion. In the presence of significant lower eyelid laxity, transverse sutures can be used instead.

Examination

The patient should undergo a careful naked eye and slit lamp examination to determine the etiology of the entropion, e.g., a corneal foreign body causing a spastic entropion, and to determine the most appropriate treatment. The conjunctiva is examined to exclude scarring, symblephara, or keratin on the posterior lamella (Fig. 3.5).

The lower lid is gently repositioned with a finger. If the eyelid remains in a normal position without blinking, the etiology is likely to be involutional rather than cicatricial, although more than one etiological factor may be present. If there is no entropion present, but the history suggests an intermittent episodic inversion of the eyelid, the patient should be asked to look down and to forcibly close the eyes. The patient should then be asked to slowly open the eyes and the eyelid should be carefully observed. An entropion may appear or the preseptal orbicularis muscle may be seen to roll upward (overriding of the preseptal orbicularis).

The eyelid margin should be observed in down gaze. Laxity, dehiscence, or disinsertion of the lower eyelid retractors is associated with a poor movement of the eyelid margin when the patient looks down. The eyelid margin is seen to ride above the inferior limbus.

The eyelid should be assessed for horizontal laxity. The eyelid should be drawn medially and laterally to determine the degree of medial and lateral canthal tendon laxity (the "distraction" test). It is unusual to have significant medial canthal tendon

laxity in lower lid entropion, and it is extremely rare for this to require surgical correction. This is in contrast to the situation with lower lid ectropion. The eyelid should be drawn away from the globe to determine the degree of laxity of the tarsus. It should only be possible to draw the eyelid approximately 2 to 3 mm from the globe. This is the "pinch" test (Fig. 3.6A and B). The eyelid is then drawn inferiorly and released. This is the "snap" test (Fig. 3.6C–E). The eyelid should return to lie in apposition to the globe without a blink. Failure to do so suggests significant eyelid laxity.

MANAGEMENT
Medical Management

In the case of acute spastic entropion, the treatment is directed to the provoking stimulus, e.g., trichiasis, blepharitis, or a dry eye. Although a bandage contact lens or botulinum-toxin injections may improve symptoms temporarily, these are rarely justified. The use of lower lid tape can be advised for use in a primary care setting while the patient is waiting to be seen by an ophthalmologist.

Surgical Management
Involutional Entropion

Although over 100 procedures have been described for the surgical repair of lower eyelid involutional entropion, very few have withstood the test of time and the majority have been abandoned. This is mainly because these procedures have failed to address the underlying etiological factors responsible for the entropion.

Although a multitude of operations are still used by many different surgeons, only those procedures which are used in the author's clinical practice are described:

1. Everting or transverse sutures
2. Lower lid retractor advancement with a lateral tarsal strip procedure
3. Lower lid retractor advancement with a lower lid wedge resection

These procedures are usually performed under local anesthesia, with or without sedation.

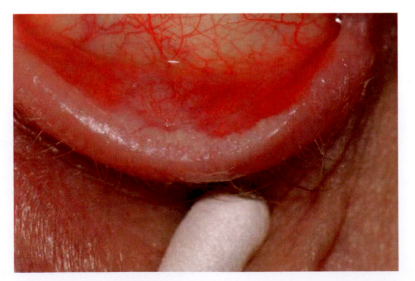

Figure 3.5 Keratin on the posterior lamella of the everted lower eyelid of a patient with Stevens Johnson syndrome.

Everting sutures are offered to all patients over the age of 70 years at the initial consultation, and are used exclusively for the following patients:

1. Elderly patients with concomitant medical problems for whom surgery is contraindicated

2. Patients who decline a more definitive surgical treatment
3. Patients who have a bleeding diathesis or who take anti-coagulants
4. Patients who are unable to cooperate with surgery

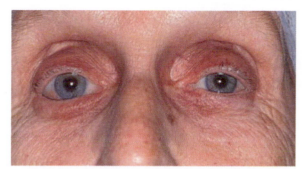
(A)

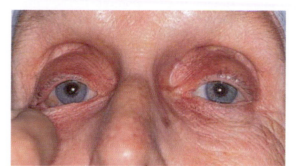
(B)

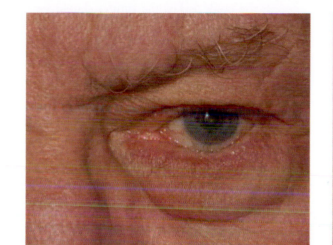
(C)

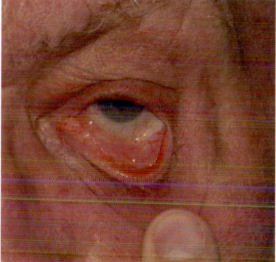
(D)

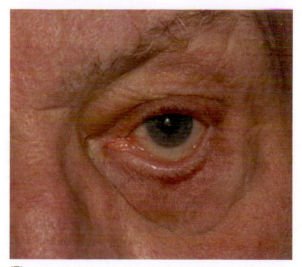
(E)

Figure 3.6 (**A**) A right lower eyelid involutional entropion. (**B**) A lower eyelid "pinch" test. (**C**) A patient with a left lower eyelid involutional entropion. (**D**) A "snap" test being performed on the left lower eyelid. (**E**) The lower eyelid has failed to return to the globe without a blink indicating that the patient has significant laxity of the eyelid.

5. Patients who are unable to lie in a semi-recumbent position for the duration of surgery
6. Patients willing to undergo a trial of everting sutures.

Everting sutures have been commonly regarded as a temporary form of treatment, but many patients achieve a long-lasting or permanent result with the sutures alone. If the entropion recurs within a relatively short period of time, the patient is then offered a more definitive surgical procedure unless surgery is contraindicated. The sutures are very quick and simple to insert in a clinic setting and provide instant relief for the patient. It is also very easy to repeat such treatment as required. If the patient has significant eyelid laxity, transverse sutures are placed rather than everting sutures to avoid the possibility of causing a secondary ectropion. For some patients with lower lid laxity everting sutures can be combined with a lateral tarsal strip procedure.

KEY POINT

Lower lid everting sutures are very quick and simple to place, and have a high success rate. They can be used as the definitive treatment of a lower lid entropion in the older patient, or they can be used as a trial treatment before considering a more invasive procedure.

For all other patients, a lower eyelid retractor advancement is performed combined with either a lateral tarsal strip procedure or, less frequently, a lower eyelid wedge resection. Wherever appropriate these procedures can be combined with a debulking of the orbicularis oculi muscle. e.g., in a patient who has very marked orbicularis hypertrophy or overaction, or with a lower eyelid blepharoplasty, e.g., in a patient with marked fat pad prolapses.

KEY POINT

If a retractor advancement is not combined with a horizontal eyelid tightening procedure there is a great potential for recurrence of the entropion, even if the degree of lower eyelid laxity is not considered significant.

A lower eyelid retractor advancement combined with a lateral tarsal strip procedure is a very convenient operation for the patient, as no sutures need to be removed postoperatively. It is preferable to avoid the procedure, however, in the patient with marked upper eyelid laxity to avoid an upper eyelid overhang at the lateral canthus. It is also preferable to avoid this procedure in the obese, hypertensive patient who is unable to discontinue the use of aspirin preoperatively. In such patients, bleeding is much easier to control with a wedge resection of the lower lid. A lower eyelid retractor advancement combined with a lower lid wedge resection takes longer to perform and has the disadvantage that the

patient must return for suture removal 2 weeks following surgery. It is also associated with the risk of dehiscence of the wedge resection wound, notching of the eyelid margin or secondary trichiasis.

Everting Sutures
Surgical Procedure
1. Proxymethacaine drops are instilled into the inferior conjunctival fornix.
2. Two to three milliliters of 0.5% Bupivacaine with 1:200,000 units of adrenaline mixed 50:50 with 2% lidocaine with 1:80,000 units of adrenaline are injected immediately under the skin in the lower eyelid, avoiding bleeding from the orbicularis muscle and a hematoma.
3. Three or four double-armed 5/0 Vicryl sutures are passed through the eyelid from the inferior fornix to emerge 2 mm apart just below the lash line (Fig. 3.7A and B). The sutures are tied tightly enough to produce a minimal degree of ectropion (Fig. 3.8). If the eyelid is lax, the sutures should instead be passed through the eyelid from just below the tarsus to emerge 2 mm apart 2 to 3 mm below the lash line (transverse sutures) (Fig. 3.7C).
4. Antibiotic ointment is instilled into the eye.

Postoperative care. The patient is discharged with instructions to place topical antibiotic ointment in the eye and on the sutures externally three times a day for 2 weeks. Cool packs can be applied intermittently for 24 to 48 hours to reduce swelling. The sutures are removed in clinic 3 weeks postoperatively if still present. The patient can, however, be discharged from the clinic as the sutures will eventually dissolve over the course of 4 to 6 weeks.

Lower Lid Retractor Advancement with Lateral Tarsal Strip Procedure
Surgical procedure
Retractor advancement
1. Proxymethacaine drops are instilled into the inferior conjunctival fornix.
2. Two to three milliliters of 0.5% Bupivacaine with 1:200,000 units of adrenaline mixed 50:50 with 2% lidocaine with 1:80,000 units of adrenaline are injected immediately under the skin in the lower eyelid and at the lateral canthus, avoiding bleeding from the orbicularis muscle and a hematoma.
3. A 4/0 Silk traction suture is placed horizontally through the gray line of the lower eyelid centrally and fixated to the head drapes using a small curved artery clip.
4. A skin incision is then made 3 to 4 mm below the eyelid margin extending from just below the inferior punctum to the lateral aspect of the lower eyelid using a Colorado needle (Fig. 3.9A).
5. Hemostasis is obtained using bipolar cautery.

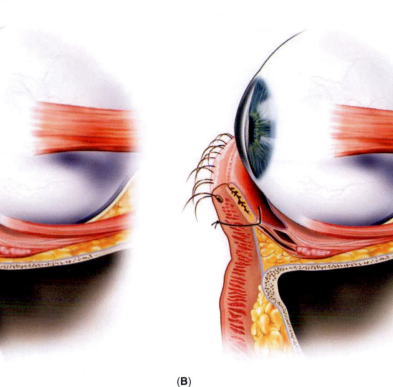

(A)   (B)

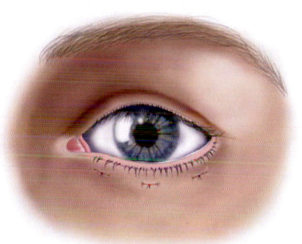

(C)

Figure 3.7 (**A**) The everting sutures are passed through the eyelid from the inferior fornix to emerge 2 mm apart just below the lash line. (**B**) Transverse sutures. (**C**) The position of the transverse sutures on the external surface of the eyelid is demonstrated.

6. The Colorado needle is then used to dissect through the orbicularis oculi muscle exposing the orbital septum. The orbicularis muscle is then dissected away from the underlying orbital septum for 2 mm.

7. The septum is then opened inferiorly with the Colorado needle or Westcott scissors 6 to 8 mm below the eyelid margin, exposing the preaponeurotic fat (Fig. 3.9B).

8. The lower eyelid retractors are identified beneath the fat.

9. The tarsus is not specifically exposed

10. The retractors are then carefully dissected from the underlying conjunctiva 1 to 2 mm below the tarsus with Westcott scissors, avoiding the inferior tarsal vascular arcade (Fig. 3.9C).

11. The retractors are then held and the patient instructed to look down (Fig. 3.10). An inferior pull on the capsulopalpebral fascia should be felt.

12. A 1 mm strip of fascia is removed with Westcott scissors, shortening the retractors vertically.

13. Next, two to three interrupted 5/0 Vicryl sutures are used to reattach the lower lid retractors to the inferior border of the tarsus, avoiding the medial

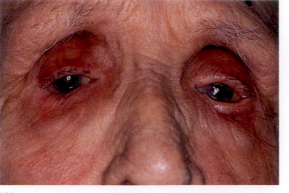
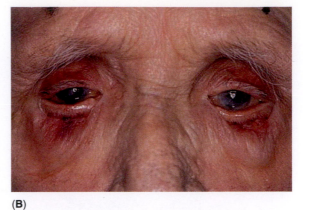

(A)   (B)

Figure 3.8 (**A**) An elderly patient with a right lower eyelid involutional entropion. Everting sutures have been placed in the left lower eyelid. (**B**) The sutures have been placed in both lower eyelids and tied tightly enough to produce a minimal degree of ectropion.

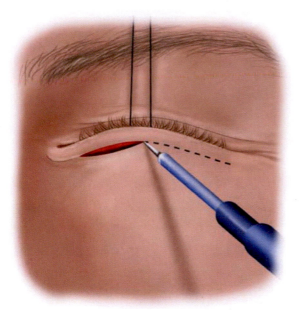
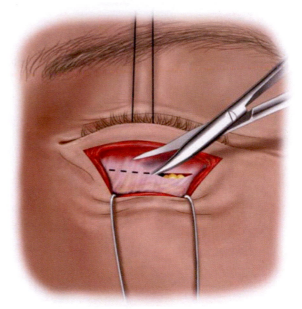

(A)   (B)

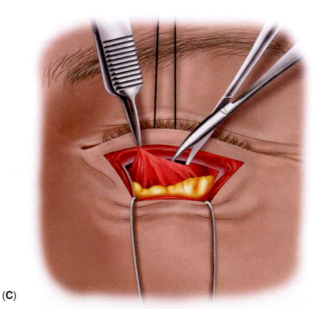

(C)

Figure 3.9 (**A**) A skin incision is made at the lower border of the tarsus. (**B**) The orbital septum is opened exposing the preaponeurotic fat. (**C**) The lower eyelid retractors are dissected from the underlying conjunctiva.

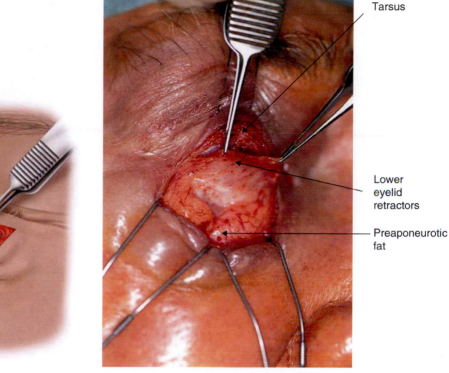

Tarsus

Lower
eyelid
retractors

Preaponeurotic
fat

(A)   (B)

Figure 3.10 (**A**) The lower eyelid retractors are held, and the patient is asked to look down. (**B**) The appearance of the lower eyelid retractors dissected from the underlying conjunctiva.

aspect of the eyelid to avoid creating a medial punctal ectropion (Fig. 3.11). When these are tied, the lower eyelid should now have a minimal degree of central and lateral ectropion. If a tarsal strip procedure is not going to be used it is important to avoid creating more than a minimal degree of overcorrection. The traction suture is removed.

14. Next a lateral tarsal strip procedure is performed (see below). The eyelid should be tightened sufficiently to bring the eyelid in apposition with the globe.

Lateral tarsal strip procedure

1. A lateral canthotomy is performed using straight blunt-tipped scissors (Fig. 3.12A). The canthotomy is extended to the lateral orbital rim. (A Colorado needle can be used instead if available.)
2. The lower eyelid is then lifted in a superotemporal direction and the inferior crus of the lateral canthal tendon is cut using blunt-tipped Westcott scissors (Fig. 3.12B and C).
3. The septum is also freed with the Westcott scissors until the eyelid becomes loose. Care is taken to avoid excessive bleeding using bipolar cautery. It is easier to perform the initial steps of this procedure sitting at the head of the patient. It is then preferable to move to the side of the patient to complete the remainder of the procedure.

4. Once the lower eyelid has been freed of its canthal attachments, the anterior and posterior lamellae are split along the gray line using Westcott scissors (Fig. 3.12D). This is aided by holding the skin and orbicularis muscle taut at the lateral end of the eyelid with Paufique forceps.
5. The lateral tarsal strip is then formed by cutting along the inferior border of the tarsus (Fig. 3.13A). Next, the eyelid margin is excised (Fig. 3.13B).
6. The tarsal strip is then drawn to the lateral orbital margin to determine the extent of any redundant tarsal strip. This is then excised.
7. The tarsal strip is then positioned over the handle of a Paufique forceps with the conjunctival side exposed and the conjunctiva scraped from the tarsal strip using a no. 15 blade (Fig. 3.13C and D). Alternatively this can be achieved by the gentle application of bipolar cautery using a sweeping motion.
8. The redundant anterior lamella is excised with the Westcott scissors (Fig. 3.14A and B).
9. Next, a double-armed 5/0 Vicryl suture on a 1/2-circle needle is passed through the periosteum of the lateral orbital wall, the needles each being passed from inside the orbital rim exiting at the rim, leaving a loop (Fig. 3.14C).
10. The end of the tarsal strip is passed through the loop. The needle is then reverse mounted and passed from the under surface of the tarsal strip exiting on the anterior surface lateral to the loop.

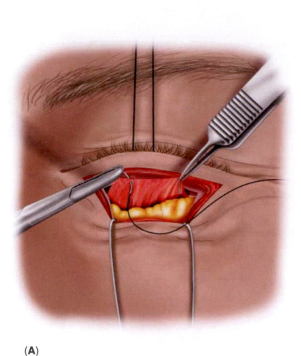

(A)

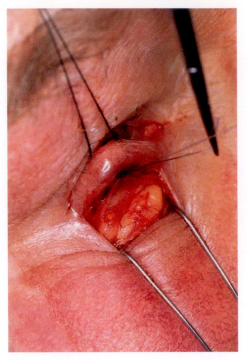

(B)

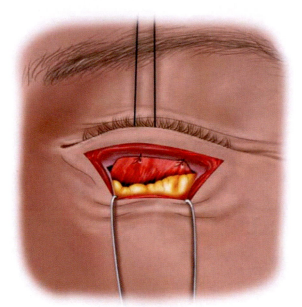

(C)

Figure 3.11 (**A**) The lower eyelid retractors are sutured to the inferior border of the tarsus. (**B**) The lower eyelid retractors have been sutured to the central area of the tarsus. (**C**) Two 5/0 Vicryl sutures have been placed: one centrally and one laterally.

This is repeated with the second needle. As the suture is pulled, the loop is then tightened, drawing the tarsal strip in a posterior direction against the globe (Fig. 3.14D and E).

11. The suture is then tied avoiding excessive tension.

12. A single 7/0 Vicryl suture is passed through the gray line at the edges of the lateral aspects of the upper and lower eyelids reforming the angle of the lateral commissure.

13. The subciliary wound is closed with interrupted 7/0 Vicryl sutures. The lateral canthal wound is then closed using 1 or 2 7/0 Vicryl sutures subcutaneously ensuring that the 5/0 Vicryl suture is

buried followed by interrupted 7/0 Vicryl sutures to the skin wound.

14. Antibiotic ointment is instilled into the eye, and if there has been much oozing, a compressive dressing can be applied.

Postoperative care. The patient is discharged with instructions to place topical antibiotic ointment along the lower eyelid and lateral canthal wound three times a day for 2 weeks. If a dressing was applied, this is removed the following day. The patient should be instructed to sleep with the head elevated for 2 weeks. Cool packs can be applied intermittently for 24 to 48 hours to reduce swelling. Any residual sutures can be

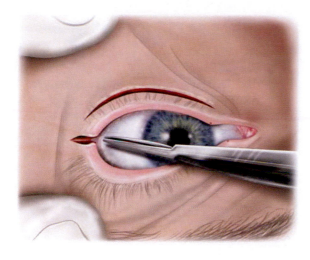

(A)

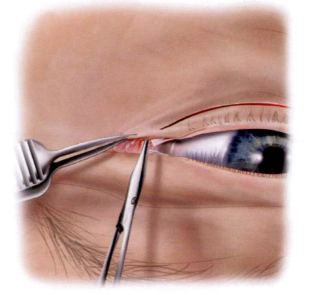

(B)

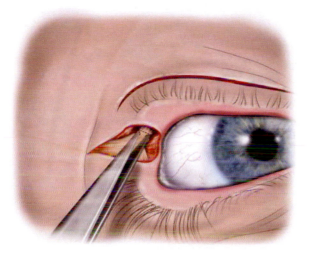

(C)

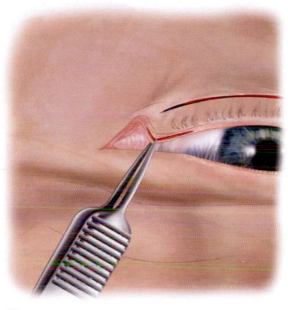

(D)

Figure 3.12 (**A**) A lateral canthotomy is performed (Surgeon's view). (**B**) The eyelid is drawn superolaterally and the attachments of the eyelid to the lateral orbital margin are cut (Surgeon's view). (**C**) This drawing shows that the inferior crus of the lateral canthal tendon is severed (Surgeon's view) (**D**) The gray line has been split (Surgeon's view).

removed in clinic 2 to 3 weeks postoperatively if still present. The patient can, however, be discharged following the surgery as the sutures will eventually dissolve over the course of 3 to 4 weeks.

Lower Lid Retractor Advancement with Lower Lid Wedge Resection
Surgical procedure

1. Proxymethacaine drops are instilled into the inferior conjunctival fornix.
2. Two to three milliliters of 0.5% Bupivacaine with 1:200,000 units of adrenaline mixed 50:50 with 2% lidocaine with 1:80,000 units of adrenaline are injected immediately under the skin in the lower eyelid avoiding bleeding from the orbicularis muscle and a hematoma.
3. The retractor dissection proceeds in the same manner as described above to the point at which the lower lid retractors have been dissected from the underlying conjunctiva.
4. Next the lower lid margin is incised vertically for 2 mm at the junction of the lateral third with the medial two-thirds of the eyelid using a no. 15 Bard Parker blade (Fig. 3.15A and B).
5. Straight iris scissors are then used to complete a vertical cut through the tarsus.
6. The edges of the eyelid wounds are then grasped with Paufique forceps and overlapped without undue tension.

7. The redundant eyelid to be removed is marked with gentian violet.
8. The eyelid margin is again incised with a no. 15 Bard Parker blade and straight iris scissors are then used to complete a vertical cut through the tarsus.
9. The scissors are then angulated at 45° to complete the wedge resection.

10. Hemostasis is obtained with bipolar cautery.
11. The tarsus is repaired using interrupted 5/0 Vicryl sutures ensuring that the sutures do not pass through the tarsal conjunctiva.
12. The first Vicryl suture is passed just below the lid margin and is tied with a single throw to ensure that the eyelid margin is correctly aligned. If this is not the case the suture is removed and replaced.

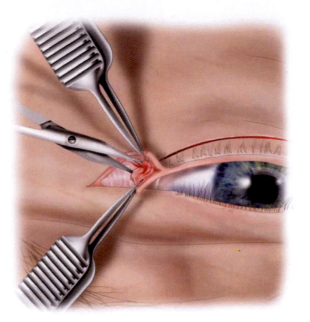

(A)

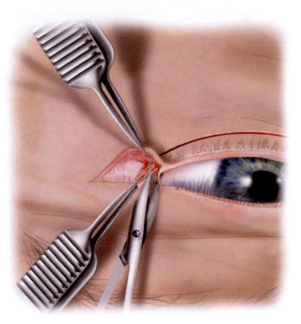

(B)

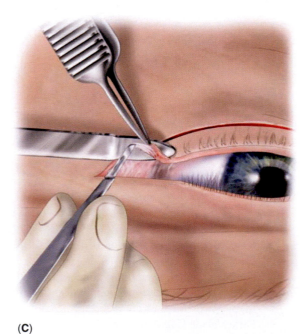

(C)

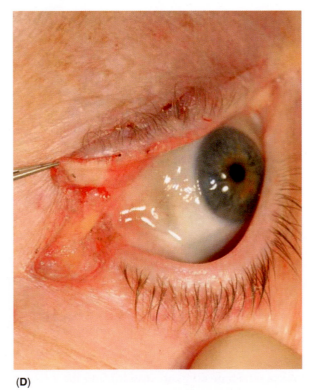

(D)

Figure 3.13 (**A**) The lateral tarsal strip is then formed by cutting along the inferior border of the tarsus (Surgeon's view). (**B**) Next, the superficial border of the tarsus is excised (Surgeon's view). (**C**) The tarsal strip is then positioned over the handle of a Paufique forceps with the conjunctival side exposed and the conjunctiva scraped from the tarsal strip using a no. 15 blade (Surgeon's view). (**D**) The appearance of the tarsal strip after the conjunctiva has been removed (Surgeon's view).

13. The Vicryl suture is then pulled up and fixated to the head drapes with a curved artery clip. This makes it easier to place the remaining tarsal sutures.

14. The rest of the tarsus is reapproximated using interrupted 5/0 Vicryl sutures.

15. The orbicularis muscle below the tarsus is also reapproximated using interrupted 5/0 Vicryl sutures.

16. Next the superior Vicryl suture is tied.

17. The eyelid margin is repaired with 2 6/0 Silk sutures passed along the lash line and along the line of the meibomian gland orifices (see also Fig. 10.10C and D) in a vertical mattress fashion.

18. The silk sutures are tied creating a slight eversion of the eyelid margin wound edges. The ends are left long.

19. Next a 1 mm strip of eyelid retractor fascia is removed with Westcott scissors, shortening the retractors vertically.

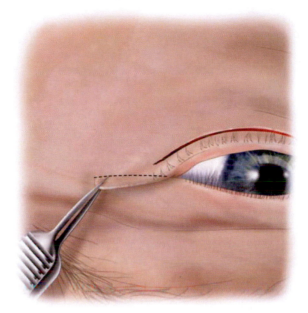

(A)

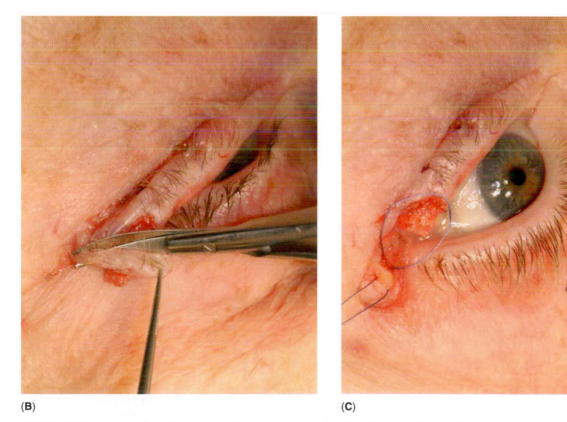

(B)   (C)

Figure 3.14 (**A**) The lid is drawn laterally and the amount of redundant anterior lamella is determined (Surgeon's view). (**B**) The redundant anterior lamella is removed (Surgeon's view). (**C**) A double-armed 5/0 Vicryl suture on a half-circle needle has been passed through the periorbita on the internal aspect of the lateral orbital margin at the lateral orbital tubercle A loop of suture has been left (Surgeon's view). (*Continued*)

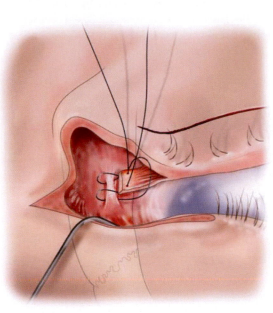

(D)

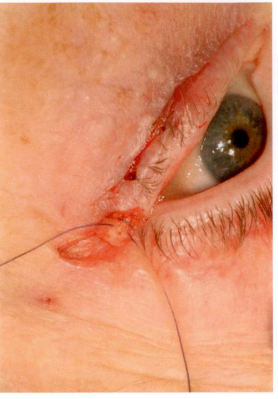

(E)

Figure 3.14 (*Continued*) (**D**) The lateral tarsal strip has been passed through the loop of suture. The suture needles have then been passed through the strip from below (Surgeon's view). (**E**) As the suture is pulled taut, the eyelid is drawn laterally and posteriorly into contact with the globe. If the eyelid is pulled anteriorly, the suture has not been positioned correctly and should be replaced (Surgeon's view).

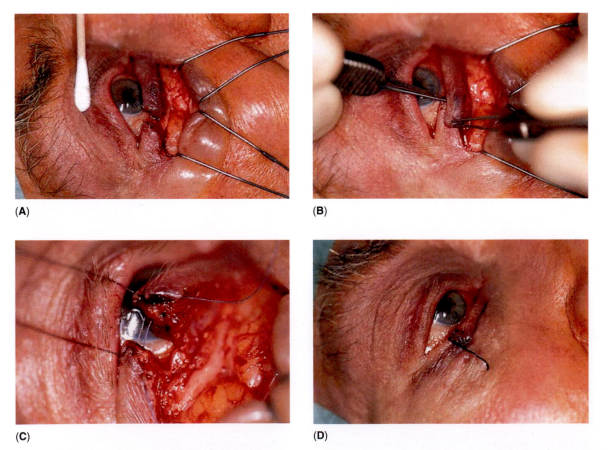

(A)

(B)

(C)

(D)

Figure 3.15 (**A**) The lower eyelid has been incised at the junction of the medial two-thirds with the lateral third. (**B**) The eyelid is overlapped to determine the amount of eyelid which can be safely removed without leaving the wound under undue tension and without causing lower eyelid retraction. (**C**) The uppermost Vicryl suture is used for traction, while the remaining Vicryl sutures are placed in the tarsus. (**D**) The appearance of the eyelid at the completion of surgery.

20. Next two to three interrupted 5/0 Vicryl sutures are used to reattach the lower lid retractors to the inferior border of the tarsus, avoiding the medial aspect of the eyelid to avoid creating a medial punctal ectropion. When these sutures are tied, the lower eyelid should be in apposition to the globe without any ectropion.
21. The subciliary skin wound is then closed using interrupted 7/0 Vicryl sutures although the remaining 6/0 Silk suture can also be used.
22. The vertical skin incision is closed with the same sutures.
23. The eyelid margin silk sutures are moistened with saline and laid over the lower lid skin. These are then incorporated into the vertical skin closure sutures to ensure that the silk suture is kept away from the cornea postoperatively.
24. A compressive dressing is applied.

Postoperative care. The patient is discharged with instructions to place topical antibiotic ointment along the lower eyelid wound three times a day for 2 weeks. The compressive dressing is removed after 24 to 48 hours. The patient should be instructed to sleep with the head elevated for 2 weeks. Cool packs can be applied intermittently for 24 to 48 hours to reduce swelling. The sutures are removed in clinic 2 weeks postoperatively.

Complications

These procedures have an extremely low recurrence rate and minimal morbidity in the hands of an experienced oculoplastic surgeon. The many potential complications of these procedures can be avoided by careful patient selection, by a good knowledge of surgical anatomy, and by attention to appropriate hemostasis and meticulous surgical technique:

1. Granuloma
2. Wound dehiscence
3. Hematoma
4. Infection
5. Ectropion
6. Lateral canthal discomfort
7. Overlapping of the upper eyelid
8. Eyelid notch
9. Trichiasis
10. Corneal ulcer
11. Recurrence of entropion
12. Lateral canthal angle deformity

A lateral canthal granuloma following a lateral tarsal strip procedure is seen when a permanent suture has been used to fixate the tarsal strip e.g., an Ethibond suture, and this has not been completely buried. This problem is very rarely seen when a dissolvable suture, e.g., a Vicryl suture, is used instead.

Before performing a wedge resection the surgeon should determine the precise amount of eyelid, which can be safely sacrificed without leaving the wound under tension. If the eyelid wound is under too much tension or if the sutures are tied too tightly causing strangulation of the wound edges, the wound is more likely to dehisce.

A hematoma or excessive postoperative edema places the wound at risk of breakdown. These are avoided by the preoperative management of hypertension, the avoidance of antiplatelet agents, meticulous dissection, and careful use of bipolar cautery, and by the postoperative use of a compressive dressing.

A notch and trichiasis are avoided by meticulous attention to the apposition of the wound edges and the use of vertical mattress sutures through the eyelid margin. A corneal ulcer is avoided by careful placement of the eyelid margin sutures.

Great care needs to be taken over the placement of the periorbital fixation suture in the lateral tarsal strip procedure. This should engage the periorbita just inside the lateral orbital wall at the junction with the upper eyelid to avoid anterior displacement of the eyelid from the globe and lateral canthal dystopia. If the upper eyelid is very lax, there may be an unsightly overlap of the upper eyelid over the lower eyelid if the lateral tarsal strip is over tightened. The patient should be warned preoperatively that the lateral canthal area will be sore and lumpy to touch for the first few weeks following surgery until the suture dissolves. The suture causes a local periostitis and a sensitive wound.

Cicatricial Entropion

The choice of surgical procedure for the management of a lower lid cicatricial ectropion is dictated by the severity of the entropion and eyelid retraction and by the underlying cause. In the case of a cicatricial entropion caused by ocular cicatricial pemphigoid, surgery should be confined to the anterior lamella wherever possible to avoid exacerbating the conjunctival disease.

The surgical procedures that may be used are:

1. Retractor advancement
2. Tarsal fracture
3. Posterior lamellar graft

Retractor Advancement

This procedure is particularly useful for patients with active conjunctival disease or ocular cicatricial pemphigoid. A retractor advancement is used alone without any horizontal eyelid shortening. The retractor advancement can be repeated if the entropion recurs.

Surgical procedure. This is as described above.

Postoperative management. This is as described above.

Tarsal Fracture

This procedure is indicated for patients with a mild cicatricial entropion with a minor degree of lower lid retraction.

Surgical procedure

1. Proxymethacaine drops are instilled into the inferior conjunctival fornix.
2. Two to three milliliters of 0.5% Bupivacaine with 1:200,000 units of adrenaline mixed 50:50 with 2% lidocaine with 1:80,000 units of adrenaline are injected immediately under the skin in the lower eyelid avoiding bleeding from the orbicularis muscle and a hematoma. A small quantity of the local anesthetic solution is also injected subconjunctivally just below the tarsus.
3. A 4/0 Silk traction suture is placed horizontally through the gray line of the lower eyelid centrally and the eyelid is everted over a Desmarres retractor.

4. A horizontal incision is made through the whole length of the tarsus on the posterior surface of the eyelid just below its center down to the deep surface of the orbicularis muscle (Fig. 3.16A).

5. Three or four double-armed 5/0 Vicryl sutures are passed through the tarsus just below the incision and through the eyelid to emerge through the skin just below the lash line (Fig. 3.16B). These sutures are tied to produce a moderate ectropion (Fig. 3.16C and D).

Postoperative care. The patient is discharged with instructions to instill topical antibiotic ointment into the eye three times a day for 2 weeks. The patient should be instructed to sleep with the head elevated for 2 weeks. Cool packs can be applied intermittently for 24 to 48 hours to reduce swelling. The sutures are removed in clinic 3 weeks postoperatively.

Posterior Lamellar Graft

A posterior lamellar graft is indicated for the patient with a more severe degree of cicatricial entropion with more marked eyelid retraction. A hard palate graft is preferred. The procedure is usually performed under general anesthesia although in carefully selected patients it can be performed under local anesthesia with sedation.

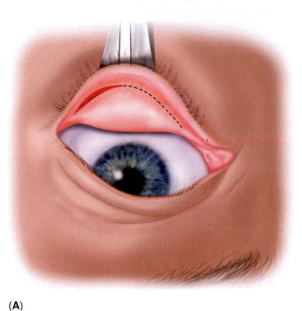

(A)

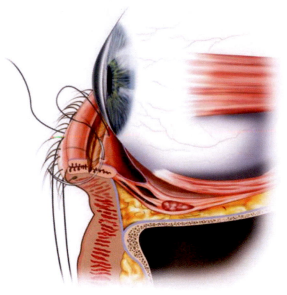

(B)

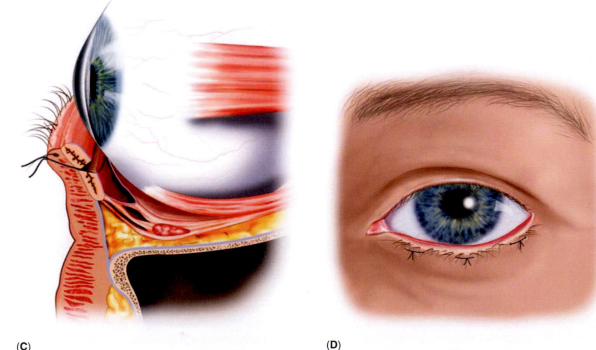

(C)   **(D)**

Figure 3.16 (A) An incision is made through the tarsal conjunctiva and tarsus down to the orbicularis muscle. (B) Double-armed 5/0 Vicryl sutures are passed through the tarsus just below the incision and through the eyelid to emerge through the skin just below the lash line. (C and D) The sutures are tied to produce a moderate ectropion.

Surgical procedure

1. Two to three milliliters of 0.5% Bupivacaine with 1:200,000 units of adrenaline mixed 50:50 with 2% lidocaine with 1:80,000 units of adrenaline are injected immediately under the skin in the lower eyelid avoiding bleeding from the orbicularis muscle and a hematoma. A small quantity of the local anesthetic solution is also injected subconjunctivally just below the tarsus.

2. A 4/0 Black silk traction suture is placed horizontally through the gray line of the lower eyelid centrally and the eyelid is everted over a Desmarres retractor.

3. A horizontal incision is made through the whole length of the tarsus on the posterior surface just below its center down to the deep surface of the orbicularis with a no. 15 blade.

4. The inferior margin of the tarsus is freed from the eyelid retractors and the orbital septum using blunt-tipped Westcott scissors.

5. The ensuing defect is measured and a slightly oversized hard palate graft is harvested.

6. The hard palate graft is carefully prepared by removing any uneven or excessive submucosal tissue with Westcott scissors.

7. Three or four double-armed 5/0 Vicryl sutures are passed in a partial thickness fashion through the hard palate graft and passed through the full thickness of the eyelid. These are tied just below the lash line to evert the eyelid margin and to maintain the graft in apposition to its bed.

8. The edges of the graft are sutured to the cut edge of the tarsus superiorly and the recessed edges of the conjunctiva inferiorly with interrupted 8/0 Vicryl sutures ensuring that the sutures are buried to avoid corneal irritation or a corneal abrasion.

9. Topical antibiotic ointment is applied to the eye and eyelids and a compressive dressing applied.

Postoperative management. The patient is discharged on an oral broad-spectrum antibiotic for 1 week. The patient should be reviewed 5 days postoperatively when the dressing is removed and the eyelids meticulously cleaned. Topical antibiotic ointment should be instilled in the eye three times a day for 2 weeks. Cool packs can be applied intermittently for 24 to 48 hours to reduce swelling. The patient should be instructed to sleep with the head elevated for 2 weeks. The 5/0 Vicryl sutures are removed 2 weeks postoperatively.

Complications

1. Corneal abrasion
2. Corneal ulcer
3. Hematoma
4. Necrosis of the hard palate graft
5. Infection
6. Recurrence of the entropion

These potential complications can be largely avoided. The cornea should be protected intraoperatively, and adequate and frequent lubrication should be applied. If the potential development of a suture abrasion is a concern, a bandage contact lens can be used. The graft should be firmly attached to its bed to prevent a hematoma from collecting beneath it. A hematoma or movement of the graft can lead to graft failure.

Congenital Entropion

A congenital entropion is managed under general anesthesia (Fig. 3.17).

Retractor Advancement

Surgical procedure

1. Two to three milliliters of 0.25% Bupivacaine are injected immediately under the skin in the lower eyelid avoiding bleeding from the orbicularis muscle and a hematoma.

2. A 4/0 Silk traction suture is placed horizontally through the gray line of the lower eyelid centrally and fixated to the head drapes using a small artery clip.

3. A skin incision is then made immediately below the lashes, as in a cosmetic lower lid blepharoplasty, extending from just below the inferior punctum to the lateral aspect of the lower eyelid using a Colorado needle.

4. Hemostasis is obtained using bipolar cautery.

5. The Colorado needle is then used to dissect through the orbicularis oculi muscle exposing

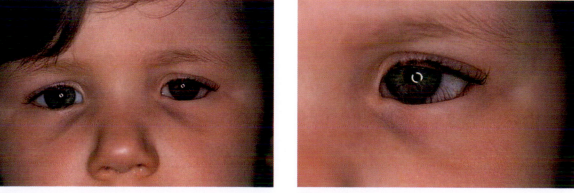

(A)   **(B)**

Figure 3.17 (**A**) A left lower eyelid congenital entropion. (**B**) A close-up photograph of the lower eyelid entropion. This should be differentiated from a lower eyelid congenital epiblepharon.

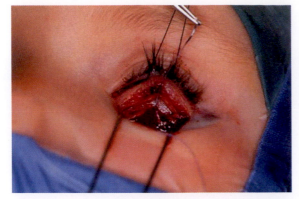

(A)

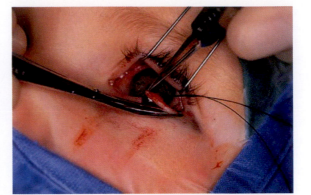

(B)

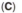

(C)

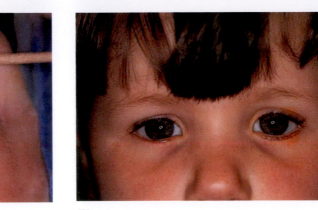

(D)

Figure 3.18 (**A**) The lower eyelid retractors are advanced and attached to the lower border of the tarsus. (**B**) A conservative skin–muscle blepharoplasty is performed. (**C**) The appearance of the eyelid at the completion of surgery. (**D**) The postoperative appearance of the eyelid 2 weeks after surgery.

the orbital septum. The orbicularis muscle is then dissected away from the underlying orbital septum for 4 to 5 mm.

6. The septum is then opened inferiorly with the Colorado needle or Westcott scissors 5 to 6 mm below the eyelid margin, exposing the preaponeurotic fat.
7. The lower eyelid retractors are identified beneath the fat. The retractors may be found to be disinserted from their attachment to the tarsus.
8. The tarsus is not specifically exposed
9. The retractors are then carefully dissected from the underlying conjunctiva 2 to3 mm below the tarsus with Westcott scissors, avoiding the inferior tarsal vascular arcade.
10. No shortening of the retractors is required.
11. Next, two to three interrupted 5/0 Vicryl sutures are used to reattach the lower lid retractors to the inferior border of the tarsus, avoiding the medial aspect of the eyelid to avoid creating a medial punctal ectropion (Fig. 3.18A). When these are tied, the lower eyelid should not have any degree of ectropion.
12. A very conservative resection of a strip of skin and orbicularis muscle may be required (Fig. 3.18B). No eyelid shortening is normally required.
13. The skin is closed with interrupted 7/0 Vicryl Rapide sutures.

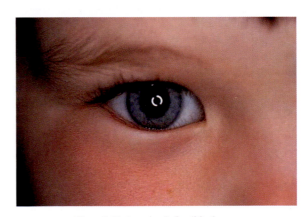

Figure 3.19 A congenital epiblepharon.

Postoperative care. No dressings are required. The parent is advised to clean the wound three times a day with cotton wool moistened with sterile saline or cooled boiled water and to apply topical antibiotic ointment three times a day until all the sutures have dropped out spontaneously. This usually takes 2 to 3 weeks.

Congenital Epiblepharon

A congenital epiblepharon is an excess fold of skin and orbicularis muscle in the medial aspect of the lower eyelid (Fig. 3.19). Epiblepharon can cause the eyelashes to invert against the globe, and can be unilateral or bilateral. The management of this condition should be conservative, as spontaneous improvement typically occurs with age, and eyelashes in an infant tend to be very soft. If, however, the child suffers from tearing, photophobia, and discomfort with corneal abrasions caused by the lashes, surgical intervention is warranted. The procedure is performed under general anesthesia.

Surgical procedure

1. One to two milliliters of 0.25% Bupivacaine are injected immediately under the skin in the lower eyelid avoiding bleeding from the orbicularis muscle and a hematoma.
2. A 4/0 Silk traction suture is placed horizontally through the gray line of the lower eyelid centrally and fixated to the head drapes using a small curved artery clip.
3. A skin incision is then made immediately below the lashes, extending from just below the inferior punctum to the junction of the lateral third with the medial two-thirds of the eyelid using a Colorado needle.
4. Hemostasis is obtained using bipolar cautery.
5. The Colorado needle is then used to dissect a 4 to 5 mm skin-muscle flap from the orbital septum.
6. The traction suture is released and reapplied with very gentle tension.
7. The skin–muscle flap is draped over the eyelid margin and the excess skin and muscle is very carefully excised with Westcott scissors, taking great care not to excise too much tissue.
8. If the eyelid margin is still inverted the eyelid retractors can be dissected free, advanced, and sutured to the lower border of the tarsal plate with a single 6/0 Vicryl suture until the eyelid margin is normally positioned.
9. The skin edges are then reapproximated with interrupted 7/0 Vicryl Rapide.

Postoperative management. This is as described above for congenital entropion.

FURTHER READING

1. Albert DM, Lucarelli MJ: Entropion. In: Clinical Atlas of Procedures in Ophthalmic Surgery, Chicago, MI: AMA Press, 2004: 257–60.
2. American Academy of Ophthalmology. Basic and Clinical Science Course: Orbit, Eyelids, and Lacrimal System, section 7.. San Francisco, CA: The American Academy of Ophthalmology, 2006/7: 201–5.
3. Anderson RL, Gordy DD. The tarsal strip procedure. Arch Ophthalmol 1979; 97: 2192–6.
4. Dutton JJ. Atlas of clinical and surgical orbital anatomy. Philadelphia, PA: WB Saunders, 1994.
5. Goldberg, et al. Entropion Repair. In: Wobig JL, Dailey RA, eds. Oculoplastic Facial Plastic Surgery: Face, Lacrimal System, and Orbit. New York, NY: Thieme, 2004: 91–7.
6. Hawes MJ, Dortzbach RK. The microscopic anatomy of the lower eyelid retractors. Arch Ophthalmol 1982; 100: 1313–18.
7. Jones LT, Rech MJ, Wobig JL. Senile entropion: a new concept for correction. Am J Ophthalmol 1972; 74: 327–9.
8. Katowitz JA, Heher KL, Hollsten DA: Involutional entropion. In: Levine MR, ed. Manual of Oculoplastic Surgery, 3rd edn. Boston, MA: Butterworth-Heinemann, 2003: 137–44.
9. Kersten RC, Kleiner FP, Kulwin DR. Tarsotomy for the treatment of cicatricial entropion with trichiasis. Arch Ophthalmol 1992; 110: 714.
10. Martin RT, Nunery WR, Tanenbaum M. Entropion, trichiasis, and distichiasis. In: McCord CD, Tanenbaum M, Nunery WR, eds. Oculoplastic Surgery, 3rd edn. New York, NY: Raven Press, 1995: 221–48.
11. Nerad JA, Carter KD, Alford MA. Entropion. In: Rapid Diagnosis in Ophthalmology—Oculoplastic and Reconstructive Surgery Philadelphia, PA: Mosby Elsevier, 2008: 92–5.
12. Penne RB. Entropion. In: Color Atlas & Synopsis of Clinical Ophthalmology: Oculoplastics. New York, NY: McGraw-Hill, 2003: 56–61.
13. Wesley RE. Cicatricial entropion. In: Levine MR, ed. Manual of Oculoplastic Surgery, 2nd edn. Boston, MA: Butterworth-Heinemann, 1996: 129–34.
14. Wesley RE. Cicatricial entropion. In: Levine MR, ed. Manual of Oculoplastic Surgery, 3rd edn. Boston, MA: Butterworth-Heinemann, 2003: 145–50.
15. Wright M, Bell D, Scott C, Leatherbarrow B. Everting suture correction of lower lid involutional entropion. Br J Ophthalmol 1999; 83: 1060–3.

4 Upper eyelid entropion

INTRODUCTION

Upper eyelid entropion is an eyelid malposition in which the upper eyelid margin is turned inward against the globe. It can be responsible for severe ocular morbidity. It is an uncommon condition in the Western World, in contrast to a number of countries in the Third World, where trachoma is endemic. It has tended to receive very little attention in standard oculoplastic texts in spite of the fact that its management can be difficult and challenging. Upper eyelid entropion may be broadly classified as congenital or acquired.

CLASSIFICATION

1. Congenital
2. Acquired

A true congenital upper lid entropion is very rare. A horizontal tarsal kink is a similar but separate entity. The upper lid tarsus in affected patients is frequently found to be abnormal and foreshortened (Fig. 4.1).

Acquired upper lid entropion can be further classified according to the underlying etiology (Table 4.1). Any cause of conjunctival scarring can lead to an acquired upper lid entropion. The entropion may be further sub-classified according to its severity as mild, moderate, or severe.

PATIENT ASSESSMENT

A careful history and meticulous clinical examination are essential to determine the etiology of the entropion. In addition to a complete ocular examination, the eyelid should be everted and the posterior lamella and the superior fornix examined. It is important to establish the presence of an upper eyelid entropion and differentiate this from simple trichiasis. The presence of an early entropion is indicated by an apparent posterior migration of the meibomian gland orifices. It is important to determine whether or not there is any keratin present on the posterior lamella. The presence and degree of eyelid retraction and lagophthalmos should be determined. If an artificial eye is present, this should be removed, and the superior fornix examined.

SURGICAL MANAGEMENT

A number of factors influence the operative management of this eyelid malposition (Table 4.2).

Congenital Upper Eyelid Entropion

In some cases the upper lid entropion resolves spontaneously but where this is causing distress or ocular complications the eyelid malposition should be corrected surgically. This is performed under general anesthesia.

Upper Lid Auricular Cartilage Graft

Surgical Procedure

1. The upper eyelid skin crease is marked with gentian violet after degreasing the skin with an alcohol wipe.

2. Two to three milliliters of 0.25% Bupivacaine with 1:200000 units of adrenaline are injected along the upper lid skin crease immediately under the skin in order to avoid bleeding from the orbicularis muscle and the development of a hematoma.
3. A 4/0 Silk traction suture is placed through the gray line of the upper eyelid centrally and the eyelid is everted over a Desmarres retractor.
4. A small quantity of the local anesthetic solution is also injected subconjunctivally just above the tarsus. The Desmarres retractor is removed.
5. A skin crease incision is made with a no. 15 Bard Parker blade.
6. The incision is carried down to the tarsus centrally using blunt-tipped Westcott scissors.
7. The whole of the anterior surface of the tarsus is exposed using the Westcott scissors down to the eyelash follicles, taking care not to damage these.
8. The eyelid retractors (the levator aponeurosis and Müller's muscle) are freed from the surface and superior margin of the tarsus with the Westcott scissors.
9. An auricular cartilage graft is harvested from the patient's ear (see chap. 13).
10. The auricular cartilage graft is shaped to mimic the size and shape of a normal tarsus.
11. This is then placed over the patient's tarsus, extending above its superior border onto the conjunctiva (Fig. 4.9). Interrupted 7/0 Vicryl sutures may be used to fixate the graft to the patient's tarsus.
12. The levator aponeurosis is then attached to the superior third of the cartilage graft with interrupted 5/0 Vicryl sutures.
13. The skin crease is reformed using interrupted 7/0 Vicryl Rapide sutures, taking a bite of the lower skin edge, then a bite of the eyelid levator aponeurosis, and finally a bite of the upper lid skin edge. This is tied tightly, creating a well-defined eyelid crease.
14. Antibiotic ointment is instilled into the eye.

Postoperative Care

The patient is discharged on topical antibiotic ointment three times per day to the eyelid wound until the sutures have dissolved, and topical lubricants for 3 to 4 weeks.

The patient seen in Figures 4.1 and 4.9 is shown before and after this surgical procedure (Fig. 4.10A,B).

Acquired Upper Eyelid Entropion

In contrast to the management of lower eyelid entropion, one of a number of different surgical procedures is selected for the individual patient based on the factors listed in Table 4.2 (see Table 4.3).

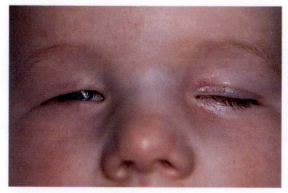
(A)

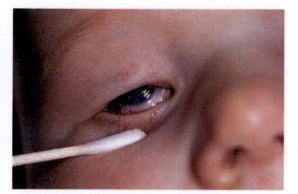
(B)

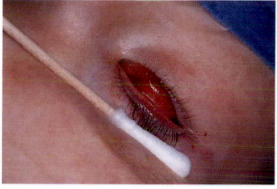
(C)

(D)

Figure 4.1 (**A**) A congenital right upper eyelid entropion. (**B**) A close-up of the right upper eyelid entropion. (**C**) The right upper eyelid everted demonstrating a small tarsus. (**D**) The left upper eyelid everted demonstrating a normal tarsus.

Table 4.1 Classification of Upper Eyelid Entropion

Congenital
Acquired
- Trachoma (Fig. 4.2)
- Chronic blepharoconjunctivitis
- Chemical burns
- Cicatrizing conjunctivitis
  - Topical glaucoma medications
  - Stevens–Johnson syndrome (Fig. 4.3)
  - Herpes zoster ophthalmicus (Fig. 4.4)
  - Ocular cicatricial pemphigoid (Fig. 4.5)
- Iatrogenic—e.g., a complication of the Fasanella–Servat procedure (Fig. 4.6A)
- Chronic anophthalmic socket inflammation (Fig. 4.6B)
- Severe eyebrow ptosis (Fig. 4.7)
- Thyroid eye disease (Fig. 4.8)

Table 4.2 Factors Influencing the Surgical Management of Upper Eyelid Entropion

- The severity of the entropion
- The thickness of the tarsal plate
- The presence or absence of keratin on the posterior lamella
- The degree of eyelid retraction
- The degree of any lagophthalmos
- The underlying etiology
- The presence of a corneal graft
- The planning of a future corneal graft
- The presence of an artificial eye

Table 4.3 The Choice of Operative Procedures in the Management of Acquired Upper Eyelid Entropion

- Anterior lamellar reposition with gray line split
- Tarsal wedge excision
- Lamellar split and posterior lamellar advancement
- Terminal tarsal rotation
- Posterior lamellar graft
- Auricular cartilage graft

Anterior Lamellar Reposition with Gray Line Split

This procedure is relatively simple to perform under local anesthesia, with or without sedation. It is used for patients with a mild upper lid entropion that is typically the result of chronic blepharoconjunctivitis (Fig. 4.11).

Surgical Procedure

1. Proxymethacaine drops are instilled into the inferior conjunctival fornix.
2. An upper lid skin crease incision is marked with gentian violet.
3. Two to three milliliters of 0.5% Bupivacaine with 1:200,000 units of adrenaline mixed 50:50 with 2% lidocaine with 1:80,000 units of adrenaline are injected along the upper lid skin crease.
4. The eyelid is held firmly and the lid margin everted slightly.

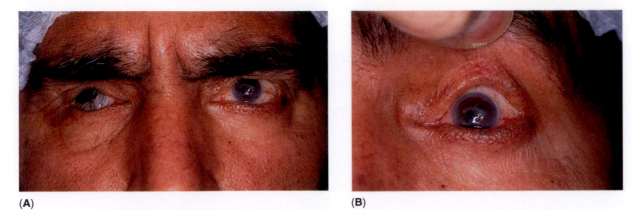

(A)   **(B)**

Figure 4.2 (**A**) A severe right upper eyelid entropion and a right lower lid cicatricial entropion and a left upper eyelid entropion as a consequence of trachoma in an Asian patient. The right cornea shows end stage scarring and the left cornea shows central scarring. The extent of the left upper lid entropion is masked by a brow ptosis. (**B**) A close up photograph of the left eyelids with the brow elevated demonstrating the extent of the upper eyelid entropion.

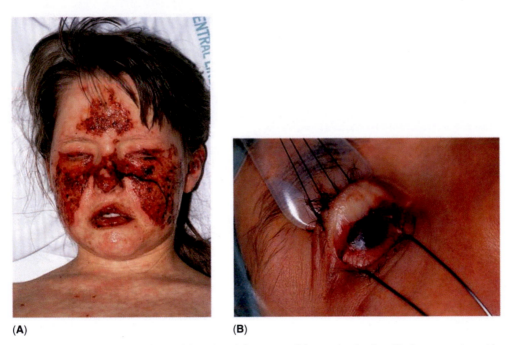

(A)   **(B)**

Figure 4.3 (**A**) A patient with acute Stevens–Johnson syndrome. (**B**) A severe right upper eyelid entropion developed in the same patient with extensive keratinisation of the posterior lamella.

5. A Beaver micro-sharp blade (7530) on a Beaver blade handle used to create a gray line split to a depth of 1 to 2 mm (Fig. 4.12). The incision should be made in a single sweep to avoid an irregular wound.

6. Next, an upper lid skin crease incision is made with a Colorado needle and the superior half of the tarsus is exposed (Fig. 4.13).

7. The upper lid retractors are dissected from the superior border of the anterior surface of the tarsus and recessed approximately 5 to 6 mm.

8. A 5/0 Vicryl suture on a 1/4 circle needle is passed through the skin and orbicularis muscle just anterior to the gray line split and then passed horizontally in a lamellar fashion through the tarsus (Fig. 4.14). The height of this suture placement determines the degree of eyelash eversion.

9. The suture is then passed anteriorly through the orbicularis muscle and skin 2 to 3 mm away from the initial suture pass and held with a bulldog clip (Fig. 4.15).

10. A series of additional sutures are placed along the length of the tarsus and then tied.

11. The skin crease is reformed with interrupted 7/0 Vicryl sutures, taking bites of the underlying levator aponeurosis (Fig. 4.16).

12. Antibiotic ointment is instilled into the eye.

Postoperative Care

Topical antibiotic ointment should be smeared along the wounds three times a day for 2 weeks. Cool packs can be applied intermittently for 24 to 48 hours to reduce swelling. The patient should be instructed to sleep with the head elevated for 2 weeks. The sutures are removed 3 to 4 weeks postoperatively, if still present.

Tarsal Wedge Excision

A tarsal wedge excision is typically used for patients with a greater degree of entropion with a thickened tarsus, an absence of posterior lamellar keratin and no lagophthalmos

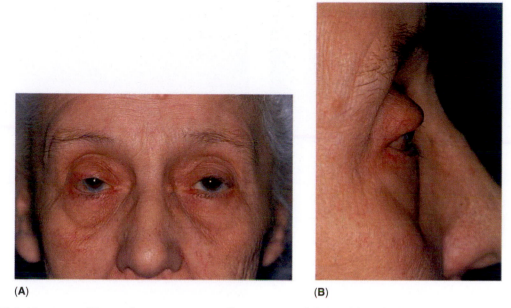

Figure 4.4 (A) A right upper eyelid entropion as a consequence of herpes zoster opthalmicus. (B) A side view of the right upper eyelid entropion.

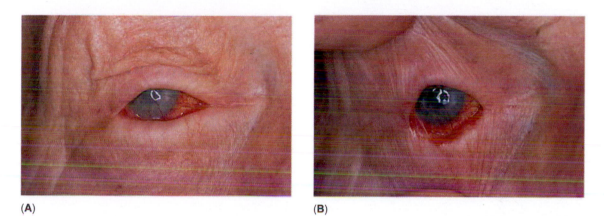

Figure 4.5 (A) A right upper and lower eyelid entropion caused by ocular cicatricial pemphigoid. Previous extensive cryotherapy has caused a loss of all lashes. (B) Extensive symblephara with obliteration of the fornices.

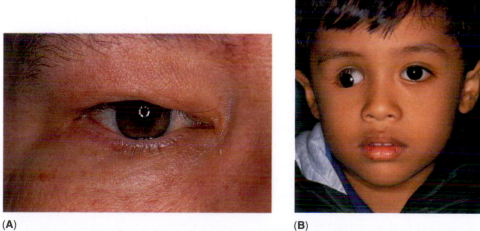

Figure 4.6 (A) A right upper eyelid entropion occurring as a complication of a Fasanella-Servat procedure. (B) A right upper eyelid entropion in a child with a contracted anophthalmic socket.

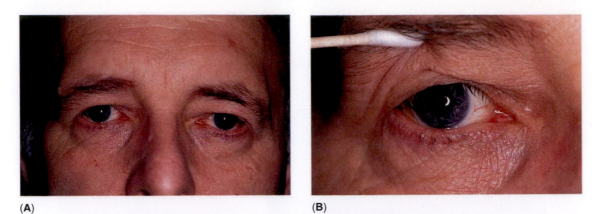

(A)   **(B)**

Figure 4.7 (**A**) A bilateral upper eyelid entropion as a consequence of a marked bilateral brow ptosis. (**B**) A close-up of the right side demonstrating the proximity of the brow to the eyelid margin.

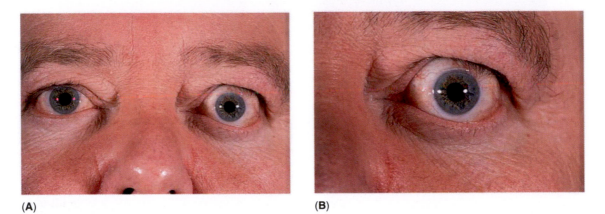

(A)   **(B)**

Figure 4.8 (**A**) A left upper eyelid entropion as a consequence of thyroid eye disease. (**B**) A close-up of the left side demonstrating the upper eyelid entropion with marked upper eyelid retraction, proptosis, and thickening of the sub-brow tissue.

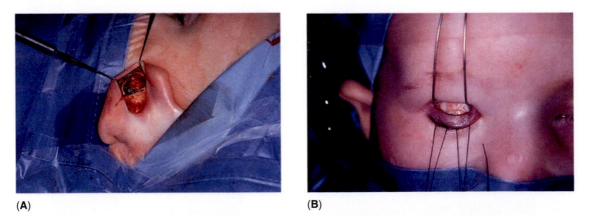

(A)   **(B)**

Figure 4.9 (**A**) An auricular cartilage graft has been harvested from the left ear. (**B**) The graft has been placed over the infant's tarsus, extending superiorly onto the conjunctiva.

on voluntary eyelid closure. This condition is typically seen in the patient who has an upper lid entropion from trachoma.

Surgical Procedure
The operation differs from the anterior lamellar reposition with gray line split only in that a horizontal wedge is removed with a blade from the anterior tarsal surface along the line of maximal thickening. The eyelid retractors are recessed to a greater degree to allow a posterior lamellar

advancement to compensate for any eyelid retraction. Failure to recess the retractors will result in worsening of eyelid retraction postoperatively. The wedge resection is closed with interrupted 5/0 Vicryl sutures before the everting sutures are placed as in the anterior lamellar reposition with gray line split (Fig. 4.17).

Postoperative Care
This is as described above.

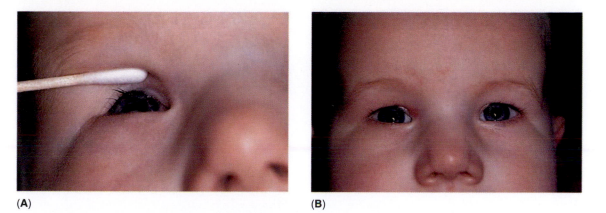

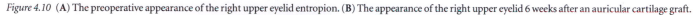

Figure 4.10 (**A**) The preoperative appearance of the right upper eyelid entropion. (**B**) The appearance of the right upper eyelid 6 weeks after an auricular cartilage graft.

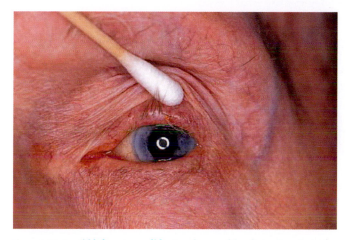

Figure 4.11 A mild left upper eyelid entropion resulting from chronic staphylococcal blepharitis.

Lamellar Split and Posterior Lamellar Advancement

This procedure is typically used for patients with a greater degree of entropion with a thin tarsus, an absence of posterior lamellar keratin and no lagophthalmos on voluntary eyelid closure. This is typically seen in the anophthalmic patient who has an upper lid entropion. This can be performed under either general anesthesia or under local anesthesia with sedation.

Surgical Procedure

Steps 1 to 5 are as described for an anterior lamellar reposition with gray line split.

1. The gray line incision is then deepened with Westcott scissors and the eyelid divided into an anterior and a posterior lamella as far as the superior fornix.
2. The eyelid retractors are recessed 5 to 6 mm and any subconjunctival scar tissue dissected from the conjunctiva to allow the posterior lamella to advance.
3. Next, four double-armed 4/0 Vicryl sutures are passed through the full thickness of the eyelid from the superior fornix to the skin crease where they are tied.
4. The posterior lamellar advancement should extend below the inferior margin of the anterior lamella by approximately 4 mm. The recessed edge of the anterior lamella is sutured to the advanced tarsus with interrupted 7/0 Vicryl sutures.

5. The raw surface of the tarsus is left to granulate (Fig. 4.18).
6. A lower lid 4/0 Nylon Frost suture is inserted and a compressive dressing is applied to keep postoperative swelling and bruising to a minimum.

Postoperative Care

The dressing is removed after 48 hours. Topical antibiotic ointment should be smeared along the wounds three times a day for 2 weeks. Cool packs can be applied intermittently for 24 to 48 hours to reduce swelling. The patient should be instructed to sleep with the head elevated for 2 weeks. The sutures are removed 3 to 4 weeks postoperatively.

Terminal Tarsal Rotation

This procedure is used for patients with an upper lid entropion with keratin on the inferior aspect of the tarsus, which typically occurs as a complication of Stevens–Johnson syndrome (Fig. 4.19). This can be performed under either general anesthesia or under local anesthesia with sedation.

Surgical Procedure

1. Proxymethacaine drops are instilled into the inferior conjunctival fornix.
2. Two to three milliliters of 0.5% Bupivacaine with 1:200,000 units of adrenaline mixed 50:50 with 2% lidocaine with 1:80,000 units of adrenaline are injected along the upper lid skin crease.
3. A 4/0 Silk traction suture is placed horizontally through the gray line of the lower eyelid centrally and the eyelid is everted over a Desmarres retractor.
4. A small quantity of the local anesthetic solution is also injected subconjunctivally just below the tarsus.
5. An incision is made with a no. 15 Bard Parker blade through the tarsus just above the keratin (Fig. 20).
6. The anterior surface of the tarsus and the conjunctiva are dissected up to the superior fornix using Westcott scissors until the posterior lamella will advance freely.
7. A vertical relieving incision is made through the eyelid margin just lateral to the punctum and at the lateral aspect of the eyelid (Fig. 4.21).

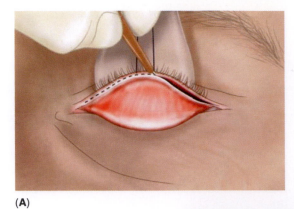

(A)

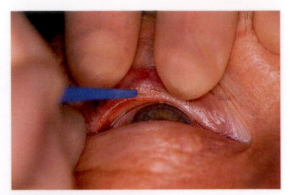

(B)

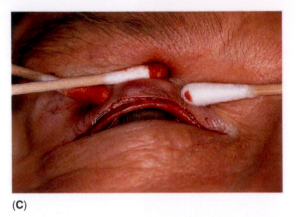

(C)

Figure 4.12 (**A, B**) A gray line split being performed with a micro-sharp blade. (**C**) The appearance of a gray line split.

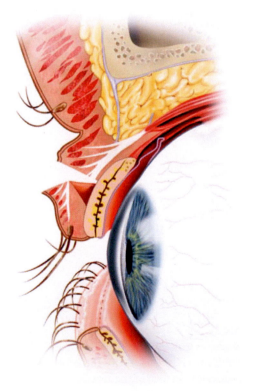

Figure 4.13 The anterior surface of the tarsus is exposed via a skin crease incision.

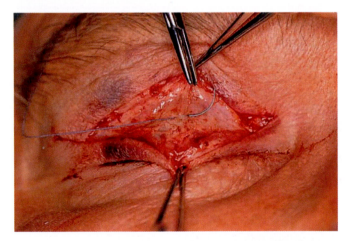

Figure 4.14 The upper lid retractors have been recessed. A 5/0 Vicryl suture is placed horizontally through the tarsus close to its upper border.

9. Next, three double-armed 4/0 Vicryl sutures are passed through the full thickness of the eyelid from the superior fornix to the desired position of the skin crease, where they are tied (Figs. 4.22B and 4.23).

10. The posterior lamellar advancement should extend below the inferior margin of the anterior lamella with its attached distal tarsal fragment by approximately 4 mm.

11. The everted fragment of tarsus is sutured to the advanced anterior tarsal surface with interrupted 7/0 Vicryl sutures. The raw surface of the tarsus is left to granulate (Fig. 4.23).

8. The anterior surface of the inferior tarsus is undermined with Westcott scissors until this fragment will rotate through 180° (Fig. 4.22A).

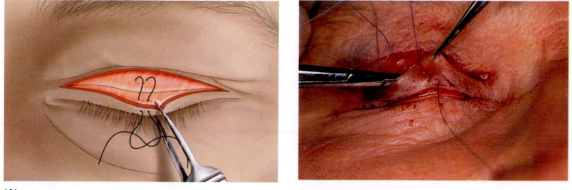

(A)   **(B)**

Figure 4.15 (**A**) The suture ends are brought through the anterior flap of skin and orbicularis muscle. (**B**) The needles emerge onto the skin surface just above the gray line split approximately 2 mm apart.

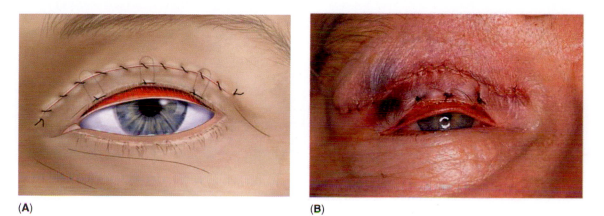

(A)   **(B)**

Figure 4.16 (**A**) A diagram demonstrating the position of the sutures. (**B**) In this patient the gray line split has been opened more than is usually required. A continuous suture was used to avoid a well defined skin crease for better symmetry in this patient.

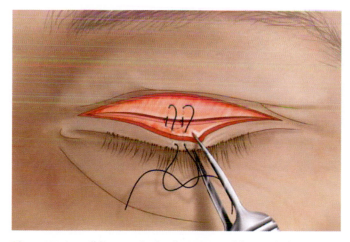

Figure 4.17 A small linear wedge has been removed from a thickened tarsus and the wedge closed with the Vicryl suture also used to open the gray line split.

12. A lower lid 4/0 Nylon Frost suture is inserted and a compressive dressing is applied to keep postoperative swelling and bruising to a minimum.

Postoperative Care

This is as described above.

Although the eyelashes are initially in an overcorrected position, these gradually return to a satisfactory position as the wound granulates (Fig. 4.24).

Posterior Lamellar Mucous Membrane Graft

A posterior lamellar mucous membrane graft is typically used for patients with a severe entropion with marked symblephara, severe lagophthalmos, and eyelid retraction. A graft is indicated if the patient requires a subsequent penetrating keratoplasty. Amniotic membrane may be used as an alternative graft if the patient agrees to the use of donor material. It is preferable to avoid the use of a hard palate graft for use in the upper eyelid as the corneal surface, which is often already compromised, can be damaged by its rougher surface.

The procedure is usually performed under general anesthesia. A throat pack is placed and the anesthetist is asked to position the endotracheal tube to one corner of the mouth to make access to the lower lip donor site easier.

Surgical Procedure

1. Two to three milliliters of 0.5% Bupivacaine with 1:200,000 units of adrenaline mixed 50:50 with 2% lidocaine with 1:80,000 units of adrenaline is injected along the upper lid skin crease.
2. A 4/0 Silk traction suture is placed horizontally through the gray line of the upper eyelid centrally and the eyelid is everted over a Desmarres retractor.
3. All symblephara are divided with Westcott scissors.
4. The conjunctiva at the upper border of the tarsus is incised and dissected free from all subconjunctival

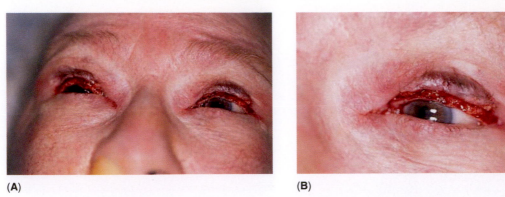

(A)   (B)

Figure 4.18 (**A**) A completed bilateral lamellar split and posterior lamellar advancement. (**B**) A close-up of the left eye.

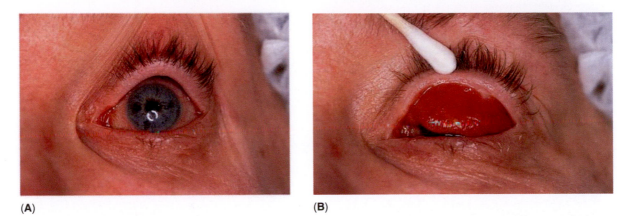

(A)   (B)

Figure 4.19 (**A**) The appearance of a keratinized left upper eyelid margin in a patient with Stevens-Johnson syndrome. (**B**) Keratin is seen extending onto the inferior aspect of the tarsus in this patient.

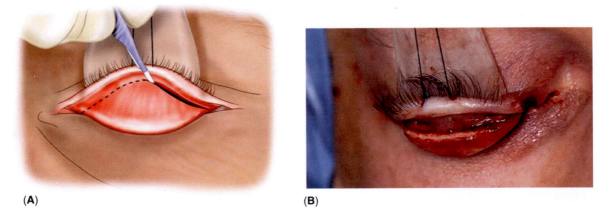

(A)   (B)

Figure 4.20 (**A**) A incision is made through the full thickness of the tarsus with a no. 15 Bard Parker blade. (**B**) The appearance of the incised tarsus.

scar tissue into the superior fornix and onto the bulbar surface of the globe.

5. At the same time, the retractors are freed from the tarsus to correct eyelid retraction.
6. Next, a template is taken of the conjunctival defect.
7. The lower lip mucosa is injected with 0.5% Bupivacaine with 1:200,000 units of adrenaline.
8. Atraumatic Babcock's bowel clamps are used to evert the lower lip.
9. The lip mucosa is dried with a swab.
10. The template is transferred to the lower lip mucosa, avoiding the vermillion border.

11. This is outlined with a sterile gentian violet marker pen.
12. The graft is harvested with a no. 15 Bard Parker blade and blunt-tipped Westcott scissors.
13. The bowel clamps are removed and the graft donor site is compressed with topical 1:1,000 adrenaline on a swab. Bipolar cautery is used to cauterize any bleeding vessels.
14. The graft is carefully shaped with Westcott scissors and sutured into place with interrupted 8/0 Vicryl sutures (Fig. 4.25).
15. A symblepharon ring of suitable size and shape is inserted (Fig. 4.26).

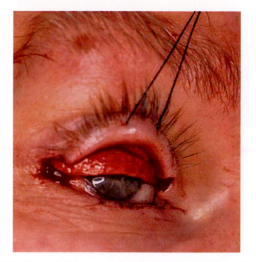

Figure 4.21 Relieving incisions are made through the eyelid margin medially and laterally.

16. Topical antibiotic ointment is instilled into the eye.
17. The silk suture is fixated to the cheek skin as a reverse Frost suture.
18. A compressive dressing is applied.

Postoperative Care

The patient is instructed to avoid any hot drinks or hot food for a period of 2 weeks. The patient is discharged on a broad-spectrum oral antibiotic for a week and an oral anti-septic mouth wash for 5 days. The dressing is removed after 4 to 5 days along with the reverse Frost suture. Topical preservative free antibiotic drops are instilled into the eye four times a day for 2 weeks. A preservative free topical lubricant is used every 2 to 3 hours. The patient should be instructed to sleep with the head elevated for 2 weeks. The symblepharon ring should be maintained in place for a minimum period of 6 to 8 weeks. The patient should be reviewed twice weekly to ensure that the symblepharon ring does not cause any corneal problems.

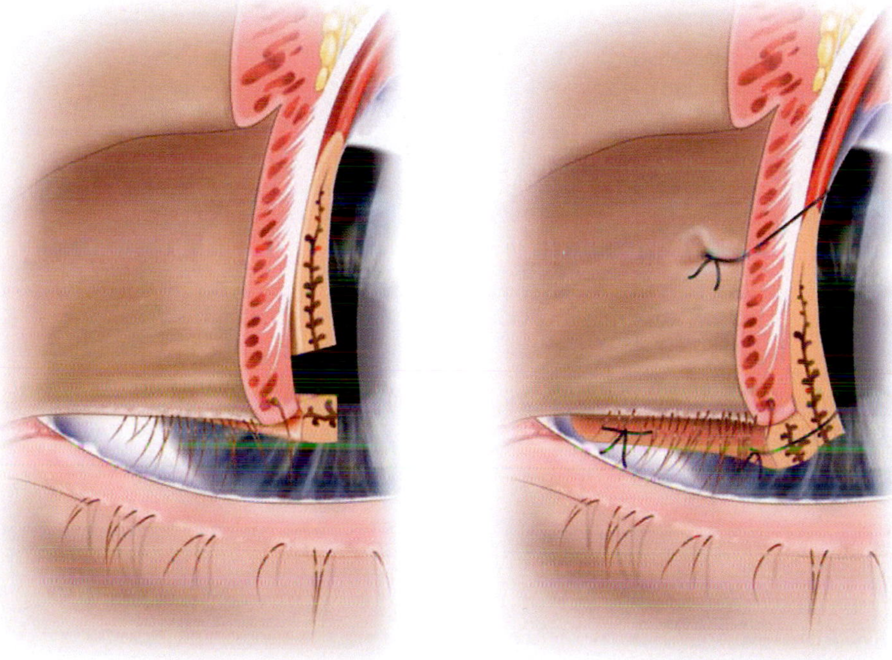

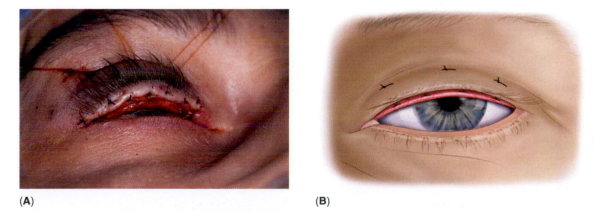

(A)   (B)

Figure 4.22 (**A**) The lower tarsal fragment is undermined anteriorly until it will rotate 180°. (**B**) The terminal tarsal fragment has been rotated and sutured to the anterior tarsal surface.

(A)   (B)

Figure 4.23 (**A**) The terminal tarsal fragment has been rotated 180° and sutured to the anterior surface of the tarsus. (**B**) Three 4/0 Vicryl sutures are tied in the skin crease to hold the posterior lamella in an advanced position.

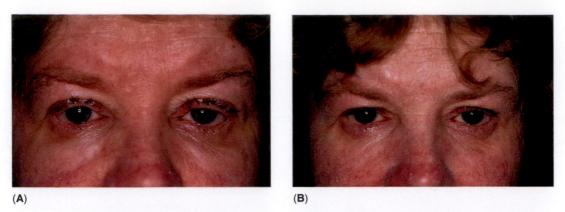

Figure 4.24 (**A**) The appearance of the eyelids 2 weeks following a terminal tarsal rotation procedure. (**B**) The appearance of the eyelids in the same patient 6 months postoperatively.

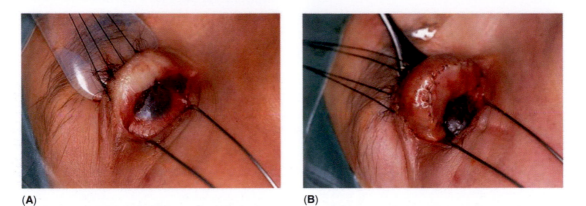

Figure 4.25 (**A**) Extensive keratinization of the posterior lamella of the upper eyelid with obliteration of the superior fornix following severe Stevens–Johnson syndrome. (**B**) The symblephara have been dissected, the keratinized area excised and a large mucous membrane graft sutured into place.

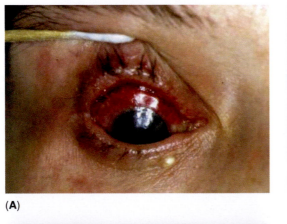
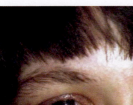
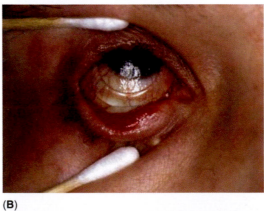
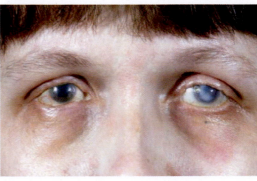

Figure 4.26 (**A**) The patient seen 6 weeks postoperatively with a symblepharon ring in place. (**B**) The symblepharon ring is seen on up gaze. (**C**) The right cornea has re-epithelialised. A left central tarsorrhaphy was required for a severe central corneal ulcer. (**D**) The same patient 15 years later.

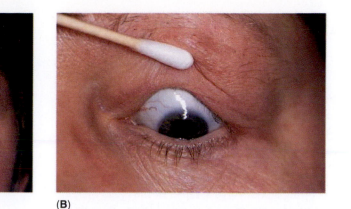

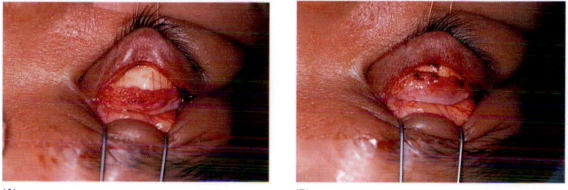

Figure 4.27 (**A**) A patient referred with a severe left upper eyelid entropion following an excessive resection of tarsus in a Fasanella servat procedures. (**B**) A close-up of the left upper eyelid entropion. Previous inappropriate cryotherapy has been performed for "trichiasis."

Figure 4.28 (**A**) An auricular cartilage graft has been scored vertically with a no. 15 Bard Parker blade to allow the graft to bend to a slightly convex configuration. It has been inserted to lie over the residual tarsal plate extending inferiorly to a position just above the lash roots. (**B**) The levator aponeurosis has been attached to the auricular cartilage graft.

Auricular Cartilage Graft

This procedure is typically required for patients with a moderate degree of upper lid entropion who have undergone an excessive excision of tarsal plate during eyelid reconstructive surgery or ptosis surgery (Fig. 4.27). The procedure is performed in the same manner as that described above for the management of a congenital upper eyelid entropion (Fig. 4.28).

FURTHER READING

1. Collin JRO. A Manual of Systematic Eyelid Surgery. New York, NY: Churchill Livingstone, 1989.

2. Goldberg RA, Joshi AR, et al. Management of severe cicatricial entropion using shared mucosal grafts. Arch Ophthalmol 1999; 117: 1255–9.

3. Jackson WB. Blepharitis: current strategies for diagnosis and management. Canc J Ophthalmol 2008; 43(2): 170–9.

4. Rhatigan MC, Ashworth JL, Goodall K, Leatherbarrow B. Correction of blepharoconjunctivitis-related upper eyelid entropion using the anterior lamellar reposition technique. Eye 1997; 11(Part 1): 118–20.

5. Tyers AG, Collin JRO. Colour Atlas of Ophthalmic Plastic Surgery, 3rd edn, Oxford, UK: Butterworth-Heinemann Elsevier, 2008: 108–15. ISBN 978-0-7506-8860-4.

6. Yaqub A, Leatherbarrow B. The use of autogenous auricular cartilage in the management of upper eyelid entropion. Eye 1997; 11(Part 6): 801–5.

5 Abnormal eyelashes

INTRODUCTION

Trichiasis refers to a condition in which aberrant eyelashes turn inward against the globe in the absence of any eyelid malposition (Fig. 5.1). It is frequently seen in association with chronic blepharoconjunctivitis or cicatrizing conjunctivitis, e.g., ocular cicatricial pemphigoid. It may also be seen following eyelid margin trauma or following a poor surgical repair of the eyelid margin, e.g., following a wedge resection of an eyelid lesion. In contrast, distichiasis refers to a condition in which accessory eyelashes arise from the lid margin in an area other than the normal ciliary line, e.g., from the meibomian gland orifices (Fig. 5.2). If eyelashes abrade the cornea the patient will experience constant irritation, photophobia, and lacrimation. Fluorescein staining of the cornea will occur. Constant corneal abrasion by ingrowing eyelashes can result in severe visual morbidity, e.g., corneal scarring seen in advanced trachoma. Very rarely, abnormal eyelashes may be seen growing from an unusual location in the eyelid (Fig. 5.3).

The management of misdirected lashes due to an eyelid malposition is addressed in chapters 3 and 4.

MANAGEMENT

1. Epilation
2. Bandage contact lens
3. Electrolysis
4. Argon laser ablation
5. Cryotherapy
6. Surgical excision

Epilation

Epilation of eyelashes provides a temporary relief from symptoms, but the symptoms are often exacerbated as the eyelashes regrow. The eyelashes are initially short and firm, and create more corneal damage. Epilation also prevents definitive treatment by electrolysis. The surgeon is unable to identify the offending eyelashes until these have begun to regrow.

Bandage Contact Lens

A temporary relief from symptoms can be obtained by the fitting of a bandage contact lens while definitive treatment is being arranged. The contact lens has to be worn continuously, which exposes the patient to a risk of bacterial keratitis.

Electrolysis

Electrolysis is an appropriate form of treatment if only a few eyelashes are present, particularly if these are located in different positions in the eyelids. The Ellman–Surgitron radiofrequency device is particularly suited for electrolysis provided the patient does not have a cardiac pacemaker (Fig. 5.4).

Surgical Procedure
1. A topical anesthetic agent is instilled into the eye.
2. One to two milliliters of 2% lidocaine with 1:80,000 units of adrenaline are injected subcutaneously and subconjunctivally into the affected eyelid.
3. The neutral plate is positioned between the patient's shoulder blades.
4. The eyelid is grasped with a pair of Paufique forceps. The electrolysis needle is inserted along the lash to a depth of approximately 2 to 3 mm to the position of lash bulb using an operating microscope.
5. The current is applied for 2 to 3 sec only using the foot pedal. Care should be taken to commence the procedure using the lowest settings on the device.
6. A gentle bubbling should be observed. The lash should either accompany the electrolysis needle as this is withdrawn or the lash should come out of the eyelid easily using epilation forceps but without any resistance. If there is any resistance the procedure should be repeated.

Postoperative Care
Antibiotic ointment is applied to the eyelid margin three times a day for a week. The patient should be warned that some lashes may fail to respond to treatment and that a further treatment session a few weeks later may be required.

Argon Laser Ablation

Argon laser ablation can be useful for a small number of darkly pigmented lashes.

Surgical Procedure
1. A topical anesthetic agent is instilled into the eye.
2. One to two milliliters of 2% lidocaine with 1:80,000 units of adrenaline is injected subcutaneously and subconjunctivally into the affected eyelid.
3. The usual laser safety precautions are observed.
4. The eyelid is everted with the surgeon's forefinger.
5. The laser aiming beam should be aimed parallel to the shaft of the eyelash by everting the eyelid margin.
6. A 50 µ spot size should be used. The initial power should be set at 300 mW for 0.5 sec and increased as required.
7. A hole is burned to an approximate depth of 1.5 to 2 mm. Great care should be taken to avoid damaging the surrounding eyelid tissue.
8. The lash should come out of the eyelid easily using epilation forceps but without any resistance. If there is any resistance the procedure should be repeated.

Postoperative Care
Antibiotic ointment is applied to the eyelid margin three times a day for a week. The patient should be warned that some lashes may fail to respond to treatment and that a further treatment session a few weeks later may be required.

Cryotherapy

Cryotherapy is an appropriate form of treatment for more extensive trichiasis or distichiasis. Before undertaking this treatment, however, it is essential to exclude the presence of an upper or lower eyelid entropion which should be addressed appropriately (see chaps. 3 and 4). The application of liquid nitrogen to the affected area is the most effective method of delivering cryotherapy. Alternatively, a nitrous oxide cryotherapy unit can be used with a block probe (Fig. 5.5), which allows a greater area of the eyelid to be treated with each application than a retinal cryotherapy probe. The temperature at the level of the eyelash follicle should be monitored with a thermocouple. The goal is to reduce the temperature to approximately –25°C, which should destroy the lash bulb without inducing tissue necrosis. A double freeze–thaw cycle is used. At this temperature level, however, pigment cells in the skin are also destroyed, leaving hypopigmentation. The patient must be warned about this. The patient should also be warned about the risk of recurrence and the potential requirement for repeated treatment.

Surgical Procedure

1. A topical anesthetic agent is instilled into the eye.
2. One to two milliliters of 2% lidocaine with 1:80,000 units of adrenaline are injected subcutaneously and subconjunctivally into the affected eyelid.
3. The globe must be protected with a *plastic* eye guard lightly coated with a lubricant ointment on the surface in contact with the globe (Fig. 5.6).

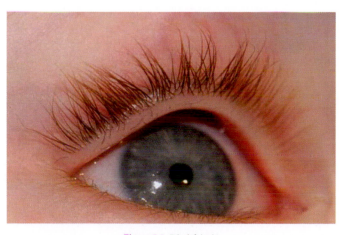

Figure 5.1 Trichiasis.

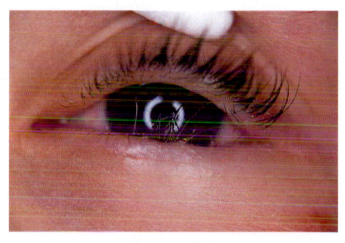

Figure 5.2 Distichiasis.

4. A sterile thermocouple is carefully inserted into the affected area of eyelid.
5. Liquid nitrogen is applied to the affected area of the eyelid using a small delivery head which assures a precise application (Fig. 5.6).
6. The liquid nitrogen is applied until the affected area becomes white (Fig. 5.6).
7. The eyelid tissues are allowed to thaw slowly before the application is repeated and again the tissues are allowed to thaw slowly.
8. If a cryoprobe is used instead, the probe is held against the lid margin in the affected area while the temperature is reduced. The application duration is usually 30 sec on the upper eyelid and 25 sec on the lower eyelid. With thin, atrophic eyelids, a shorter freeze time should be used to avoid the risk of inducing necrosis of the eyelid.
9. The probe should be allowed to thaw slowly before it is removed. A double freeze–thaw cycle is again undertaken.
10. The lash should come out of the eyelid easily using epilation forceps but without any resistance.

Postoperative Care

Antibiotic ointment is applied to the eyelid margin three times per day for a week. The patient should be warned that some lashes may fail to respond to treatment and that a further treatment session a few weeks later may be required.

KEY POINT

It is essential to protect the globe with a plastic and not a metal eye guard in order to insulate the globe from the effects of cryotherapy.

Surgical Excision

A localized area of trichiasis in a patient with eyelid laxity may be more conveniently managed by a wedge excision of the affected area and direct closure of the defect (see discussion on "wedge resection" in chap. 6). Although it is feasible to expose

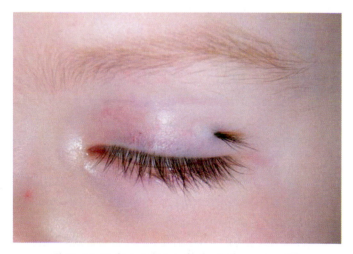

Figure 5.3 An abnormal crop of lashes in the upper eyelid.

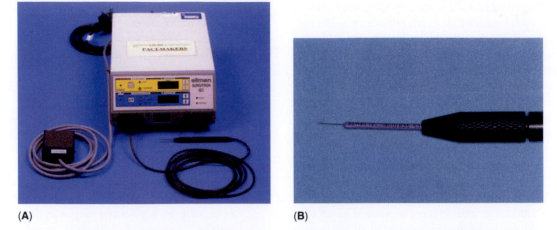

Figure 5.4 (**A**) The Ellman radiofrequency device. (**B**) The Ellman probe with electrolysis needle.

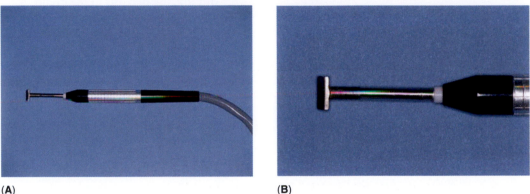

Figure 5.5 (**A**) An eyelid cryoprobe. (**B**) A close-up photograph of the end of the cryoprobe.

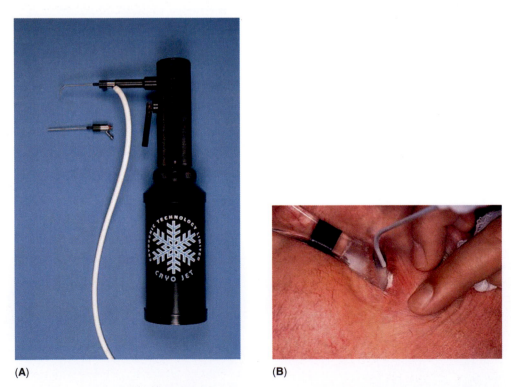

Figure 5.6 (**A**) A "Cryojet" cryotherapy device which utilizes liquid nitrogen. A series of interchangeable delivery heads are available. (**B**) The globe is protected with a plastic eyeguard when the cryotherapy is applied to the eyelids.

and individually remove eyelash roots and bulbs via an upper eyelid skin crease or lower eyelid subciliary incision, this is a tedious exercise and rarely required.

Distichiasis is managed by splitting the eyelids along the gray line and by applying cryotherapy to the posterior lamella of the eyelid. The procedure can be performed under local

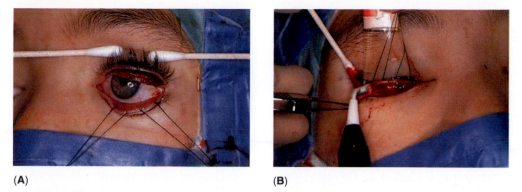

(A)   **(B)**

Figure 5.7 (**A**) The upper eyelid has been separated into anterior and posterior lamellae. (**B**) Cryotherapy is being applied to the posterior lamella of the lower eyelid.

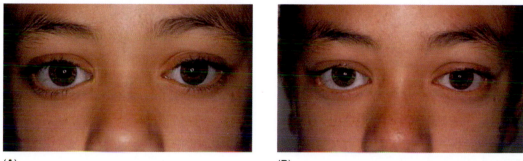

(A)   **(B)**

Figure 5.8 (**A**) A patient with distichiasis affecting the upper and lower eyelids bilaterally. (**B**) The patient following eyelid splitting and cryotherapy to the posterior lamellae. The upper eyelid lashes have survived but there is extensive loss of eyelashes in the lower eyelids.

anesthesia with or without sedation, or under general anesthesia. The patient should be warned about the likelihood of severe postoperative eyelid edema which can take some weeks to resolve.

Surgical Procedure

1. A topical anesthetic agent is instilled into the eye.
2. One to two milliliters of 2% lidocaine with 1:80,000 units of adrenaline are injected subcutaneously along the upper eyelid skin crease in the upper eyelid and along the subciliary border in the lower eyelid.
3. The eyelid is split along the gray line with an angled micro-sharp blade on a Beaver blade handle.
4. The eyelids are then carefully divided into anterior and posterior lamellae with blunt-tipped Westcott scissors (Fig. 5.7A).
5. This dissection is carried as far as the superior fornix in the upper eyelid and the inferior fornix in the lower eyelid.
6. Cryotherapy is then selectively applied to the posterior lamella only (Fig. 5.7B). This is as described above.
7. The eyelid retractors are recessed a few millimeters.
8. The posterior lamella is then advanced 2 mm and the anterior lamella is sutured to the anterior surface of the posterior lamella in a recessed postion to avoid any subsequent contracture and lid retraction or entropion.

Although the goal of this approach is to avoid damage to the normal eyelashes, many of these rarely survive, particularly in the lower eyelids (Fig. 5.8). It is important that the patient is suitably counseled about this beforehand.

Postoperative Care
Antibiotic ointment is applied to the eyelid margin three times per day for a week.

FURTHER READING

1. American Academy of Ophthalmology. Basic and Clinical Science Course: Orbit, Eyelids, and Lacrimal System, section 7. San Francisco, CA: The American Academy of Ophthalmology, 2006/7: 201–5.
2. Anderson RL, Harvey JT. Lid splitting and posterior lamella cryosurgery for congenital and acquired distichiasis. Arch Ophthalmol 1981; 99: 631–3.
3. Anderson RL, Wood JR. Complications of cryosurgery. Arch Ophthalmol 1981; 90: 460–3.
4. Bartley GB, Lowry JC. Argon laser treatment of trichiasis. Am J Ophthalmol 1992; 113: 71–4.
5. Martin RT, Nunery WR, Tanenbaum M. Entropion, trichiasis and distichiasis. In: McCord CD, Tanenbaum M, Nunery WR, eds. Oculoplastic Surgery, 3rd edn. New York, NY: Raven Press, 1995: 230–48.
6. Rose GE, Collin JRO. Management of entropion and trichiasis. In: American Academy of Ophthalmology Monographs, Surgery of the Eyelid, Orbit, and Lacrimal System, Vol. 2. 1994: 34–52.
7. Sullivan JH, Beard C, Bullock JD. Cryosurgery for treatment of trichiasis. Am J Ophthalmol 1976; 82: 117–21.
8. Boynton R, Naugle T. Trichiasis and distichiasis. In: Levine MR, ed. Manual of Oculoplastic Surgery, 3rd edn. Boston, MA: Butterworth-Heinemann, 2003: 181–9.
9. Nerad JD, Carter KD, Alford MA. Trichiasis, marginal entropion, and other causes. In: Rapid Diagnosis in Ophthalmology-Oculoplastic and Reconstructive Surgery. Philadelphia, PA: Mosby Elsevier, 2008: 96–9.
10. Jeffrey AN. Techniques in Ophthlmic Plastic Surgery—A Personal Tutorial. Philadelphia, PA: Elsevier Inc. 2010: 113–26. ISBN 978-1-4377-0008-4.

6 Lower eyelid ectropion

INTRODUCTION
Eyelid ectropion is an eyelid malposition in which the eyelid margin is turned away from its normal apposition to the globe. This more frequently affects the lower eyelid. Upper eyelid ectropion is more unusual. The condition may be classified into four categories according to the underlying etiology.

CLASSIFICATION
1. Involutional ectropion (Fig. 6.1A)
2. Cicatricial ectropion (Fig. 6.1B)
3. Paralytic ectropion (Fig. 6.2A)
4. Mechanical ectropion (Fig. 6.2B)

It should be recognized, however, that more than one etiological factor may be present in an individual patient: e.g., in a patient with a chronic facial palsy and a lower lid ectropion, all four etiological factors may coexist (Fig. 6.3). An ectropion affecting the upper eyelid is less commonly encountered and may be seen following eyelid trauma, herpes zoster ophthalmicus, icthyosis, and burns (Fig. 6.4).

It is important to be able to classify the type of ectropion that is seen so that the correct treatment is directed at the underlying cause. Involutional ectropion is by far the most common type of ectropion but a cicatricial cause of lower lid ectropion is often overlooked (Fig. 6.5). Such an ectropion will only respond to the addition or recruitment of skin into the lower eyelid using a full thickness skin graft, a mid-face lift, or with the use of soft tissue expansion.

Failure to recognize this leads to poor results from inappropriately selected surgical procedures (Fig. 6.6).

KEY POINT
A cicatricial cause of lower lid ectropion should not be overlooked.

The initial sign of a lower lid ectropion is inferior punctal eversion (Fig. 6.7).

This can lead to a vicious cycle of secondary events and needs to be addressed early. Eversion of the inferior punctum leads to exposure and drying of the punctum, which becomes stenosed. Epiphora ensues, which may lead to excoriation and contracture of the skin of the lower eyelid that further exacerbates the ectropion. In addition, the patient tends to continually wipe the tears from the lower eyelid, which in turn results in eyelid and medial canthal tendon laxity that further exacerbates the lower eyelid ectropion. If the condition is neglected, the tarsal conjunctiva becomes exposed and eventually thickened and keratinized (Fig. 6.8). Lower lid ectropion often results in a corneal epitheliopathy, especially in the inferior third of the cornea.

PATIENT EVALUATION
The patient's history may point to a number of dermatological disorders which may be responsible for a cicatricial ectropion, e.g., eczema, lamellar icthyosis (Fig. 6.9). A drug history may reveal topical medications the patient may be taking to which there may be an allergy with a secondary chronic dermatitis, e.g., topical glaucoma medications (Fig. 6.10). This is not an infrequent cause of lower lid ectropion in elderly patients attending glaucoma clinics and is frequently overlooked or misdiagnosed.

Patients who have previously undergone a lower eyelid blepharoplasty, laser skin resurfacing, or a chemical peel may be reluctant to divulge such information (Fig. 6.11).

KEY POINT
A chronic allergic dermatitis is not an infrequent cause of a lower lid ectropion in elderly patients attending glaucoma clinics and is frequently overlooked or misdiagnosed.

When examining the patient, the whole of the patient's face should be scrutinized for evidence of a dermatological disorder, connective tissue disorder, facial weakness, scars from previous surgery or trauma, or evidence of malignant cutaneous lesions (Figs. 6.12–6.14).

The degree of eyelid laxity is assessed by drawing the eyelid away from the globe and releasing it (the "snap" test) (Fig. 6.15).

The distance that the lid can be pulled away from the globe using the thumb and forefinger can also be measured in millimeters using a ruler (the "pinch" test).

The eyelid is drawn laterally and the position of the punctum is observed (the "lateral distraction" test). If the punctum can be drawn lateral to the medial limbus with the globe in the primary position, the medial canthal tendon will probably require attention during the surgical repair of the ectropion (Fig. 6.16). Rounding of the lateral canthus indicates lateral canthal tendon laxity or dehiscence.

If a cicatricial component of the ectropion is not obvious, the lower eyelid skin should be observed for tension lines seen when the patient blinks. The patient is asked to look up and to open the mouth to see whether or not these maneuvers exacerbate the ectropion (Fig. 6.17).

KEY POINT
Failure to recognize a cicatricial component is a common cause of surgical failure in the management of lower lid ectropion.

MANAGEMENT
It is important to recognize dermatological causes of cicatricial ectropion that may be amenable to medical management

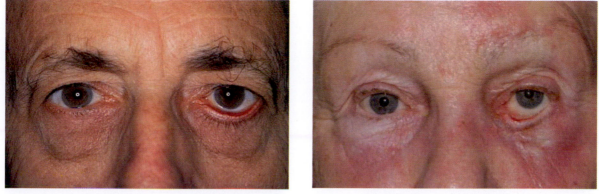

(A)   **(B)**

Figure 6.1 (**A**) A left lower eyelid involutional ectropion. (**B**) A left lower eyelid cicatricial ectropion.

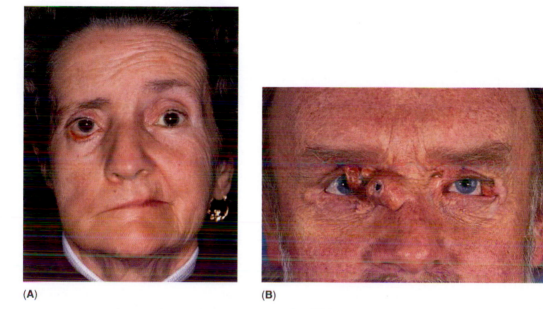

(A)   **(B)**

Figure 6.2 (**A**) A right lower eyelid paralytic ectropion. (**B**) A left lower eyelid mechanical ectropion.

alone, e.g., chronic contact or allergic dermatitis. Removal of the offending substance, e.g., replacement of a topical glaucoma medication with a preservative-free preparation along with a short course of a weak topical steroid cream to the eyelid skin, may be all that is required.

The choice of surgical procedure depends on a number of factors:

1. The degree of ectropion
2. The location of the ectropion
3. The degree of laxity of the medial and lateral canthal tendons
4. The horizontal laxity of the eyelid
5. The tone of the orbicularis muscle
6. The nature of any cicatricial forces
7. The presence of any mechanical force
8. The age and general health of the patient

The surgical procedure(s) should be selected to address these factors in each individual patient. Although an abundance of

surgical procedures has been described for the management of lower eyelid ectropion, the choice of procedure can in practice be made from a relatively small number. The procedures utilized in the author's practice are:

1. Retropunctal cautery
2. Medial spindle
3. Medial spindle with medial wedge resection
4. Medial canthal tendon plication
5. Medial canthal resection
6. Lateral wedge resection
7. Lateral wedge resection with skin–muscle blepharoplasty
8. Lateral tarsal strip procedure
9. Z-plasty
10. Lateral wedge resection or lateral tarsal strip with skin graft
11. Posterior approach retractor reinsertion with medial spindle with lateral tarsal strip

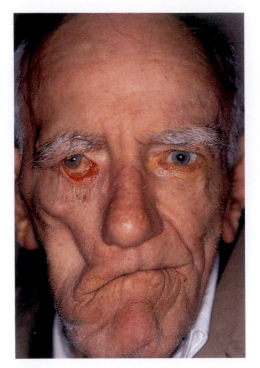

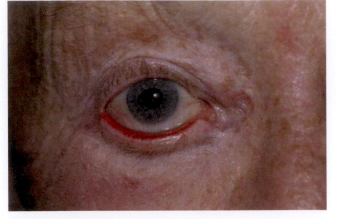

Figure 6.5 A right lower lid cicatricial ectropion due to photo-damaged, aged, and "weather-beaten" skin.

Figure 6.3 A right lower eyelid ectropion in a patient with a chronic lower motor neuron facial palsy. In this patient all the etiological factors coexist and should be addressed in his management.

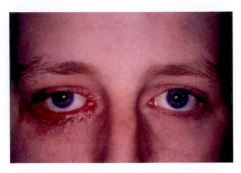

Figure 6.6 A disastrous result from a K–Z procedure inappropriately performed on a patient who presented with epiphora and a medial ectropion. His mild cicatricial ectropion was due to eczema.

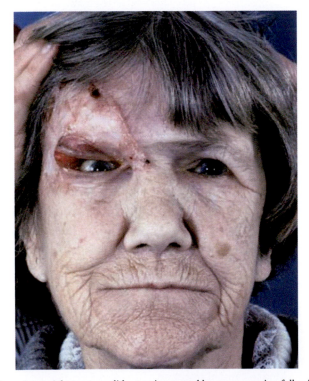

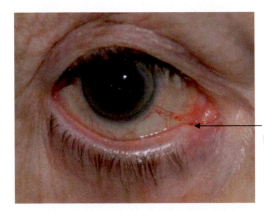

Inferior punctum

Figure 6.7 Punctal eversion of the right lower eyelid.

Figure 6.4 A right upper eyelid ectropion caused by severe scarring following herpes zoster ophthalmicus.

12. Fascia lata sling
13. Removal of lesion causing mechanical ectropion
14. Local tissue flap
15. Mid-face lift
16. Soft tissue expansion with local tissue flap

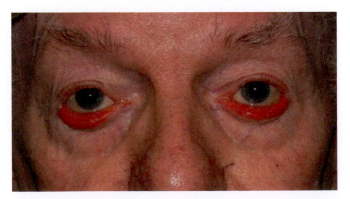

Figure 6.8 A patient with a bilateral complete tarsal ectropion with keratinization of the chronically exposed conjunctiva.

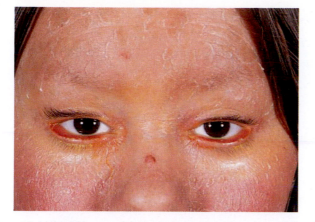

Figure 6.9 A bilateral lower eyelid cicatricial ectropion in a patient with lamellar ichthyosis.

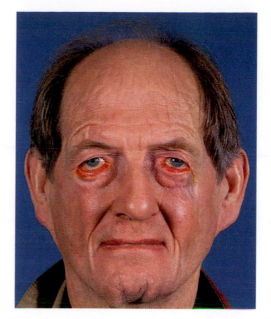

Figure 6.12 A patient with a bilateral lower eyelid ectropion. The patient has Ehlers–Danlos syndrome.

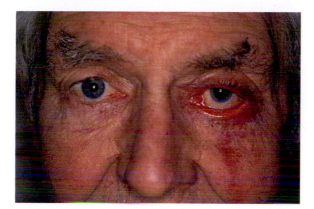

Figure 6.10 A patient with a left lower eyelid cicatricial ectropion. The patient was allergic to the topical glaucoma medication prescribed for the left eye only. The ectropion (and ptosis) resolved completely after a short course of topical steroid applied to the periocular skin.

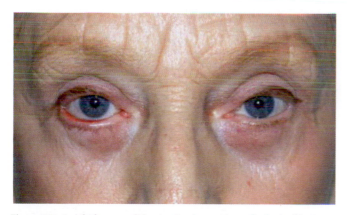

Figure 6.11 A right lower eyelid ectropion in a patient who had undergone a 4-lid blepharoplasty with laser skin resurfacing 10 years previously by a plastic surgeon. The secondary hollowing of the lower eyelids from excessive fat removal and the smooth lower lid skin contrasting with the rest of the periorbital skin texture are tell tale signs that indicate the reason for the development of the lower lid cicatricial ectropion.

Involutional Ectropion

Involutional ectropion can be further classified into the following subtypes:

1. Punctal ectropion
2. Medial ectropion without horizontal eyelid laxity

3. Medial ectropion with horizontal eyelid laxity
4. Medial ectropion with medial canthal tendon laxity
5. Ectropion of the whole length of the lower eyelid
6. Complete tarsal ectropion

Punctal Ectropion
Retropunctal Cautery
Where the lower lid ectropion is very early, it is simple to apply retropunctal cautery.

Surgical procedure
1. One to two milliliters of 2% lidocaine with 1:80,000 units of adrenaline are injected subcutaneously and subconjunctivally into the medial aspect of the lower eyelid.
2. Using a disposable cautery device, deep burns are applied to the conjunctiva 3 to 4 mm below the punctum. The effect on the punctal position is observed and titrated by the number of burns applied and the depth of the burn. Great care should be taken when using such a device close to the globe, and inflammable swabs should be kept away from the surgical field.
3. Antibiotic ointment is instilled into the eye

Postoperative care. Antibiotic drops are instilled into the eye three times per day for a week.

Medial Ectropion Without Horizontal Eyelid Laxity
Medial Spindle Procedure
Where the punctal ectropion is more pronounced, a medial spindle procedure is performed. It is usually necessary to dilate the punctum with a Nettleship dilator at the same time, as this is often stenosed. It is not usually appropriate

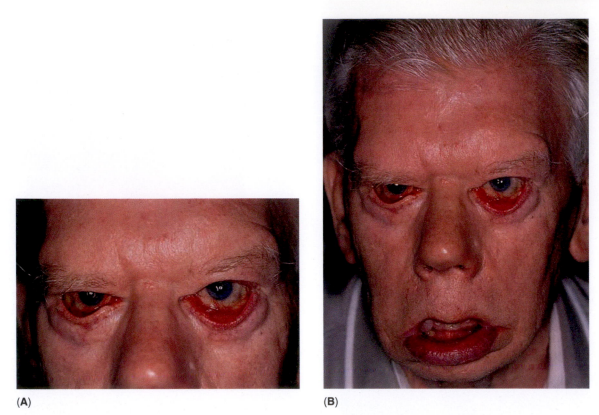

(A)   **(B)**

Figure 6.13 (**A**) A patient with a severe bilateral lower eyelid ectropion. He also has a bilateral brow ptosis. (**B**) An examination of his whole face reveals a severe bilateral lower facial weakness. He also had a bilateral abduction weakness of both eyes. The patient has Möbius syndrome.

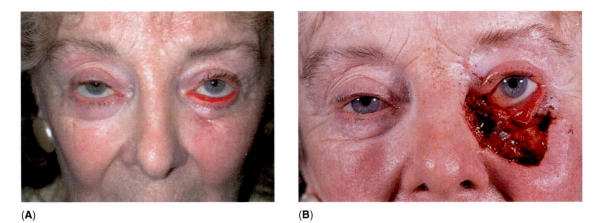

(A)   **(B)**

Figure 6.14 (**A**) This patient's left lower eyelid ectropion was due to a lower eyelid morphoeic basal cell carcinoma. (**B**) The patient's appearance following a Mohs' micrographic surgical excision of the tumor.

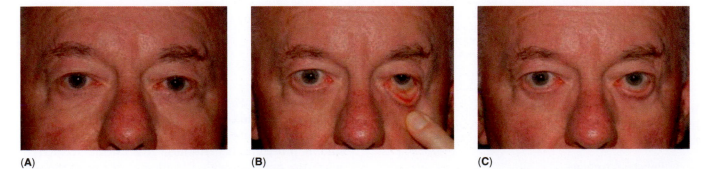

(**A**)   (**B**)   (**C**)

Figure 6.15 (**A**) A patient with a punctal ectropion. (**B**) A "Snap" test being performed. (**C**) Positive "snap" test: the eyelid fails to return to the globe without a blink

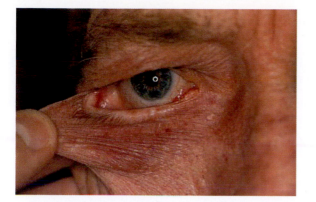

Figure 6.16 Medial canthal tendon laxity demonstrated with a lateral distraction test.

to perform any destructive procedures on the punctum, e.g., a 3-snip punctoplasty, as the punctum, may resume its normal appearance and function once it has been repositioned against the globe. Alternatively, a perforated punctal plug, or a Crawford bi-canalicular or mono-canalicular stent can be placed temporarily to maintain patency of the punctum. If a stenosed punctum needs to be surgically enlarged, it is preferable to do this using a Kelly punch.

Surgical procedure

1. One to two milliliters of 2% lidocaine with 1:80,000 units of adrenaline are injected subcutaneously and subconjunctivally into the medial aspect of the lower eyelid.

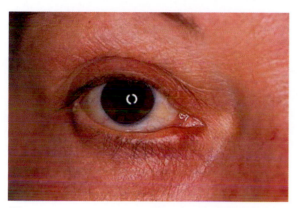

(A)

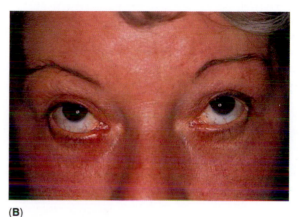

(B)

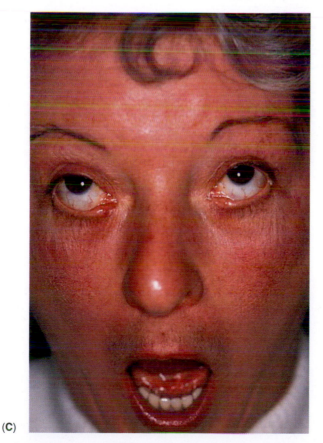

(C)

Figure 6.17 (**A**) A lower eyelid punctal ectropion in a patient referred with epiphora. (**B**) The punctal ectropion is exaggerated by asking the patient to look up. (**C**) The punctal ectropion is further exaggerated by asking the patient to open her mouth.

2. A 00 Bowman probe is inserted into the inferior canaliculus. This step is omitted when experience has been gained.

3. The conjunctiva is lifted just below the inferior punctum using Paufique forceps. A diamond-shaped excision of conjunctiva is performed using Westcott scissors. A cut is made through the tented conjunctiva in a horizontal plane medial and then lateral to the forceps creating a diamond-shaped excision (Fig. 6.18).

4. A double-armed 5/0 Vicryl suture on a 1/4-circle needle is passed through the lower eyelid retractors at the base of the conjunctival wound, with the needle being rotated toward the globe.

5. The needle is then reverse mounted and passed away from the globe through the superior edges of the conjunctival wound on either side of the apex of the diamond.

6. Again the needle is reverse mounted and is then passed back through the inferior edges of the conjunctival wound on either side of the apex of the diamond and out through the skin of the lower lid at the junction of eyelid and cheek skin (Fig. 6.19). The effect of the suture is to attach the inferior retractors to the superior aspect of the wound, to pull the punctum posteriorly against the globe, and to close the wound. The tension on the suture is titrated against the effect on the position of the punctum. Ideally the punctum should be slightly over-inverted against the globe.

Postoperative care. Postoperatively topical antibiotic ointment is prescribed three times a day for 2 weeks and the patient is instructed not to pull the eyelid down to instill this. The ointment should simply be smeared across the medial aspect of the eyelid. The suture should be removed in clinic after 2 to 3 weeks.

Medial Ectropion with Horizontal Eyelid Laxity
Medial Spindle Procedure with a Medial Wedge Resection
In this situation a medial spindle procedure is combined with a medial wedge resection of the lower eyelid (Fig. 6.20). The wedge resection is positioned to remove thickened keratinized conjunctiva. It is important that sufficient eyelid is left medial to the resection to enable vertical mattress sutures to be placed across the eyelid margin without risking damage to the punctum or to the inferior canaliculus.

Surgical procedure
1. One to two milliliters of 2% lidocaine with 1:80,000 units of adrenaline are injected subcutaneously

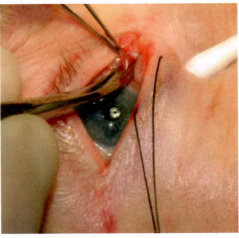
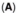

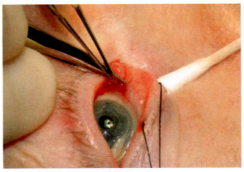
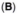

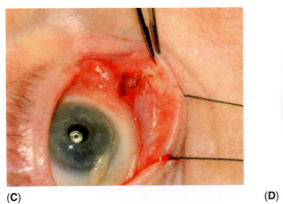

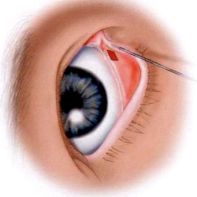

Figure 6.18 (**A**) The conjunctiva is lifted with a pair of Paufique forceps and cut. (**B**) A further cut is made from the opposite side while keeping hold of the conjunctiva with the forceps. (**C**) A diamond-shaped tissue defect remains. (**D**) A diagrammatic representation of the location of the diamond-shaped excision of conjunctiva. A 00 Bowman probe has been inserted into the inferior canaliculus to protect this during the conjunctival resection.

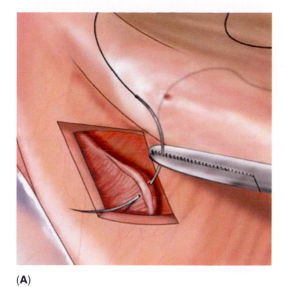

(A)

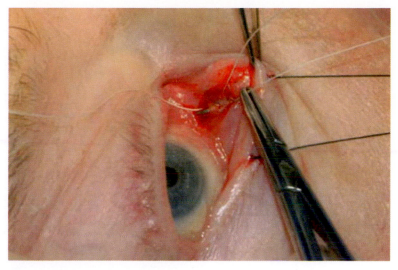

(B)

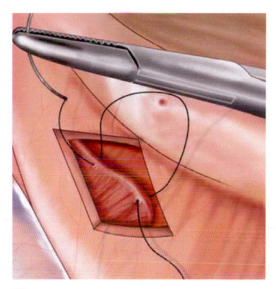

(C)

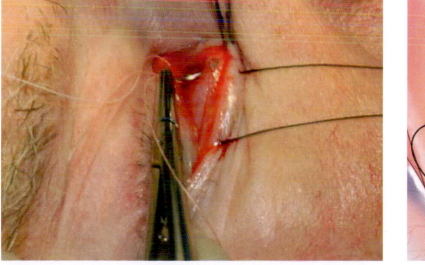

(D)

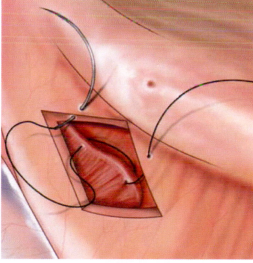

(E)

Figure 6.19 (**A–C**) The double-armed 5/0 Vicryl suture is passed through the eyelid retractors. (**D,E**) The needle is reversed and passed through the superior edges of the diamond-shaped conjunctival wound. (*Continued*)

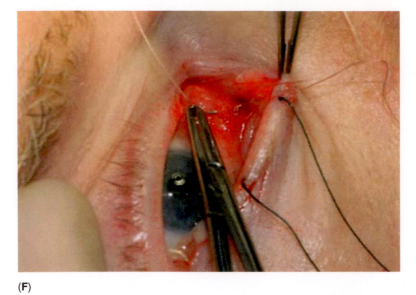

(F)

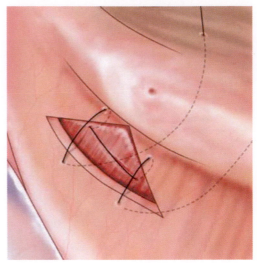

(G)

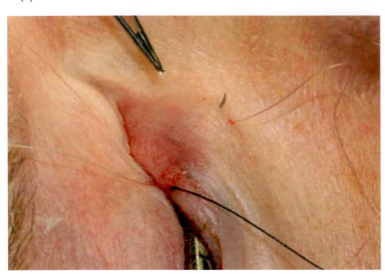

(H)

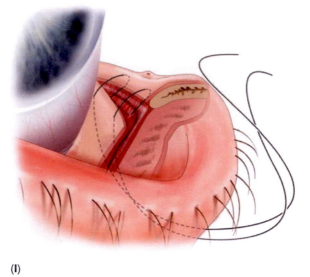

(I)

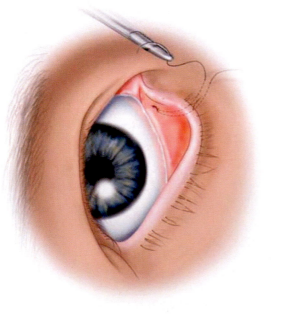

(J)

(K)

Figure 6.19 (Continued) (**F,G**) The needle is kept reversed and passed through the inferior edges of the diamond-shaped conjunctival wound. (**H,I**) The sutures are brought out through the skin at the lid-cheek junction. (**J,K**) The suture is pulled until the diamond is closed and the punctum is brought back into contact with the lacus lacrimalis.

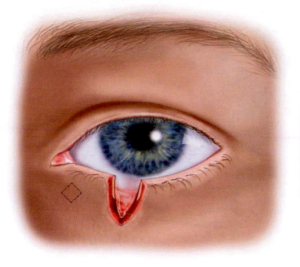
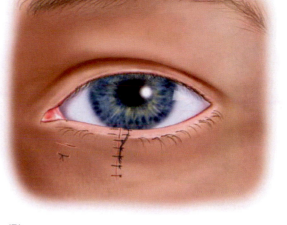

(A)   **(B)**

Figure 6.20 (**A**) A wedge resection is performed just lateral to the position of the medial spindle. (**B**) The wedge resection closure is performed after the closure of the medial spindle.

and subconjunctivally into the medial aspect of the lower eyelid.

2. The medial spindle procedure is performed first but the suture is not tied until the wedge resection has been performed.

3. The eyelid margin is held with Paufique forceps and a vertical incision is made with a no. 15 Bard Parker blade through the eyelid margin to a depth of approximately 2 mm. The blade is passed away from the globe for safety.

4. A vertical incision is then made to the base of the tarsus using straight iris scissors.

5. Hemostasis is achieved using bipolar cautery.

6. A second pair of Paufique forceps is then used to overlap the medial and lateral edges of the cut eyelid in order to assess the amount of eyelid that can safely be removed without placing undue tension on the wound.

7. The eyelid margin is again held with Paufique forceps and another vertical incision made with the no. 15 Bard Parker blade through the eyelid margin at the point of overlap.

8. A vertical incision is then made to the base of the tarsus using straight iris scissors.

9. The wedge excision is completed by angling the iris scissors at 45° at the base of the eyelid wounds and cutting inferomedially and inferolaterally.

10. A 5/0 Vicryl suture on a half circle needle is then passed through the tarsus just below the eyelid margin ensuring that the suture lies above the surface of the conjunctiva posteriorly and just beneath the skin anteriorly. The suture is tied with a single throw and the alignment of the eyelid checked. If it is not satisfactory, the suture is replaced. Once the alignment is satisfactory, the suture is loosened and used for traction by fixating it to the head drape using an artery clip. This elongates the wound making it easier to place further sutures in the tarsus.

11. Further 5/0 Vicryl sutures are placed horizontally through the tarsus and orbicularis muscle below the tarsus and tied.

12. The initial suture is now tied.

13. A 6/0 black silk suture is now passed horizontally through the gray line 2 to 3 mm from the wound edge and brought out through the gray line a similar distance from the wound edge. The needle is then reverse mounted and passed back as a horizontal mattress suture through the wound edges. The suture is tied causing the wound edges to evert slightly. A further 6/0 black silk suture is passed in the same way through the lash line and tied. The suture ends are cut leaving these long. The ends are incorporated in the skin closure sutures to keep the suture ends away from the cornea.

14. The skin edges are closed with interrupted 7/0 Vicryl sutures or with the 6/0 black silk sutures.

15. Antibiotic ointment is instilled into the eye.

Postoperative care. Postoperatively topical antibiotic ointment is prescribed three times a day for 2 weeks and the patient is instructed not to pull the eyelid down to instill this. The ointment should simply be smeared across the medial aspect of the eyelid. The sutures should not be removed for at least 2 weeks.

Medial Ectropion with Medial Canthal Tendon Laxity
In the majority of elderly patients with medial canthal tendon laxity, no specific measures are necessary to address this. A moderate degree of lateral punctal displacement is well tolerated and it may be inappropriate to subject the patient to a longer operative procedure. Where the degree of medial canthal tendon laxity is very pronounced, however, this can be addressed with a medial canthal resection procedure. In general, medial canthal tendon plication procedures do not tend to achieve adequate long-lasting results but may be attempted in those deemed fit enough to tolerate the surgery.

Medial Canthal Tendon Plication

Surgical procedure

1. One to two milliliters of 2% lidocaine with 1:80,000 units of adrenaline are injected subcutaneously and subconjunctivally into the medial aspect of the lower eyelid and plica semilunaris, and a further 1 to 2 mls are given as a regional infratrochlear nerve block.
2. A conjunctival incision is made with Westcott scissors between the caruncle and the plica semilunaris and extended to the medial end of the inferior tarsal plate (Fig. 6.21).
3. Stevens tenotomy scissors are then used to dissect bluntly down to the posterior lacrimal crest. Small Wright's retractors are then used to aid visualization of the periosteum of the crest.
4. A double-armed 5/0 Ethibond suture on a 1/2-circle needle is passed through the posterior lacrimal crest (Fig. 6.22).
5. Next, each needle of the Ethibond suture is passed through the exposed medial aspect of the tarsal plate (Fig. 6.23). The Ethibond suture is tied, bringing the eyelid into contact with the globe.
6. 7/0 Vicryl sutures are positioned across the conjunctival wound and tied to ensure that the Ethibond suture is not left exposed.
7. Antibiotic ointment is instilled into the eye.
8. Tincture of benzoin is applied to the cheek and forehead skin and a firm compressive dressing is applied. Tape is applied to the cheek and drawn superomedially to ensure that tension is reduced on the wound.

Postoperative care. The dressing is not removed for 4 to 5 days. Antibiotic ointment is prescribed three times a day for 2 weeks, and the patient is instructed not to pull the eyelid down to instill this. The ointment should simply be smeared across the medial aspect of the eyelid. Suture removal is not required.

Medial Canthal Resection

Surgical procedure

1. One to two milliliters of 0.5% Bupivacaine with 1:200,000 units of adrenaline mixed 50:50 with 2% lidocaine with 1:80,000 units of adrenaline are injected subcutaneously and subconjunctivally into the medial aspect of the lower eyelid.
2. A full-thickness vertical incision is made through the eyelid adjacent to the caruncle (Fig. 6.24).
3. A conjunctival incision is made with Westcott scissors between the caruncle and the plica semilunaris and extended to the medial end of the inferior tarsal plate (Fig. 6.21).
4. Stevens tenotomy scissors are then used to bluntly dissect down to the posterior lacrimal crest. Small Wright's retractors are then used to aid visualization of the periosteum of the crest.
5. A double-armed 5/0 Ethibond suture on a 1/2-circle needle is passed through the posterior lacrimal crest (Fig. 6.22).
6. Next, a triangular section of medial eyelid is removed, sufficient to allow the wound to be closed without undue tension (Fig. 6.25).

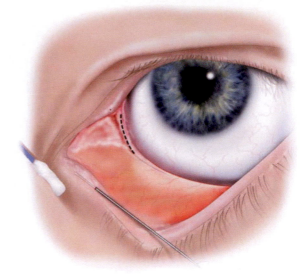

Figure 6.21 A conjunctival incision is made between the caruncle and the plica semilunaris.

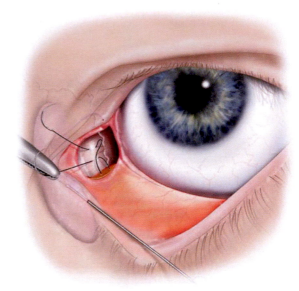

Figure 6.22 A double-armed 5/0 Ethibond suture on a 1/2-circle needle is passed through the medial aspect of the tarsus and through the periosteum of the posterior lacrimal crest.

7. The canaliculus is opened and marsupialized into the conjunctiva sac using interrupted 8/0 Vicryl sutures.
8. A Crawford style mono-canalicular silicone stent can be passed into the canaliculus.
9. Next, each needle of the Ethibond suture is passed through the cut end of the tarsus and tied, bringing the eyelid into contact with the globe.
10. 7/0 Vicryl sutures are positioned across the conjunctival wound and tied to ensure that the Ethibond suture is not left exposed.
11. The skin is then closed with interrupted 6/0 silk sutures to aid in support of the wound.
12. Antibiotic ointment is instilled into the eye.
13. Tincture of benzoin is applied to the cheek and forehead skin and a firm compressive dressing is applied. Tape is applied to the cheek and drawn

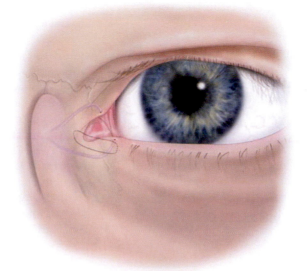

(A)

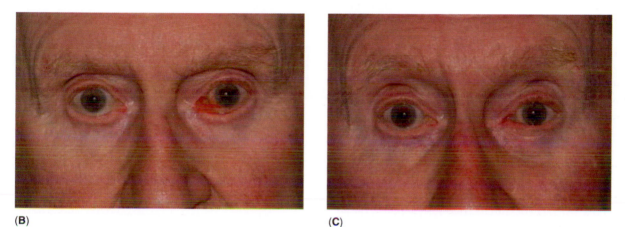

(B) (C)

Figure 6.23 (**A**) The suture is tied and the medial aspect of the eyelid is repositioned against the globe. (**B**) A patient with a left medial ectropion and laxity of the medial canthal tendon. He also has dry skin with cicatricial changes. (**C**) The postoperative appearance following a medial canthal tendon plication procedure which was combined with a small lower lid skin graft.

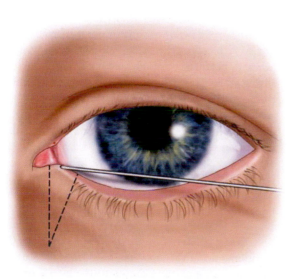

Figure 6.24 The extent of the excision in a medial canthal resection is demonstrated.

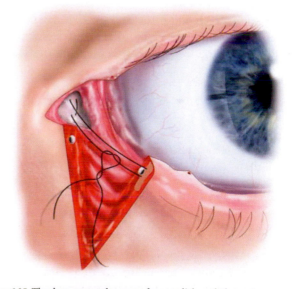

Figure 6.25 The deep suture placement for a medial canthal resection procedure is illustrated.

superomedially to ensure that tension is reduced on the wound.

Postoperative care. The dressing is not removed for 4 to 5 days. Antibiotic ointment is prescribed three times a day for 2 weeks and the patient is instructed not to pull the eyelid down to instill this. The ointment should simply be smeared across the medial aspect of the eyelid. The sutures are removed after 2 weeks.

Ectropion of the Whole Length of the Lower Eyelid with Lateral Canthal Tendon Laxity

The choice of procedure for a more extensive lower eyelid ectropion depends on a consideration of the following factors:

1. The degree of rounding of the lateral canthus
2. The presence of excess lower eyelid skin
3. The degree of horizontal eyelid laxity
4. The degree of upper eyelid laxity
5. The general health of the patient

If there is significant lateral canthal tendon laxity with rounding of the lateral canthus and a narrowing of the horizontal palpebral aperture, a wedge resection of the lateral aspect of the eyelid will further exaggerate the problem and will not address the underlying anatomical abnormality. A lateral tarsal strip procedure is preferable for such a patient. A lateral tarsal strip procedure is also more convenient as this avoids the need for suture removal but may leave an unsatisfactory overlap of the upper lid at the lateral canthus if the upper eyelid is very lax. The lateral tarsal strip procedure is also more problematic to perform in the obese, hypertensive patient, or in the patient who is unable to discontinue the use of aspirin preoperatively. If the patient has excess lower eyelid skin, a lateral wedge resection or a lateral tarsal strip procedure can be combined with a lower lid skin–muscle blepharoplasty or a skin pinch blepharoplasty.

These procedures can also be combined with a medial spindle procedure for a punctal ectropion that is not corrected by a lateral eyelid-tightening procedure. The medial spindle procedure should be performed prior to completing the repair of any lateral eyelid-tightening procedure.

Lateral Wedge Resection

The wedge resection is performed at the junction of the lateral third with the medial two-thirds of the eyelid. It is important to ensure that a retraction of the lower eyelid is not caused by too aggressive a resection of eyelid tissue.

Surgical Procedure
This is as described above.

Lateral Wedge Resection with Skin–Muscle Blepharoplasty
The vertical cutaneous scar created by a simple wedge resection can be avoided by creating a skin–muscle blepharoplasty flap and performing the wedge resection beneath this.

Surgical procedure
1. Two to three milliliters of 0.5% Bupivacaine with 1:200,000 units of adrenaline mixed 50:50 with 2% lidocaine with 1:80,000 units of adrenaline are injected subcutaneously along the entire length of the eyelid.

2. A 4/0 silk traction suture is placed through the gray line and fixated to the head drapes using an artery clip.
3. A subciliary skin incision is made with a Colorado needle extending inferolaterally at the lateral canthus in a skin crease.
4. A skin–muscle flap is dissected inferiorly from the orbital septum for approximately 8 to 9 mm and extended laterally.
5. The traction suture is now removed.
6. Next, a wedge resection of the underlying posterior lamella is performed and the wound closed as described above.
7. The skin–muscle flap is drawn laterally and the excess skin and muscle are resected as a base-down triangle.
8. The subciliary skin incision is closed with interrupted 7/0 Vicryl sutures (Fig. 6.26).
9. The 6/0 silk sutures are sewn to the skin of the lower eyelid with interrupted 7/0 Vicryl sutures.

Postoperative care. Postoperatively topical antibiotic ointment is prescribed three times a day for 2 weeks and the patient is instructed not to pull the eyelid down to instill this. The ointment should simply be smeared across the eyelid margin. The sutures should not be removed for at least 2 weeks. Cool packs can be applied intermittently for 24 hours.

Lateral Tarsal Strip Procedure
Surgical procedure
1. Three to four milliliters of 0.5% Bupivacaine with 1:200,000 units of adrenaline mixed 50:50 with 2% lidocaine with 1:80,000 units of adrenaline are injected subcutaneously into the lateral aspect of the upper and lower eyelids and into the lateral canthus.
2. A lateral canthotomy is performed using straight blunt-tipped scissors (Fig. 6.27). The canthotomy is extended to the lateral orbital rim. (A Colorado needle can be used instead if available.)
3. The lower eyelid is then lifted in a superotemporal direction and the inferior crus of the lateral canthal tendon is cut using blunt-tipped Westcott scissors (Fig. 6.28).
4. The septum is also freed with the Westcott scissors until the eyelid becomes loose. Care is taken to avoid excessive bleeding by using bipolar cautery. It is easier to perform the initial steps of this procedure sitting at the head of the patient. It is then preferable to move to the side of the patient to complete the remainder of the procedure.
5. Once the lower eyelid has been freed of its canthal attachments, the anterior and posterior lamellae are split along the gray line using Westcott scissors (Fig. 6.29). This is aided by holding the skin and orbicularis muscle taut at the lateral end of the eyelid with Paufique forceps.
6. The lateral tarsal strip is then formed by cutting along the inferior border of the tarsus (Fig. 6.30). Next, the eyelid margin of the tarsal strip is excised (Fig. 6.31).
7. The tarsal strip is then drawn to the lateral orbital margin to determine the extent of any redundant tarsal strip. This is then excised (Fig. 6.32).

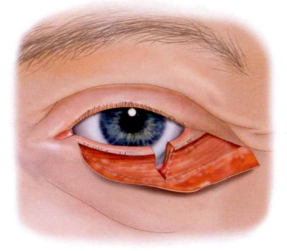

(A)

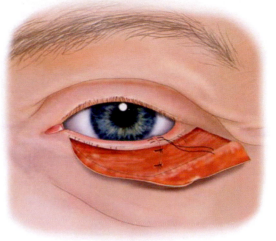

(B)

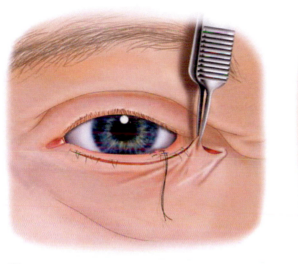

(C)

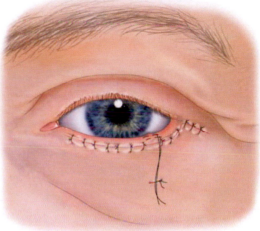

(D)

Figure 6.26 (**A**) A skin–muscle flap is raised and a lateral wedge resection performed. (**B**) The wedge resection is repaired. (**C**) The skin muscle flap is drawn laterally and the excess skin and muscle are resected as a base-down triangle. (**D**) The lateral skin wound and the subciliary incision wound are closed with 7/0 Vicryl sutures.

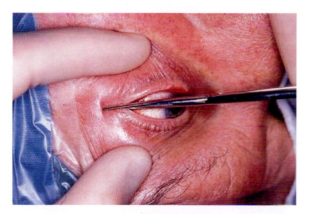

Figure 6.27 A lateral canthotomy is performed using straight blunt-tipped scissors (surgeon's view).

8. The tarsal strip is then positioned over the handle of a Paufique forceps with the conjunctival side exposed and the conjunctiva scraped from the tarsal strip using a no. 15 blade (Fig. 6.33). Alternatively

this can be achieved by the gentle application of bipolar cautery using a sweeping motion.

9. The redundant anterior lamella is excised with the Westcott scissors (Fig. 6.34).

10. Next, a double-armed 5/0 Vicryl suture on a 1/2-circle needle is passed through the periosteum of the lateral orbital wall, the needles each being passed from inside the orbital rim exiting at the rim, leaving a loop (Fig. 6.35A).

11. The end of the tarsal strip is passed through the loop. The needle is then reverse mounted and passed from the under surface of the tarsal strip exiting on the anterior surface lateral to the loop. This is repeated with the second needle. As the suture is pulled, the loop is then tightened, drawing the tarsal strip in a posterior direction against the globe (Fig. 6.35B,C).

12. The suture is then tied avoiding excessive tension.

13. A single 7/0 Vicryl suture is passed through the gray line at the edges of the lateral aspects of the upper

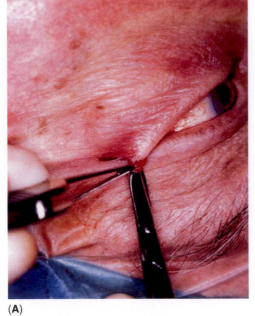

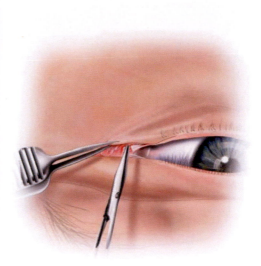

(A)   (B)

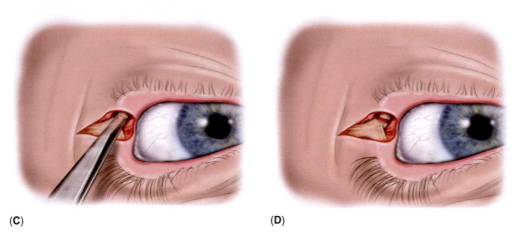

(C)   (D)

Figure 6.28 (**A**) The lower eyelid is then lifted in a superotemporal direction and the inferior crus of the lateral canthal tendon is cut using blunt-tipped Westcott scissors. (**B**) All residual attachments of the eyelid to the lateral orbital margin are released by cutting all tissues between the skin and the conjunctiva laterally. (**C**) This drawing shows that the inferior crus of the lateral canthal tendon is severed. (**D**) This drawing shows the effect of the inferior cantholysis. The eyelid should now be loose and freely mobile when drawn laterally.

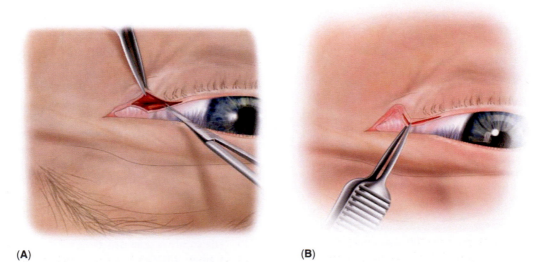

(A)   (B)

Figure 6.29 (**A**) The anterior and posterior lamellae are split along the gray line using sharp-tipped scissors. (**B**) The gray line has been split.

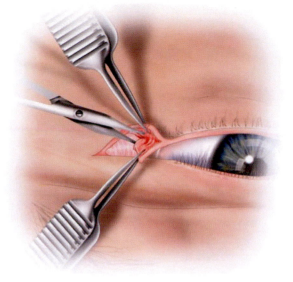

Figure 6.30 The lateral tarsal strip is then formed by cutting along the inferior border of the tarsus.

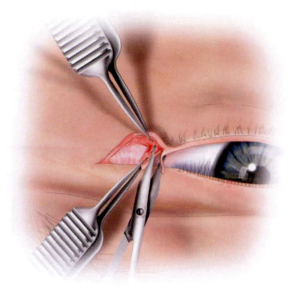

Figure 6.31 Next, the posterior eyelid margin is excised from the tarsal strip.

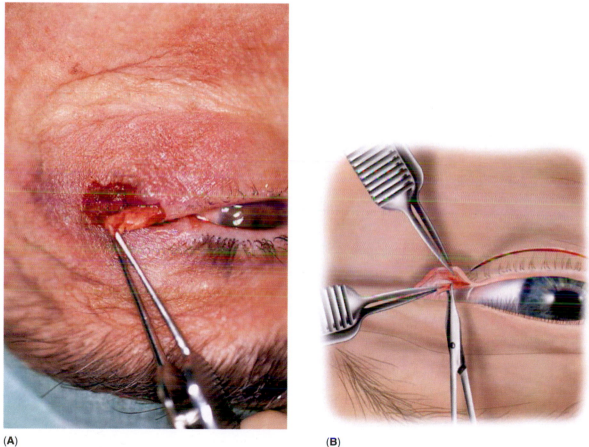

(A)   (B)

Figure 6.32 (A) The tarsal strip is drawn laterally to determine if some redundant tarsus needs to be excised. (B) The tarsal strip is shortened as required.

and lower eyelids reforming the angle of the lateral commissure.

14. The lateral canthotomy wound is then closed using interrupted 7/0 Vicryl sutures subcutaneously ensuring that the 5/0 Vicryl suture is buried, followed by interrupted 7/0 Vicryl sutures to the skin wound (Figs. 6.35D and 6.36).

The lateral tarsal strip procedure can also be combined with a skin–muscle blepharoplasty or a lateral skin pinch blepharoplasty procedure where necessary.

Postoperative care. Postoperatively topical antibiotic ointment is prescribed three times a day for 2 weeks, and the patient is instructed not to pull the eyelid down to instill this.

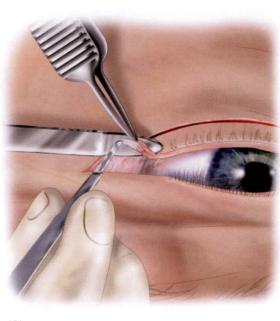

(A)

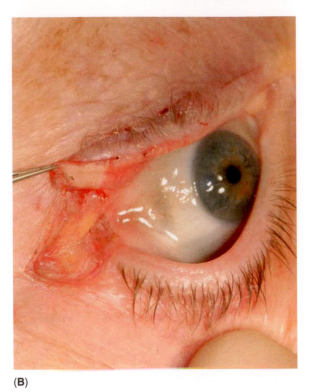

(B)

Figure 6.33 (**A**) The tarsal strip is then positioned over the handle of a Paufique forceps with the conjunctival side exposed and the conjunctiva scraped from the tarsal strip using a no. 15 blade. (**B**) The appearance of the tarsal strip after the conjunctiva has been removed.

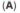

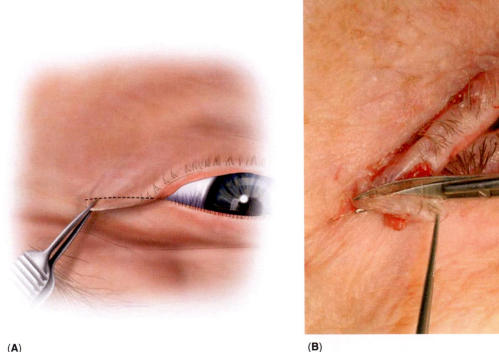

(A)   (B)

Figure 6.34 (**A**) The lid is drawn laterally and the amount of redundant anterior lamella is determined. (**B**) The redundant anterior lamella is removed.

The ointment should simply be smeared across the eyelid margin. Any remaining sutures can be removed after 2 weeks. Cool packs can be applied intermittently for 24 hours.

Complete Tarsal Ectropion
This type of lower eyelid ectropion, in which the tarsal plate is completely everted, is rare. The diagnosis is reserved for those patients who have no cicatricial element and little horizontal eyelid laxity. The condition is thought to be due to disinsertion of the lower eyelid retractors from the lower border of the tarsal plate. The malposition is managed by a combination of a posterior approach retractor reinsertion, a medial spindle procedure and a lateral tarsal strip procedure.

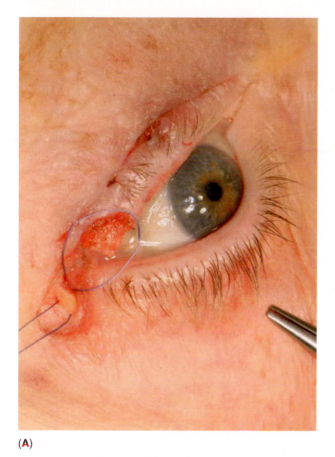

(A)

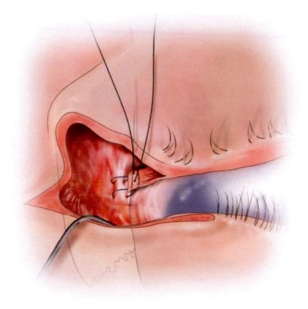

(B)

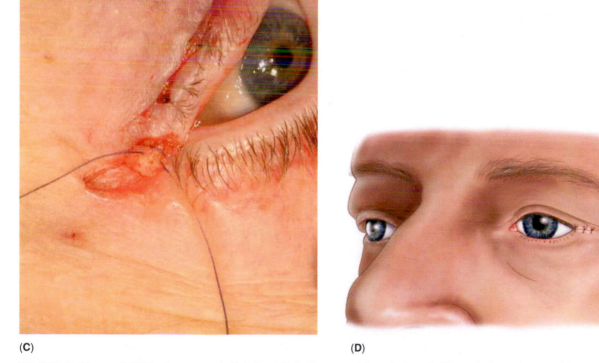

(C)   (D)

Figure 6.35 (**A**) A double-armed 5/0 Vicryl suture on a half-circle needle has been passed through the periorbita on the internal aspect of the lateral orbital margin at the lateral orbital tubercle. A loop of suture has been left. (**B**) The lateral tarsal strip has been passed through the loop of suture. The suture needles have then been passed through the strip from below. (**C**) As the suture is pulled taut, the eyelid is drawn laterally and posteriorly into contact with the globe. If the eyelid is pulled anteriorly, the suture has not been positioned correctly and should be replaced. (**D**) The lateral canthal wound is closed with interrupted 7/0 Vicryl sutures.

Posterior Approach Retractor Reinsertion with Medial Spindle with Lateral Tarsal Strip Procedure
Surgical procedure

1. Three to four milliliters of 0.5% Bupivacaine with 1:200,000 units of adrenaline mixed 50:50 with 2% lidocaine with 1:80,000 units of adrenaline are injected subcutaneously and subconjunctivally into the lower eyelid along its entire length.

2. A 4/0 silk traction suture is placed through the gray line and the eyelid is everted over a medium sized Desmarres retractor.

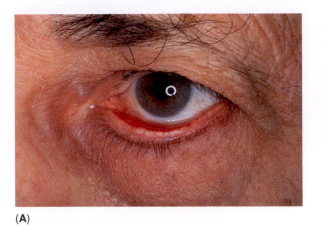

(A)

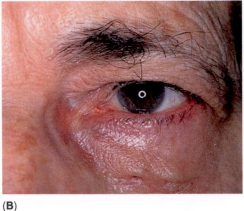

(B)

Figure 6.36 (**A**) A lower eyelid involutional ectropion. (**B**) The appearance 2 weeks following a lateral tarsal strip procedure.

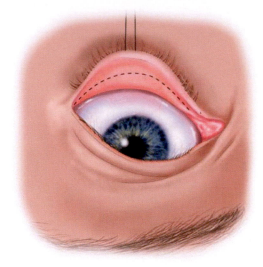

(A)

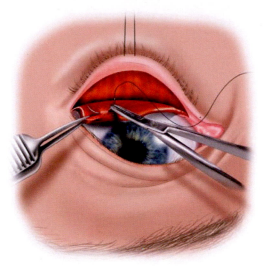

(B)

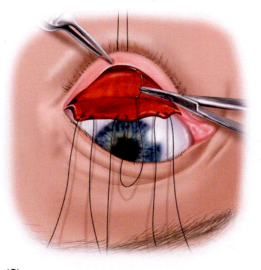

(C)

Figure 6.37 (**A**) A conjunctival incision is made at the lower border of the tarsus. (**B**) The lower eyelid retractors are dissected free and sutures passed through the retractors as shown in the drawing. (**C**) The lower eyelid retractors are advanced and sutured to the inferior border of the tarsus.

3. A conjunctival incision is made with either a no. 15 Bard Parker blade extending from a point 2 to 3 mm lateral to the punctum to the lateral canthus. The conjunctiva is undermined inferiorly for 6 to 7 mm using blunt-tipped Westcott scissors.

4. The lower eyelid retractors are now visible and are dissected from the orbital septum and orbicularis muscle with Westcott scissors.

5. Next, the retractors are advanced and reattached to the inferior border of the tarsal plate with interrupted 5/0 Vicryl sutures (Fig. 6.37).

6. The conjunctival flap is repositioned and closed with interrupted 7/0 Vicryl sutures, taking care to bury the sutures beneath the conjunctival wound (Fig. 6.38).

Next, a medial spindle procedure is performed followed by a lateral tarsal strip procedure as described above (Fig. 6.39).

Antibiotic ointment is instilled into the eye and a compressive dressing is applied.

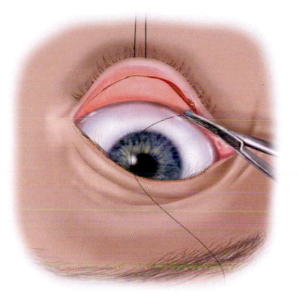

Figure 6.38 The conjunctival wound is closed ensuring that the suture knots are buried.

Postoperative care. The dressing is removed after 48 hours. Postoperatively topical antibiotic ointment is prescribed three times a day for 2 weeks, and the patient is instructed not to pull the eyelid down to instill this. The ointment should simply be smeared across the eyelid margin. The sutures are removed after 2 weeks. Cool packs can be applied intermittently for 24 hours.

Cicatricial Ectropion

A cicatricial lower eyelid ectropion is caused by scarring or contracture of the skin and/or orbicularis muscle, causing a vertical shortening of the eyelid. The causes are numerous:

1. Actinic damage from chronic sun exposure
2. Acute/chronic dermatitis, e.g., allergy to topical glaucoma medications, eczema
3. Morphoeic basal cell carcinoma of the lower eyelid/ medial canthus (Fig. 6.14)
4. Tumor irradiation therapy
5. Thermal/chemical burns
6. Specific dermatological disorders, e.g., lamellar ichthyosis
7. Trauma
8. Iatrogenic, e.g., following lower lid blepharoplasty or laser skin resurfacing/chemical peel, blowout fracture repair with scarring of the orbicularis muscle/orbital septum to the orbital margin, over-correction of lower eyelid entropion (Fig. 6.40).

Medical treatment alone may suffice for some of the many causes of cicatricial ectropion, e.g., discontinuation of topical glaucoma drops causing allergic dermatitis and the short-term application of topical steroid cream to the affected periocular skin. Although some patients will benefit from soft tissue rearrangement techniques for a very specific localized scar, e.g., a Z-plasty, such situations are not encountered very frequently. A full-thickness skin graft is more often required. A mid-face lift can recruit skin into the lower eyelid in some patients who have a mid-face ptosis. This procedure is preferable to a skin graft in patients who would find the postoperative appearance of the skin graft unacceptable.

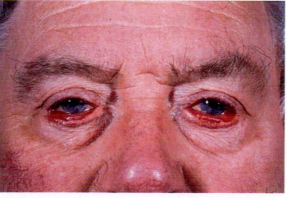

(A)

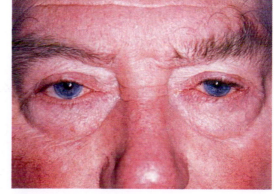

(B)

Figure 6.39 (**A**) A bilateral lower lid tarsal ectropion. (**B**) The postoperative appearance following a posterior approach retractor advancement, a medial spindle procedure, and a lateral tarsal strip procedure.

A small medial ectropion will usually require a small skin graft alone, although this can be combined with a medial spindle procedure. Where the ectropion is more extensive a horizontal eyelid-shortening procedure, either a wedge resection or a lateral tarsal strip, should be combined with the skin graft, to prevent a recurrence of the ectropion. A cicatricial ectropion affecting children is an exception to this rule.

A skin graft may be taken from a variety of sites:

1. The upper eyelid
2. The preauricular region
3. The postauricular region
4. The supraclavicular fossa
5. The upper inner arm

Each site has its advantages and disadvantages. The upper eyelid skin provides the best quality skin. It provides a good color match. It is easy to remove and has no subcutaneous fat. It is therefore very quick to prepare. The wound is simple to close. The upper lid, however, may not be a suitable site in some patients. It may show extensive actinic damage. There may be insufficient skin available to remove without risking a secondary lagophthalmos. It may leave an obvious asymmetry. It may exaggerate an associated brow ptosis.

The hairless preauricular also provides a good color match and is an easy site to access. The site may not, however, yield sufficient skin. It may also be affected by actinic damage. The postauricular site provides good skin but is unsuitable for patients who wear a hearing aid. The wound is rather more problematic to close because of difficulties with easy access and closure may alter the position of the ear.

The supraclavicular fossa skin tends to be rather pale. It can leave an unsightly scar and is best avoided in female patients who wear open-necked clothing.

The upper inner arm skin is pale but can yield a good result, particularly if the grafts are placed bilaterally. The skin is protected from solar damage. It is easy to access and large grafts can be harvested. The wound edges can be undermined to facilitate easy closure. If the wound breaks down, it can be left to heal by secondary intention. The scar is then far less obtrusive. The additional advantage is that the skin graft harvesting and the wound closure can be performed by a surgical assistant while the surgeon is working on the eyelid. This can save a great deal of valuable surgical time.

Lateral Wedge Resection or Lateral Tarsal Strip Procedure with Skin Graft
Surgical procedure
1. Three to four milliliters of 0.5% Bupivacaine with 1:200,000 units of adrenaline mixed 50:50 with 2% lidocaine with 1:80,000 units of adrenaline are injected subcutaneously into the lower eyelid along its entire length, and at the lateral aspect of the upper lid.
2. Seven to ten milliliters of the same solution are injected subcutaneously at the skin graft donor site.
3. Two 4/0 silk traction sutures are placed through the gray line and fixated to the head drapes using artery clips.
4. A subciliary skin incision is made with a no. 15 Bard Parker blade from a point 2 to 3 mm medial to the

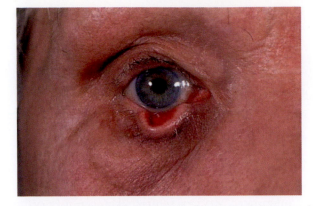

Figure 6.40 A marked cicatricial ectropion following the use of a Wies procedure for a lower eyelid involutional entropion.

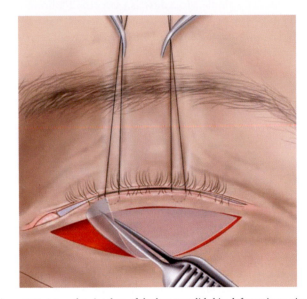

Figure 6.41 A template is taken of the lower eyelid skin defect using a piece of Steridrape.

punctum to a point 3 to 4 mm lateral to the lateral commissure.
5. A skin flap is dissected inferiorly from the orbicularis muscle using blunt-tipped Westcott scissors for a distance of approximately 7 to 8 mm. The eyelid margin should now rise with the pull from the traction sutures. If there is scarring at a deeper level, however, the eyelid will remain in the same position. Westcott scissors are now used to dissect the scar tissue away from the eyelid retractors or from the conjunctiva if the retractors are scarred.
6. The traction sutures are released.
7. Next, a wedge resection of the underlying posterior lamella is performed or, alternatively, a lateral tarsal strip procedure is performed as described above
8. The traction sutures are gently tightened again using the artery clips, exaggerating the anterior lamellar defect.
9. Next, a template is taken of the skin defect using a piece of Steridrape and a gentian violet marker pen (Fig. 6.41).
10. The template is transferred to the skin graft donor site and outlined with a gentian violet marker pen (Fig. 6.42A).

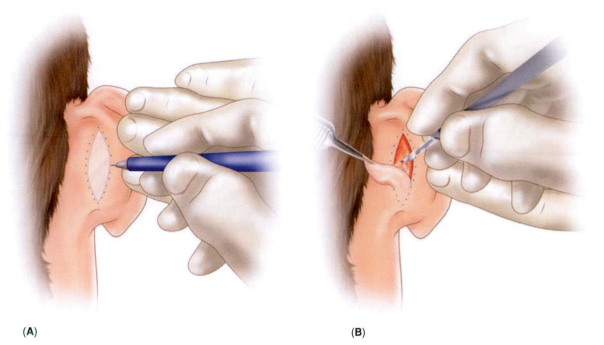

(A)   **(B)**

Figure 6.42 (**A**) The template has been transferred to the postauricular area and outlined with gentian violet. (**B**) The skin graft is harvested using a no. 15 Bard Parker blade.

11. The skin is incised with a no. 15 Bard Parker blade along the mark.

12. The skin graft is then raised at one end with a skin hook or forceps while counter traction is applied. The graft is then peeled away using a sweeping action with the blade (Fig. 6.42B).

13. The donor site is closed with a continuous interlocking 4/0 nylon suture. If the wound is under tension, the margins are undermined, and interrupted 4/0 nylon sutures are placed in a vertical mattress fashion. Antibiotic ointment is applied to the wound and a sterile dressing is applied.

14. The skin graft is placed over the tip of the surgeon's forefinger. Westcott scissors are used to remove all subcutaneous tissue meticulously until the "rete pegs" are visible (Fig. 6.43).

15. The graft is then transferred to the lower eyelid and sutured into the defect using four 6/0 silk bolster sutures. Interrupted 7/0 Vicryl sutures are placed in between the silk sutures (Fig. 6.44A).

16. The graft is then covered in topical antibiotic ointment, a piece of Jelonet and a piece of sterile sponge shaped from the template. The bolster sutures are tied over the sponge with only a moderate degree of tension (Fig. 6.44B). The bolster sutures can be omitted in small grafts, and a piece of rolled up Jelonet applied to the graft instead.

17. Tincture of benzoin is painted on the forehead and allowed to dry. The lower lid traction sutures are fixated to the forehead with Steri-strips. The suture is folded down and further Steri-strips are applied. The suture is folded up and yet further Steri-strips are applied.

18. Topical antibiotic ointment is liberally applied to the eyelids.

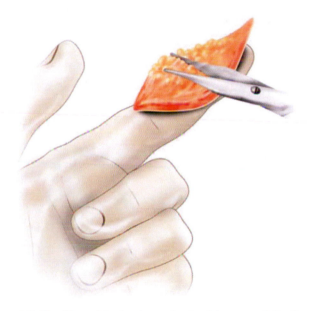

Figure 6.43 The skin graft is placed over the tip of the surgeon's forefinger with the subcutaneous surface uppermost. Westcott scissors are used to remove all subcutaneous tissue meticulously.

19. A firm compressive dressing with a supporting bandage is applied.

Postoperative care. The bandage is removed by the patient after 48 hours, but the underlying dressing is not removed until 5 days postoperatively, along with the donor site dressing. The silk bolster sutures are carefully removed. Topical antibiotic ointment is prescribed three times a day for 2 weeks and the patient is instructed to smear this across the graft. The Vicryl sutures are removed after 2 weeks, along with the donor site sutures. The patient is then instructed to commence massage to the skin graft in a horizontal and upward direction for

3 min, three times a day for at least 6 to 8 weeks after applying Lacrilube ointment to the graft. A silicone gel may be applied to help to prevent any thickening of the graft e.g., Kelocote or Dermatix, but this adds expense (Fig. 6.45).

Mid-face Lift
This is described in chapter 15 on "Blepharoplasty".

Soft Tissue Expansion
This is described in chapter 12 on "Eyelid Reconstruction".

Mechanical Ectropion
The diagnosis of mechanical lower eyelid ectropion is made where a mass lesion or a mid-face ptosis is responsible for pushing or pulling the eyelid out of its normal position. The ectropion is managed by directing treatment at the underlying cause (Fig. 6.46).

If a mid-face ptosis is causing the ectropion, as may be seen in a chronic facial palsy, the ptosis itself may be addressed in a number of ways, depending on the individual circumstances.

Treatment may be by facial suspension techniques, e.g., fascia lata graft suspension, temporalis muscle transfer, or by nerve substitution techniques, e.g., facial hypoglossal nerve anastomosis, or cross facial nerve grafting with gracilis or pectoralis muscle transplantation, performed by plastic surgery or ENT colleagues. Alternatively, the cheek may be raised by a suborbicularis oculi fat lift or a subperiosteal mid-face lift procedure, performed via a swinging lower eyelid approach and combined with a lateral tarsal strip procedure (see chap. 15).

In elderly patients, the mid-face ptosis can instead be accepted and the ectropion, whose etiology may be multifactorial, may be addressed by means of a combination of eyelid procedures only, e.g., a medial spindle, a posterior approach retractor recession, a full-thickness skin graft, and a lateral tarsal strip procedure (Fig. 6.47).

Paralytic Ectropion
The surgical management of paralytic ectropion depends on the degree of ectropion, and on the additional etiological factors that may be responsible for the ectropion,

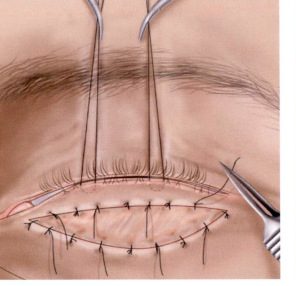
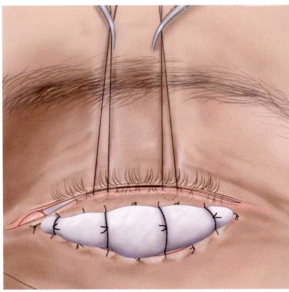

(A)   (B)

Figure 6.44 (**A**) The skin graft is anchored into place with interrupted 6/0 silk sutures, and interrupted 7/0 Vicryl sutures are placed in between. (**B**) The silk sutures are then tied over a sponge bolster.

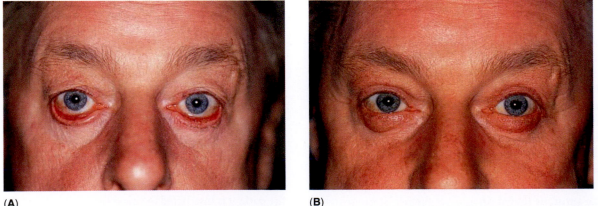

(A)   (B)

Figure 6.45 (**A**) A patient with a bilateral lower eyelid cicatricial ectropion. (**B**) The postoperative appearance 3 months following placement of lower eyelid skin grafts combined with a bilateral medial spindle procedure and a bilateral lateral tarsal strip procedure. The surgery was performed on one eyelid at a time separated by a period of 2 weeks.

e.g., cicatricial changes from chronic epiphora, mechanical changes from a mid-face ptosis. A mild degree of paralytic ectropion in a patient with exposure keratopathy may benefit from a simple lateral tarsorrhaphy. A mild degree of ectropion alone may be managed with a lateral tarsal strip procedure. A chronic paralytic ectropion with medial canthal tendon laxity would be best managed with a medial canthal tendon resection procedure.

A mild degree of paralytic medial ectropion can be managed by means of a simple medial canthoplasty.

Medial Canthoplasty
Surgical procedure

1. A vertical incision is marked just medial to the medial commissure using a gentian violet marker pen (Fig. 6.48A).
2. One to two milliliters of 0.5% Bupivacaine with 1:200,000 units of adrenaline mixed 50:50 with 2% lidocaine with 1:80,000 units of adrenaline are injected subcutaneously into the medial aspects of the upper and lower eyelids.

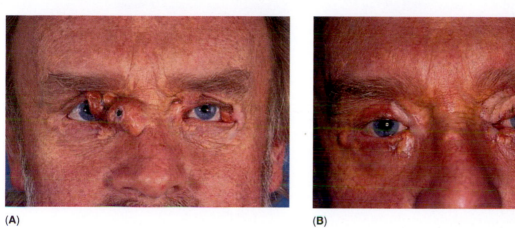

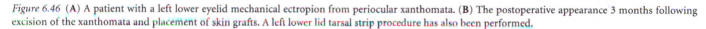

(A)   **(B)**

Figure 6.46 (**A**) A patient with a left lower eyelid mechanical ectropion from periocular xanthomata. (**B**) The postoperative appearance 3 months following excision of the xanthomata and placement of skin grafts. A left lower lid tarsal strip procedure has also been performed.

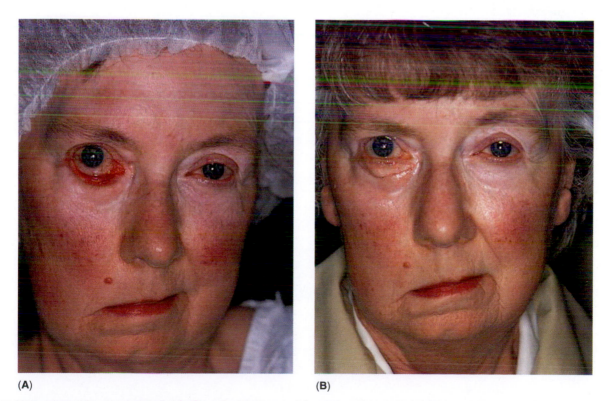

(A)   **(B)**

Figure 6.47 (**A**) A patient with a chronic right facial palsy and a right lower eyelid ectropion. The ectropion is due to a combination of factors. It is paralytic, involutional, cicatricial, and mechanical. (**B**) The ectropion has been addressed by means of a posterior approach lower lid retractor recession, a lower eyelid skin graft and a lateral tarsal strip procedure, and a medial spindle procedure. The mid-face ptosis has not been addressed in this patient.

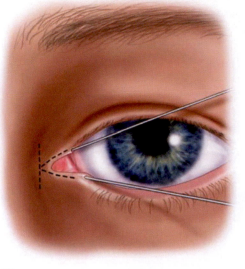

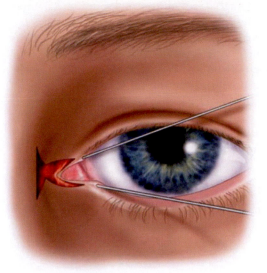

(A)   (B)

Figure 6.48 (**A**) A vertical incision is marked just medial to the medial commissure using gentian violet. (**B**) The eyelid skin is incised medial to the puncta and anterior to the canaliculi using a no. 15 Bard Parker blade. The canaliculi are protected by inserting 00 Bowman probes.

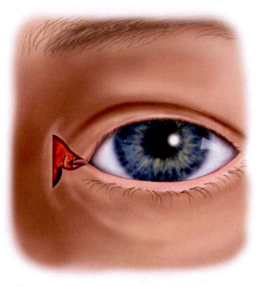

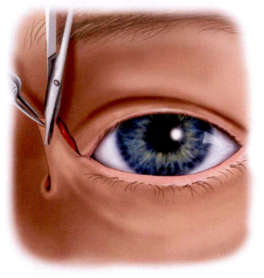

(A)   (B)

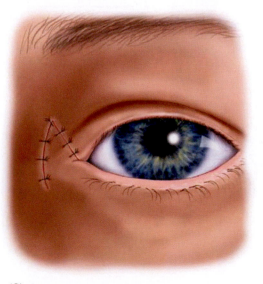

(C)

Figure 6.49 (**A**) Two 7/0 Vicryl sutures are passed though the pericanalicular tissue and tied. (**B**) The inferior skin flap is drawn medially and the dog-ear removed with Westcott scissors. (**C**) The skin is closed with interrupted 7/0 Vicryl sutures.

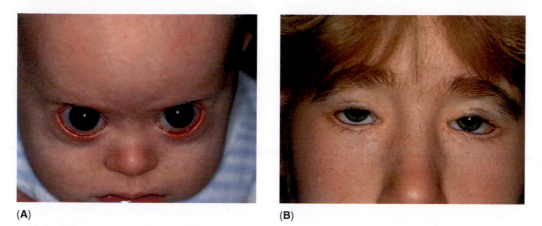

(A)					**(B)**

Figure 6.50 (**A**) An infant with a bilateral congenital lower eyelid ectropion due to a vertical skin shortening. The infant has Down's syndrome. (**B**) A patient with a bilateral lateral cicatricial ectropion. The patient has a blepharophimosis syndrome. She had undergone medial canthal surgery and ptosis surgery elsewhere.

3. The eyelid skin is incised medial to the puncta and anterior to the canaliculi using a no. 15 Bard Parker blade and Paufique forceps. The canaliculi are protected by inserting 00 Bowman probes (Fig. 6.48B).

4. The skin is undermined using blunt-tipped Westcott scissors.

5. A vertical relieving incision is made inferiorly at the medial aspect of the inferior skin flap.

6. Two 7/0 Vicryl sutures are passed though the pericanalicular tissue and tied (Fig. 6.49A).

7. The inferior skin flap is drawn medially and the dog-ear removed with Westcott scissors (Fig. 6.49B).

8. The skin is closed with interrupted 7/0 Vicryl sutures (Fig. 6.49C).

Postoperative care. Postoperatively topical antibiotic ointment is prescribed three times a day for 2 weeks. The sutures can be removed after 2 weeks.

Congenital Lower Eyelid Ectropion

The majority of patients with congenital ectropion of the lower eyelid have additional facial abnormalities, e.g., patients with Down's syndrome (Fig. 6.50A), blepharophimosis-ptosis-epicanthus inversus syndrome (Fig. 6.50B), Möbius syndrome (Fig. 6.13), or lamellar ichthyosis (Fig. 6.9). The patient's ectropion is usually either cicatricial or paralytic in etiology. The majority of such patients require a full-thickness skin graft in conjunction with a lateral tarsal strip procedure. The cosmetic results of such surgery are poor in comparison to the results in adults as skin grafts tend to thicken and be much more obtrusive in young patients.

FURTHER READING

1. American Academy of Ophthalmology. Basic and Clinical Science Course: Orbit, Eyelids, and Lacrimal System, section 7. San Francisco: The American Academy of Ophthalmology, 2006/7: 201–5.

2. Anderson RL, Gordy DD. The tarsal strip procedure. Arch Ophthalmol 1979; 97: 2192–6.

3. Bosniak SL, Zilkha MC. Ectropion. In: Nesi FA, Lisman RD, Levine MR, eds. Smith's Ophthalmic, Plastic and Reconstructive Surgery, 2nd edn. St Louis: Mosby, 1987: 290–307.

4. Dutton JJ. Atlas of clinical and surgical orbital anatomy. Philadelphia, PA: WB Saunders, 1994.

5. Fong KCS, Mavrikakis I, Sagili S, Malhotra R. Correction of involutional lower eyelid medial ectropion with transconjunctival approach retractor plication and lateral tarsal strip. ACTA Ophthalmol Scand 2006; 84: 246–9.

6. Gilbard SM. Involutional and paralytic ectropion. In: Bosniak S, ed. Principles and Practice of Ophthalmic Plastic and Reconstructive Surgery, Vol 1. Philadelphia, PA: WB Saunders, 1996: 422–37.

7. Giola VM, Linberg JV, McCormick SA. The anatomy of the lateral canthal tendon. Arch Ophthalmol 1987; 105: 529–32.

8. Goldberg et al. Ectropion repair. In: Wobig JL, Dailey RA, eds. Oculofacial Plastic Surgery, Face, Lacrimal System, and Orbits. New York, NY: Thieme, 2004: 97–102.

9. Jordan DR, Anderson RL. The lateral tarsal strip revisited: the enhanced tarsal strip. Arch Ophthalmol 1989; 107: 604–6.

10. Kahana A, Lucarelli MJ. Adjunctive transcanthotomy lateral suborbicularis fat lift and orbitomalar ligament resuspension in lower eyelid ectropion repair. Ophthal Plast Reconstr Surg 2009; 25: 1–6.

11. Marshall JA, Valenzuela AA, Strutton GM, Sullivan TJ. Anterior lamella actinic changes as a factor in involutional eyelid malposition, Ophthal Plast Reconstr Surg 2006; 22(3): 192–4.

12. Nerad JA, Carter KD, Alford MA. Ectropion. In: Rapid Diagnosis in Ophthalmology: Oculoplastic and Reconstructive Surgery. Philadelphia, PA: Mosby Elsevier, 2008: 80–91.

13. Nowinski TS, Anderson RL. The medial spindle procedure for involutional medial ectropion. Arch Ophthal 1985; 103: 1750–3.

14. Penne RB. Ectropion. In: Color Atlas and Synopsis of Clinical Ophthalmology: Oculoplastics. New York, NY: McGraw-Hill, 2003: 62–9.

15. Robinson FO, Collin JRO. Ectropion. In: Yanoff M, Duker J, eds., Ophthalmology. Philadelphia, PA: Mosby, 2004: 676–83.

16. Tse DT. Ectropion repair. In: Levine MR, ed. Manual of Oculoplastic Surgery, 2nd edn. Boston, MA: Butterworth-Heinemann, 1996: 147–56.

7 Blepharoptosis

INTRODUCTION

The term "ptosis" refers to the drooping of any body part, e.g., eyebrow ptosis, mid-face ptosis, lash ptosis. In this chapter, the term will be used to refer to a drooping of the upper eyelid (a blepharoptosis). A ptosis can affect all age groups and may be congenital or acquired. The causes of ptosis are numerous. It is important to appreciate that ptosis itself is merely a physical sign, and not a diagnosis. Therefore, before any therapeutic decision is made for the management of a patient with a ptosis, it is essential to determine the underlying cause. It is particularly important to bear in mind that a ptosis can be the presenting sign of a serious life-threatening systemic disorder. In considering the causes, it is useful to use a classification of ptosis which is based upon etiological factors (Table 7.1). This should be borne in mind when examining a patient who presents with a ptosis.

CLASSIFICATION

The classification of ptosis aims to provide some insight into the pathological processes involved. A pseudoptosis should be differentiated from a true ptosis. A true ptosis, in turn, can be categorized as neurogenic (due to an abnormality of the innervation of the levator palpebrae superioris or of Müller's muscle), myogenic (due to an abnormality of the levator muscle itself), aponeurotic (due to a defect within the levator aponeurosis or in the attachment of the aponeurosis to the tarsus), or mechanical (due to the mechanical effects of adhesions in the superior conjunctival fornix or of a mass in the upper eyelid or anterior superior orbit). These etiological mechanisms may be found in all age groups but with varying frequency. Congenital "dystrophic" ptosis and involutional aponeurotic ptosis are by far the most common types of ptosis encountered in clinical practice.

Pseudoptosis

Pseudoptosis (Table 7.2) refers to a condition that mimics a true ptosis.

> **KEY POINT**
>
> It is particularly important that a pseudoptosis is clearly recognized and that a neurological or myogenic cause of ptosis requiring further evaluation or an alternative therapeutic approach is excluded before ptosis surgery is embarked upon.

Contralateral Eyelid Retraction

Contralateral upper eyelid retraction may lead to diagnostic confusion, with the normal eyelid appearing to be ptotic. A patient presenting with unilateral eyelid retraction, e.g., from undiagnosed thyroid eye disease, may complain of a ptosis affecting the fellow eyelid (Fig. 7.1).

Hemifacial Spasm

This condition is characterized by unilateral, involuntary, intermittent, and irregular contractions of the muscles of facial expression (Fig. 7.2). The orbicularis muscle is usually the first facial muscle to be involved. In some patients the early signs may be quite subtle. The patient will typically complain of a droopy eyelid but, in addition to an apparent blepharoptosis, the position of the lower eyelid will be seen to be higher than the fellow eyelid causing an even greater vertical narrowing of the palpebral aperture. In some cases, the cause is compression of the facial nerve in the posterior cranial fossa by an aberrant artery. In these cases, neurosurgical decompression of the nerve may be successful in controlling the spasms when these are severe but the risks of such invasive surgical intervention should be considered very carefully. Injections of botulinum toxin into the medial and lateral aspects of the upper and lower eyelids can be very successful in controlling the associated blepharospasm but may lead to significant orbicularis weakness with the need to use very frequent topical lubricants to prevent exposure keratopathy symptoms and signs. In addition, such injections are associated with the risk of diplopia from extension of the toxin to the inferior oblique muscle, and with the risk of a true blepharoptosis from extension of the toxin to the levator muscle.

Aberrant Reinnervation of the Facial Nerve

Aberrant reinnervation of the facial nerve may occur following a peripheral lower motor neuron facial nerve palsy. This condition is characterized by involuntary eyelid closure stimulated by the use of other facial muscles, e.g., on smiling or whistling (Fig. 7.3). The involuntary eyelid closure may be controlled by local injections of botulinum toxin as described above. Ptosis surgery is usually contraindicated.

> **KEY POINT**
>
> It is important to exclude the possibility of aberrant regeneration in any patient referred with an acquired ptosis who gives a prior history of a facial palsy.

Post-enucleation Socket Syndrome

Ptosis (or indeed eyelid retraction in some patients) may be seen as one of the features which typify the post-enucleation socket syndrome (Fig. 7.4). It is thought to be due to the loss of the fulcrum for the action of the levator palpebrae superioris. This is corrected by addressing a socket volume deficit by means of an orbital implant. A similar situation is seen in a patient with an orbital volume expansion following an untreated orbital wall blowout fracture.

Double Elevator Palsy

A ptosis which occurs in conjunction with a hypotropic eye (e.g., a double elevator palsy), may resolve completely once the

Table 7.1 Classification of Ptosis

Pseudoptosis
True ptosis
   Neurogenic
   Myogenic
   Aponeurotic
   Mechanical

Table 7.2 Pseudoptosis

Contralateral eyelid retraction
Hemifacial spasm
Aberrant reinnervation of the facial nerve
Post-enucleation socket syndrome
Double elevator palsy
Dermatochalasis/brow ptosis
Duane's retraction syndrome

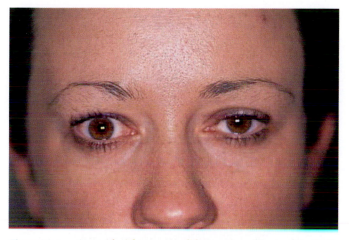

Figure 7.1 A patient with right upper eyelid retraction who complained of a left ptosis. The patient had undiagnosed thyrotoxicosis.

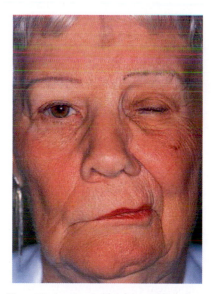

Figure 7.2 A patient with left hemifacial spasm.

eye has been repositioned surgically, usually using a Knapp procedure (Fig. 7.5). The Knapp procedure is useful for treating a double elevator palsy, especially when there is no mechanical restriction to elevation. This technique employs an upward

shift of the medial and lateral rectus muscles to a point adjacent to the borders of the insertion of the superior rectus muscle.

A cover test should be performed on all patients presenting with a history of a congenital ptosis to exclude the possibility of such a pseudoptosis (Fig. 7.6).

Dermatochalasis/brow Ptosis
Dermatochalasis (an age-related redundancy and excess of upper eyelid skin) and/or a brow ptosis may mimic an upper lid ptosis that resolves once a blepharoplasty and/or a brow lift have been performed (Fig. 7.7).

Duane's Retraction Syndrome
Narrowing of the palpebral fissure may be associated with ocular movements. Patients may present with a complaint of ptosis, but a careful examination of the patient's ocular motility reveals the true diagnosis (Fig. 7.8).

TRUE PTOSIS
Neurogenic Ptosis
For a classification of neurogenic ptosis, see Table 7.3.

Oculomotor Nerve Palsy (Third Cranial Nerve Palsy)
A third nerve palsy is characterized by a variable degree of ptosis associated with deficits of adduction, elevation, and depression of the eye due to weakness of the levator muscle, the superior, inferior and medial rectus muscles, and the inferior oblique muscle (Fig. 7.9). The pupillary fibers of the third cranial nerve may be affected or spared depending on the underlying cause. Lesions confined to the superior division of the third nerve result in a ptosis and weakness of the superior rectus muscle only. The Bell's phenomenon is typically absent or poor. Myasthenia may mimic a third nerve palsy when the pupil is spared and this should be considered.

Cyclic oculomotor nerve palsy is a rare phenomenon characterized by alternating paresis and spasm of the extraocular and intraocular muscles. These cyclic phenomena are usually noted in early childhood and may be evident at birth.

Third nerve palsy may be caused by neoplastic, inflammatory, vascular, or traumatic lesions, any of which may affect the nerve in its course from the midbrain to the orbit. Associated symptoms and signs help to localize the underlying lesion. Damage to the third nerve within the subarachnoid space produces an isolated third nerve palsy. The main causes are compression of the nerve by an expanding aneurysm of the posterior communicating artery or the basilar artery, and ischemic vasculopathy. There will usually be pain in aneurysmal compression and pupillary involvement is typical, though there have been infrequent cases of aneurysmal compression that did not initially affect pupillary function. In ischemic vascular third nerve palsies, pain is infrequent and the pupil is typically normal and reactive. The major of ischemic vascular third nerve palsies resolve spontaneously and show a gradual recovery over a period of 3 to 6 months.

Damage to the third nerve in the cavernous sinus, superior orbital fissure, or posterior orbit is unlikely to present as an isolated third nerve palsy due to the confluence of other structures in these areas. Cavernous sinus involvement may also include pareses of the fourth and sixth cranial nerves, the ophthalmic division of the 5th nerve, and an ipsilateral Horner's

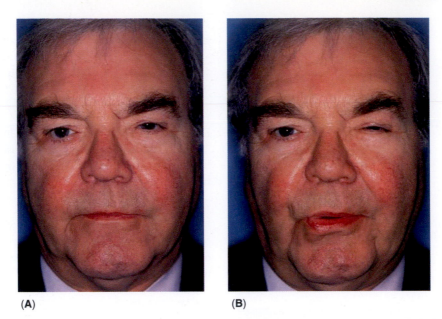

(A)   (B)

Figure 7.3 (**A**) A patient following recovery from a Bell's palsy. There is an apparent left ptosis. The lower eyelid position is also high, further narrowing the palpebral aperture. (**B**) The same patient demonstrating aberrant reinnervation of the facial nerve with a narrowing of the palpebral aperture on pursing his lips to blow.

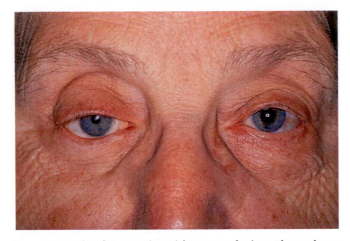

Figure 7.4 A patient demonstrating a right post-enucleation socket syndrome.

syndrome. The most common causes of damage to the third nerve in these areas include metastatic disease, orbital inflammatory disease, herpes zoster, a carotid artery aneurysm, a pituitary adenoma and pituitary apoplexy, and a sphenoid wing meningioma.

In complicated third nerve palsies where other neural structures are involved, the patient should undergo an MRI scan. In isolated third nerve palsies with no pupillary involvement, where the patient is over 50 years of age, MRI scanning, investigations for the cause of a vasculopathy, and a daily pupillary evaluation are indicated.

For patients under the age of 50 years presenting with an isolated pupil-sparing third nerve palsy, intracranial angiography is indicated as an ischemic vasculopathy is far less likely to occur in this age group than is an aneurysm. If an adult patient of any age presents with a complete or incomplete isolated third nerve palsy with pupillary involvement, this should be considered to be a medical emergency and the patient should undergo urgent intracranial angiography. In these cases, the cause is likely to be a life-threatening subarachnoid aneurysm. The majority of third nerve palsies presenting in children are traumatic or congenital.

> **KEY POINT**
>
> If an adult patient of any age presents with a complete or incomplete isolated third nerve palsy with pupillary involvement, this should be considered to be a medical emergency and the patient should undergo urgent intracranial angiography.

Treatment of the ptosis associated with a third nerve palsy is problematic due to the impaired Bell's phenomenon with a risk of exposure keratopathy. A frontalis suspension procedure may be undertaken after strabismus surgery has been performed to realign the globe in the primary position. A frontalis suspension procedure may be undertaken prior to strabismus surgery in infants to treat amblyopia. It is wise to use a 4/0 polypropylene suture for the frontalis suspension as this can easily be removed and the procedure reversed if the patient develops exposure keratopathy.

> **KEY POINT**
>
> Myasthenia gravis has the ability to mimic virtually any cranial neuropathy, including isolated third nerve palsies. Myasthenia gravis must remain a possible diagnosis when encountering a third nerve palsy, when the clinical course is variable or atypical.

Horner's Syndrome (Oculosympathetic Paresis)

Horner's syndrome is characterized by a ptosis of 1 to 2 mm with good levator function and a raised skin crease, a pupillary miosis, and an apparent enophthalmos. It is occasionally associated with facial anhidrosis depending on the site of the lesion. The eyelid features are due to interference with the sympathetic nerve supply to Müller's muscle in the upper eyelid and to its smooth muscle counterpart in the lower eyelid, and to the dilator pupillae muscle. The resultant anisocoria is accentuated in dim illumination. The apparent enophthalmos is due to the decrease in the vertical height of the palpebral aperture. Iris heterochromia may also be seen if it occurs

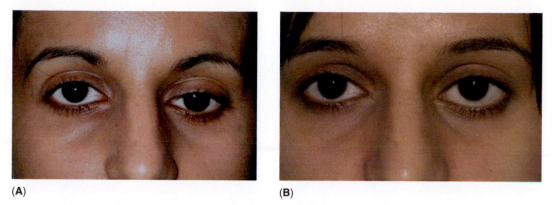

(A)   **(B)**

Figure 7.5 (**A**) A patient with a left hypotropia and a pseudoptosis. (**B**) The same patient following a left Knapp procedure showing a complete resolution of the apparent ptosis (but with postoperative lower lid retraction).

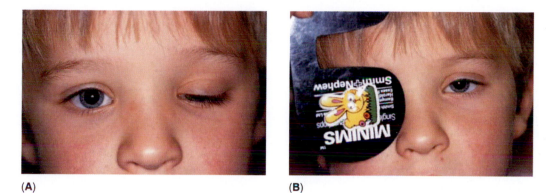

(A)   **(B)**

Figure 7.6 (**A**) A child with an apparent left ptosis. The underlying globe is hypotropic. (**B**) On cover testing, the left eye is forced to take up fixation. The apparent ptosis has resolved. The right eye under the occluder is now in a hypertropic position. The patient has a left double elevator palsy.

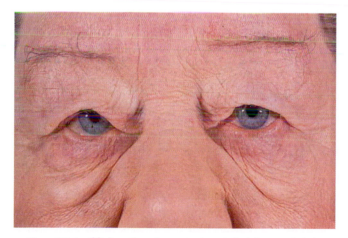

Figure 7.7 An elderly patient demonstrating marked dermatochalasis.

before 2 years of age. Iris pigmentation, which is under sympathetic control during early development, is completed by the age of two, making heterochromia an uncommon finding in a Horner's syndrome acquired later in life. Old photographs can aid the clinician in distinguishing a congenital Horner's syndrome from an acquired Horner's syndrome by documenting heterochromia present at, or close to, birth.

A Horner's syndrome may be caused by a lesion which interrupts the course of the sympathetic neurons anywhere from their origin in the hypothalamus to the orbit (Fig. 7.10). There are three orders of neuron carrying the sympathetic innervation to the orbit. The first neuron commences in the hypothalamus and descends and travels between the levels of the eighth cervical and fourth thoracic vertebrae (C8-T4) of the spinal cord, synapsing with the second neuron in the intermediolateral cell column. There, the preganglionic cell bodies of the second order neurons give rise to axons. These axons pass over the apex of the lung and across the neck of the first rib, and then ascend behind the carotid sheath, entering the sympathetic chain in the neck. They synapse with the third neuron in the superior cervical ganglion, which lies in front of the lateral mass of the atlas and axis. There, cell bodies of third order neurons give rise to postganglionic axons that travel to the eye via the cavernous sinus. These sympathetic nerve fibers course anteriorly through the uveal tract and join the fibers of long posterior ciliary nerves to innervate the dilator of the iris. Postganglionic sympathetic fibers also innervate Müller's muscle in the upper eyelid. Postganglionic sympathetic fibers, responsible for facial sweating, follow the external carotid artery and its branches to the sweat glands and blood vessels of the neck, face, and head. Interruption at any location along this pathway (preganglionic or postganglionic) will induce an ipsilateral Horner's syndrome.

The common etiologies of an acquired preganglionic Horner's syndrome include trauma, aortic dissection, carotid artery dissection, tuberculosis, and a Pancoast tumor. Common etiologies of a postganglionic Horner's syndrome include trauma, cluster migraine headache, and iatrogenic following surgical procedures on the neck. An isolated Horner's syndrome is typically vascular in nature.

The diagnosis of Horner's syndrome is made clinically but may be confirmed with pharmacological testing by the

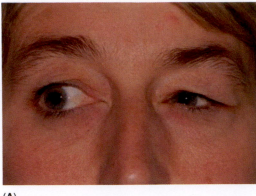

(A)   (B)

Figure 7.8 (**A**) A patient with Duane's retraction syndrome demonstrating an apparent left ptosis on looking to the right due to co-contraction of the horizontal recti. The palpebral aperture has narrowed due to retraction of the globe. (**B**) The palpebral aperture has opened on looking to the left.

Table 7.3 Neurogenic Ptosis
Oculomotor nerve palsy
Horner's syndrome
Myasthenia gravis
Synkinetic ptosis
Marcus–Gunn jaw-winking phenomenon
Aberrant reinnervation of the oculomotor nerve
Guillain–Barré syndrome
Cerebral ptosis
Spread of botulinum toxin to the levator muscle following periocular injection
Botulism

instillation of 5% cocaine solution into both eyes. Cocaine acts as an indirectly acting sympathomimetic agent by inhibiting the re-uptake of noradrenaline at the nerve ending. A Horner's pupil, in contrast to the normal pupil, will fail to dilate, or will dilate poorly, because of the absence of endogenous noradrenaline at the nerve ending. The pupils should be evaluated 30 minutes after the instillation of the drops to ensure accuracy. The cocaine test is used to confirm or deny the presence of a Horner's syndrome. A positive cocaine test does not, however, localize the lesion.

In order to localize the lesion as either preganglionic or postganglionic, 1% hydroxyamphetamine solution can be instilled into the eye after waiting for a further 48 hours. (It is important to delay this test as cocaine can inhibit the uptake of hydroxyamphetamine into the presynaptic vesicle). Hydroxyamphetamine displaces noradrenaline from the presynaptic vesicles. If the third neuron is damaged, there will be no endogenous noradrenaline and the pupil will not dilate, thus indicating a postganglionic lesion. Dilation indicates a first- or second-order neuron lesion. There is currently no method of pharmacological testing which can differentiate a first-order preganglionic lesion from a second-order preganglionic lesion. The differentiation between a first-order and a second-order neuron lesion is based upon the neurological signs associated with a first-order neuron lesion.

The instillation of a weak solution of phenylephrine (1%) may demonstrate denervation hypersensitivity, resulting in a temporary resolution of the ptosis and restoration of a normal skin crease (Fig. 7.10).

KEY POINT

It is important to differentiate a preganglionic from a postganglionic Horner's syndrome as lesions which result in a postganglionic Horner's syndrome are usually benign (usually vascular in nature) in contrast to those resulting in a preganglionic Horner's syndrome.

In general, the treatment for a Horner's syndrome depends upon the underlying cause. In many cases there is no treatment that improves or reverses the condition. Treatment in acquired cases is directed toward eradicating the lesion that is responsible for the syndrome.

The ptosis may be treated surgically either by means of a Müller's muscle resection or by means of a levator aponeurosis advancement procedure. It is very difficult to improve the slightly elevated position of the lower eyelid surgically.

Myasthenia Gravis

Myasthenia gravis is an autoimmune disorder caused by antibodies to the acetylcholine receptors of the motor endplate of voluntary muscles. The antibodies block access of the neurotransmitter acetylcholine to the receptors. The hallmarks of the disorder are variable muscular weakness and fatigue on exercise. Myasthenia may be generalized and may threaten the muscles of respiration, or it may be localized to the eyes (ocular myasthenia). Approximately 30% of patients present with ocular signs and symptoms (ptosis and diplopia), whereas 80% to 90% of patients have ocular signs at the time of diagnosis. Thyroid disorders may be seen in as many as 10% of patients with myasthenia gravis, and symptoms of hyperthyroidism or hypothyroidism may also be present.

If the symptoms and signs remain confined to the eyes for 3 years, progress to generalized myasthenia is unlikely. Ptosis is the most common clinical manifestation of myasthenia. It may be unilateral or bilateral. Exercise of the levator or sustained up gaze may provoke or worsen a ptosis. Attempted rapid saccades from down gaze to the primary position may provoke an overshoot of the upper eyelid above the superior limbus with a gradual fall of the lid to its original position (Cogan's twitch sign). There may be an associated weakness of the orbicularis oculi muscle and the Bell's phenomenon may be poor.

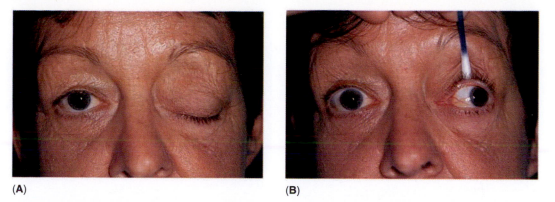

Figure 7.9 (**A**) A patient with a complete left ptosis due to an oculomotor nerve palsy. (**B**) The same patient with the eyelid mechanically elevated demonstrating a divergent left eye due to the unopposed action of the unaffected lateral rectus muscle.

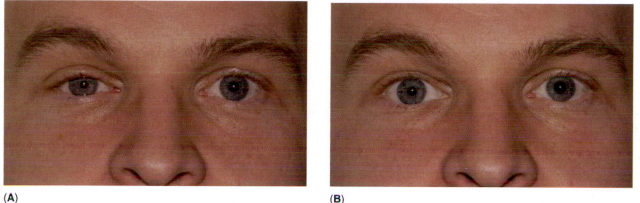

Figure 7.10 (**A**) A patient demonstrating a right Horner's syndrome. Note the high position of the right lower eyelid, which, together with the upper eyelid ptosis gives the impression of a right enophthalmos. The patient also shows a compensatory right frontalis overaction. (**B**) The same patient 2 minutes following the instillation of 1% phenylephrine into the right eye. The ptosis has resolved and the lower eyelid has returned to a normal position. The compensatory right frontalis overaction has also diminished.

The diagnosis of myasthenia should be contemplated in any patient with an acquired ptosis and normal pupils. The diagnosis may be confirmed by means of a Tensilon test (edrophonium chloride) (Fig. 7.11). Tensilon is a short-acting anticholinesterase agent that increases the amount of acetylcholine available at the motor endplate when administered intravenously. In the majority of cases it will temporarily and dramatically overcome the muscle weakness of myasthenia. Failure to do so, however, does not exclude the diagnosis. Precautions should be taken prior to performing the Tensilon test. Resuscitation equipment should be available and an intravenous cannula placed for venous access because, very occasionally, edrophonium can cause a significant bradycardia, heart block, and asystole. Monitoring of vital signs should be performed prior to and during the test. Atropine should be drawn up ready to administer in the event of the development of any of these adverse systemic events. A small intravenous test dose (2 mg) of Tensilon should be given and the response observed, prior to injection of a further 8 mg, to ensure there are no adverse side effects.

Other confirmatory tests can be performed, such as an acetylcholine receptor antibody assay, standard electromyography, single-fiber electromyography, and repetitive nerve stimulation electromyography showing decremental responses. A simple clinical test to perform is the ice pack test. Cooling may improve neuromuscular transmission. In a patient with myasthenia gravis who has a ptosis, placing ice in a surgical glove that is wrapped in a surgical towel over the eyelid for 2 minutes can lead to improvement of the ptosis.

The treatment of the patient with myasthenia should be undertaken by a neurologist. The treatment may involve the use of anticholinesterase agents, systemic steroids, immunosuppressants, or plasmapheresis. A CT scan or an MRI of the chest is highly accurate in detecting a thymoma. Every patient with myasthenia gravis should be screened for a thymoma. Thymectomy may be beneficial in some cases.

The ophthalmologist plays a role in the management of ptosis and/or diplopia unresponsive to medical therapy. The ptosis may be treated by the use of ptosis props if the Bell's phenomenon is absent and if the orbicularis function is poor. Patients with normal orbicularis function rarely tolerate ptosis props. The surgical management depends upon the levator function. If this is better than 4 to 5 mm, a levator aponeurosis advancement procedure may be used. If the levator function is less than 4 mm, a frontalis suspension procedure will be required. The risk of exposure keratopathy must be considered carefully before embarking on such surgery.

KEY POINT

The diagnosis of myasthenia should be contemplated in any patient with an acquired ptosis and normal pupils.

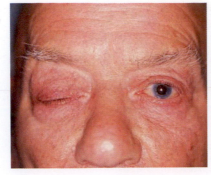
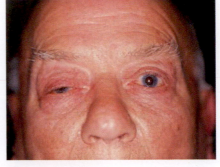
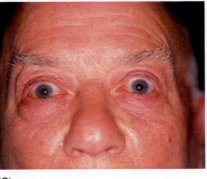

Figure 7.11 (**A**) A patient referred with a history of an acquired variable right ptosis and diplopia. (**B**) The same patient following a test dose of Tensilon. (**C**) The same patient following the injection of 10 mg of Tensilon.

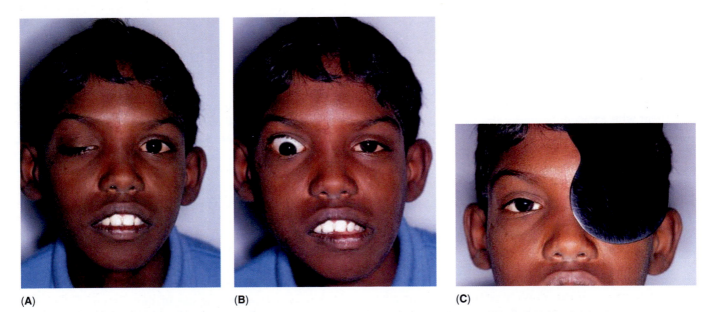

Figure 7.12 (**A**) A patient with a right ptosis and hypotropia. (**B**) The same patient demonstrating an external pterygoid-levator synkinesis on moving his mandible to the left. (**C**) The right ptosis in the resting position resolves on occluding the left eye, as the patient has an associated right double elevator palsy.

Synkinetic Ptosis

A synkinesis is simultaneous movement of muscles supplied by different nerves or by separate branches of the same nerve. It can be congenital or acquired.

Marcus Gunn Jaw Wink phenomenon (Congenital trigemino-oculomotor synkinesis). In this disorder, there is a central anomalous innervational pattern between the oculomotor and trigeminal nerves. The phenomenon is characterized by eyelid synkinesis with jaw movement (Fig. 7.12). Characteristically, a unilateral ptosis of variable degree is noted shortly after birth. The ptotic eyelid is noted to open and close as the infant feeds. The phenomenon accounts for approximately 5% of congenital ptosis cases, and may be associated with amblyopia, anisometropia, and strabismus. It may also be associated with a superior rectus palsy or a double elevator palsy (Fig. 7.12).

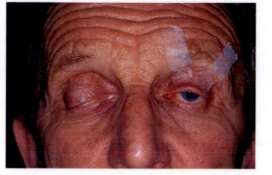

(A)   (B)

Figure 7.13 (**A**) A patient with cerebral ptosis. (**B**) The patient had resorted to the use of Micropore tape to enable him to see.

There are two major groups of trigemino-oculomotor synkinesis:

1. External pterygoid-levator synkinesis in which the lid elevates when the jaw is thrust to the opposite side, when the jaw is projected forward, or when the mouth is widely opened
2. Internal pterygoid-levator synkinesis in which the lid elevates on teeth clenching

In some patients, the abnormal movements are only provoked by sucking.

A rare condition in which the lid falls as the mouth opens has been referred to as the inverse Marcus Gunn jaw wink phenomenon.

The treatment of this phenomenon is difficult. It is important to ascertain whether the wink, the ptosis or both are of concern to the patient or the parents. If the wink is mild and not of major concern, the ptosis can be treated according to the usual criteria applied to the management of ptosis, i.e., determined by the degree of levator function. If the wink is of concern, it can be treated either by an extirpation of the levator and a frontalis suspension procedure, performed unilaterally or, more controversially, bilaterally, or by means of a Lemagne procedure (see Page 168). The success of a Lemagne procedure relies on the patient having good preoperative levator function.

It can be very difficult to explain the pros and cons of this approach to the parents of a child with this condition. Naturally, most parents are reluctant to consent to surgery on the normal side. Although frontalis suspension surgery performed bilaterally can provide good symmetry, it is important for the parents to appreciate that this will nevertheless result in an abnormal symmetry, with lag of both eyelids on down gaze. The extirpation of the levator muscle can be undertaken either as an anterior approach, with direct suturing of autogenous fascia lata to the tarsus, or as a posterior approach, with the fascia lata placed as a closed technique (see Page 166).

Aberrant reinnervation of the oculomotor nerve. In this disorder, there is an innervational anomaly within the neural sheath between the eyelid and other targets of the oculomotor nerve. It is characterized by inappropriate eyelid and extraocular muscle synkinesis. The disorder typically follows trauma or compression of the oculomotor nerve. The management of this disorder is particularly difficult. The aberrant eyelid movements can be halted by extirpating the

Table 7.4 Myogenic Ptosis

Congenital " dystrophy" of the levator muscle
Myotonic dystrophy
Chronic progressive external ophthalmoplegia
Muscle trauma

levator muscle, which is followed by placement of a frontalis sling. The absence of a Bell's phenomenon, however, places the patient at risk of exposure keratopathy.

Guillain–Barré Syndrome
This rare disorder, which may be generalized or may present as a bulbar variant, usually follows a febrile illness. Ptosis, which is usually of mild degree, is symmetrical and occurs in the context of a rapidly progressive bilateral ophthalmoplegia and facial diplegia. Classically, the cerebrospinal fluid (CSF) shows a raised protein level in the absence of a cellular response. A more limited form of Guillain–Barré syndrome, the Miller–Fisher variant, consists of bilateral ptosis and ophthalmoplegia associated with ataxia and areflexia but with no systemic weakness.

Cerebral Ptosis
A moderate to severe bilateral ptosis may be seen following acute damage to the right cerebral hemisphere. The ptosis may be asymmetric. A conjugate ocular deviation is also seen in this condition (Fig. 7.13).

Botulism
Botulinum toxin blocks neuromuscular transmission and is commonly used therapeutically in the treatment of essential blepharospasm. It is being increasingly used by a variety of medical and non-medical practitioners for the cosmetic improvement of periocular lines and wrinkles, and to produce a brow lift. Blepharoptosis is a potential complication of the use of periocular botulinum toxin injections. The ptosis, which is usually partial when it occurs, is temporary and resolves completely after approximately 3 to 4 months as the effects of the botulinum toxin wear off. Patients undergoing periocular botulinum toxin injections should be warned about this risk. The ptosis may respond to the temporary topical administration of Iopidine, an α-agonist, but the patient must be warned of the potential side effects of this glaucoma medication.

Botulism, acquired through food poisoning, is a very rare neurological disorder characterized by ptosis and ophthalmoplegia, followed by dysarthria and dysphagia, and then by weakness of the extremities.

Myogenic Ptosis
For a classification of myogenic ptosis, see Table 7.4.

Congenital 'Dystrophy' of the Levator Muscle
In this condition, the levator muscle is replaced to a variable extent by fibrous and fatty tissue. The levator function varies from good to poor. The degree of ptosis can vary from minimal to severe and may interfere with visual development. Amblyopia associated with a congenital ptosis may be due to occlusion from the ptosis if this is severe enough to occlude the visual axis, but may also be due to an undiagnosed refractive error or strabismus. The eyelid typically shows lag on down gaze (Fig. 7.14).

A congenital "dystrophic" ptosis may occur in isolation (simple congenital "dystrophic" ptosis) or it may be associated with a weakness of the superior rectus muscle (Fig. 7.15). It may also be seen in the blepharophimosis-ptosis-epicanthus-inversus syndrome (BPES) or in congenital ocular fibrosis syndromes.

The BPES is an autosomal dominant disorder, which comprises bilateral ptosis, usually with poor levator function, blepharophimosis, telecanthus, epicanthus inversus (a fold of skin running upward and inward from the lower eyelid), and high arched eyebrows (Fig. 7.16). Two clinical subtypes have been described in which Type 1, but not Type 2, is associated

with infertility due to primary ovarian failure. Patients may also have a lateral lower lid ectropion. Such patients often require a bilateral frontalis suspension procedure, usually following surgery to address the telecanthus and the epicanthus inversus. Patients with this disorder often have independent control of each eyebrow, which can pose particular cosmetic difficulties following a frontalis suspension procedure.

The extraocular fibrosis syndromes are congenital ocular motility disorders that arise from dysfunction of the oculomotor, trochlear, and abducens nerves and/or the muscles that they innervate. Each is marked by a specific form of restrictive paralytic ophthalmoplegia with or without ptosis. Individuals with the classic form of congenital fibrosis of the extraocular muscles (CFEOM1) are born with bilateral ptosis and a restrictive infraductive external ophthalmoplegia. The absence of a Bell's phenomenon leaves such patients at risk of exposure keratopathy from a frontalis suspension procedure.

Myotonic Dystrophy
Myotonic dystrophy is a rare autosomal dominant myopathic process that may be associated with a mild degree of symmetrical ptosis with a fair to poor degree of levator function. It is characterized by a progressive symmetrical external ophthalmoplegia, a myopathy with atrophy affecting the musculature of the face, neck and limbs, and classical cataracts (Fig. 7.17). These consist of small, colored crystalline opacities, or posterior, subcortical, and spoke-like opacities. Classically, these patients demonstrate myotonia, a delayed relaxation after contraction, which is most noticeable on shaking hands when greeting the patient. Males may show frontal balding and testicular atrophy.

KEY POINT

Patients with myotonic dystrophy typically have a poor Bell's phenomenon and orbicularis oculi muscle weakness. They are at particular risk of exposure keratopathy following surgery. They are more likely to tolerate ptosis props compared to other patients as their orbicularis muscle is weakened.

Other ocular signs associated with myotonic dystrophy include pupillary light-near dissociation, ocular hypotonia, dry eyes, and a retinal pigmentary degeneration.

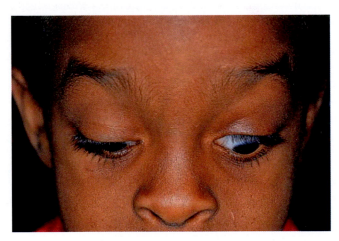

Figure 7.14 A patient with a congenital 'dystrophic' ptosis, demonstrating left lid lag on down gaze.

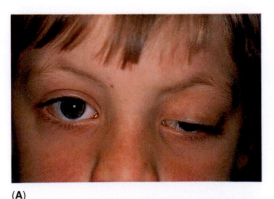 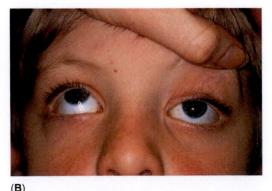

(A)   (B)

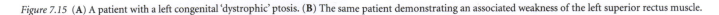

Figure 7.15 (**A**) A patient with a left congenital 'dystrophic' ptosis. (**B**) The same patient demonstrating an associated weakness of the left superior rectus muscle.

Chronic Progressive External Ophthalmoplegia (CPEO)
CPEO is a rare, slowly progressive disorder that is characterized by a progressive, symmetric paralysis of the extraocular muscles, which do not respond to oculocephalic movements

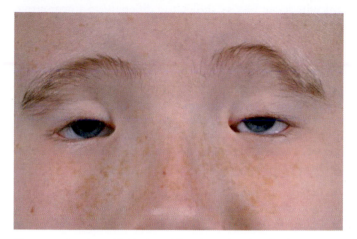

Figure 7.16 A patient with blepharophimosis-ptosis-epicanthus inversus syndrome (BPES).

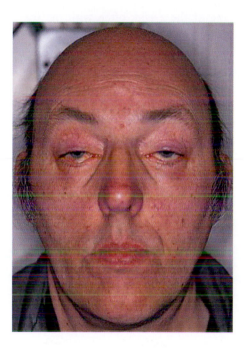

Figure 7.17 A patient with myotonic dystrophy.

or to caloric stimulation. It may affect patients of all ages, but typically manifests in the young adult years. Among the mitochondrial myopathies, CPEO is the most common manifestation, estimated at two-thirds of all incidences of mitochondrial-associated myopathies. Patients typically present with ptosis, which is often the presenting symptom (Fig. 7.18). The first presenting symptom of ptosis is often unnoticed by the patient until the lids droop to the point of producing a visual field defect. Often, patients will adopt an abnormal head posture, with a chin elevation, to compensate for the progressing ptosis. As the ptosis becomes more severe, the patients will show marked frontalis overaction. The ptosis is typically bilateral, but may be unilateral for a period of months to years before the fellow lid becomes involved.

As the ophthalmoplegia is usually symmetric, diplopia is not often a complaint of these patients. In fact, the progressive ophthalmoplegia is often unnoticed until decreased ocular motility limits peripheral vision. Often, the ocular motility restriction is drawn to the patient's attention by someone else. Patients tend to move their heads to adjust for the loss of peripheral vision caused by the horizontal ophthalmoplegia. Although all directions of gaze are affected, down gaze tends to be the least affected. Weakness of other muscle groups, including the orbicularis oculi muscle, facial and limb muscles, may be present in up to 25% of patients with CPEO. Frontalis muscle weakness may exacerbate the ptosis. Facial muscles may be involved which leads to atrophy of facial muscle groups producing a thin, expressionless face. Neck, shoulder, and extremity weakness with atrophy may affect some patients and can be mild or severe.

Mitochondrial DNA, which is maternally inherited, encodes proteins that are critical to the respiratory chain required to produce adenosine triphosphate (ATP). Deletions or mutations to segments of mitochondrial DNA lead to defective function of oxidative phosphorylation. This may be made evident in highly oxidative tissues like skeletal muscle and heart tissue. However, the extraocular muscles contain a volume of mitochondria that is several times greater than any other muscle group. As such, this results in the severe ocular symptoms of CPEO.

The diagnosis of CPEO is confirmed by muscle biopsy. An examination of muscle fibers stained with Gomori trichrome stain reveals an accumulation of enlarged mitochondria. This produces a dark red staining of the muscle fibers, referred to as "ragged red fibers". Although ragged red fibers are seen in

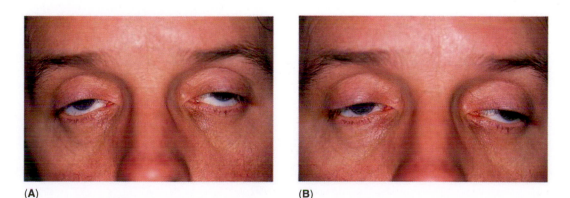

(A)   **(B)**

Figure 7.18 (**A**) A patient with chronic progressive external ophthalmoplegia (CPEO). (**B**) The same patient trying to look to an extreme left gaze position.

normal aging, levels exceeding normal aging provide a diagnosis of a mitochondrial myopathy. In addition, polymerase chain reaction (PCR), from a sample of a patient's blood or muscle tissue, can determine a mutation of the mitochondrial DNA.

There is currently no defined treatment to improve the muscle weakness of CPEO. Ptosis associated with CPEO may be managed by means of a levator advancement procedure if the levator function is preserved but a brow suspension procedure may be required. Surgery has to be undertaken with great caution, however, as progressive weakness of the orbicularis oculi muscle, coupled with an absent Bell's phenomenon, can place the patient at risk of exposure keratopathy.

The term *ophthalmoplegia plus* has been used to refer to a range of abnormalities which may be found with chronic progressive ophthalmoplegia. These abnormalities may be manifestations of associated neurodegenerative disorders. The Kearns–Sayre syndrome (KSS) refers to a condition characterized by chronic progressive ophthalmoplegia, a retinal pigmentary degeneration, cardiac conduction defects often leading to complete heart block, and elevated CSF protein. This can affect young adults. It is important to perform dilated fundoscopy to determine if there is a pigmentary retinopathy that may signify KSS. It is important to identify the cardiac conduction defect in such a patient by means of an electrocardiogram (ECG), as a cardiac pacemaker may be life-saving.

Oculopharyngeal muscular dystrophy is an autosomal dominant disorder, which manifests in the sixth decade of life, in patients with a mutation on the PABPN1 gene. Affected patients typically demonstrate a bilateral ptosis, and a progressive external ophthalmoplegia. Dysphagia, facial weakness, and proximal limb weakness develop later on as the disorder progresses. A large number of such patients are of French-Canadian descent. The management of the ptosis is similar to that of ptosis-complicating myasthenia (see above).

KEY POINT

A levator aponeurosis advancement procedure for CPEO is best performed via a posterior eyelid approach. This affords a greater control of the final eyelid position and offers greater protection of the cornea in the early postoperative period as the eyelid is initially low and the degree of postoperative lagophthalmos is less than that with an anterior approach.

Muscle Trauma

A myogenic ptosis can occur following eyelid or orbital trauma, e.g., a "blow-in" fracture of the orbital roof. Where the levator muscle has previously been transected following penetrating trauma resulting in complete ptosis with no levator function, it can be very difficult to differentiate a neurogenic ptosis from a myogenic ptosis.

Aponeurotic Ptosis

For a classification of aponeurotic ptosis, see Table 7.5.

Aponeurotic ptosis is the result of a defect in the aponeurotic linkage between the levator muscle and the tarsal plate. It may be the result of a frank disinsertion of the aponeurosis from the tarsal plate, or a dehiscence in the aponeurosis, or involutional stretching and redundancy of the aponeurosis. The typical features of an aponeurotic ptosis are:

1. A ptosis that is constant in all positions of gaze
2. A lid drop as opposed to a lid lag on down gaze (Fig. 7.19)
3. Good levator function
4. A high skin crease
5. An upper lid sulcus
6. Thinning of the eyelid, often with the iris visible through the closed eyelid (Fig. 7.20).

KEY POINT

Particular care should be taken when making a skin crease incision in a patient with an aponeurotic ptosis, as the eyelid may be extremely thin. A corneal protector should be used.

Patients typically notice worsening of the ptosis towards the end of the day and this history of variability may lead to the suspicion of myasthenia.

Table 7.5 Aponeurotic Ptosis

Involutional
Post surgical, e.g. cataract surgery
Post eyelid trauma
Post eyelid edema, e.g. blepharochalasis
Post long term contact lens wear
Floppy eyelid syndrome
Chronic eyelid rubbing

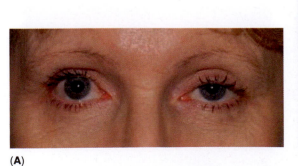

(A)

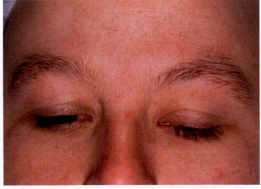

(B)

Figure 7.19 (**A**) A patient with a left contact lens-induced aponeurotic dehiscence. The patient is wearing a gas permeable contact lens in her left eye. (**B**) A patient with a left levator aponeurosis dehiscence following contact lens wear demonstrating a raised skin crease and a typical lid drop on down gaze.

Mechanical Ptosis

For a classification of mechanical ptosis, see Table 7.6.

A variety of eyelid lesions can result in a secondary mechanical ptosis (Figs. 7.21 and 7.22), the management of which depends on the nature of the lesion, e.g., an upper lid capillary hemangioma, which may respond satisfactorily to the local injection of steroids, or the use of systemic Propranolol (Fig. 7.23). Orbital lesions may present with a secondary mechanical ptosis (Figs. 7.24 and 7.25). Adhesions between the eyelid and the globe, e.g., in mucous membrane pemphigoid, may also result in a mechanical ptosis (Fig. 7.26).

KEY POINT

It is essential to palpate around the eyelids, to evert the eyelids, and to examine the superior fornices to exclude mechanical causes of a ptosis.

PATIENT ASSESSMENT

The purpose of a careful assessment of the patient by means of a good history and physical examination, in some cases followed by specific investigations/diagnostic tests, is to determine the diagnosis and classification of the ptosis and thereby decide on the most appropriate therapeutic intervention.

Table 7.6 Mechanical Ptosis

Eyelid tumors
Orbital lesions
Cicatrizing conjunctival disorders
Foreign bodies

History

One should establish the age of onset of the ptosis, the presence of any known predisposing factors, e.g., trauma, previous ocular or eyelid surgery, any variability, associated symptoms, e.g., jaw-winking, diplopia, muscle weakness, dysphagia, and any family history (Table 7.7). A past ophthalmic history, including contact lens wear or previous refractive surgery, and a past medical and surgical history are not to be overlooked. A patient with an acquired ptosis should be directly questioned about the prior use of periocular botulinum toxin injections as such information may not be volunteered.

Examination

A complete ophthalmic examination should be undertaken. Where appropriate, a general physical and neurological examination should also be performed. In all cases, the following examination should be undertaken:

1. The palpebral apertures should be measured in the primary position to determine the degree of ptosis (Fig. 7.27). If the lower lid is abnormally positioned, however, the degree of ptosis can instead be measured using the margin reflex distances (MRD1 and MRD2). MRD1 is the distance between the centre of the pupillary light reflex and the upper eyelid margin with the eye in primary gaze. A measurement of 4 to 5 mm is considered normal. MRD-2 is the distance between the center of the pupillary light reflex and the lower eyelid margin with the eye in primary gaze.

   Frontalis overaction by the patient should be prevented by applying direct pressure over the brows. Frontalis action can be marked in some patients, particularly those with bilateral ptosis.

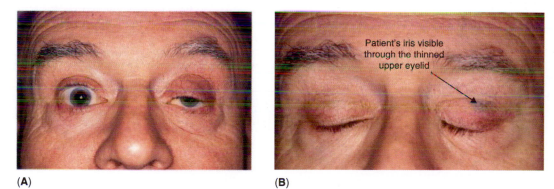
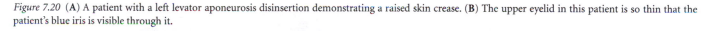

(A)   (B)

Figure 7.20 (A) A patient with a left levator aponeurosis disinsertion demonstrating a raised skin crease. (B) The upper eyelid in this patient is so thin that the patient's blue iris is visible through it.

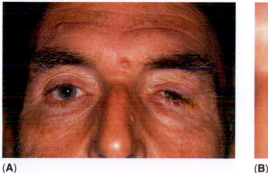
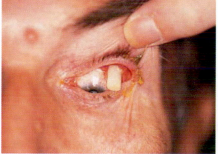

(A)   (B)

Figure 7.21 (A) Patient referred with a left ptosis. (B) Raising of the left upper lid revealed an extruding retinal explant to be the cause of the ptosis.

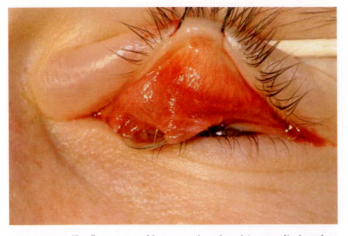

Figure 7.22 A "lost" gas permeable contact lens found in a medical student who had presented with a left ptosis of gradual onset.

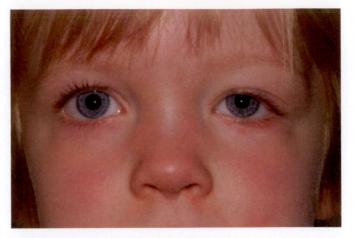

Figure 7.24 A patient with a left ptosis due to the presence of a previously undiagnosed plexiform neurofibroma.

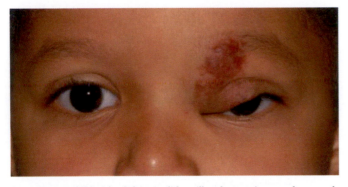

Figure 7.23 A child with a left upper lid capillary hemangioma and a secondary mechanical ptosis.

KEY POINT

In unilateral cases, the ptotic lid should be manually elevated and the contralateral eyelid observed. The contralateral eyelid may be seen to drop spontaneously, following Hering's law of equal innervation (Fig. 7.28). This maneuver may unmask a bilateral asymmetric ptosis. In some patients, the use of 2.5% phenylephrine drops, instilled into the eye on the ptotic side, may cause the lid to rise and may similarly unmask a contralateral ptosis. It is particularly seen in involutional aponeurotic ptosis and it is important that the patient's attention is drawn to this preoperatively. Failure to observe this phenomenon can lead to unexpected postoperative disappointment and a "seesaw" effect as the contralateral eyelid drops postoperatively, and when this is subsequently raised the first eyelid becomes ptotic again. For this reason, such patients are better managed by means of a bilateral levator advancement. If staged unilateral surgery is performed instead, it is important to deliberately overcorrect the more ptotic eyelid first by approximately 1.5 to 2 mm in such patients. It is important to fully explain the rationale of the treatment to the patient at the initial assessment.

2. Perform a cover test to exclude a hypotropia and pseudoptosis and observe any abnormal head posture. It is important to ensure an infant with a congenital ptosis undergoes a complete orthoptic evaluation and a cycloplegic refraction. Most infants

with a ptosis develop amblyopia from undetected strabismus and untreated refractive errors (Fig. 7.29). Twenty percent of infants with a congenital ptosis will have concurrent strabismus, of which 50% have a concurrent vertical deviation.

3. The levator function should be very carefully assessed. This will not usually be possible to do in infants below the age of 4 years. The maximum excursion of the lid margin from down gaze to up gaze is measured, ensuring that the frontalis muscle is prevented from assisting the lid movement by pressing on the brow with a thumb (Fig. 7.30). Normal levator function is approximately 15 to 18 mm. Levator function is graded as good (9–18 mm), fair (5–8 mm), poor (1–4 mm) and absent (0 mm). In addition to the excursion of the eyelid, the quality of the movement should also be noted, e.g., this might be quite sluggish, suggesting a myopathic process. This assessment is purely qualitative.

4. The lid position on down gaze is noted. This will demonstrate lid lag in congenital dystrophic ptosis in which the "dystrophic" muscle will neither contract nor relax normally (Fig. 7.31). Lid lag may also be seen where previous surgery has been performed or where there has been previous trauma with adhesions. In contrast, a lower position of the eyelid compared to the fellow upper eyelid is seen on down gaze in patients with an aponeurotic ptosis (Fig. 7.19).

5. The skin crease height above the lid margin should be measured. The presence of a good skin crease in an infant with ptosis is a guide to the presence of at least fair levator function; conversely, the absence of a skin crease suggests poor levator function (Fig. 7.32). A high skin crease suggests an aponeurotic defect (Fig. 7.19). In adults, any excess upper lid skin and any degree of eyebrow ptosis should be noted.

6. The Bell's phenomenon should be assessed. Its absence should be taken into consideration in recommending ptosis surgery, as the risk of postoperative corneal exposure is increased. At the same time, the orbicularis function should be determined and

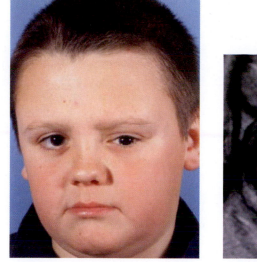

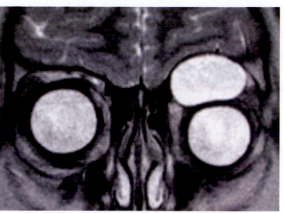

(A)   **(B)**

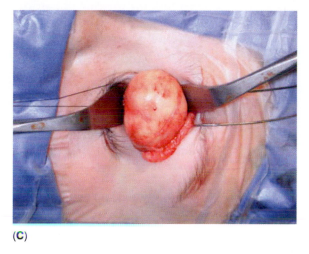

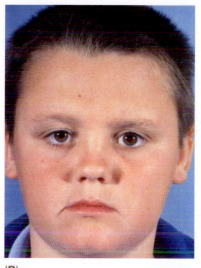

(C)

(D)

Figure 7.25 (**A**) A patient referred to for the management of a left "congenital" ptosis. A left hypoglobus was noted which had gone unrecognized previously. (**B**) A preoperative MRI demonstrated a large smooth mass with internal imaging characteristics consistent with diagnosis of a dermoid cyst. (**C**) The dermoid cyst was removed via an anterior orbitotomy. (**D**) The postoperative appearance.

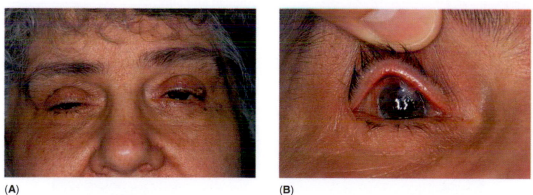

(A)   **(B)**

Figure 7.26 (**A**) A patient referred with a severe right ptosis. (**B**) Raising of the right upper lid revealed a symblepharon.

the extent of any lagophthalmos recorded (Fig. 7.33). The extent of the reflex blink should also be assessed on slit lamp examination.

7. The ocular movements should be assessed, looking specifically for a superior rectus weakness or aberrant eyelid movements (Fig. 7.34).

8. Jaw winking should be looked for by asking the patient to open and close the mouth, and to thrust the jaw from side to side. An infant can be observed feeding and a child can be observed sucking a sweet. In some patients, the phenomenon is only manifest when sucking (Fig. 7.35).

9. The pupils should be examined to exclude the possibility of a Horner's syndrome.

10. Myasthenia should always be considered in acquired ptosis. Examine for fatigability, and a Cogan's twitch. Consider a Tensilon test where appropriate (after informed consent has been obtained and all necessary safety precautions taken). An ice pack test can also be performed.

11. Evert the upper eyelid and examine the tarsus. Document the height of the tarsal plate and exclude any giant papillary conjunctivitis, amyloid lesions, etc. (Figs. 7.36–7.40). Undue laxity of the upper eyelid with a papillary conjunctivitis and a lash ptosis should raise the suspicion of a "floppy eyelid syndrome" (Figs. 7.38 and 7.39).

12. Examine the superior fornix and exclude any symblephara, or lesions such as a salmon patch typically seen in patients with orbital lymphoma (Fig. 7.37). A thin-walled cystic trabeculectomy drainage bleb may be at risk of perforation unless great care is taken during ptosis surgery (Fig. 7.41). In addition, it may be wise to undercorrect a ptosis in a patient with such a bleb.

13. Palpate the upper lid and lacrimal gland to exclude any masses (Fig. 7.37).

14. Examine the fundi for pigmentary retinopathy seen in some patients with chronic progressive external ophthalmoplegia.

15. Determine the presence of normal corneal sensation (prior to any instillation of a topical anesthetic agent for tonometry) and exclude a dry eye or tear film abnormality, which may be aggravated by ptosis surgery.

16. Consider a phenylephrine test. A drop of 2.5% phenylephrine is instilled into the affected eye. Some surgeons consider a good response to indicate that the patient is more likely to respond well to a posterior approach Müller's muscle resection. The test can actually be of more practical use in demonstrating to the patient the effect of contralateral eyelid drop.

Table 7.7 History

Parameter	Ptosis category
Age of onset	Congenital vs. acquired
Any known abnormal lid movements	Jaw wink
Previous ocular surgery	Aponeurotic ptosis
Variability	Myasthenia
Diplopia, muscle weaknesses	Myasthenia
Previous contact lens wear	Aponeurotic ptosis or mechanical ptosis from giant papillary conjunctivitis (GPC)
Previous trauma	Aponeurotic ptosis
Atopy	Mechanical ptosis from GPC
Previous facial palsy	Aberrant reinnervation/brow ptosis

It is always helpful to examine old photographs of the patient whenever these are available.

Applied Anatomy
See chapter 2.

MANAGEMENT
The major determining factor in deciding the most appropriate surgical procedure for the correction of ptosis is the degree

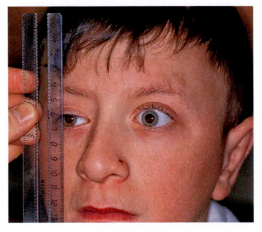

Figure 7.27 A patient undergoing measurements of the palpebral aperture, MRD-1 and MRD-2.

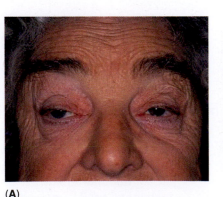
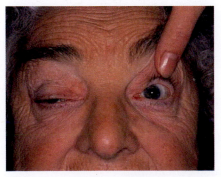

(A)   (B)

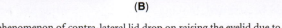

Figure 7.28 A patient demonstrating the phenomenon of contra-lateral lid drop on raising the eyelid due to Hering's Law of equal innervation.

of levator function (Table 7.8). Most cases of ptosis can be adequately managed by means of a levator aponeurosis advancement procedure. This should be performed under local anesthesia with or without intravenous sedation in adults, as intraoperative patient cooperation permits the most accurate and consistent results. It should be performed under general anesthesia in children.

In children, the extent of advancement of the aponeurosis, or of resection of the levator muscle, has been determined by various formulae advocated by different surgeons over the years. Although a variety of formulae have been described to assist in the estimation of how much of a resection to perform, these formulae often relate to levator muscle resections where Whitnall's ligament has not been preserved. A simpler rule of thumb to remember is: the eyelid height achieved intraoperatively with this procedure tends to remain relatively stable postoperatively in patients with a preoperative levator function of approximately 8 mm. If the levator function is 4 to 7 mm, the lid position will drop postoperatively and therefore an intraoperative overcorrection should be planned. If the levator function is 9 mm or better, the lid position will tend to be slightly higher postoperatively and the intraoperative lid position should be adjusted accordingly.

Where the levator function is good and the extent of the ptosis is 2 mm or less, a Müller's muscle resection may be performed. (The Fasanella–Servat procedure, a destructive procedure, which has been advocated by many surgeons for many years, should be avoided). For children with borderline levator function (3–4 mm), an internal Whitnall's sling procedure can be considered. For patients with poor levator function, a frontalis suspension procedure is required using either autogenous (usually fascia lata) or non-autogenous materials (e.g., polypropylene, silicone tubing, supramid, or vicryl/polypropylene mesh).

In patients with an acquired myopathy who have an absent Bell's phenomenon and poor orbicularis function, and /or a dry eye, ptosis props should be considered.

> **KEY POINT**
>
> For patients in whom ptosis surgery would be potentially dangerous, e.g., myotonic dystrophy with an absent Bell's phenomenon, poor orbicularis function, and/or a dry eye, ptosis props should be considered.

It is important to document the ptosis with photographs in the primary position and in up and down gaze prior to surgery.

Fasanella–Servat Procedure

This procedure has been advocated by many surgeons for many years for the management of minimal degrees of ptosis in patients with good levator function, e.g., Horner's syndrome. The Fasanella–Servat procedure is a simple but crude procedure that is best avoided as it sacrifices both a portion of the tarsal plate, which is important for the structural integrity of the upper eyelid, and conjunctival tear secretor glands (Figs. 7.42 and 7.43).

In this procedure, two curved artery clips are placed at least 4 mm from the eyelid margin to include equal amounts of tarsus and palpebral conjunctiva (Fig. 7.42A). These artery clips are angulated slightly away from the eyelid margin. A 6/0 Nylon suture is passed through the eyelid medially and run just above the artery clips taking five to six bites. The suture is brought out of the eyelid laterally after cutting along the crush marks created by the artery clips using blunt-tipped Westcott scissors. The ends of the suture are taped to the skin and removed 7 days postoperatively.

The Fasanella–Servat procedure has the disadvantage that it does not allow for graded adjustment. It does not take into

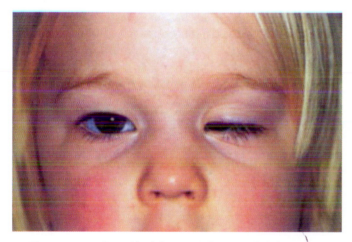

Figure 7.29 A patient with a left congenital ptosis and a left esotropia.

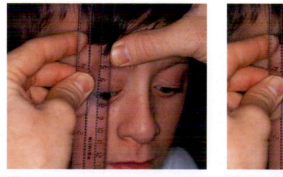

(A)   (B)

Figure 7.30 (A) A patient undergoing measurements of levator function. The eyebrow is fixated using the examiner's thumb. The patient is asked to look downward as much as possible. (B) The patient is then asked to look upward as much as possible.

account the variable height of the tarsal plate and is often used for inappropriate cases by general ophthalmic surgeons because of its simplicity. The recurrence rate is high. It may cause corneal problems from exposed posterior sutures. It can be difficult to correct postoperative contour defects and aponeurotic surgery, required to manage a recurrence, is much more difficult to perform later because of the loss of a portion of the tarsal plate. A Müller's muscle resection procedure is much preferred for the management of small degrees of ptosis in patients with good levator function.

KEY POINT

The Fasanella–Servat procedure should be avoided. It is a crude and destructive procedure. It sacrifices a variable amount of tarsus and conjunctiva. It has a high recurrence rate. Further surgery undertaken to manage a recurrence is more difficult due to the loss of part of the tarsus.

Müller's Muscle Resection

This posterior approach procedure is particularly useful for a small degree of ptosis (1–2 mm) in patients who have good levator function. It is also an excellent procedure to consider

for the majority of patients with an anophthalmic ptosis (Fig. 22.25, Page 512). It is preferable to the Fasanella–Servat procedure as only a portion of Müller's muscle is excised, leaving the rest of the upper eyelid anatomy intact. It may be useful to apply the 2.5% phenylephrine eye drop test preoperatively to help to determine patient suitability for this procedure and to demonstrate the potential effect of the surgery to the patient. The procedure can be performed under either local or general anesthesia, as patient cooperation with intraoperative suture adjustments is not generally required.

Surgical Procedure
1. Proxymethacaine is instilled into both eyes and Lacrilube ointment is instilled into the non-operated eye to help to prevent drying of the cornea or an inadvertent corneal abrasion if the patient opens the eye.
2. About 1 to 1.5 ml of 0.5% Bupivacaine with 1:200,000 units of adrenaline mixed 50:50 with 2% lidocaine with 1:80,000 units of adrenaline is injected into the upper eyelid immediately under the skin along the skin crease using a 1-inch orange needle. The injection is given slowly from the temporal side of the patient ensuring that the tip of the needle is kept in a horizontal plane in case the patient moves or sneezes. The local anesthetic solution is injected as the needle is advanced. If possible, a single needle pass should be used to minimize the risk of causing a hematoma.
3. The patient is prepped and draped leaving the face fully exposed. A damp 4×4 inch swab is placed over the non-operated eye.
4. A 4/0 silk suture is placed through the gray line of the upper eyelid and the eyelid is everted over a medium Desmarres retractor. The silk suture is fixated to the surgical drapes around the patient's forehead using a small curved artery clip.
5. A further 0.5 to 1 ml of local anesthetic solution is injected subconjunctivally and pressure applied to the closed eye with a swab. A few minutes should be allowed for the adrenaline to take effect.

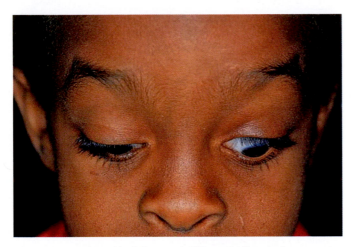

Figure 7.31 A patient with a left congenital "dystrophic" ptosis, demonstrating lid lag on down gaze.

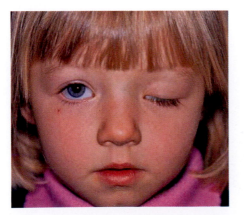

Figure 7.32 A patient with a left congenital "dystrophic" ptosis with very poor levator function. Note the absence of any skin crease.

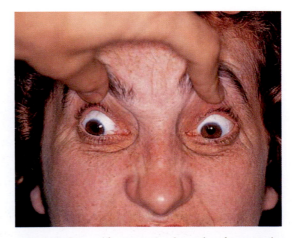

Figure 7.33 A patient with myotonic dystrophy demonstrating poor orbicularis function on attempted forced closure of the eyelids and an absent Bell's phenomenon.

6. The Desmarres retractor is replaced and a conjunctival incision is made with a no. 15 Bard–Parker blade just above the superior aspect of the tarsus.
7. The conjunctiva is grasped with Paufique forceps and drawn anteriorly. An incision is made with blunt-tipped Westcott scissors through Müller's muscle, exposing the avascular space between Müller's muscle and the levator aponeurosis (Fig. 7.44). This plane is then dissected superiorly with blunt-tipped Westcott scissors for a distance of 8 to 10 mm until a white line is seen. This represents the junction of the levator aponeurosis and the orbital septum.

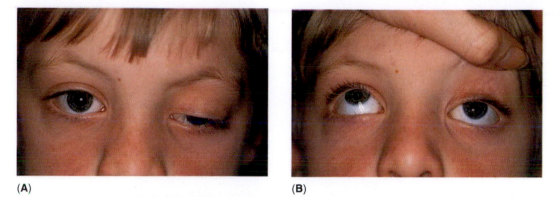

(A)   (B)

Figure 7.34 (**A**) A patient with a left congenital ptosis. (**B**) The same patient demonstrating left superior rectus under action.

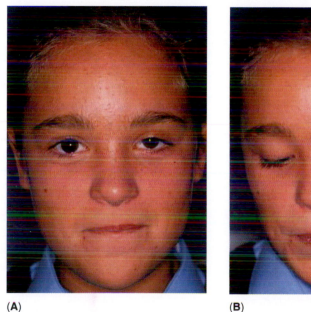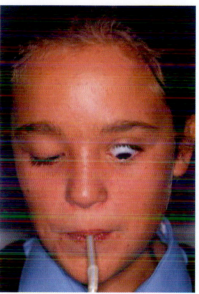

(A)   (B)

Figure 7.35 (**A**) A patient referred with a mild left ptosis. (**B**) Synkinetic movements of the left upper lid have been provoked by sucking on a straw.

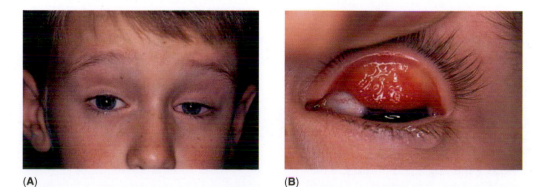

(A)   (B)

Figure 7.36 (**A**) A child referred with a bilateral ptosis. (**B**) Eversion of this child's eyelids revealed vernal catarrh.

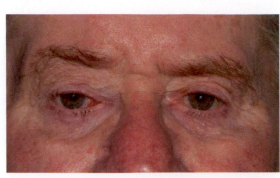
(A)

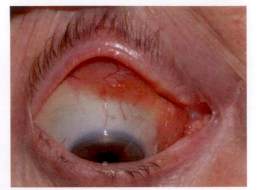
(B)

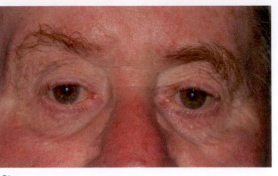
(C)

Figure 7.37 (**A**) A patient referred with a right acquired ptosis. (**B**) Raising his upper eyelid revealed a "salmon patch" lesion. A biopsy of the lesion confirmed the diagnosis of lymphoma. (**C**) The same patient following a course of orbital radiotherapy.

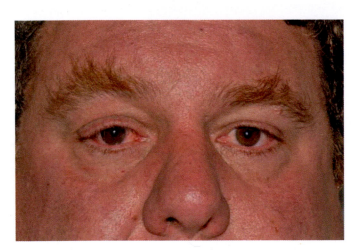

Figure 7.38 A patient with a right acquired ptosis who complained of an irritable eye with a mucoid discharge. He weighed 110 kg. Note the typical lash ptosis.

8. The Desmarres retractor is then removed and two 4/0 silk traction sutures are placed in the medial and lateral aspects of the conjunctiva and these are clipped to the face drapes using small curved artery clips. Müller's muscle is then separated from the underlying conjunctiva with blunt-tipped Westcott scissors using a peeling action with the tips of the scissors held slightly apart (Fig. 7.45).

9. A 5 to 6 mm strip of Müller's muscle is then carefully resected after applying bipolar cautery to prevent bleeding (Fig. 7.46). It is important to avoid removing a greater extent of Müller's muscle or

great difficulty will be encountered in placing sutures through the remaining strip of muscle.

10. Interrupted 7/0 vicryl sutures are then passed through the stump of Müller's muscle and through the posterior aspect of the most superior part of the tarsus to ensure that the sutures are buried (Fig. 7.47). The knots are cut short ensuring that no suture ends are left which may abrade the cornea. Three to four sutures should be placed (Fig. 7.48). No sutures should be passed through the most medial aspect of Müller's muscle, as this will cause an abnormal medial eyelid peak.

11. The traction sutures are then removed and the height and contour of the eyelid checked. The sutures can be removed and replaced if the eyelid contour is not satisfactory. No conjunctiva is excised and the conjunctiva is reposited into the superior fornix. The conjunctival wound is left unsutured.

12. Topical antibiotic ointment is instilled into the eye.

Postoperative Care
Antibiotic drops are instilled into the eye 4 times per day for 2 weeks. Lacrilube ointment is used as required for comfort for a few days.

A postoperative overcorrection or contour defect can be managed by eyelid traction. The patient is instructed to grasp the edge of the eyelid between the thumb and forefinger at the peak of the eyelid and to pull the eyelid downward while looking upward. This traction should be performed for a minimum period of 3 to 4 minutes three to four times per day until the desired height and contour of the eyelid have been achieved.

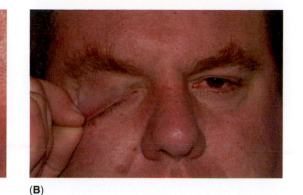

(A)   **(B)**

Figure 7.39 (**A**) The right upper eyelid everts extremely easily and demonstrates a subtarsal papillary conjunctivitis with a mucoid discharge. (**B**) The right upper eyelid is extremely lax and can be easily distracted from the globe. This patient has a typical floppy eyelid syndrome. This should be managed by a lateral upper eyelid wedge resection. The ptosis should be managed by a levator aponeurosis advancement performed secondarily. The patient should be referred to a sleep physician for assessment of obstructive sleep apnoea.

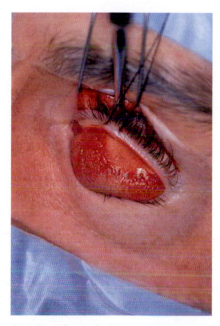

Figure 7.40 Multiple "pseudo-papillae" in a patient referred with a unilateral acquired ptosis. This is localized conjunctival amyloidosis and was a cause of spontaneous bleeding from the eyelid.

Levator Aponeurosis Advancement Procedure

KEY POINT

It is important to have a very good understanding of eyelid and orbital anatomy before embarking upon surgery on the levator muscle or its aponeurosis.

Anterior Approach

This is the most common type of ptosis surgery performed. It can be combined with an upper lid blepharoplasty if necessary. In adults, wherever possible, the procedure should be performed under local anesthesia, with or without sedation, in order to achieve a greater degree of accuracy in adjusting the height and contour of the upper eyelid. Short-acting intravenous sedation provided by an anesthetist is particularly useful to avoid problems when patient cooperation is required during the adjustment of the eyelid. The patient should be advised that an intraoperative overcorrection of the lid height will be the goal, as the lid position will drop postoperatively, and that

postoperative topical lubricants will be necessary to avoid exposure keratopathy until the denervated orbicularis oculi muscle regains normal function (usually after 4–6 weeks). The patient should be placed on an operating table or operating trolley, which permits the patient to be easily brought into a sitting position during the course of surgery.

Surgical Procedure

1. A skin crease incision is marked at the desired level in the upper eyelid using a cocktail stick dipped into a gentian violet marker block, after degreasing the skin with an alcohol wipe. Detailed attention should be paid to the normal shape of the upper lid skin crease remembering that the lateral aspect of the crease is higher than the medial aspect. Proxymethacaine is instilled into both eyes and Lacrilube ointment is instilled into the non-operated eye to help to prevent drying of the cornea or an inadvertent corneal abrasion if the patient opens the eye.

2. About 1 to 1.5 ml of 0.5% Bupivacaine with 1:200,000 units of adrenaline mixed 50:50 with 2% lidocaine with 1:80,000 units of adrenaline is injected into the upper eyelid immediately under the skin along the skin crease using a 1-inch orange needle. The needle should be inserted at the lateral aspect of the eyelid skin crease and it is advanced holding the syringe between forefinger and middle finger with the thumb over the plunger. The needle should be inserted parallel to the surface of the eyelid in order to avoid inadvertent trauma to the globe should the patient sneeze and the anesthetic solution should be slowly injected as the needle is advanced. It is important to avoid a deeper injection and multiple injections in order to prevent a hematoma, and to minimize the effect on the levator function. Pressure should be maintained on the eyelid with a swab for a few minutes. The patient is prepped and draped, taking care to ensure that the drapes do not apply any pressure to the eyebrows.

3. A 4/0 silk traction suture is placed through the gray line of the upper lid at the desired location of the peak of the eyelid and fixated to the face drapes

Table 7.8 Surgical Procedures for the Management of Ptosis

Müller's muscle resection
Levator aponeurosis advancement
Levator muscle resection
Whitnall's sling procedure
Frontalis suspension procedure
Lemagne procedure

using a small curved artery clip (Fig. 7.49). This straightens the marked incision line making the incision easier to perform.

4. An upper eyelid skin crease incision is made using a Colorado needle to minimize bleeding and to aid identification of the tissue planes (Fig. 7.50).

5. The Colorado needle is used to dissect down through the orbicularis oculi muscle to the orbital

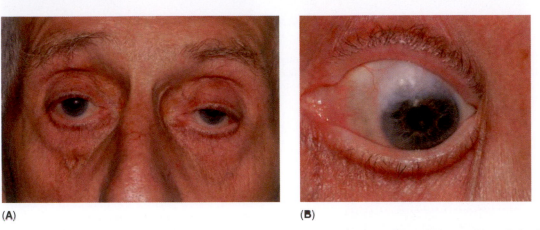

(A)   (B)

Figure 7.41 (**A**) An elderly patient with a left involutional ptosis. (**B**) Retraction of this patient's left upper eyelid revealed a very thin-walled cystic drainage bleb encroaching onto his cornea.

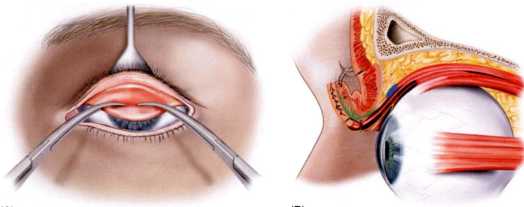

(A)   (B)

Figure 7.42 (**A**) This diagram demonstrates the method of placement of the artery clips in a Fasanella-Servat procedure. (**B**) A diagram demonstrating the tissue resected in a Fasanella-Servat procedure. This does not usually include the levator aponeurosis.

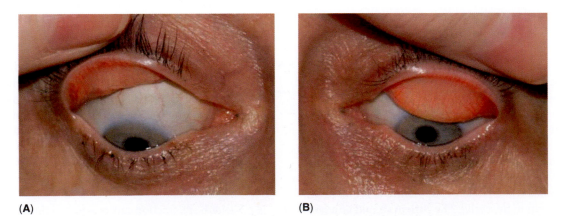

(A)   (B)

Figure 7.43 (**A**) The foreshortened right upper lid tarsus of a patient who has previously undergone a Fasanella-Servat procedure. (**B**) The normal tarsal plate of the left upper eyelid in the same patient.

septum. This is readily seen as a pale structure in contrast to the brown color of the orbicularis muscle. The orbicularis is then dissected from the orbital septum superiorly for 4 to 5 mm to avoid inadvertent injury to the levator aponeurosis (Fig. 7.51A).

6. The orbital septum is then opened with the Colorado needle throughout the entire length of the incision and the preaponeurotic fat exposed (Fig. 7.51B). Using the Colorado needle it will be appreciated that the septum is multilayered. In order to confirm that the fat seen is preaponeurotic fat and not fat within a degenerative levator muscle or Müller's muscle, pressure can be applied to the globe through the lower eyelid with a finger causing preaponeurotic fat to prolapse.

7. The preaponeurotic fat is carefully dissected from the underlying levator aponeurosis using either the Colorado needle or blunt-tipped Westcott scissors. This is facilitated by drawing the fat upward, away from the underlying aponeurosis, with Paufique forceps.

8. A Jaffe lid speculum is then placed in the incision site to provide complete exposure of the levator aponeurosis and the elastic band fixated to the surgical drapes around the patient's forehead using a curved

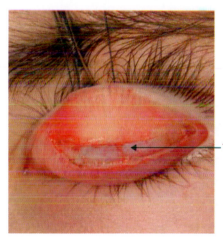

Figure 7.44 The eyelid is everted over a Desmarres retractor and an incision made through the conjunctiva and Müller's muscle exposing the levator aponeurosis.

artery clip (Fig. 7.52). A curved artery clip lies flat and does not interfere with surgical maneuvers.

9. Two skin hooks are then placed under the orbicularis muscle inferiorly and the upper 1/3 of the tarsus is bared using the Colorado needle.

10. If a dehiscence in the aponeurosis is identified, this is repaired with a 5/0 Vicryl suture; otherwise, the edge of the levator aponeurosis is identified and dissected off the tarsus throughout the entire length of the incision using blunt-tipped Westcott scissors, taking care to avoid the superior tarsal vascular arcade.

11. The levator aponeurosis is dissected from the underlying Müller's muscle, taking care not to damage the levator horns or Whitnall's ligament (Fig. 7.53). The dissection is kept to a minimum, with the aim of disrupting normal structures as little as possible. This minimizes the risk of a lateral shift of the tarsus, particularly in older patients in whom the medial levator horn is quite fragile.

12. A double-armed 5/0 Vicryl suture is passed in a lamellar fashion through the tarsus at the junction of the upper 1/3 with the lower 2/3 of the tarsus in a transverse orientation taking care to protect the underlying globe (Fig. 7.54A). The needle should be passed in a strictly parallel fashion with the flat of the needle against the tarsus to avoid cutting the tarsus with the side of the needle. The lid should be lifted off the underlying globe with Paufique forceps before passing the suture. The eyelid should then be everted using the traction suture and the Paufique forceps to ensure that the suture has not passed through the full thickness of the tarsus. This initial suture is placed just above the silk traction suture to ensure the maximum peak is at this position.

13. Both arms of the 5/0 Vicryl suture are passed through the levator aponeurosis at a suitable distance from the tarsus (Fig. 7.55A) and tied in a loop fashion (Fig. 7.55B). The height and contour of the lid is checked with the patient placed into a sitting position (Fig. 7.56). The eyelid should be overcorrected by 1 to 1.5 mm.

14. Excess levator aponeurosis is excised and two additional 5/0 Vicryl sutures are passed through

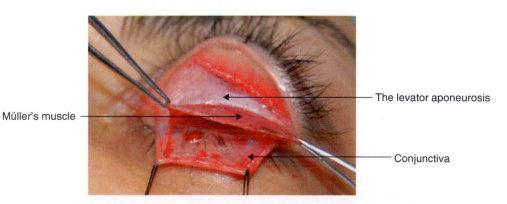

Figure 7.45 Müller's muscle has been dissected from the underlying conjunctiva.

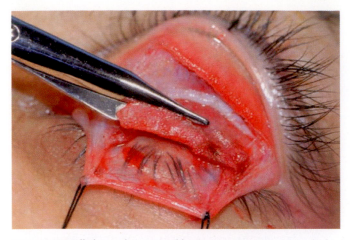

Figure 7.46 Müller's muscle is resected leaving a 2–3 mm stump attached to the levator aponeurosis.

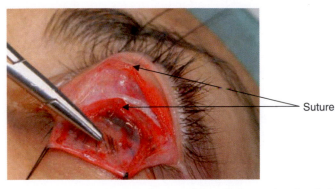

Figure 7.47 A 7/0 Vicryl suture is then passed through the cut edge of Müller's muscle and then through the internal aspect of the superior edge of the tarsus.

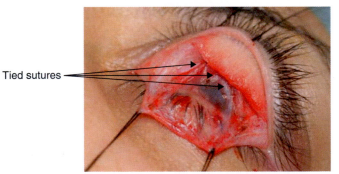

Figure 7.48 Three 7/0 Vicryl sutures are placed and tied attaching the resected edge of Müller's muscle to the superior edge of the tarsus, avoiding the medial aspect of the tarsus in order to avoid an unsatisfactory peak.

the tarsus and through the aponeurosis in a vertical fashion, and the lid position is checked again, with the patient in a sitting position.

15. Once the height and contour are found to be acceptable, the skin edges are reapproximated using interrupted 7/0 Vicryl sutures, incorporating the levator aponeurosis to reform the skin crease. Topical antibiotic ointment is instilled into the eye.

16. If there has been much bleeding encountered during the surgery, it is preferable to place a 4/0 Nylon Frost suture through the gray line of the lower eyelid, which is fixated to the forehead skin using Steristrips, ensuring that the cornea is fully

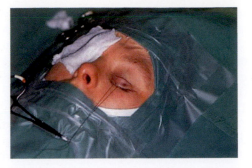

Figure 7.49 The basic set up for a levator aponeurosis advancement procedure under general anesthesia. The set-up for the procedure under local anesthesia with sedation is shown in Figure 7.56.

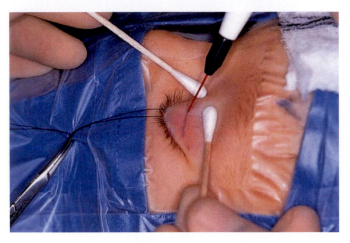

Figure 7.50 A Colorado needle being used to make a skin crease incision. Placing the eyelid on traction with a suture straightens the incision, making this procedure easier to perform.

protected. A compressive dressing is then applied for 24 to 48 hours. Otherwise, cool packs should be applied intermittently for 24 to 48 hours. An alternative to the use of a Frost suture is the subcutaneous injection of air into the lower eyelid, which raises the lower eyelid temporarily and affords protection of the cornea until the effects of the local anesthetic on the orbicularis muscle have worn off.

Postoperative Care

Postoperatively, the patient is prescribed a topical antibiotic ointment to the upper lid wounds three times a day for 2 weeks and Lacrilube ointment 1 to 2 hourly to the eyes for 48 hours and at bedtime. The Lacrilube ointment is then changed to preservative-free topical lubricant drops to be used hourly during the day and Lacrilube is continued at bedtime until the degree of lagophthalmos has improved. The frequency of the lubricants is then gradually reduced over the course of the next few weeks. The patient is instructed to keep the head of the bed elevated for 4 weeks and to avoid lifting any heavy weights for 2 weeks. Clean cool packs are gently applied to the eyelids intermittently for 48 hours. The patient should be reviewed in clinic within 2 weeks and again within 4 to 6 weeks. The upper lid skin sutures are removed after 2 weeks.

Postoperative adjustments for an unsatisfactory height and contour can be made within the first few days after surgery but

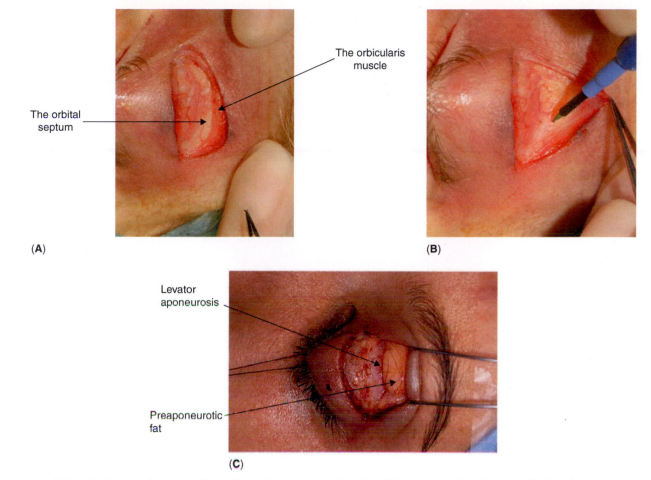

Figure 7.51 (**A**) The orbicularis muscle has been dissected from the orbital septum for a few millimeters using the Colorado needle which helps to define the plane. (**B**) The orbital septum is now opened carefully with the Colorado needle exposing the preaponeurotic fat. (**C**) Preaponeurotic fat exposed.

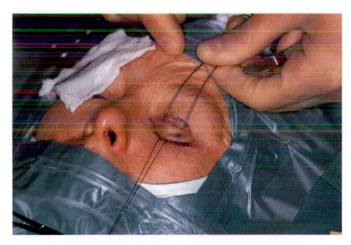

Figure 7.52 The placement of a Jaffe eyelid retractor.

are rarely necessary with attention to detail at the primary procedure. Postoperative eyelid massage can be commenced 2 to 3 weeks after surgery for any residual minor overcorrection. There is no requirement to remove any sutures in children. The skin crease is cleaned with sterile saline solution three times per day and antibiotic ointment applied.

The patient should be advised that the final result following surgery will not be seen for approximately 2 to 3 months as it often takes this amount of time for the postoperative pretarsal edema to completely resolve (Fig. 7.57).

Posterior Approach

This alternative approach has the advantage that it is more adjustable postoperatively and, as there is no incision made through the orbicularis oculi muscle, there is less postoperative lagophthalmos than is seen with the anterior approach. Any skin excess can be removed at a later stage by means of an upper eyelid blepharoplasty. It should be avoided in patients with dry eyes, contact lens wearers, and patients with a tarsus with a small vertical dimension. For these reasons, the anterior approach is preferable in the majority of patients.

The surgical procedure is as described below under levator muscle resection, posterior approach.

Levator Muscle Resection

Anterior Approach

The anterior approach is performed for congenital "dystrophic" ptosis where the levator function is between 5 and 8 mm. This procedure differs from a levator aponeurosis advancement in that the levator aponeurosis is dissected along with Müller's muscle from the conjunctiva and the levator muscle is exposed above Whitnall's ligament. Müller's muscle should be dissected from the conjunctiva until the common sheath of the levator muscle and the superior rectus muscle are encountered. The horns of the levator are cut very carefully with blunt-tipped Westcott scissors taking great care not to cut Whitnall's ligament and the levator muscle is advanced beneath Whitnall's ligament if possible. A double-armed

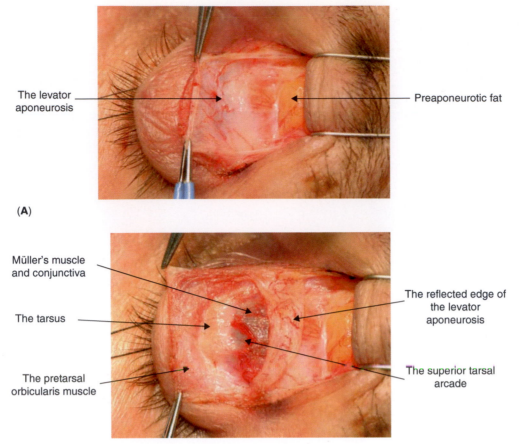

(A)

(B)

Figure 7.53 (**A**) The levator aponeurosis has been dissected free and is being held in an advanced position with forceps. (**B**) The levator aponeurosis has been reflected to expose the tarsus and the underlying Müller's muscle and conjunctiva, along with the superior tarsal arcade.

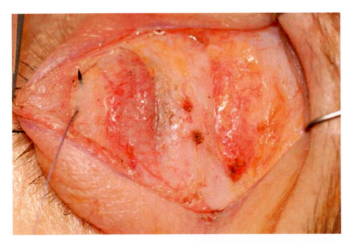

Figure 7.54 The 5/0 Vicryl needle is passed through the tarsus in a lamellar fashion at the junction of the superior 1/3 with the inferior 2/3. Great care should be taken to protect the globe from inadvertent injury from the needle.

5/0 vicryl suture is placed through the tarsus at the desired position of the peak of the eyelid at the junction of the upper 1/3 with the lower 2/3 of the tarsus and then through the advanced levator muscle and Müller's muscle at a position which is estimated to be sufficient to raise the lid to the desired position (depending on the preoperative degree of ptosis and the patient's levator function). The suture is tied with a temporary slipknot and the position of the lid assessed. If this is satisfactory, a section of levator muscle and Müller's muscle

below the suture is resected using blunt-tipped Westcott scissors. The medial and lateral edges of the muscle complex are then sutured to the tarsus medially and laterally with two further 5/0 Vicryl sutures. The skin edges are reapproximated with interrupted 7/0 Vicryl sutures, incorporating a bite of the levator muscle to recreate a skin crease.

It is very difficult to achieve accurate results in levator muscle resection procedures and parents should be warned preoperatively that a further procedure might be required within 1 to 2 weeks if the eyelid height achieved is not satisfactory.

Posterior Approach

The posterior approach can be technically demanding for the inexperienced surgeon, but it offers particular advantages to patients at risk of exposure keratopathy, e.g., patients with chronic progressive external ophthalmoplegia. Such patients are also exquisitely sensitive to the effects of local anesthetic agents, which cause a marked decline in levator function intraoperatively, making eyelid height adjustments via the anterior approach under local anesthesia particularly difficult. This approach does not involve an incision that transects the orbicularis muscle and its motor innervation, and does not therefore cause the same degree of postoperative lagophthalmos associated with the anterior approach. In addition, the eyelid height is lower in the immediate postoperative period, with a gradual rise in the eyelid height occurring over the first few days, which also affords greater corneal protection. The wound can be manipulated by the patient very early in the

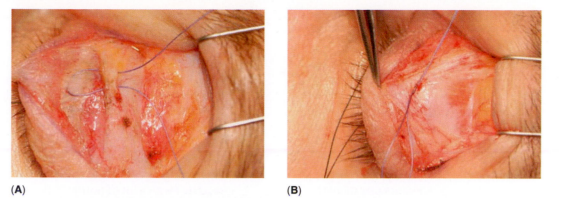

(A)   **(B)**

Figure 7.55 (**A**) The suture is then passed through the levator aponeurosis at the desired level. (**B**) The suture is tied and the patient is then placed into a sitting position to determine whether or not the height and contour of the eyelid are satisfactory.

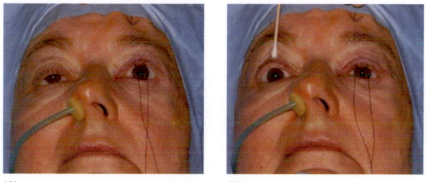

(A)   **(B)**

Figure 7.56 (**A**) The patient is placed into a sitting position and the height and contour of the eyelid are checked. Note that in this patient the left upper eyelid appears to be overcorrected and the right upper eyelid has become ptotic due to Herring's law of equal innervation. (**B**) The right upper eyelid has been raised with a cotton-tipped applicator and the left upper eyelid has immediately assumed a lower position.

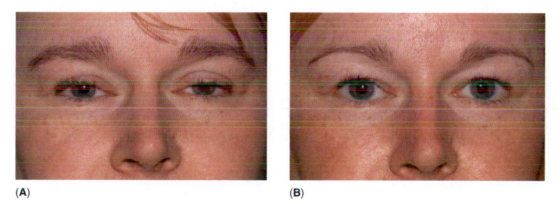

(A)   **(B)**

Figure 7.57 (**A**) A patient with a bilateral levator aponeurosis dehiscence and a history of contact lens wear. (**B**) The same patient 3 months following a bilateral anterior approach levator aponeurosis advancement.

postoperative period to adjust the height and contour of the eyelid. It does not, however, permit any removal of associated dermatochalasis, although this can be addressed at a later stage with a blepharoplasty.

Surgical Procedure

1. The skin crease is marked at the desired level in the upper eyelid using a cocktail stick dipped into a gentian violet block after degreasing the skin with an alcohol wipe. Proxymethacaine is instilled into both eyes and Lacrilube ointment is instilled into the non-operated eye to help to prevent drying of the cornea or an inadvertent corneal abrasion if the patient opens the eye. The patient is prepped and draped leaving the face fully exposed. A damp 4×4 inch swab is placed over the non-operated eye.

2. About 1 to 1.5 ml of 0.5% Bupivacaine with 1:200,000 units of adrenaline mixed 50:50 with 2% lidocaine with 1:80,000 units of adrenaline is injected into the upper eyelid immediately under the skin along the skin crease using a 1-inch orange needle. The injection is given slowly from the temporal

side of the patient ensuring that the tip of the needle is kept in a horizontal plane in case the patient moves or sneezes. The local anesthetic solution is injected as the needle is advanced. If possible, a single needle pass should be used to minimize the risk of causing a hematoma.

3. A 4/0 silk traction suture is placed through the gray line of the upper lid at the desired location of the peak of the eyelid and the lid everted over a medium Desmarres retractor. A further 0.5 to 1 ml of local anesthetic solution is injected subconjunctivally and pressure applied to the closed eye with a swab. A few minutes should be allowed for the adrenaline to take effect.

4. The Desmarres retractor is replaced and the conjunctiva is incised along the superior margin of the tarsus with a no. 15 blade.

5. The conjunctiva and Müller's muscle are dissected from the levator aponeurosis until a white line is located. An incision is made just above the white line with blunt-tipped Westcott scissors, exposing the levator aponeurosis and the preaponeurotic fat pad (Fig. 7.58A and B).

6. Müller's muscle is dissected from the conjunctiva until the common sheath is reached and both the levator aponeurosis and Müller's muscle are advanced from beneath Whitnall's ligament after carefully releasing the medial and lateral horns of the levator.

7. Three double-armed 6/0 silk sutures are placed through the levator muscle and Müller's muscle, through the conjunctiva (Fig. 7.58C), and through the superior edge of the tarsus (Fig. 7.58D) and brought through into the skin crease (Fig. 7.59A) and tied loosely with slipknots.

8. The height and contour of the lid are inspected. If these are unsatisfactory, the sutures are replaced in a different location through the eyelid retractors. Once the result is satisfactory, the redundant Müller's muscle and levator muscle are resected and the sutures are tied over cotton wool bolsters (Fig. 7.59B and C). The suture tension can be adjusted to achieve the desired contour of the eyelid.

9. Topical antibiotic is instilled into the eye. A lower lid 4/0 Nylon Frost suture is placed and a compressive dressing applied for 48 hours, as this approach is associated with a lot of postoperative swelling.

Postoperative Care

The eyelid is inspected after the dressing has been removed. If the eyelid is still low, the sutures are left in position and the patient is reviewed after a further 5 days and the sutures are removed. Eyelid traction/massage is commenced if the eyelid rises above its desired level (Fig. 7.60).

The postoperative care is otherwise as described above for a Müller's muscle resection procedure.

Whitnall's Sling Procedure

The Whitnall's sling procedure offers a potential advantage for the child with "borderline" levator function (3–5 mm) where a frontalis suspension is not desired. In this procedure, the eyelid is very carefully dissected to ensure that Whitnall's ligament attachments are maintained intact (Fig. 7.61). The tarsus is sutured directly to Whitnall's ligament after resecting redundant levator aponeurosis and Müller's muscle (Fig. 7.61). An example of a patient who has undergone this procedure is shown in Figure 7.62. This is, however, associated with a rather static eyelid with marked lag on down gaze.

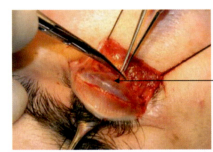

The levator aponeurosis

(A)

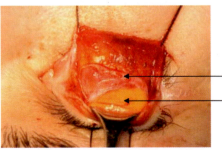

The cut edge of the levator aponeurosis

The preaponeurotic fat

(B)

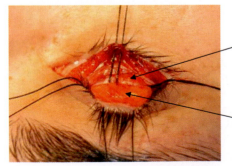

The levator muscle

The preaponeurotic fat

(C)

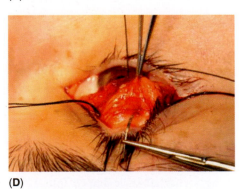

(D)

Figure 7.58 (**A**) The surgeon's view of the levator aponeurosis is being opened at the level of the "white line". (**B**) The levator aponeurosis has been opened exposing the preaponeurotic fat. (**C**) A double-armed 6/0 black silk suture has been passed through the advanced levator muscle and Müller's muscle and through the edge of the conjunctiva. (**D**) The suture is then passed through the tarsus just above the incision line.

Frontalis Suspension Procedure

The purpose of a frontalis sling procedure is to harness the action of the frontalis muscle to elevate the eyelid(s). The normal frontalis muscle has 10 to 15 mm of action, which can be transferred directly to the eyelid if it is connected to the eyelid with either autogenous tissue or non-autogenous material. It can yield very good functional and cosmetic results when performed bilaterally but is less successful if the procedure is performed unilaterally for a unilateral ptosis.

It is essential that the patient is examined immediately preoperatively and the frontalis action observed. The surgical incision markings in the forehead should take into consideration

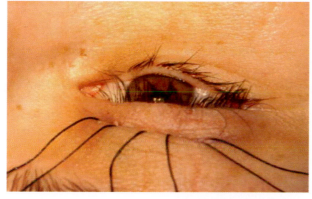

(A)

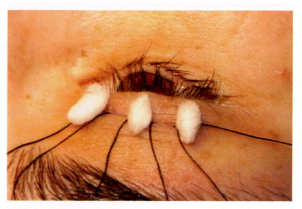

(B)

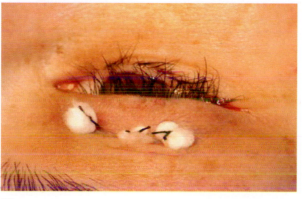

(C)

Figure 7.59 (A) The sutures are brought out through the upper lid skin crease. (B) Small cotton wool bolsters are prepared. (C) The sutures are tied over the cotton wool bolsters adjusting the height and contour of the eyelid by adjusting the tension on the sutures.

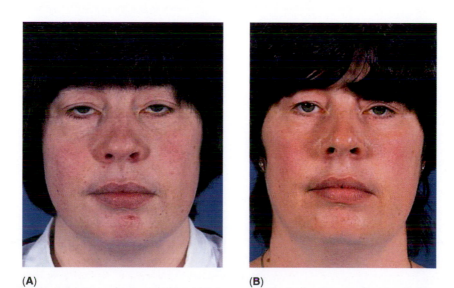

(A)   (B)

Figure 7.60 (A) A patient with myotonic dystrophy and a bilateral ptosis. (B) The patient following a bilateral posterior approach levator resection.

the shape and direction of movement of the brows, as well as any asymmetries.

Autogenous tissue such as fascia lata is preferable for this procedure but non-autogenous materials can be used; e.g., in infants from whom fascia lata cannot be harvested (it is usually necessary to wait until the age of approximately 5 years for a child's leg to be sufficiently developed to harvest fascia lata), and whose ptosis is so marked as to cause amblyopia; in older patients in whom it is less desirable to harvest fascia lata (patients over the age of 60 years with systemic co-morbidities who pose a risk of deep vein thrombosis); and in patients with progressive myopathies as the procedure is essentially irreversible in the event that the patient develops exposure keratopathy. There is a variety of non-autogenous suspensory material (Table 7.9) which can be used, but all materials have the disadvantages of potential infection, extrusion, breakage, or foreign body granuloma formation. Silicone, with the use of an adjustable sleeve, provides an advantage in patients with muscular dystrophies, as the degree of lagophthalmos is not as great.

Polypropylene has the advantage of being very quick and easy to insert and very easy to remove or cut, if necessary, in contrast to Mersilene mesh. It does not biodegrade. Other autogenous materials have been used, e.g., temporalis fascia, palmaris longus tendon, but fascia lata remains the most popular choice. Immense care needs to be exercised when harvesting a palmaris longus tendon for fear of inadvertent trauma to the median nerve. For this reason, the author considers its use inappropriate.

Surgical Techniques
The Fox pentagon is one of the simplest techniques which requires the least material and is preferred for non-autogenous material.

The Crawford double triangle technique gives the best control of the eyelid contour and height and is usually used with autogenous fascia lata. It gives the best long-term results. This technique can, however, be used with non-autogenous material to gain the best possible contour of the eyelid in selected cases.

Trapezoid-Pentagon (Fox) Technique
Closed approach
Surgical procedure
1. Two 1-mm incisions are marked 1 to 2 mm above the lash line, one in line with the medial limbus and

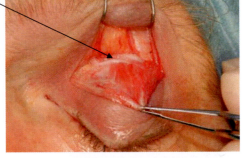

Whitnall's ligament

Figure 7.61 Whitnall's ligament has been exposed.

Table 7.9 Examples of Non-Autogenous Materials Used for Frontalis Suspension

Material	Description
Stored fascia lata	Irradiated or lyophilized
Prolene	Monofilament polypropylene
Supramid	Sheathed polyamide
Mersilene mesh	Flexible interwoven polyester fiber mesh
Silicone	Silicone cord or 240 retinal band
Gore-Tex	Polytetrafluoroethylene (PTFE)
Polypropylene/Vicryl mesh	Composite mesh of monofilament polypropylene and Vicryl

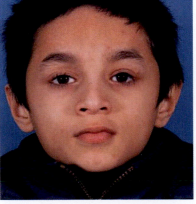

(A)   (B)

Figure 7.62 (**A**) A patient with a left congenital ptosis with only 3 mm of levator function. (**B**) The same patient 4 weeks following an internal Whitnall's sling procedure.

the other in line with the lateral limbus with the eye in primary gaze, using a cocktail stick dipped into a gentian violet marker block.

2. Three 1-mm brow incisions are then marked in the forehead, as shown in Figure 7.63. About 0.2 ml of 0.5% Bupivacaine with 1:200,000 units of adrenaline mixed 50:50 with 2% lidocaine with 1:80,000 units of adrenaline is injected subcutaneously at each mark. A further 1 to 2 mls of the same solution is injected subcutaneously just above the lid margin and also into the lower eyelid. A 4/0 silk traction suture is placed through the gray line of the upper lid and used for traction.

3. The brow incisions are made as stab incisions using a no. 15 blade.

4. The eyelid incisions are made as careful nicks with the blade down to the tarsus, ensuring that the globe is protected.

5. When using a polypropylene suture, the needle is passed through the lid incisions, engaging a partial thickness of the tarsal plate, and taking care to protect the globe with an eyelid guard lubricated with Lacrilube ointment. The eyelid is everted to ensure that the needle has not passed through the full thickness of the tarsus.

6. The needle is then carefully passed from the lid to the lowermost brow incision, passing behind the orbital septum. The other end of the suture is then passed from the lid to the other lowermost brow incision using a Wright's ptosis needle (Fig. 7.63). (When using a Supramid suture, the ski needles are used to engage the tarsus and to pass the suture from the lid to the brow. When using Mersilene mesh, Vicryl/polypropylene mesh, or stored fascia lata, the material is threaded subcutaneously in the eyelid in front of the tarsus using a Wright's ptosis needle and then passed behind the orbital septum using the same needle).

7. The suture is then brought through the central brow incision. The suture is tied with a single throw and the lid is brought to the desired height, which will depend on the requirements of the individual patient, taking into consideration the Bell's phenomenon and orbicularis function, e.g., in a patient with CPEO, the patient should be able to close the eye passively when relaxing the frontalis but should be able to clear the visual axis with moderate frontalis effort.

8. The contour is then adjusted by adjusting the tension on each limb of the suture.

9. A locking Castroviejo needle holder is applied to the suture immediately below the single throw, and the suture is tied using a surgeon's knot. In the case of a polypropylene suture, multiple throws are added. The suture end without the needle is trimmed.

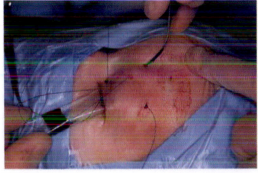

(A)

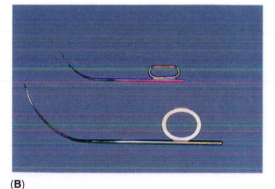

(B)

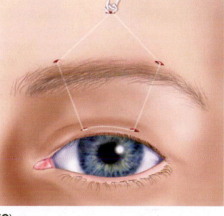

(C)

Figure 7.63 (**A**) A polypropylene frontalis suspension using a Fox pentagon technique. The globe is protected with an eyelid guard lubricated with ointment. A Wright's ptosis needle is being used to withdraw the suture from the eyelid to the medial brow incision. (**B**) Wright's ptosis needles – adult and paediatric sizes. (**C**) The suture is tied and adjusted to ensure an adequate eyelid height and satisfactory contour.

10. Using blunt-tipped Westcott scissors, a small tunnel is fashioned from the central brow incision superiorly.

11. The needle is then passed into the tunnel and out of the skin of the forehead. The suture is pulled superiorly, drawing the knot deep into the subcutaneous tunnel. The suture is then cut flush with the forehead skin.

12. The forehead wounds are closed using interrupted 7/0 Vicryl sutures. The eyelid wounds are left unsutured.

13. Antibiotic ointment is instilled into the eye and applied to the eyelid and forehead wounds.

14. A lower eyelid Frost suture is placed and a compressive dressing applied for 24 to 48 hours.

Postoperative care.   Postoperatively, the patient is prescribed a topical antibiotic ointment for the upper lid and wounds three times a day for 2 weeks and Lacrilube ointment 1 to 2 hourly to the eyes for 48 hours and at bedtime. The Lacrilube ointment is then changed to preservative-free topical lubricant drops to be used hourly during the day and Lacrilube is continued at bedtime until the degree of lagophthalmos has improved. The frequency of the lubricants is then gradually reduced over the course of the next few weeks. The patient is instructed to keep the head of the bed elevated for 4 weeks and to avoid lifting any heavy weights for 2 weeks. Clean cool packs are gently applied to the eyelids intermittently for 48 hours. The patient should be reviewed in clinic within 1 to 2 weeks and again within 4 to 6 weeks. The brow skin sutures are removed after 2 weeks. In the case of children, these can be left to fall out spontaneously.

Open approach.   If silicone tubing is used for a frontalis sling, a skin crease incision can be made and the tarsus exposed. The silicone can be sutured directly to the tarsus using a non-absorbable Mersilene suture to ensure greater stability of the silicone, reducing the risk of migration. In addition, the contour of the eyelid can be adjusted more accurately. There is, however, more swelling associated with this approach and a risk of a lash ptosis. The superior forehead wound can be made slightly larger to accommodate an adjustable sleeve. Although this allows the possibility of a postoperative adjustment, this has to be weighed against the risk of exposure and extrusion of the sleeve.

The Double Triangle (Crawford) Technique
Closed approach.   The Crawford technique is a very popular procedure that usually uses autogenous fascia lata. The technique can be performed in children or adults but a child's leg has to be sufficiently developed to harvest the fascia (usually over 4–5 years of age).

Surgical procedure
1. Two 1-mm incisions are marked 1 to 2 mm above the lash line, one in line with the medial limbus and the other in line with the lateral limbus, using a cocktail stick dipped into a gentian violet marker block. A third incision is marked in line with the pupil with the eye in primary gaze.

2. Three 1-mm brow incisions are then marked in the forehead, as shown in Figure 7.64. The markings should take into consideration the patient's individual brow action. Local anaesthetic solution is injected subcutaneously at each mark and into the upper and lower eyelids as described above. A 4/0 silk traction suture is placed through the gray line of the upper lid and used for traction.

3. The brow incisions are made as stab incisions using a no. 15 blade.

4. The eyelid incisions are made as careful nicks with the blade down to the tarsus, ensuring that the globe is protected.

5. The fascia lata material is threaded subcutaneously between the eyelid incisions using a Wright's ptosis needle and then behind the orbital septum to the medial and lateral brow incisions, taking care to protect the globe with a lid guard coated in Lacrilube ointment. The lid guard must be pushed firmly against the superior orbital margin in the superior conjunctival fornix, before the ptosis needle is pushed towards the eyelid from the brow incisions.

6. The fascia is then tied with a single throw and the eyelid is brought to a height corresponding to the superior limbus or until the eyelid comes away from the globe, and the contour is adjusted. The fascia is then tied using a surgeon's knot and the knot reinforced with a 5/0 Vicryl suture (Fig. 7.64). The longest remaining strips of fascia are brought through the central brow incision and again tied and reinforced.

7. The knots are carefully buried subcutaneously.

8. The forehead wounds are closed using interrupted 7/0 Vicryl sutures. The eyelid incisions are left unsutured.

9. Antibiotic ointment is instilled into the eye and applied to the eyelid and forehead wounds.

10. A lower eyelid Frost suture is placed and a compressive dressing applied for 24 to 48 hours.

Postoperative care.   This is as described above.

Open approach.   An alternative technique involves making a skin crease incision and exposing the tarsus to which the fascia is sewn directly using 5/0 Vicryl sutures. Although more time consuming, this technique permits the creation of a more natural skin crease that can be adjusted with a small additional blepharoplasty, if necessary (Figs. 7.65 and 7.66). The closed technique creates a very low skin crease that cannot be easily adjusted, and which may require a revision blepharoplasty at a later date.

Harvesting Autogenous Fascia Lata
Surgical Procedure
1. A 3-cm incision is marked over the lateral aspect of the thigh, just above the lateral condyle of the knee, along an imaginary line connecting the head of the fibula and the anterior superior iliac spine (Fig. 7.67).

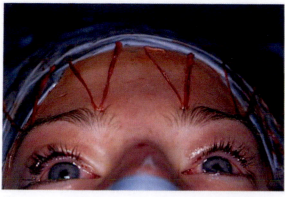
(A)

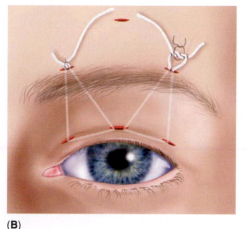
(B)

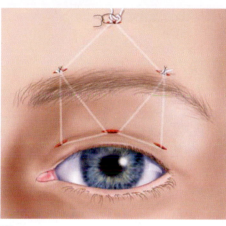
(C)

Figure 7.64 (**A**) An autogenous fascia lata brow suspension using the closed Crawford double triangle technique. (**B**) A diagram demonstrating the re-enforcement of the knots in the fascia using 5/0 vicryl sutures. (**C**) A diagram demonstrating the reinforcement of the central forehead knot in the fascia using a 5/0 Vicryl suture.

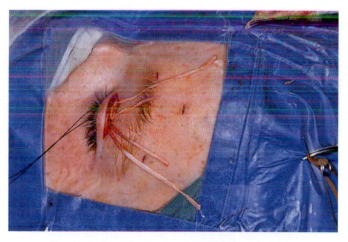

Figure 7.65 Fascia lata strips sutured directly to the tarsus.

2. A 10-ml subcutaneous injection of 0.5% Bupivacaine with 1:200,000 units of adrenaline is given.
3. A skin incision is made using a no. 15 blade.
4. Blunt dissection using Stevens scissors is used to expose the fascia lata.
5. Horizontal fascia overlying the fascia lata is bluntly dissected away with toothed forceps.
6. Two small parallel vertical incisions are then made in the fascia lata, 10 mm apart, with small straight blunt-tipped scissors. These incisions are then extended subcutaneously along the thigh with long straight blunt-tipped scissors (Nelson scissors), if a Moseley fasciotome is being used to remove the fascia. It is vital that the incisions are made as parallel as possible. This step is unnecessary if a Crawford stripper is used. The Crawford stripper has a side cutting mechanism and also has the advantage of offering a scale to measure the length of fascia to be removed (Fig. 7.68).
7. The fascia is then divided at the inferior aspect of the wound and inserted into the fascia lata stripper, which is passed up the thigh for a distance of approximately 15 cm toward the anterior superior iliac spine (Fig. 7.69).
8. The stripper's guillotine mechanism is activated and the fascia removed.
9. The leg wound is then closed with subcutaneous 4/0 Vicryl sutures and the skin closed using interrupted 4/0 nylon vertical mattress sutures.
10. The fascia is cleaned of any fat and then carefully divided into four symmetric lengths using a no. 15 Bard Parker blade and straight iris scissors. The fascia is kept moistened with saline until ready for use (Fig 7.70).

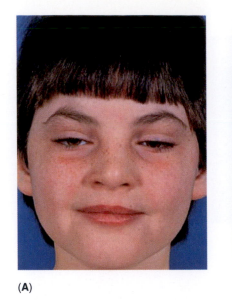
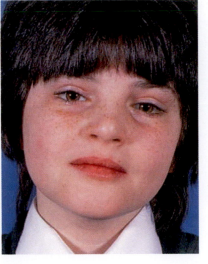

(A)   **(B)**

Figure 7.66 (**A**) A patient with a bilateral congenital ptosis with poor levator function and frontalis over action. (**B**) The same patient, three weeks following a bilateral autogenous fascia lata brow suspension using the open skin crease approach.

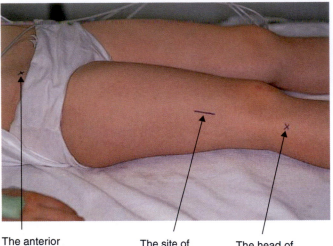

The anterior   The site of   The head of
superior iliac spine   the incision   the fibula

Figure 7.67 The incision for the removal of fascia lata lies on a line running between the anterior superior iliac spine and the head of the fibula.

Postoperative Care

Antibiotic ointment is applied to the wound. A sterile dressing is applied to the wound and the lateral thigh is covered with large soft dressings. A bandage is applied from the toes to the inguinal area. The bandage and dressings are removed the following day. The patient should be encouraged to ambulate as soon as possible following surgery. The sutures are removed after 10 to 14 days.

Lemagne Procedure

This is a two-stage unilateral procedure for the treatment of patients with a Marcus Gunn jaw-winking phenomenon who have a significant ptosis, marked aberrant movements of the eyelid, and have moderate to good levator function. Muscular neurotization is thought to occur in the transposed levator muscle from the underlying frontalis muscle, permitting some levator function to be restored. The maximal degree of levator function may not be achieved for a period of 12 months following the first stage of surgery. The procedure is successful

in abolishing aberrant eyelid movements. It requires a second-stage levator advancement procedure after 12 months to achieve a satisfactory improvement in the ptosis.

Surgical Procedure

1. The initial steps are as described for a levator resection above.
2. A 2-cm horizontal skin incision is marked just above the central aspect of the eyebrow.
3. One to two milliliters of 0.5% Bupivacaine with 1:200,000 units of adrenaline mixed 50:50 with 2% lidocaine with 1:80,000 units of adrenaline is injected subcutaneously above the eyebrow.
4. The levator muscle is isolated above Whitnall's ligament and a strabismus hook placed beneath it, ensuring that the superior rectus muscle is not inadvertently included (Fig. 7.71A).
5. The muscle is dissected to the orbital apex and where it is transected with blunt-tipped Westcott scissors (Fig. 7.71B).
6. A double-armed 5/0 Vicryl suture is placed through the cut end of the muscle (Fig. 7.71C). The levator aponeurosis and Whitnall's ligament are left undisturbed.
7. A 2-cm incision is made just above the central aspect of the eyebrow with a no. 15 Bard Parker blade. This incision and the eyelid crease incision are joined by blunt dissection with Stevens tenotomy scissors.
8. The levator muscle is transposed to lie above the frontalis muscle to which it is sutured (Fig. 7.71D). A levator advancement is then performed 12 months later.

COMPLICATIONS OF PTOSIS SURGERY

The majority of complications (Table 7.10) of ptosis surgery can be avoided by:

1. A thorough knowledge of eyelid anatomy
2. A careful preoperative evaluation of the patient
3. Selection of the most appropriate surgical procedure

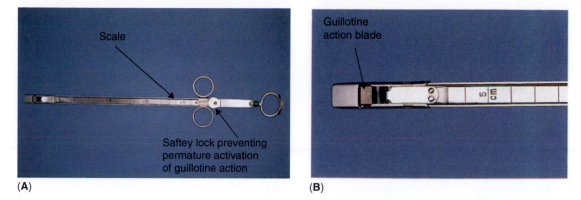

(A)   **(B)**

Figure 7.68 (**A**) A Crawford fascia lata stripper. (**B**) A close-up photograph of the Crawford fascia lata stripper demonstrating the guillotine action blade.

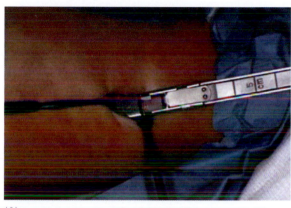

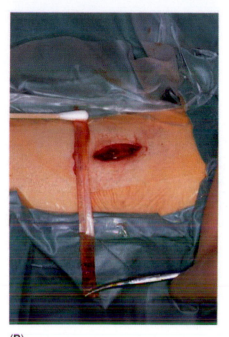

(A)   **(B)**

Figure 7.69 (**A**) The cut inferior end of the fascia is inserted into the fascia lata stripper. (**B**) The 1 cm × 15 cm strip of fascia is removed.

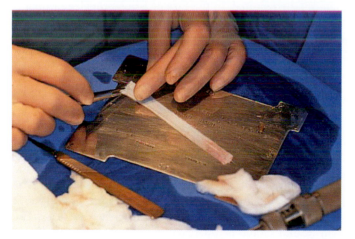

Figure 7.70 The fascia is being cleaned on a graft board before being divided into 2 mm strips.

4. Preoperative and intraoperative precautions to prevent excessive bleeding
5. Meticulous surgical technique
6. Good postoperative care

Undercorrection

Levator Aponeurosis Advancement/Levator Resection

An undercorrection may be the desired result in patients who are at high risk of exposure keratopathy. An unplanned undercorrection can have a variety of causes:

- An inadequate levator aponeurosis advancement/ levator muscle resection
- Cheese wiring of sutures placed too superficially in the tarsus
- Loosening of incorrectly tied sutures
- Placement of sutures through a very thinned levator aponeurosis
- Cheese wiring of sutures following excessive eyelid edema or hematoma

When this procedure has been performed in adults, it is preferable to explore the levator aponeurosis within a week of surgery and readvance the aponeurosis under local anesthesia with sedation. In children, this will require another general anesthetic. If there is excessive postoperative edema or hematoma, however, it is preferable to await resolution and perform a formal reoperation at a later date.

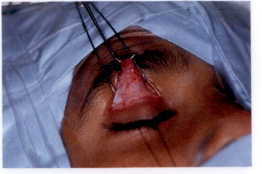

(A)

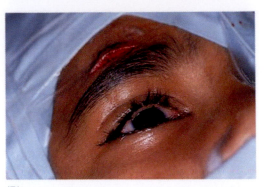

(B)

(C)

(D)

Figure 7.71 (**A**) The levator muscle is isolated and hooked with a strabismus hook. (**B**) The full length of the levator muscle is exposed. (**C**) The muscle is transacted at the orbital apex and a double armed 5/0 vicryl suture is placed through the muscle stump. (**D**) A brow incision is made just above the eyebrow and the levator muscle is transposed to lie over the frontalis muscle.

Table 7.10 Complications of Ptosis Surgery

Under-correction
Over-correction
Lagophthalmos/exposure keratopathy
Eyelid contour defects
Skin crease defects
Conjunctival prolapse
Upper lid entropion/ectropion
Eyelash ptosis
Loss of eyelashes
Posterior lamellar granuloma/suture exposure
Extrusion/infection of frontalis suspension material
Diplopia
Hemorrhage

Whitnall's Sling

An undercorrection may be cosmetically and functionally acceptable and preferable to a unilateral frontalis suspension. It may be possible to repeat the procedure within a week of surgery unless there is excessive eyelid swelling or a hematoma. An unsatisfactory result, however, will usually require a frontalis suspension to provide an adequate height to the eyelid.

Frontalis Suspension

An undercorrection can have a variety of causes:

- Cheese wiring of a suture, e.g., a polypropylene suture which did not engage the tarsus
- Cheese wiring of sutures following excessive eyelid edema or hematoma

- Loosening of inadequately reinforced fascial knots
- Failure to raise the eyelid sufficiently prior to burying the fascial knots

An undercorrection following a frontalis suspension procedure will usually require early reintervention. In the case of a fascia lata frontalis suspension, the forehead wounds should be reopened within a few days of the surgery and the fascial knots tightened and resutured. Otherwise, a reoperation at a later date will be required. In the case of a polypropylene frontalis suspension, the suture will need to be removed and the procedure repeated. If there is excessive postoperative edema or hematoma, however, it is preferable to await resolution and perform a formal reoperation at a later date.

Overcorrection

Levator Aponeurosis Advancement/Levator Resection

An overcorrection is rarely encountered following surgery for congenital "dystrophic" ptosis. In such cases, it is likely that the lid position will improve spontaneously and lubrication of the cornea is all that is required. If a marked overcorrection has been caused following an anterior approach procedure, a reoperation should be undertaken without undue delay. The skin wound should be opened and the levator resutured in a more recessed position. If too much levator aponeurosis or muscle has been resected, a temporalis fascial graft may need to be used as a "spacer" graft, sutured between the levator muscle and the tarsus. "Hang back" sutures can be used as an alternative but these are less reliable.

An overcorrection is more commonly encountered following surgery for an aponeurotic ptosis, especially if this has

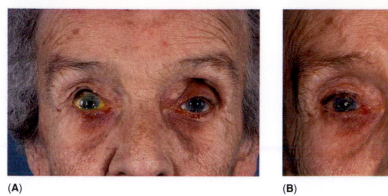

(A)   (B)

Figure 7.72 (**A**) An elderly patient with marked right upper eyelid retraction due to an overcorrected levator aponeurosis advancement which was performed under general anesthesia. (**B**) The same patient following a posterior approach levator aponeurosis recession performed under local anesthesia.

been performed under general anesthesia (Fig. 7.72). A marked overcorrection can be addressed early by a reoperation as described above. Postoperative downward eyelid traction may be performed as soon as the sutures have been removed when the levator surgery has been performed via a posterior approach. The patient should be carefully instructed about the technique. The patient should look down and then grasp the edge of the upper eyelid and eyelashes firmly between the thumb and forefinger at the position of the peak of the eyelid. The patient should then pull the eyelid downward firmly whilst looking upward. This maneuver should be undertaken for a few minutes three to four times per day until a satisfactory height and contour have been achieved and maintained. The patient should be reassured that this maneuver cannot suddenly reverse the effects of the surgery. Downward traction cannot be performed so soon following anterior approach surgery without risking a skin wound dehiscence. Downward traction has to be deferred for at least three to four weeks.

Overcorrections, which do not respond to more conservative measures, will require a levator tenotomy or a formal levator recession performed as soon as all the postoperative eyelid edema has completely resolved. In the case of an adult, this should be performed under local anesthesia with sedation wherever possible to ensure the most accurate result, but under general anesthesia in a child. The eyelid is everted over a Desmarres retractor using a gray line 4/0 silk traction suture and a transconjunctival incision is made at the upper border of the tarsus. The levator aponeurosis is dissected with Westcott scissors and the lid position inspected at intervals after removing the retractor (see Page 182 in chap. 8). The lid position should be slightly overcorrected to allow for postoperative wound contracture. No sutures are required. Downward eyelid traction in an adult is commenced as soon as the lid height is satisfactory to prevent a recurrence. In the case of children, it can be difficult to achieve the desired degree of correction under general anesthesia and the child cannot usually cooperate with postoperative eyelid traction. The parents should therefore be counseled about the possible requirement for more than one operation to achieve the desired outcome.

Whitnall's Sling
The management of an overcorrection following a Whitnall's sling procedure is as described above.

Frontalis Suspension
If synthetic material has been used, this will have to be explored and adjusted, or removed, and the procedure repeated. If a silicone band has been used with a sleeve, the sleeve can be exposed and adjusted. Such intervention, however, increases the risk of infection and extrusion. If autogenous material has been used, the bands can be divided above the skin crease once they have scarred into position, usually after a few weeks. In the case of an adult, this can be performed under local anesthesia with sedation. A gray line traction suture is placed and the lid is stretched inferiorly. The bands are then easily palpated and can be divided with Westcott scissors after making a small stab incision in the skin overlying the appropriate band using a no. 15 Bard Parker blade. This is continued until the lid has a satisfactory height and contour. The traction suture is left in place as a reverse Frost suture and taped to the cheek for 24 hours.

Lagophthalmos/Exposure Keratopathy
Patients should be warned preoperatively that their reflex blink will be incomplete following ptosis surgery and even voluntary eyelid closure may be compromised, albeit temporarily. Frequent lubrication should be used to prevent exposure keratopathy. In cases where conservative treatment fails to control the symptoms and signs of exposure, the eyelid(s) will have to be lowered as described above under overcorrection. Patients who are at increased risk of exposure keratopathy, e.g., patients with CPEO with an absent Bell's phenomenon, should be monitored very closely following ptosis surgery (Fig. 7.73). Overcorrections should be avoided.

Eyelid Contour Defects
Eyelid contour defects usually occur from improper placement of tarsal sutures during levator surgery or from improper tightening of suspension material during a frontalis suspension procedure (Fig. 7.74). Minor defects can respond to massage applied selectively to areas of overcorrection. More severe defects usually require a formal surgical correction with appropriate placement of sutures to adjust the contour if the eyelid is too low, or with a posterior approach levator recession if the eyelid is too high. A contour defect following an autogenous fascia lata sling can be adjusted by a selective division of the sling as described above.

Skin Crease Defects

Skin crease defects can mar an otherwise satisfactory result (Fig. 7.75). They can occur for a variety of reasons:

- Failure to measure out and mark the new proposed skin crease prior to surgery (Fig. 7.75)
- Failure to reform the skin crease by passing the interrupted skin sutures through the levator following levator surgery
- Failure to perform an upper lid blepharoplasty when there is excess upper lid skin

- A low skin crease is an inherent disadvantage of a closed frontalis suspension procedure (Fig. 7.76)
- A lowering of the skin crease is an inherent disadvantage of the Fasanella–Servat procedure

An unsatisfactory skin crease can usually be addressed by a formal blepharoplasty. In some cases, passing three to four double-armed 5/0 Vicryl sutures through the eyelid from the conjunctival surface at the upper border of the tarsus and tying them in the skin at the desired position will create scarring and a skin crease (Pang sutures).

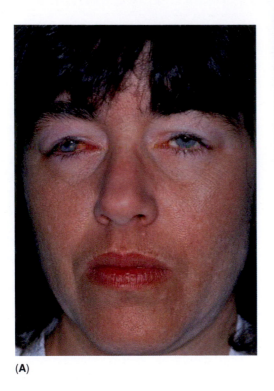

(A)

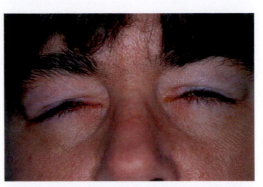

(B)

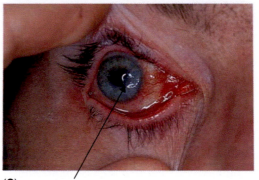

(C) Corneal ulcer

Figure 7.73 (**A**) A patient with CPEO following a bilateral autogenous fascia lata frontalis suspension presenting with a red right eye. (**B**) The same patient demonstrating lagophthalmos and an absent Bell's phenomenon. (**C**) The same patient demonstrating a medial right corneal ulcer. The ulcer perforated a few days later.

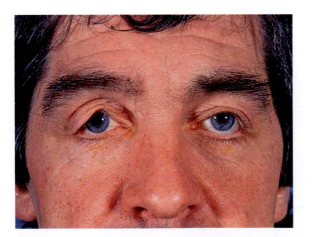

Figure 7.74 A patient with a marked right upper eyelid contour defect following a levator aponeurosis advancement.

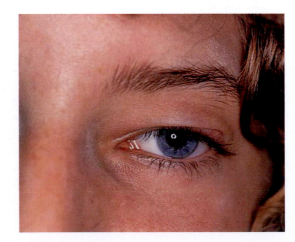

Figure 7.75 A patient with a left skin crease defect following a levator aponeurosis advancement.

Conjunctival Prolapse

A conjunctival prolapse usually occurs in severe cases of congenital "dystrophic" ptosis where the dissection has been taken above the superior fornix, causing the suspensory ligaments of the conjunctival fornix to be separated (Fig. 7.77). It may also occur as a result of excessive postoperative edema. Conservative treatment with simple topical lubrication may suffice. An attempt to reposition the prolapsed conjunctiva can be made with the use of a muscle hook, but if this fails Pang sutures can be passed through the prolapsed conjunctiva and tied in the skin crease. Rarely, if the prolapse is chronic, the prolapsed conjunctiva will require a formal excision to be performed.

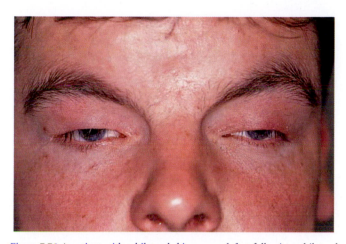

Figure 7.76 A patient with a bilateral skin crease defect following a bilateral autogenous fascia lata frontalis suspension.

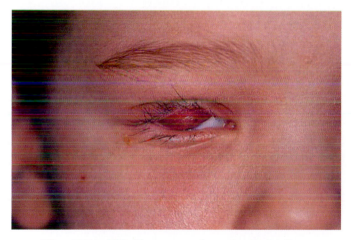

Figure 7.77 A child with a postoperative conjunctival prolapse.

Upper Lid Entropion/Ectropion

Entropion of the upper eyelid following ptosis surgery can occur in the following circumstances:

- Following an excessive tarsal resection during a Fasanella–Servat procedure (Fig. 7.78)
- Following excessive levator resections
- Following an autogenous fascia lata frontalis suspension procedure if the anterior lamellar dissection has been overly aggressive and the fascia has been sutured too low on the tarsus

Where an excessive tarsal resection has been performed, a posterior lamellar graft may have to be undertaken (see Page 94 in chap. 4). Following an excessive levator resection procedure, the eyelid position will usually improve with a release of the tarsal sutures. If an upper lid entropion occurs following a frontalis suspension procedure, the eyelid will need to be explored, scar tissue released and a more formal upper eyelid entropion procedure may be required (see chap. 4).

Ectropion of the upper eyelid following ptosis surgery is very rare. It can occur if the levator is advanced too far on the tarsus or if fascia is overly tightened during the course of a frontalis suspension procedure. This malposition should normally improve with massage or suture release.

Eyelash Ptosis

An eyelash ptosis can occur following an overly aggressive dissection of the orbicularis muscle from the tarsus along with a suturing of the levator aponeurosis or muscle at too high a position on the tarsus (Fig. 7.79). If the lash ptosis persists following resolution of pretarsal edema, the levator aponeurosis or muscle will need to be advanced on the tarsus if there is an associated blepharoptosis. This may have to be combined with a gray line split using a guarded supersharp blade on a Beaver blade handle (see chap. 4), and a formal skin crease reformation ensuring that the skin edges are sutured tightly to the underlying levator aponeurosis or to the tarsus.

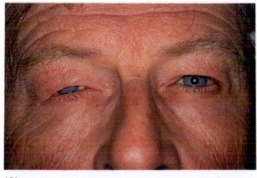

(A)

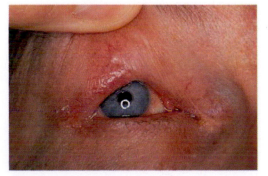

(B)

Figure 7.78 (**A**) A patient with a severe right upper eyelid entropion following a Fasanella-Servat procedure. (**B**) A close-up photograph of the right upper eyelid with the brow elevated manually demonstrating the severity of the entropion.

Loss of Eyelashes

Loss of eyelashes is caused by an overly aggressive dissection of the orbicularis muscle from the tarsus (Fig. 7.80). It is only necessary to expose the superior 1/3 of the tarsus during ptosis surgery. A severe loss of eyelashes will require individual eyelash grafting to be performed. This is a difficult, laborious, and very time-consuming procedure.

Posterior Lamellar Granuloma/suture Exposure

A foreign body granuloma as a reaction to sutures is a common complication following posterior approach levator surgery. The granuloma can be removed with Westcott scissors and the base cauterized. Occasionally, sutures erode through the conjunctiva if non-dissolvable sutures have been used (Fig. 7.81). The occurrence of a granuloma should provoke a search for such suture material.

Extrusion/Infection of Frontalis Suspension Material

Infection, foreign body reaction, and extrusion are a risk whenever non-autogenous material is used for frontalis suspension (Fig. 7.82). Once this has occurred, the material will usually have to be removed. Occasionally, the postoperative scarring can itself assist in frontalis suspension, obviating the need for further surgery.

It is important to ensure that frontalis suspension material is completely buried subcutaneously and that the wounds are closed meticulously. A strictly aseptic surgical technique should be employed with the area prepped as for an intraocular procedure. It is also important to ensure that the material is passed posterior to the orbital septum wherever possible or the material will be visible through the skin (Fig. 7.83). Visibility through the skin is, however, an inherent problem of this procedure in patients with an upper eyelid sulcus defect. In

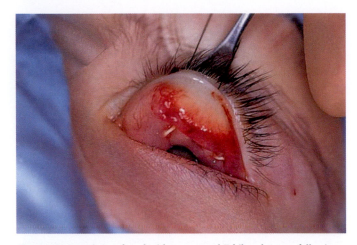

Figure 7.81 A patient referred with an exposed Ethibond suture following a levator resection.

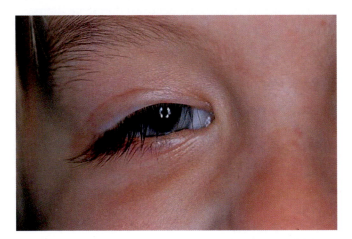

Figure 7.79 A patient with a severe right upper eyelid lash ptosis following a levator resection.

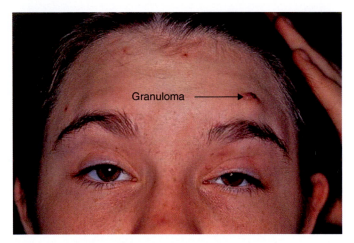

Figure 7.82 A patient with a foreign body granuloma following a Mersilene mesh frontalis suspension.

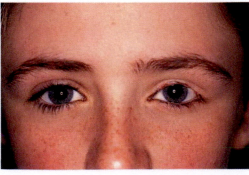

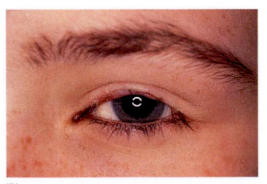

(A)   **(B)**

Figure 7.80 (A) A patient with a loss of upper eyelid lashes in the left upper eyelid following a levator resection. (B) A close-up photograph of the patient's left upper eyelid.

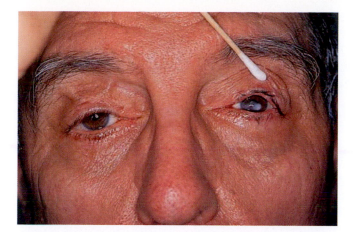

Figure 7.83 A patient with a silicone band visible through the skin in the right upper eyelid following a frontalis suspension procedure. The left eye has had the band removed following the development of severe exposure keratopathy and corneal scarring.

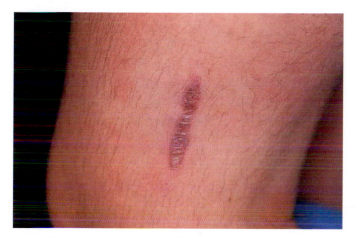

Figure 7.84 A patient with an unsightly leg scar following the harvesting of fascia lata.

carefully selected patients, this problem can be overcome with the use of fat grafting to the upper eyelid using pearls of fat harvested from the peri-umbilical area.

Although the results of autogenous fascia lata brow suspension are usually very good, the patient should also be warned that the scar on the leg may be unsightly as the wound tends to widen postoperatively (Fig. 7.84).

Diplopia

Diplopia should be an extremely rare complication following ptosis surgery. It usually occurs due to inadvertent injury to the superior rectus muscle or to the superior oblique tendon. Such a complication should not occur if the surgeon has an adequate knowledge of upper eyelid anatomy.

Hemorrhage

Hemorrhage can adversely affect the outcome of ptosis surgery. Precautions should be taken to prevent intraoperative and postoperative hemorrhage:

- The patient should discontinue aspirin and any other anti-platelet drugs at least 2 weeks prior to surgery wherever possible

- Any patient on anticoagulants should undergo surgery in consultation with a hematologist
- Any patient with hypertension should take their usual anti-hypertensive agents on the day of surgery and the hypertension should be under control
- Local anesthetic injections in the eyelids should be given just under the surface of the skin and not into the orbicularis muscle or deeper
- The surgery should be performed with the patient in a reverse Trendelenburg position
- Meticulous hemostasis should be performed at all stages of surgery
- A lower lid Frost suture and a compressive dressing should be applied postoperatively wherever possible

FURTHER READING

1. Albert DM, Lucarelli MJ. Ptosis. In: Clinical Atlas of Procedures in Ophthalmic Surgery. Chicago, IL: AMA Press, 2004.
2. Allen CE, Rubin PAD. Blepharophimosis-ptosis-epicanthus inversus syndrome (BPES): clinical manifestation and treatment. Int Ophthalmol Clin 2008; 48(2): 15–23.
3. Anderson RL, Beard C. The levator aponeurosis. Arch Ophthalmol 1977; 95: 1437–41.
4. Anderson RL, Dixon RS. Aponeurotic ptosis surgery. Arch Ophthalmol 1979; 97: 1123–8.
5. Anderson RL. Age of aponeurotic awareness. Ophthal Plast Reconstr Surg 1985; 1: 77–9.
6. Anderson RL, Jordan DR, Dutton JJ. Whitnall's sling for poor function ptosis. Arch Ophthalmol 1990; 108: 1628–32.
7. Baroody M, Holds JB, Vick VL. Advances in the diagnosis and treatment of ptosis [Review]. Curr Opin Ophthalmol. 2005; 16(6): 351–5.
8. Beard C. A new classification of blepharoptosis. Int Ophthal Clin 1989; 29: 214–16.
9. Beard C. Ptosis. St. Louis, MO: CV Mosby, 1981.
10. Ben Simon GJ, Lee S, Schwarcz RM, et al. Muller's muscle-conjunctival resection for correction of upper eyelid ptosis: relationship between phenylephrine testing and the amount of tissue resected with final eyelid position. Arch Facial Plas Surg 2007; 9(6): 413–17.
11. Berry-Brincat A, Willshaw H. Paediatric blepharoptosis: a 10 year review. Eye (Lond) 2009; 23(7):1554–9.
12. Bowyer JD, Sullivan TJ. Management of Marcus Gunn jaw winking synkiesis. Ophthal Plast Reconstr Surg 2004; 20(2): 92–8.
13. Buckman G, Levine MR. Treatment of prolapsed conjunctiva. Ophthal Plast Reconstr Surg 1986; 2: 33–9.
14. Carroll RP. Preventable problems following the Fasanella–Servat procedure. Ophthal Surg 1986; 11: 44–51.
15. Cetinkaya A, Brannan PA. What is new in the era of focal dystonia treatment? Botulinum injections and more. Curr Opin Ophthalmol 2007; 18: 424–9.
16. Cetinkaya A, Brannan PA. Ptosis repair options and algorithm. Curr Opin Ophthalmol 2008; 19: 428–34.
17. Codere F, Tucker NA, Renaldi B. The anatomy of Whitnall ligament. Ophthalmology 1995; 102: 2016–19.
18. Collin JR. Complications of ptosis surgery and their management: a review. J R Soc Med 1979; 72: 25–6.
19. Dresner SC. Further modification of the Müller's muscle: conjunctival resection procedure for blepharoptosis. Ophthal Plast Reconstr Surg 1991; 7: 114–22.
20. Dutton JJ. Atlas of clinical and surgical orbital anatomy. Philadelphia, PA: WB Saunders, 1994.
21. Edmunds B, Manners RM, Weller RO, Steart P, Collin JR. Levator palpebrae superioris fibre size in normals and patients with congenital ptosis. Eye 1998; 12: 47–50.
22. Fasanella RM, Servat J. Levator resection for minimal ptosis, with indications and reappraisal. Int Ophthal Clin 1970; 10: 117–30.
23. Ficker LA, Collin JR, Lee JP. Management of ipsilateral ptosis with hypotropia. Br J Ophthalmol 1986; 70: 732–6.
24. Frueh BR. The mechanistic classification of ptosis. Ophthalmology 1980; 87: 1019–21.

25. George A, Haydar AA, Adams WM. Imaging of Horner's syndrome. Clin Radiol 2008; 63: 499–505.

26. Georgescu D, Vagefi MR, McMullan TFW, McCann JD, Anderson RL. Upper eyelid myectomy in blepharospasm with associated apraxia of lid opening. Am J Ophthalmol 2008; 145: 541–7.

27. Jordan DR, Anderson RL. The aponeurotic approach to congenital ptosis. Ophthal Surg 1990; 21: 237–44.

28. Juel VC, Massey JM. Myasthenia gravis. Orphanet J Rare Dis 2007; 2: 44.

29. Khooshabeh R. Baldwin HC. Isolated Muller's muscle resection for the correction of blepharoptosis. Eye. 2008; 22(2): 267–72. Comment in: Eye (Lond) 2009; 23(5): 1236; author reply 1236–7; PMID: 18497831.

30. Koursh DM, Modjtahedi SP, Selva D, Leibovitch I. The blepharochalasis syndrome. Surv Ophthalmol 2009; 54(2): 235–44.

31. Lane CM, Collin JR. Treatment of ptosis in chronic progressive external ophthalmoplegia. Br J Ophthalmol 1987; 71: 290–4.

32. Leibovitch I, Selva D. Floppy eyelid syndrome: clinical features and the association with obstructive sleep apnea. Sleep Med 2006; 7:117–22.

33. Leone CR Jr., Shore JW. The management of the ptosis patient: Part I. Ophthal Surg 1985; 16: 666–70.

34. Manners RM, Rosser P, Collin JR. Moorfields Eye Hospital, London, UK. Levator transposition procedure: a review of 35 cases. Eye 1994; 10: 539–44.

35. Manners RM, Tyers AG, Morris RJ. The use of Prolene as a temporary suspensory material for brow suspension in young children. Eye 1994; 8: 346–8.

36. Martin JJ Jr., Tenzel RR. Acquired ptosis: dehiscences and disinsertions. Are they real or iatrogenic? Ophthal Plast Reconstr Surg 1992; 8: 130–2; discussion 133.

37. McCord C, ed. Complications of ptosis surgery and their management. In: Eyelid Surgery Principles and Techniques. Philadelphia, PA: Lippincott-Raven, 1995a: 144–55.

38. McCord C, ed. Decision making in ptosis surgery. In: Eyelid Surgery Principles and Techniques. Philadelphia, PA: Lippincott-Raven, 1995b: 139–43.

39. McNab AA. The eye and sleep. Clin Exp Ophthalmol 2005; 33: 117–25.

40. McNab AA. The eye and sleep apnea. Sleep Med Rev 2007; 11: 269–76.

41. Meyer DR, Linberg JV, Wobig JL, McCormick SA. Anatomy of the orbital septum and associated eyelid connective tissues. Implications for ptosis surgery. Ophthal Plast Reconstr Surg 1991; 7: 104–13.

42. Michels KS, Vagefi MR, Steele E, et al. Müller muscle-conjunctiva resection to correct ptosis in high-risk patients. Ophthal Plast Reconstr Surg 2007; 23(5): 363–6.

43. Nerad JA, Carter KD, Alford MA. Disorders of the eyelid: blepharoptosis and eyelid retraction. In: Rapid Diagnosis in Ophthalmology-Oculoplastic and Reconstructive Surgery. Philadelphia, PA: Mosby Elsevier, 2008: 102–15.

44. Ortisi E, Henderson HWA, Bunce C, Xing W, Collin JRO. Blepharospasm and hemifacial spasm: a protocol for titration of Botulinum toxin dose to the individual patient and for the management of refractory cases. Eye 2006; 20: 916–22.

45. Putterman AM. Müllers muscle-conjunctival resection ptosis procedure. Austral NZ J Ophthalmol 1985; 13: 179–83.

46. Putterman AM. Muller's muscle-conjunctival resection. In: Levine MR, ed. Manual of Oculoplastic Surgery, 3rd edn. Boston, MA: Butterworth-Heinemann, 2003: 117–23.

47. Shore JW, Bergin DJ, Garrett SN. Results of blepharoptosis surgery with early postoperative adjustment. Ophthalmology 1990; 97: 1502–11.

48. Striph GG, Miller NR. Disorders of eyelid function caused by systemic disease. In: Bosniak S, ed. Principles and Practice of Ophthalmic Plastic and Reconstructive Surgery. Philadelphia, PA: WB Saunders, 1996: pp.72–93.

49. Woog JJ. Obstructive sleep apnea and the floppy eyelid syndrome. Am J Ophthalmol 1990; 110: 314–6.

50. Wong VA, Beckisale PS, Oley CA, Sullivan TJ. Management of myogenic ptosis. Am Acad Ophthalmol 2002; 109: 1023–31.

51. Yanovitch T, Buckley E. Diagnosis and management of third nerve palsy. Curr Opin Ophthal 2007; 18: 373–8.

8   The management of thyroid-related eyelid retraction

INTRODUCTION

The appropriate management of eyelid retraction in Graves' disease depends on an understanding of the pathophysiological mechanisms responsible for the eyelid malposition. Attention to the pathophysiology of the eyelid malposition permits the selection of the most appropriate intervention and improves the predictability of the outcome. In the upper and lower eyelids the pathophysiological mechanisms are:

- Adrenergic stimulation of Müller's muscle and its smooth muscle equivalent in the lower eyelid
- Pseudoproptosis due to axial myopia
- Proptosis
- Inflammation and fibrosis of the upper and lower eyelid retractors
- Inflammation and fibrosis of the anterior orbital fascial septa
- Fibrosis of the tensor intermuscularis
- Inflammation and fibrosis of the inferior rectus muscle

These mechanisms may occur singly or in combination and with varying degrees of asymmetry.

Mild degrees of eyelid retraction caused by increased sensitivity of Müller's muscle and its smooth muscle equivalent in the lower eyelid to circulating catecholamines may resolve with treatment of the hyperthyroid state.

Axial myopia is commonly overlooked as a cause of eyelid retraction. High myopia can compound other mechanisms of eyelid retraction and make the surgical management particularly challenging (Fig. 8.1).

Proptosis, similarly, acts as a wedge between the eyelids. In many patients, treatment of the proptosis by orbital decompression surgery can relieve the eyelid retraction, particularly lower eyelid retraction (Fig. 8.2), but eyelid retraction will only improve in those patients in whom proptosis is the major cause of the retraction.

Inflammation and fibrosis of the upper and lower eyelid retractors can be responsible for marked degrees of eyelid retraction (Fig. 8.3). Downward traction applied by the examiner to the upper eyelid margin will be met with marked resistance.

Inflammation and fibrosis of the anterior orbital fascial septa also play a part in eyelid retraction in some patients. This is evident at surgery, when lid retraction may persist in spite of a satisfactory degree of eyelid retractor recession having been achieved.

Fibrosis of the tensor intermuscularis, the muscle fibers lying circumferentially within the superolateral intermuscular septum, may account for the disproportionate lateral lid retraction seen in Graves' disease.

Inflammation and fibrosis of the inferior rectus muscle may cause a hypotropia with a compensatory overaction of the superior rectus/levator complex causing eyelid retraction. The degree of eyelid retraction should be assessed and compared in downgaze and upgaze. Upper eyelid retraction which worsens on upgaze is due to fibrosis of the inferior rectus muscle (Fig. 8.4). Such patients also demonstrate a rise in intraocular pressure on upgaze. A recession of the inferior rectus muscle with adjustable sutures should be considered for such patients and should be undertaken after an orbital decompression procedure but before any eyelid lengthening procedure. An inferior rectus recession can cause an increase in proptosis and can result in worsening of lower eyelid retraction.

PATIENT EVALUATION

The patient should be carefully evaluated to determine the following:

- The degree of activity of the disease
- The mechanisms responsible for the eyelid retraction
- The severity of any exposure keratopathy
- The degree of eyelid retraction
- The variability of the eyelid retraction

The patient's upper eyelid margin and eyelashes should be grasped between the examiner's forefinger and thumb and downward traction applied. The degree of resistance should be noted. Marked resistance is indicative of fibrosis within the upper lid retractors, the anterior orbital fascial septa and/or the tensor intermuscularis. Surgery on such patients will be more difficult and will have a less predictable outcome.

In some patients the degree of upper eyelid retraction can be underestimated due to the presence of a brow ptosis and dermatochalasis or upper eyelid swelling. The brows should be gently elevated to ascertain the true position of the upper eyelids (Fig. 8.5).

TIMING OF SURGICAL INTERVENTION

Surgery to manage eyelid retraction in thyroid eye disease should be deferred until the disease has entered a quiescent phase, unless exposure keratopathy unresponsive to medical therapy requires more urgent intervention. Eyelid retraction surgery undertaken during the active phase can compromise the outcome. In general, the thyroid status and eyelid position should be stable for a minimum period of 6 months before any eyelid surgery is undertaken. When such surgery has to be postponed due to active thyroid eye disease, chemodenervation-induced ptosis using botulinum toxin injections can be considered (10–20 units of Dysport can be injected subconjunctivally into Müller's muscle or transcutaneously into the levator muscle and repeated as required after 10 days), or a temporary lateral tarsorrhaphy can be performed.

> **KEY POINT**
>
> As a general rule, eyelid surgery should be undertaken after orbital decompression surgery and any strabismus surgery, should these be required.

**ORBITAL DECOMPRESSION VERSUS
EYELID SURGERY**

It can be difficult to counsel a patient with significant proptosis about the relative merits of orbital decompression surgery versus eyelid repositioning surgery in the absence of other clear indications for orbital decompression, e.g., compressive optic neuropathy unresponsive to medical therapy. In the presence of a significant degree of proptosis, unilateral proptosis or asymmetric proptosis, there is no question that eyelid repositioning surgery alone will not achieve a good cosmetic result for the patient (Fig. 8.6). Orbital decompression surgery is, however, far more invasive than eyelid surgery alone and is associated with a number of risks. The decision should be made on an individual basis.

A patient must be carefully counseled about the aims, risks, and potential complications of surgery. Unrealistic

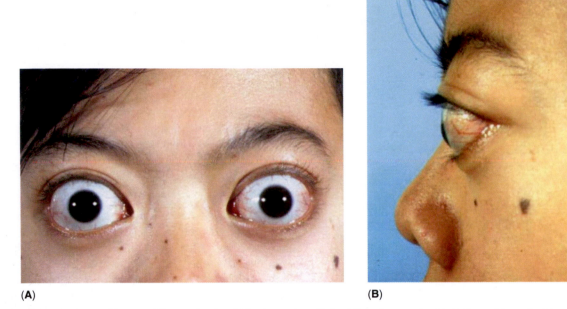

(A)   **(B)**

Figure 8.1 (**A**) Bilateral upper and lower eyelid retraction in a Malaysian patient. He has bilateral proptosis with shallow orbits and axial myopia (axial lengths 29 mm). (**B**) Lateral view demonstrating marked proptosis.

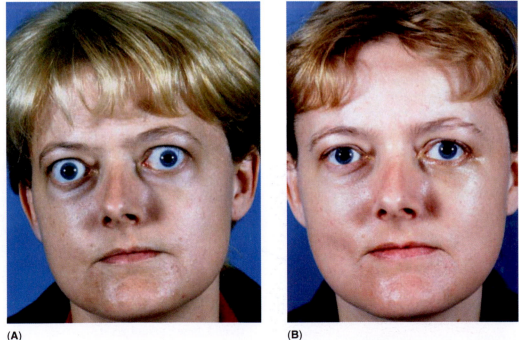

(A)   **(B)**

Figure 8.2 (**A**) Bilateral upper eyelid retraction in a patient with moderate proptosis. (**B**) The early postoperative appearance of the same patient following a bilateral 2 wall orbital decompression procedure performed via a swinging lower eyelid flap approach. No eyelid repositioning surgery was required.

expectations will lead to an unhappy patient postoperatively. The patient should be prepared for the possibility of multiple surgical procedures to achieve the desired end result. Many patients also seek blepharoplasty surgery hoping to restore their appearance to that which preceded the onset of their thyroid eye disease. Such patients should understand that this

is rarely achieved and that infiltration of the eyelid by glycos-aminoglycans with sub-brow eyelid thickening is not amenable to complete surgical correction. They also need to appreciate that an upper lid blepharoplasty runs the risk of postoperative lagophthalmos or an incomplete blink with exacerbation of dry eye symptoms.

UPPER EYELID RETRACTION

The upper eyelid, in contrast to the lower eyelid, does not require the use of spacers to achieve the desired postoperative position.

Methods of Upper Eyelid Lowering

A variety of surgical procedures have been described to manage upper eyelid retraction in Graves' disease. All these procedures aim to reduce upper eyelid retractor tone. The choice of procedure depends on the degree of eyelid retraction and the degree of resistance to downward traction of the upper eyelid. The aim is to achieve a satisfactory lowering of the eyelid without a temporal flare, which can mar the cosmetic result. The procedures that are used by the author are:

- Müllerectomy (1–2 mm of retraction)
- Posterior approach levator recession and Müllerectomy (2–3 mm of retraction)

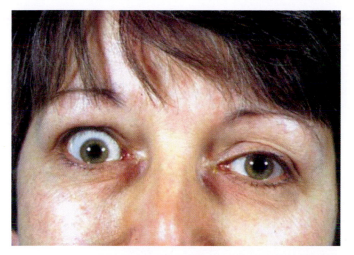

Figure 8.3 Severe right upper eyelid retraction in a patient with thyroid eye disease. There was marked resistance to inferior traction applied to the eyelid.

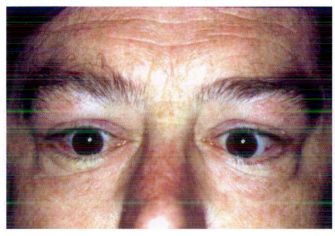

(A)

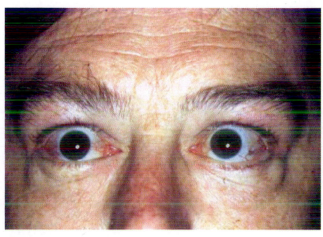

(B)

Figure 8.4 This patient's upper eyelid retraction increases on upgaze due to inferior rectus contracture.

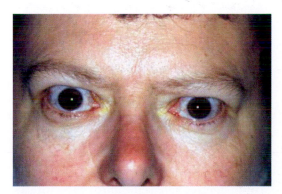

(A)

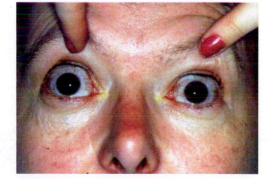

(B)

Figure 8.5 This patient's upper eyelid retraction is partially masked by her bilateral brow ptosis.

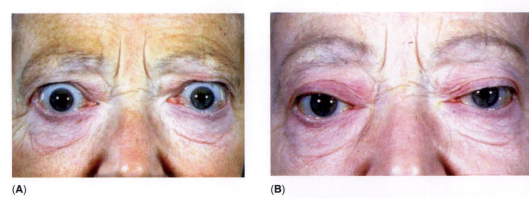

(A)   (B)

Figure 8.6 (**A**) Bilateral upper eyelid retraction in a patient with bilateral symmetric proptosis. (**B**) The patient is seen following a bilateral upper eyelid retractor recession performed without addressing the proptosis. A typically abnormal eyelid contour with lateral flare is the inevitable consequence of performing this surgery in the presence of untreated proptosis.

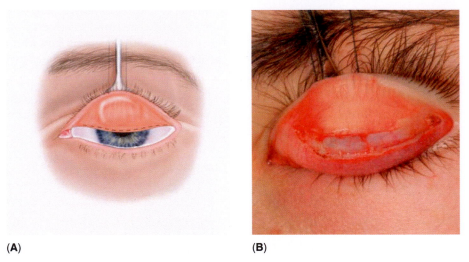

(A)   (B)

Figure 8.7 (**A**) The conjunctival incision is made at the upper border of the tarsus with the eyelid everted over a Desmarres retractor. (**B**) The incision is extended through Müller's muscle to the levator aponeurosis.

Müller's muscle
overlying the
conjunctiva

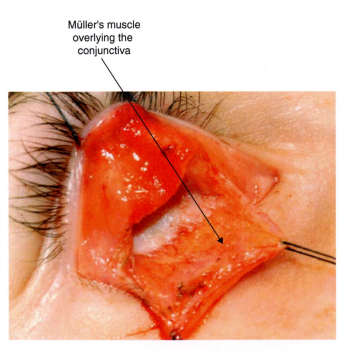

Figure 8.8 Müller's muscle showing fatty infiltration.

- Posterior approach levator recession with partial division of lateral levator horn and Müllerectomy (2–3 mm of retraction)
- Anterior approach levator recession with division of lateral levator horn and Müllerectomy (3–4 mm of retraction)
- Anterior approach Z-myotomy with division of lateral levator horn and Müllerectomy (>4 mm of retraction)

Müllerectomy

A Müllerectomy is a relatively simple surgical procedure that is useful for small degrees of eyelid retraction (1–2 mm). It can be performed under local anesthesia with or without intravenous sedation, or under general anesthesia as no intraoperative patient cooperation is required.

Surgical Procedure
1. 1 to 1.5 ml of 0.5% Bupivacaine with 1:200,000 units of adrenaline mixed 50:50 with 2% Lidocaine with 1:80,000 units of adrenaline, is injected subcutaneously into the upper eyelid.

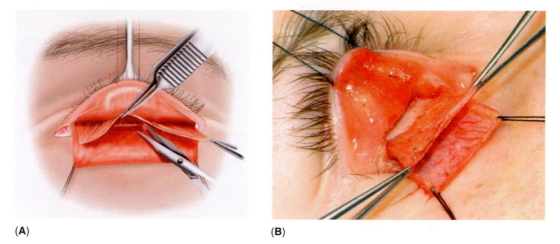

(A)   **(B)**

Figure 8.9 (**A**) Müller's muscle is dissected from the underlying conjunctiva using blunt-tipped Westcott scissors using a stripping motion with the tips slightly apart. (**B**) Müller's muscle has been dissected free and is seen attached to the levator aponeurosis at the "white line."

2. A 4/0 silk suture is placed through the gray line of the upper eyelid and the eyelid is everted over a medium Desmarres retractor. The silk suture is fixated to the surgical drapes around the patient's forehead using a small curved artery clip.

3. A further 1 ml of local anesthetic solution is injected subconjunctivally. The retractor is removed and pressure is applied for 5 minutes.

4. A conjunctival incision is made using a no. 15 Bard Parker blade across the whole of the upper eyelid just above the upper border of the tarsus (Fig. 8.7).

5. The conjunctival edge is lifted with Paufique forceps and the underlying Müller's muscle is opened with blunt-tipped Westcott scissors. The surgical space between the levator aponeurosis and Müller's muscle is dissected open with the Westcott scissors for a distance of approximately 10 to 12 mm. Müller's muscle will contain fatty tissue and will bleed (Fig. 8.8). Bipolar cautery will be required frequently, taking great care to protect the cornea from any damage from the cautery.

6. Sutures of 4/0 silk traction are passed through the medial and lateral edges of the conjunctiva with a double pass and the sutures are fixated to the face drapes with small curved artery clips, ensuring that the sutures are drawn medially and laterally away from the cornea.

7. 0.5 to 1.0 ml of local anesthetic solution is carefully injected into Müller's muscle and left for a few minutes.

8. An incision is then made through Müller's muscle close to the traction sutures using blunt-tipped Westcott scissors (Fig. 8.9A).

9. Using Castroviejo 0.3 mm toothed forceps and blunt-tipped Westcott scissors, Müller's muscle is dissected from the underlying conjunctiva with a blunt stripping motion from the cut edge of the conjunctiva to its superior origin from the levator.

10. Müller's muscle is excised, leaving a small residual strip nasally to avoid a medial ptosis (Fig. 8.10).

11. The traction sutures are then removed.

Sutures are unnecessary and risk causing discomfort or a corneal abrasion.

Postoperative Care

Postoperatively the patient is prescribed a topical antibiotic ointment to the eye three times a day for a week. The patient is instructed to keep the head of the bed elevated for 4 weeks and to avoid lifting any heavy weights for 2 weeks. The patient should be reviewed in clinic within a week and the antibiotic ointment discontinued and antibiotic drops prescribed instead for a further week. If the eyelid begins to rise above the desired position, the patient should be instructed to commence eyelid traction to maintain the desired height and contour of the upper eyelid. The patient should grasp the edge of the eyelid and lashes at the peak of the eyelid while looking down, and should then pull the eyelid down firmly while looking up. This can be continued for 2 to 3 minutes three times a day for a period of 4 to 6 weeks.

Posterior Approach Levator Recession with Müllerectomy

This approach can be performed under local anesthesia with intraoperative monitoring of the eyelid position, with or without intravenous sedation as required.

Advantages

1. No sutures are required.

2. The height and contour of the eyelid can be manipulated postoperatively with eyelid traction.

3. The absence of a skin incision reduces the degree of postoperative eyelid edema and permits a more rapid postoperative recovery.

4. The absence of an incision through the orbicularis muscle avoids temporary denervation of the orbicularis muscle and secondary lagophthalmos.

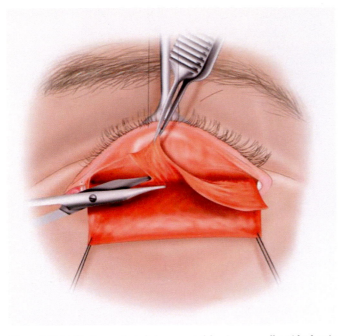

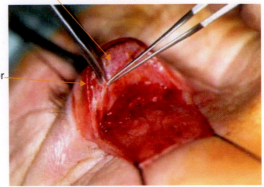

Levator aponeurosis

Superior border
of tarsus

Figure 8.11 The levator aponeurosis is carefully stripped away from the superior border of the tarsus temporally. Müller's muscle has been removed leaving a residual stump (for the purpose of illustration).

Figure 8.10 Müller's muscle is being resected leaving a small residual strip undisturbed medially.

Postoperative Care
The postoperative care is as described for Müllerectomy above.

Posterior Approach Levator Recession with Partial Division of the Lateral Levator Horn and Müllerectomy
Surgical Procedure
The initial aspects of this approach are identical to stages 1 to 11, as described for a posterior approach levator recession and Müllerectomy.

Disadvantages
1. This approach does not permit as satisfactory a degree of exposure of the lateral horn of the levator muscle as the anterior approach.
2. The skin crease cannot be adjusted or any excess upper eyelid skin removed.
3. Intraoperative bleeding following division of the lateral horn can be more difficult to control with a more limited view than that gained via an anterior transcutaneous approach.
4. There is a greater risk of trauma to the globe from the surgical dissection or from the use of bipolar cautery.

Surgical Procedure
The initial aspects of this approach are identical to stages 1 to 10, as described above for a Müllerectomy.

11. The levator aponeurosis is stripped away from the superior border of the tarsus using blunt-tipped Westcott scissors commencing temporally (Fig. 8.11).
12. The patient is placed into a sitting position and the height and contour of the upper eyelid are assessed. This is repeated as required.
13. The stripping of the levator aponeurosis fibers is continued until the desired end point is reached. (This is usually a 1 to 1.5 mm overcorrection. A greater degree of overcorrection risks a postoperative ptosis. It is much easier to undertake a further levator recession for an undercorrection than it is to have to undertake ptosis surgery for an overcorrection.)
14. The traction sutures are removed.

Sutures are unnecessary and risk causing discomfort or a corneal abrasion.

12. If the desired eyelid height has not been achieved the levator aponeurosis is opened at the "white line," exposing the preaponeurotic fat as in a posterior approach levator advancement.
13. The lateral horn of the levator can then be gently divided taking great care to avoid damage to the lacrimal gland. The lateral horn of the levator should be cauterized and divided in small steps with blunt-tipped Westcott scissors. Great care should be taken as such maneuvers increase the risk of postoperative overcorrection and hemorrhage.
14. The patient is placed into a sitting position and the height and contour of the upper eyelid are reassessed. This is repeated as required until the desired end point is reached. This is usually a 1 to 1.5 mm overcorrection.
15. The traction sutures are removed.

Sutures are unnecessary and risk causing discomfort or a corneal abrasion.

Postoperative Care
The postoperative care is as described for Müllerectomy above.

In determining the desired end point, it is important to contrast symmetrical upper eyelid retraction with asymmetrical or unilateral upper eyelid retraction. As the upper eyelids obey Hering's law, alterations to the position of one eyelid will have an influence on the position of the fellow eyelid. This can create a challenge in achieving symmetry. In addition, the eyelid position is further influenced by the patient's own voluntary effort, by the effects of adrenaline and by the effects of edema. It is always preferable to aim for an undercorrection (Fig. 8.12).

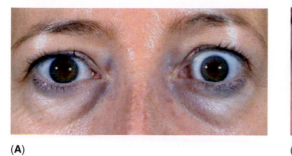
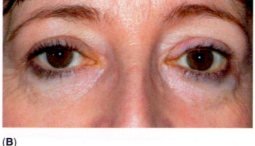

(A)   **(B)**

Figure 8.12 (**A**) A patient with bilateral asymmetrical dysthyroid upper eyelid retraction. (**B**) The postoperative appearance of the same patient following a bilateral posterior approach levator recession with Müllerectomy and division of the lateral levator horn on the left side.

> **KEY POINT**
>
> It is much easier to undertake a further levator recession for an undercorrection than it is to have to undertake ptosis surgery for an overcorrection. A patient will be far more dissatisfied with a postoperative ptosis than with an improved but undercorrected eyelid retraction.

Anterior Approach Levator Recession with Division of the Lateral Levator Horn and Müllerectomy

This approach is required for greater degrees of eyelid retraction and can be combined with a Z-myotomy of the levator aponeurosis and muscle. It can be performed under local anesthesia, although intravenous sedation is usually required. General anesthesia may be preferred for the more anxious patient, particularly as the degree of fibrosis within the eyelid requiring this surgical approach makes it more difficult to provide effective local anesthesia.

Advantages

1. This approach is familiar to surgeons performing anterior approach levator surgery for the management of ptosis.
2. It allows better access to the lateral horn of the levator and to the more proximal aspect of the levator muscle.
3. It is easier to control the desired height and contour of the eyelid intraoperatively.
4. It allows the skin crease to be set at the desired level.
5. It allows an upper lid blepharoplasty to be performed simultaneously.
6. The globe is well protected during the course of the surgery.

Disadvantages

1. This approach is associated with a longer postoperative recovery period with significant pretarsal eyelid edema.
2. The upper eyelid incision temporarily denervates the orbicularis oculi muscle, causing lagophthalmos.
3. This approach requires more surgical time.

Surgical Procedure

1. A skin crease incision is marked at the desired level in the upper eyelid using gentian violet and a cocktail stick after cleansing the skin with an alcohol wipe. If a blepharoplasty is planned, the excess skin should be marked out very carefully, ensuring that the eyelid can be closed passively by the patient while gently pinching the upper lid skin excess. If general anesthesia is to be used, the marking should be done prior to the induction of general anesthesia.
2. 1 to 1.5 ml of 0.5% Bupivacaine with 1:200,000 units of adrenaline mixed 50:50 with 2% Lidocaine with 1:80,000 units of adrenaline, is injected subcutaneously into the upper eyelid along the marked skin crease incision. It is important to avoid a deeper injection in order to prevent a hematoma and to minimize the effect of the local anesthetic on the levator function.
3. A 4/0 silk traction suture is placed through the gray line of the upper lid and fixated to the face drapes using a small curved artery clip.
4. An upper eyelid skin crease incision is made using a Colorado needle. If a blepharoplasty is to be performed, skin should only be removed leaving the orbicularis muscle intact to avoid exacerbating postoperative lagophthalmos.
5. The Colorado needle is used to dissect down through the orbicularis oculi muscle to the orbital septum. The orbicularis muscle is dissected from the orbital septum superiorly to avoid inadvertent injury to the levator aponeurosis.
6. The orbital septum is then opened with the Colorado needle throughout the entire length of the incision and the preaponeurotic fat exposed. The preaponeurotic fat is dissected from the underlying levator aponeurosis.
7. A Jaffe lid speculum is then placed in the incision site to provide complete exposure of the levator aponeurosis.
8. The levator aponeurosis is dissected from the underlying Müller's muscle, commencing 2 to 3 mm above the superior aspect of the tarsus. Great care should be taken to avoid inadvertent bleeding from the superior tarsal vascular arcade. The medial attachment of the levator to the tarsus should be left undisturbed if possible to avoid a low position of the medial aspect of the eyelid with temporal flare (Fig. 8.13).
9. 0.5 to 1.0 ml of 0.5% bupivacaine with 1:200,000 units of adrenaline is carefully injected into Müller's muscle and left for a few minutes taking care to protect the globe.

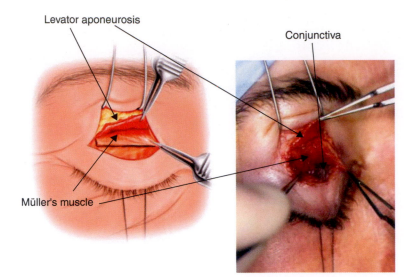

Figure 8.13 (**A**) The levator aponeurosis is opened above the superior tarsal arcade to avoid bleeding. (**B**) Müller's muscle is exposed and excised.

10. Using Castroviejo 0.3 mm toothed forceps and blunt-tipped Westcott scissors, Müller's muscle is dissected from the underlying conjunctiva with a blunt upward stripping motion with the blades of the scissors slightly apart, from just above the superior tarsal arcade to its superior origin from the levator.

11. Müller's muscle is excised.

12. Westcott scissors are then used to strip away any subconjunctival scar tissue, again using a blunt upward stripping motion.

13. The levator aponeurosis is dissected to the common sheath with the superior rectus muscle. The common sheath is recognized as a white tissue beneath the levator muscle.

14. If the procedure is being performed under local anesthesia, the patient is placed into a sitting position and the height and contour of the eyelid are assessed. This is repeated as required.

15. The lateral horn of the levator is then divided to overcome temporal flare, taking great care not to damage the lacrimal gland. The lateral horn of the levator should be cauterized and divided in small steps with blunt-tipped Westcott scissors. Great care should be taken as such maneuvers increase the risk of postoperative overcorrection and hemorrhage.

16. Once the desired position has been achieved, the edges of the recessed levator aponeurosis are attached to the subconjunctival tissue using interrupted 7/0 Vicryl sutures, taking care to ensure that the sutures do not pass through the full thickness of the conjunctiva and abrade the cornea (Fig. 8.14).

17. Preaponeurotic and sub-dermal fat can be carefully removed as required using the Colorado needle, taking great care to ensure adequate hemostasis with bipolar cautery as larger vessels are exposed.

18. The skin crease is reformed by firmly attaching the skin edges to the superior border of the tarsus with interrupted 7/0 Vicryl sutures.

19. The traction suture is removed.

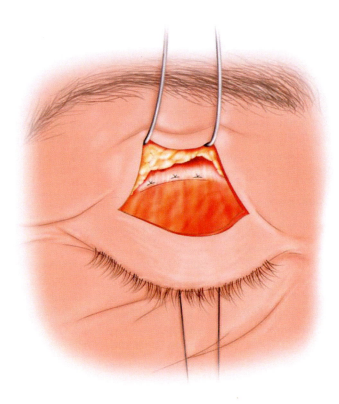

Figure 8.14 The recessed edge of the levator aponeurosis is sutured to the conjunctiva.

The end point of the surgery is the attainment of the desired eyelid height and contour, as the eyelid should remain at its intraoperative height. If the operation has been performed under general anesthesia, adjustable 5/0 Vicryl sutures can be placed and the height and contour of the eyelid adjusted later the same day following recovery from the anesthesia. It is preferable, however, to perform the necessary adjustments intraoperatively under local anesthesia.

Again, it is preferable to aim for an undercorrection rather than risk an overcorrection.

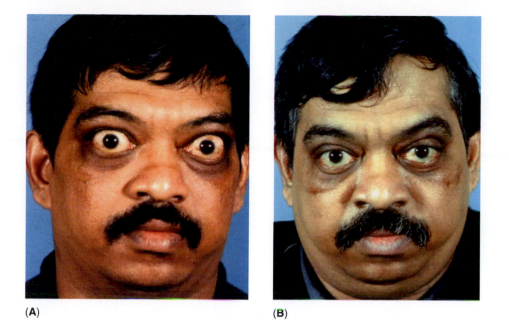

(A) **(B)**

Figure 8.15 (A) A patient with a bilateral symmetric proptosis and severe upper eyelid retraction. (B) The postoperative appearance of the same patient following a bilateral, medial, and lateral orbital wall decompression with fat excision, and a bilateral anterior approach levator recession with a Müllerectomy and a division of the lateral levator horns.

Postoperative Care

Postoperatively the patient is prescribed a topical antibiotic ointment three times a day to the upper eyelid wound for 2 weeks and Lacrilube ointment 1 to 2 hourly to the eye for 48 hours and at bedtime. The Lacrilube ointment is then changed to a preservative-free topical lubricant gel to be used hourly during the day and Lacrilube is continued at bedtime until the degree of lagophthalmos has improved. The frequency of the lubricants is then gradually reduced over the course of the next few weeks. The patient is instructed to keep the head of the bed elevated for 4 weeks and to avoid lifting any heavy weights for 2 weeks. Clean cool packs are gently applied to the eyelid intermittently for 48 hours. The patient should be reviewed in clinic within a week and again within 3 weeks. The upper eyelid skin sutures are removed at the second clinic visit.

An example of a patient who has undergone this procedure following an orbital decompression is shown in Fig. 8.15.

Anterior Approach Z-Myotomy with Division of the Lateral Levator Horn and Müllerectomy

This procedure is reserved for patients with severe degrees of upper eyelid retraction. The surgery is normally performed with the patient under general anesthesia, as the dissection can be difficult. Severe degrees of retraction are associated with widespread fibrosis, fatty infiltration, and bleeding of the upper eyelid tissues. The initial aspects of this approach are identical to stages 1 to 13, as described for an anterior approach levator recession.

14. The lateral horn of the levator is divided completely, taking great care not to damage the lacrimal gland. The lateral horn of the levator should be cauterized and divided in small steps with blunt-tipped Westcott scissors. Great care should be taken as

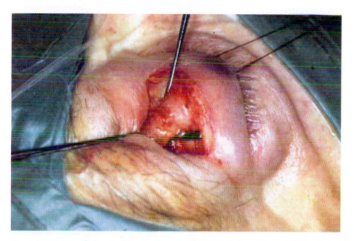

Figure 8.16 Muscle hooks have been passed beneath the enlarged belly of the levator muscle.

such maneuvers increase the risk of postoperative overcorrection and hemorrhage.

15. Whitnall's ligament is divided medially and laterally.
16. A muscle hook is passed beneath the belly of the levator muscle and the levator muscle is pulled forward (Fig. 8.16).
17. The levator muscle is partially transected from one side of the muscle and from the opposite side at a higher level using the Colorado needle to prevent bleeding.

The operation is completed as for an anterior approach levator recession. The eyelid is usually overcorrected postoperatively but should not be adjusted. The eyelid will gradually rise over the course of the next 6 to 12 weeks and no further adjustments should be made until all postoperative edema has subsided and the eyelid position is static (Fig. 8.17).

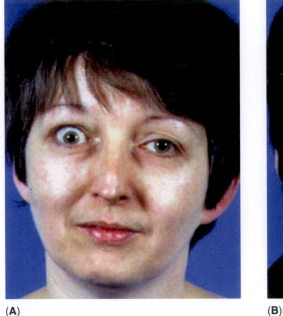
(A)

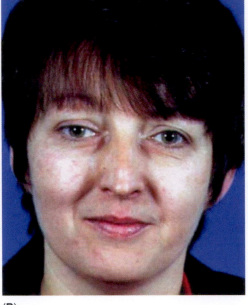
(B)

Figure 8.17 (**A**) A patient with severe right upper eyelid retraction (>5 mm) and marked resistance to downward traction. (**B**) The postoperative result 3 months following an anterior approach Z-myotomy with division of the lateral levator horn and Müllerectomy showing a slight residual ptosis and flattening of the eyelid contour. The day after surgery she was overcorrected by 3 mm.

Postoperative Care
The postoperative care is as described for an anterior approach levator recession with division of the lateral levator horn and Müllerectomy above.

Graded Full-thickness Anterior Blepharotomy
Graded full-thickness anterior blepharotomy is not a surgical procedure undertaken by the author, but the procedure should be included in the options for the management of upper lid retraction in thyroid eye disease. This simple procedure involves the use of a skin crease incision followed by a dissection through all layers of the eyelid. The dissection is then continued in a graded manner with the patient in a sitting position, until the eyelid height and contour are satisfactory. The skin is then sutured. The procedure is quick and simple to perform but is associated with a risk of the development of an eyelid fistula.

LOWER EYELID RETRACTION
Surgery for the management of lower eyelid retraction is not required as frequently as that for upper eyelid retraction. Patients do not tend to be as concerned about lower eyelid retraction, as they do about upper eyelid retraction, which has much more of a profound effect on a patient's ocular function and cosmesis. Surgery for lower eyelid retraction is rarely required following successful orbital decompression surgery.

The lower eyelid, in contrast to the upper eyelid, usually requires the use of a spacer to achieve the desired position. Although a variety of surgical procedures have been described to manage lower eyelid retraction in Graves' disease, the underlying principles are based on:

- Division of the orbital septum
- Recession of the inferior retractor complex and conjunctiva
- Placement of a spacer between the recessed inferior retractors and conjunctiva, and the inferior border of the tarsus

A number of spacers are available. The ideal spacer should be sufficiently rigid to counteract the effects of gravity without adding bulk to the eyelid, and should have a mucosal surface to allow maximal recession of the conjunctiva as well as the inferior retractors.

Spacers
- Hard palate
- Upper eyelid tarsus

Both of these spacers meet the required criteria. Ear cartilage, or a nasal septal cartilage graft, are not as satisfactory in this situation. A dermal graft may also be used. Non-autogenous materials, e.g. Alloderm, must be covered by the inferior palpebral conjunctiva and risk exposure and foreign body reactions. Donor sclera is no longer an acceptable material for use as a spacer because of the risk of transmissible disease.

The patient's hard palate is examined to determine its suitability for use as a spacer. Alternatively the patient's upper eyelids are everted and the height of the tarsus is assessed to determine whether or not the upper eyelid tarsus is suitable for use as a spacer. If a hard palate graft is to be used the surgery should ideally be performed under general anesthesia whereas the surgery may be performed under local anesthesia if upper lid tarsus is to be used.

In general, upper eyelid retraction should be addressed first and the management of lower eyelid retraction deferred until a satisfactory result has been obtained from upper eyelid surgery.
Lower Lid Retractor Recession with Hard Palate Graft Spacer
Surgical Procedure
The surgeon should be familiar with the anatomy of the greater and lesser palatine vessels. It is much easier to harvest the graft in the edentulous patient.

The hard palate graft is harvested first. The anesthetist is asked to place the endotracheal tube in the midline. A throat pack is placed and its presence recorded to ensure that this is removed prior to extubation.

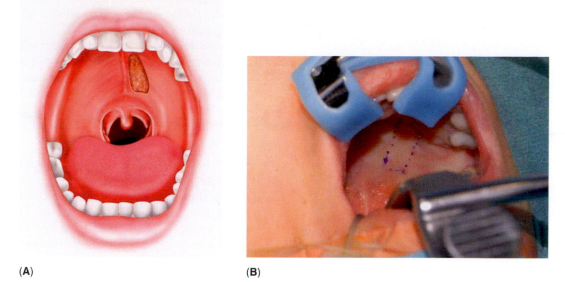

(A)   (B)

Figure 8.18 (**A**) A drawing showing the location of a hard palate graft donor site. (**B**) A hard palate graft has been outlined with gentian violet.

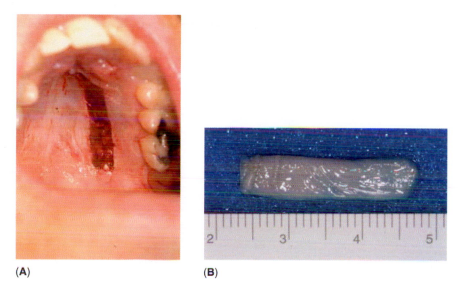

(A)   (B)

Figure 8.19 (**A**) The appearance of a hard palate graft donor site following removal of the hard palate graft. (**B**) A photograph of a hard palate graft.

1. The hard palate is injected with 3 to 5 ml of 0.5% bupivacaine with 1:200,000 units of adrenaline. A Boyle–Davies retractor is placed, taking great care not to damage the teeth or to disturb the endotracheal tube.
2. The graft, measuring approximately 20 to 25 mm × 4 to 5 mm is outlined on the hard palate, avoiding the midline raphé and the soft palate (Fig. 8.18).
3. The hard palate is incised with a no. 15 Bard Parker blade.
4. The graft is then dissected out in the plane of the submucosa using a no. 66 Beaver blade, leaving the underlying mucoperiosteum undisturbed (Fig. 8.19).
5. The dissection can then be completed with blunt-tipped Westcott scissors.
6. The submucosa of the graft is then thinned with the Westcott scissors and then wrapped in a saline-soaked gauze swab and kept in a safe location by the scrub nurse until it is required.
7. Neurosurgical patties moistened with 1:1,000 adrenaline solution are placed over the hard palate wound for 5 minutes.
8. The wound is then inspected and bipolar cautery applied to any bleeding vessels.

Next, attention is directed to the lower eyelids:

1. Two milliliters of 0.5% Bupivacaine with 1:200,000 units of adrenaline mixed 50:50 with 2% Lidocaine with 1:80,000 units of adrenaline are injected subconjunctivally into the lower eyelid.
2. Two 4/0 silk traction sutures are placed through the gray line of the lower eyelid and the lid is everted over a medium Desmarres retractor.

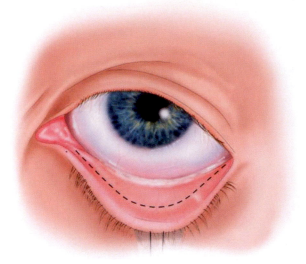

Figure 8.20 A conjunctival incision is made at the lower border of the tarsus.

3. A conjunctival incision is made with a no. 15 Bard Parker blade at the lower border of the tarsus (Fig. 8.20).
4. The conjunctiva is dissected into the inferior fornix and onto the globe using blunt-tipped Westcott scissors and Paufique forceps. (A lateral canthotomy and inferior cantholysis can be combined with this approach to enable a lateral tarsal strip procedure to be performed if there is significant lower eyelid laxity.)

5. The lower lid retractors, which lie immediately beneath the conjunctiva, are then undermined from the orbicularis muscle with Westcott scissors and dissected from the lower border of the tarsus.
6. The retractors are then dissected free into the inferior fornix and the orbital septum opened, exposing the lower eyelid preaponeurotic fat (Fig. 8.21).

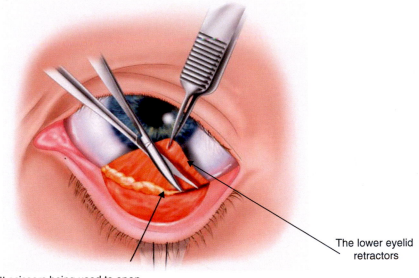

The lower eyelid retractors

Westcott scissors being used to open the orbital septum exposing fat

Figure 8.21 The lower eyelid retractors are dissected free.

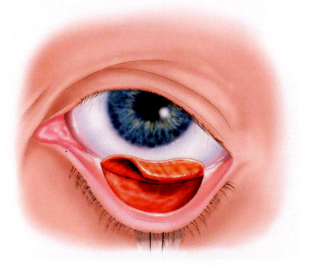

Figure 8.22 The inferior aspect of the hard palate graft is first sutured to the superior border of the recessed lower eyelid retractors.

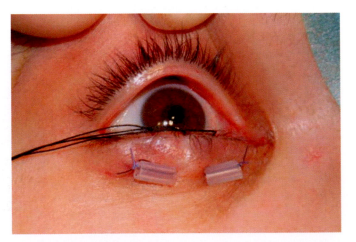

Figure 8.23 The hard palate graft has been secured in place with two double-armed 5/0 vicryl sutures tied over silicone bolsters.

The lower lid should now rise above the inferior limbus with gentle traction.

7. The hard palate graft is placed into the inferior fornix with the mucosal surface facing the globe and sutured to the recessed inferior retractors and conjunctival edge with interrupted 8/0 Vicryl sutures (Fig. 8.22).

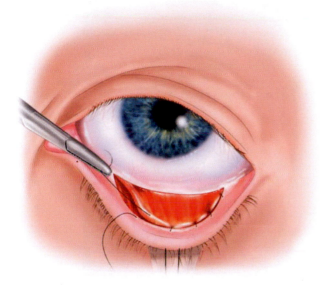

Figure 8.24 The superior aspect of the hard palate graft is then sutured to the inferior margin of the tarsus.

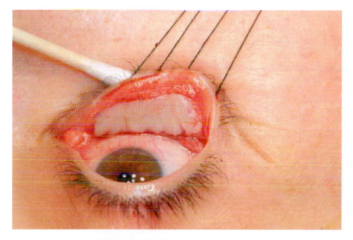

Figure 8.25 The hard palate graft sutured into place in the lower eyelid.

8. Two to three interrupted 5/0 Vicryl sutures are then passed from the submucosa of the mid-portion of the graft through the full thickness of the eyelid and tied over silicone bolsters (Fig. 8.23).

9. The superior margin of the graft is sutured to the inferior border of the tarsus using interrupted 8/0 Vicryl sutures that are buried to prevent any corneal irritation (Figs. 8.24 and 8.25).

10. The traction sutures are removed.

Postoperative Care

Postoperatively the patient is prescribed a topical antibiotic ointment three times a day for 2 weeks. The patient should be prescribed an antiseptic oral rinse twice a day for 7 days and should have a soft bland diet until the hard palate wound has healed. This normally takes 2 to 3 weeks.

The patient is instructed to keep the head of the bed elevated for 4 weeks and to avoid lifting any heavy weights for 2 weeks. Clean cool packs are gently applied to the eyelid intermittently for 48 hours. The patient should be reviewed in clinic within a week and again within 2 weeks. The 5/0 Vicryl sutures and the bolsters are removed after 2 weeks.

An example of an early postoperative result following this surgical procedure is shown in Fig. 8.26.

Lower Lid Retractor Recession with Free Tarsal Graft Spacer

The tarsal graft is harvested from the upper eyelid, ensuring that a minimum of 3.5 mm of tarsus above the eyelid margin is left undisturbed. This is described in chapter 13. The graft is used in a similar fashion to a hard palate graft.

This surgical technique is better reserved for the management of lower eyelid retraction due to causes other than thyroid eye disease.

THE ROLE OF A LATERAL TARSORRHAPHY IN THYROID EYE DISEASE

A lateral tarsorrhaphy can be used as an urgent procedure to protect an exposed cornea in a patient with thyroid eye disease prior to a more definitive procedure, e.g. an orbital decompression or an eyelid lengthening procedure. It is not a satisfactory procedure when performed alone as it tends to become stretched and unsightly or it may cause the lower eyelid to be drawn upwards, creating a cosmetic deformity (Fig. 8.27).

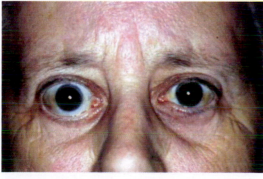
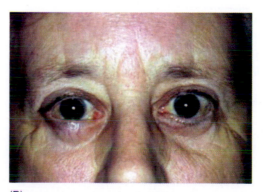

(A)   (B)

Figure 8.26 (**A**) A patient with right upper and lower eyelid retraction. (**B**) The postoperative appearance 6 weeks following a right upper eyelid posterior approach levator recession and Müllerectomy, and a lower eyelid retractor recession with a hard palate graft and a lateral tarsal strip procedure.

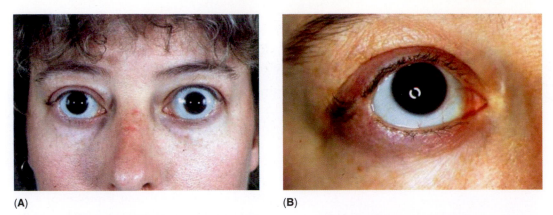

(A)   **(B)**

Figure 8.27 (**A**) A patient with proptosis and bilateral upper and lower eyelid retraction who has been inappropriately managed with lateral tarsorrhaphies alone. (**B**) A close-up of the right eye demonstrating a stretched lateral tarsorrhaphy.

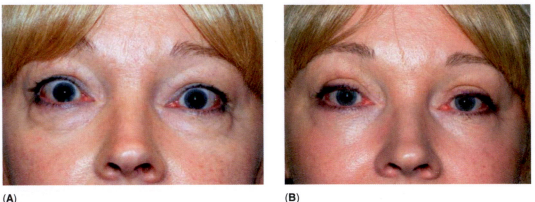

(A)   **(B)**

Figure 8.28 (**A**) A patient with thyroid eye disease with bilateral upper lid retraction who requested cosmetic eyelid surgery and bilateral upper lid lowering. (**B**) The postoperative appearance of the patient 4 months after undergoing a bilateral anterior approach levator recession with division of the lateral levator horns and Müllerectomy combined with a bilateral upper lid blepharoplasty with debulking of the central and medial fat pads with a skin crease reformation and a bilateral lower lid transcutaneous blepharoplasty with central and medial fat repositioning over the inferior orbital margins and a conservative lateral fat pad debulking with a bilateral orbicularis oculi muscle sling.

A small lateral tarsorrhaphy can, however, be very useful when used as an adjunct to an orbital decompression or to eyelid lengthening procedures.

The lateral tarsorrhaphy should only extend for 3 to 4 mm for the optimal cosmetic result. Although a variety of methods for performing the tarsorrhaphy in this situation have been described, it is preferable to undertake a very simple procedure that can be reversed if required.

Surgical Technique
1. The lateral aspects of the upper and lower lids are injected with 1 to 2 ml of 0.5% Bupivacaine with 1:200,000 units of adrenaline mixed 50:50 with 2% Lidocaine with 1:80,000 units of adrenaline
2. The eyelid is held taut centrally and laterally with Paufique forceps.
3. A micro-sharp blade mounted in a Beaver blade handle is used to make a shallow incision for 4 to 5 mm along the gray line of each eyelid.
4. Using the same blade, two incisions are made at 90° to the gray line incision posteriorly. Next, using a Castroviejo 0.3 mm toothed forceps and a sharp-tipped Westcott scissors, a 0.5-mm strip of eyelid margin tissue is carefully removed posteriorly.

5. An interrupted 5/0 Vicryl suture on a 1/4-circle needle is passed horizontally through the tarsal plates of the upper and lower lids and tied with the knot placed anteriorly away from the cornea.
6. Interrupted 7/0 Vicryl sutures are placed through the anterior lips of the gray line incisions.

There is no requirement for any external bolsters. Topical antibiotic ointment is applied for 2 weeks. The eyelids fuse laterally. This procedure does not sacrifice normal eyelashes.

BLEPHAROPLASTY IN THYROID EYE DISEASE
Upper and lower lid blepharoplasty is the final surgical procedure to be undertaken in the functional and cosmetic rehabilitation of the patient with Graves' ophthalmopathy. In the upper eyelid a very conservative blepharoplasty with fat removal or debulking can be combined with upper lid lowering procedures, or can be undertaken at a later stage following eyelid repositioning (Fig. 8.28). The surgical procedure is outlined in detail in chapter 15. Great care should be taken not to exacerbate any lagophthalmos or incomplete blink in such a patient. The patient's expectations must also be realistic as sub-brow infiltration and thickening are not very amenable to surgical correction.

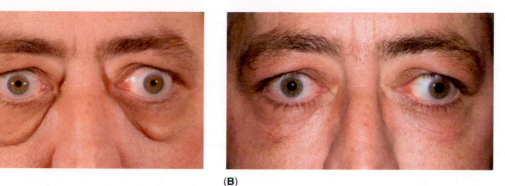

(A)   **(B)**

Figure 8.29 (**A**) A patient with thyroid eye disease and lower lid "festoons." (**B**) The patient 4 months after direct excision of the "festoons". His left exotropia (and amblyopia) preceded his thyroid eye disease and did not concern him. He was unconcerned about his upper lid retraction but very concerned about the appearance of the lower eyelid "festoons."

Lower eyelid blepharoplasty can be performed alone or can be combined with orbital decompression surgery. The surgical procedure is outlined in detail in chapter 15. Great care should be exercised when performing a transcutaneous lower eyelid blepharoplasty to avoid removing too much skin to avoid the complication of lower eyelid retraction or ectropion. It is preferable to debulk lower lid fat prolapses via a transconjunctival approach in the absence of any significant lower eyelid skin laxity or excess.

Lower lid "festoons" are particularly difficult to manage. In the majority of cases it is preferable to perform a direct excision of the festoon as this yields a better result with little risk of eyelid retraction or ectropion than would be the case attempting to address this problem via a transcutaneous lower eyelid blepharoplasty (Fig. 8.29).

FURTHER READING

1. Bartley GB. The differential diagnosis and classification of eyelid retraction. Ophthalmology 1996; 103: 168–76.
2. Beatty RC, Harris G, Bauman GR, Mills MP. Intraoral palatal mucosal graft harvest. Ophthal Plast Reconstr Surg 1993; 9: 120–4.
3. Cohen MS, Shorr N. Eyelid reconstruction with hard palate mucosal grafts. Ophthal Plast Reconstr Surg 1992; 8:183–95.
4. Gardner TA, Kennerdell JS, Buerger GE. Treatment of dysthyroid lower eyelid retraction with autogenous tarsus transplants. Ophthal Plast Reconstr Surg 1992; 8: 26–31.
5. Goodall KL, Jackson A, Leatherbarrow B, Whitehouse RW. Enlargement of the tensor intermuscularis muscle in Graves' ophthalmopathy. Arch Ophthalmol 1995; 113: 1286–9.
6. Kersten PC, Kulwin DP, Levartovksy S, et al. Management of lower eyelid retraction with hard palate mucosal grafting. Arch Ophthalmol 1990; 108: 1339–43.
7. Lemke BN. Anatomic considerations in upper eyelid retraction. Ophthal Plast Reconstr Surg 1991; 7: 158–66.
8. Putterman AM. Surgical treatment of thyroid related upper eyelid retraction: Graded Müller excision and lessor recession. Ophthalmology 1981; 88: 507–12.
9. Hintschich C, Haritoglou C. Full thickness eyelid transection (blepharotomy) for upper eyelid lengthening in lid retraction associated with Graves' disease. Br J Ophthalmol 2005; 89(4): 413–6.
10. Elner V, Hassan A, Frueh B. Graded full-thickness anterior blepharotomy for upper eyelid retraction. Trans Am Ophthalmol Soc 2003; 101: 67–75.

9 Facial palsy

INTRODUCTION

The ophthalmologist may be the first clinician to see a patient who presents with an acute facial nerve palsy. Under such circumstances the ophthalmologist should make every effort to establish the underlying cause of the facial palsy and should ensure that the patient's cornea is adequately protected. Many patients presenting with a facial palsy are automatically assumed to have a Bell's palsy and many clinicians incorrectly use the term "Bell's palsy" synonymously with the term "facial palsy." A Bell's palsy is an idiopathic facial palsy and a diagnosis of exclusion.

KEY POINT

Approximately 10% of patients presenting with an acute facial palsy have a treatable lesion

The ophthalmologist should be aware of:

1. The varied disorders which may cause a facial palsy (Table 9.1)
2. The detailed evaluation of the patient with a facial palsy
3. The various medical and surgical treatments available

A number of other disciplines may be involved in the care of the patient with a facial palsy, e.g., an ENT (ear, nose and throat) surgeon, a neurosurgeon, a neurologist, a plastic surgeon, a physician.

KEY POINT

It is essential that effective communication exist between such clinicians for the optimal care of the patient. The ophthalmologist must be made aware of the prognosis for recovery of facial nerve function, e.g. following the removal of an acoustic neuroma, and of any plans for surgery by other colleagues, e.g. facial reanimation surgery.

The ophthalmologist should be involved in the care of any patient in whom a facial palsy may be anticipated postoperatively, e.g., acoustic neuroma surgery. In the early postoperative period following acoustic neuroma surgery, periorbital swelling can cause a patient with a complete facial palsy to have apparently normal eyelid closure. As the swelling subsides such a patient develops severe lagophthalmos, which may be compounded by a reduced or absent corneal sensation, decreased tear production, and a poor Bell's phenomenon.

KEY POINT

The priority for any clinician involved in the management of a patient with a facial palsy is prevention of exposure keratopathy. It is much simpler to prevent corneal ulceration from exposure than it is to treat this once it has occurred (Fig. 9.1).

A facial palsy can have a devastating effect on a patient. It is associated with a number of potential problems that need to be addressed on an individual basis:

1. Visual defects from corneal exposure or its medical and surgical management
2. Ocular pain or discomfort
3. Chronic lacrimation and epiphora from corneal exposure, paralytic ectropion, and lacrimal pump failure
4. Cosmetic disfigurement
5. Difficulties with speech/drooling

These problems can affect a patient's ability to work, drive, and to interact socially. Patients may lose self-esteem and become discouraged and depressed.

HISTORY AND EXAMINATION

History

A full history should be taken and a comprehensive examination performed to determine the cause of the facial palsy. Specific questions should be asked about the following:

1. Onset and duration of the palsy
2. Any prior trauma
3. Any past ENT history
4. Any symptoms of hearing loss or hyperacusis
5. Any symptoms of ear pain or discharge
6. Any symptoms of other cranial nerve dysfunction, e.g., diplopia, anosmia, difficulty swallowing, neurosensory facial deficits
7. Past medical history, e.g., diabetes, sarcoidosis, myasthenia
8. Any skin rashes

The patient's presenting ocular complaints should be noted.

The patient should be carefully observed during the history taking. An incomplete blink may be noted as well as any facial asymmetry or loss of the nasolabial fold or forehead creases.

Examination

The patient should undergo a complete ophthalmic examination. The patient should be examined systematically:

1. The muscles of facial expression should be tested to determine if the patient has a facial nerve paresis or a complete paralysis. In a chronic palsy, signs of aberrant reinnervation should also be sought.
2. The degree of facial motor nerve palsy can be graded using the House–Brackmann scoring system (Table 9.2) to assist in monitoring the return of facial nerve function. In general, the temporal branches of the facial nerve are the most severely affected and the last to return.

3. The frontalis muscle should be tested to differentiate an upper motor neuron (intact frontalis action) from a lower motor neuron lesion (impaired frontalis action).
4. The extent of voluntary passive and forced eyelid closure should be determined and the degree of lagophthalmos measured (Fig. 9.2).
5. Any upper eyelid retraction is noted (Fig. 9.2). (The upper eyelid retracts in chronic facial palsy due to the unopposed action of the levator muscle. In some patients there is a chronic shortening of the anterior lamella, which further aggravates lagophthalmos.)

Table 9.1 The More Common Causes of Facial Palsy

- Bell's palsy
- Ramsay Hunt syndrome
- Otitis media
- Mastoiditis
- Cholesteatoma
- Trauma
- Acoustic neuroma surgery
- Sarcoidosis
- Parotid tumor
- Lymphoma
- Nasopharyngeal carcinoma
- Metastatic carcinoma
- Congenital

6. The corneal sensation must be tested before the instillation of any topical anesthetic agents and the sensation in the distribution of the branches of the trigeminal nerve is also tested.
7. The tear film and the tear meniscus are examined and a Schirmer's test performed to determine tear production.
8. The cornea is examined using a slit lamp and fluorescein is instilled into the conjunctival sac (Fig. 9.3). Any exposure keratopathy is recorded.
9. The fluorescein dye disappearance can also be observed and compared with the fellow eye. The patient's blink should also be observed using the slit lamp, noting whether this is complete or incomplete.
10. The presence or absence of a Bell's phenomenon is determined (Fig. 9.4).
11. The lower eyelid should be examined for any retraction or frank ectropion (Figs. 9.2 and 9.5).
12. The position and patency of the inferior punctum is determined.
13. The ocular motility should be carefully tested. This is important as the abducens nerve lies in close anatomical proximity intracranially to the facial nerve nucleus and fascicles.
14. The patient's hearing should be tested and the ear examined for any skin lesions affecting the external auditory meatus, e.g., herpes zoster (Ramsay–Hunt syndrome) (Fig. 9.6).

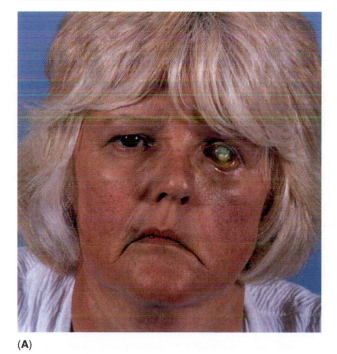

(A)

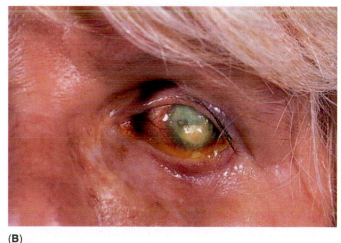

(B)

Figure 9.1 (**A**) A patient referred with a complete left lower motor neuron facial palsy and a painful left eye. (**B**) A close-up photograph of the patient's left eye. She had marked lagophthalmos and a dry eye. Her neglected exposure keratopathy had resulted in a secondary corneal abscess and endophthalmitis. The eye had to be eviscerated.

Table 9.2 The House–Brackmann Score

Grade	Description	Measurement	Function (%)	Estimated function (%)
I	Normal	8/8	100	100
II	Slight	7/8	76–99	80
III	Moderate	5/8–6/8	51–75	60
IV	Moderately Severe	3/8–4/8	26–50	40
V	Severe	1/8–2/8	1–25	20
VI	Total	0/8	0	0

The House–Brackmann score is a score used to grade the degree of nerve damage in a facial palsy. The score is determined by measuring the upward movement of the mid-portion of the eyebrow, and the lateral movement of the angle of the mouth. Each reference point scores 1 point for each 0.25 cm movement, up to a maximum of 1cm. The scores are then added together, to give a number out of 8.

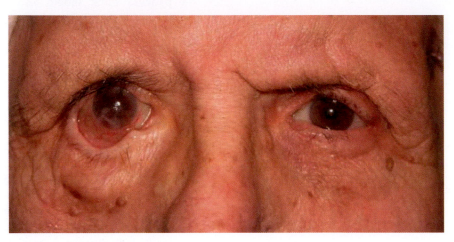

Figure 9.2 A patient with a right lower motor neuron facial palsy demonstrating right upper eyelid retraction, a right lower eyelid paralytic ectropion, and chronic inferior exposure keratopathy.

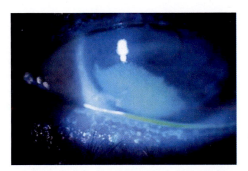

Figure 9.3 A patient with exposure keratopathy highlighted by the use of fluorescein.

15. The parotid glands should be palpated for masses.
16. The preauricular, submandibular, and cervical lymph nodes should be palpated.
17. The oropharynx should be examined.

Although the patient's visual acuity should be recorded, this can be inaccurate due to the presence of ophthalmic ointments, which may have been instilled into the eye for corneal protection.

GENERAL TREATMENT CONSIDERATIONS

The patients who are at high risk of exposure keratopathy and corneal ulceration should be identified early. The following are significant risk factors:

1. Absence of corneal sensation
2. Severe lagophthalmos

3. An absent Bell's phenomenon
4. A dry eye

Patients may have more than one risk factor that further compounds the problem.

KEY POINT

Loss of corneal sensation indicates a severely guarded prognosis for patients with facial palsy and demands urgent and aggressive treatment.

Other factors must also be considered in determining the most appropriate medical or surgical treatment of an individual patient. These include the patient's age, general health, and ability to comply with medical therapy regimens and frequent follow-up visits.

MEDICAL TREATMENT

A number of relatively simple medical therapies can be applied, particularly for a limited time in the patient who has a good prognosis for the recovery of facial nerve function and who has no risk factors for the development of exposure keratopathy. These include:

1. The use of frequent preservative free topical lubricants
2. The avoidance of ocular irritants
3. The use of spectacle side shields or moisture chamber goggles
4. Taping the eye closed at night

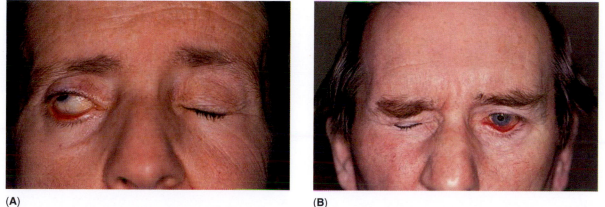

(A)   (B)

Figure 9.4 (**A**) A patient with lagophthalmos but a good Bell's phenomenon. (**B**) A patient with lagophthalmos and an absent Bell's phenomenon.

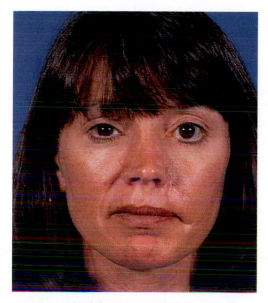

Figure 9.5 A patient with a left post-traumatic facial palsy. Her widened left palpebral aperture is due to both upper and lower eyelid retraction.

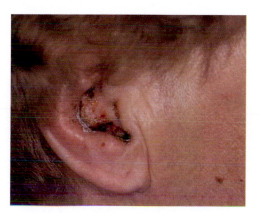

Figure 9.6 A patient with Ramsay Hunt syndrome.

5. Upper eyelid botulinum toxin injections
6. The application of external eyelid weights

The most common ophthalmic treatment for facial palsy is the use of frequent lubricants. The lubricants should be used at least on an hourly basis during the day and should be preservative free to avoid corneal toxicity from such frequent exposure to preservatives. The use of preservative free lubricant ointment e.g., Lacrilube, provides more efficient corneal protection than drops with a much reduced frequency of instillation but with more blurring of vision. Patients should avoid ocular irritants wherever possible, e.g., tobacco smoke.

Most patients do not tolerate moisture chamber goggles or plastic wrap occlusive dressings but spectacle side shields are relatively unobtrusive and well tolerated.

The upper eyelid can be taped closed over the eye at night using Micropore tape but it is essential to ensure that the eye is fully closed to prevent further trauma to the cornea by the tape.

Botulinum toxin can be injected into the levator muscle to induce a ptosis for a patient with a temporary facial palsy

(Fig. 9.7). This is, however, expensive and commits the patient to monovision for a period of 8 to 12 weeks before spontaneous recovery occurs. Some patients can develop problems with fusion and suffer diplopia following the use of botulinum toxin. In addition, as the superior rectus can be weakened, the Bell's phenomenon may be adversely affected, creating more problems with exposure keratopathy during the recovery phase.

An external eyelid weight may be applied to the upper eyelid with a tissue adhesive. The weight is flesh colored to make it less conspicuous. Such weights are useful for a temporary facial palsy but can also be used for a trial period before subjecting a patient to an upper eyelid gold weight implant.

Patients with the onset of a true Bell's palsy should be treated within 72 hours of the onset of the palsy with a high dose of oral corticosteroids to improve the rate of recovery. The use of antiviral medications is more controversial for these patients, but the current evidence appears to suggest that these medications are ineffective.

SURGICAL TREATMENT

Oculoplastic surgical treatment in the management of the patient with facial palsy has a number of indications and aims:

1. The prevention or management of corneal exposure
2. The correction of lower eyelid ectropion
3. The management of brow ptosis
4. The management of chronic epiphora

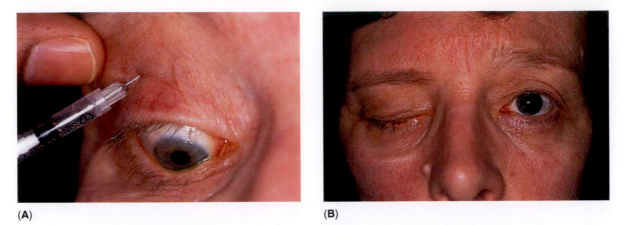

(A)   **(B)**

Figure 9.7 (**A**) The technique of botulinum toxin injection into the levator muscle. (**B**) A patient with a right facial palsy 3 days following an upper eyelid botulinum toxin injection. She had a complete right ptosis.

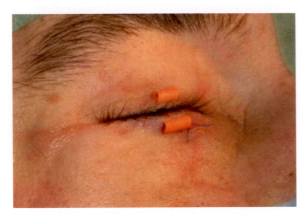

Figure 9.8 A temporary suture tarsorrhaphy.

The surgical planning should take into consideration any plans for surgery by other clinicians, e.g., facial reanimation surgery.

The Prevention or Management of Corneal Exposure

Punctal Occlusion

In patients with decreased tear production who cannot be managed adequately with topical lubricants alone, punctal occlusion is beneficial. This can be achieved temporarily with the use of silicone punctal plugs. If these are tolerated without secondary epiphora, surgical punctal occlusion can be performed under local anesthesia. A simple disposable cautery device is used with a brief application to the puncta. This method does not prevent the reopening of the puncta at a later stage if necessary. A more permanent occlusion of the lacrimal drainage pathway can be achieved by inserting an electrolysis needle, attached to a Colorado needle hand-piece, into the inferior canaliculus for a few millimeters and pressing the coagulation button for 2 to 3 seconds.

Temporary Suture Tarsorrhaphy

A temporary suture tarsorrhaphy can be used for the patient who has an acute facial palsy and who is unsuitable to undergo any other procedure or who is unable to instill lubricant drops or ointment e.g., the patient who has undergone major neurosurgery and who will be in a bed in

intensive care for a few days. A 4/0 nylon suture is passed through the gray line of the upper and lower eyelids and tied over silicone or rubber bolsters (Fig. 9.8). The suture can be tied with a slipknot enabling the tarsorrhaphy to be opened to examine the eye.

Lateral Tarsorrhaphy

A lateral tarsorrhaphy has been the time-honored simple surgical method of providing adequate corneal protection in the management of the patient with a facial palsy.

Advantages
1. Simple and quick to perform
2. Inexpensive
3. Reversible

Disadvantages
1. Cosmetic disfigurement
2. Limitation of visual field
3. Secondary complications, e.g., trichiasis

It is preferable to perform a more extensive tarsorrhaphy than is thought to be required as it is easier to partially open the tarsorrhaphy at a later date than to have to extend the tarsorrhaphy if it proves to be inadequate. In a patient with absent corneal sensation who is at risk of developing a neurotrophic ulcer, the lateral tarsorrhaphy should be very extensive and, unless the corneal sensation recovers, may have to be permanent.

Surgical Procedure
1. The upper and lower lids are injected subcutaneously with 2 to 3 ml of 0.5% Bupivacaine with 1:200,000 units of adrenaline mixed 50:50 with 2% lidocaine with 1:80,000 units of adrenaline.
2. The lower eyelid is held taught by an assistant who should grasp the eyelid just medial to the proposed medial limit of the tarsorrhaphy and at the most lateral aspect of the eyelid with 2 pairs of Paufique forceps (Fig. 9.9A).
3. An incision is then made 2 to 3 mm deep along the gray line of the lower eyelid using a Beaver

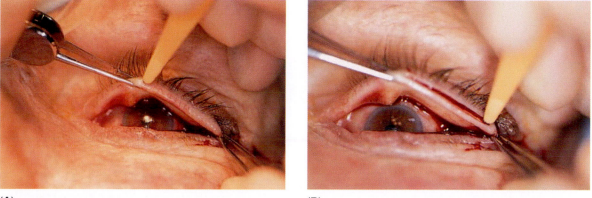

(A) **(B)**

Figure 9.9 (**A**) The upper eyelid is being held taught with toothed forceps. (**B**) The positioning of the eyelid enables a linear incision to be made using a micro-sharp blade.

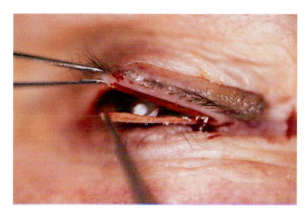

Figure 9.10 A strip of eyelid margin is excised from the posterior aspect of the eyelid margin.

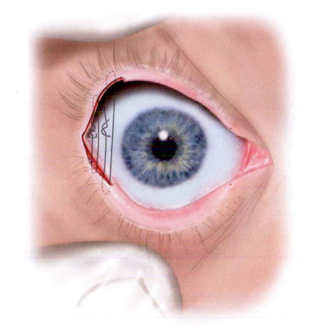

Figure 9.12 (**A**) The sutures are tied ensuring that the suture knots are away from the cornea.

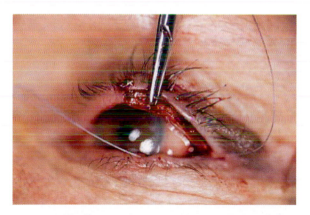

Figure 9.11 A 5/0 Vicryl suture is being passed horizontally through the tarsus, taking a partial-thickness bite.

micro-sharp blade (7530) mounted in a Beaver blade handle (Fig. 9.9B).

4. Using the same blade, two small relieving incisions are made at 90° to the gray line incision in a posterior direction.

5. Next, using a pair of Castroviejo 0.12 toothed forceps and a pair of sharp-tipped Westcott scissors, a very superficial strip of eyelid margin tissue is carefully removed posterior to the gray line incision (Fig. 9.10).

6. Next, the same procedures are undertaken in the upper eyelid.

7. Two separate interrupted 5/0 Vicryl sutures on a 1/4-circle needle are passed horizontally through the tarsal plates of the upper and lower lids and tied with the knot placed anteriorly away from the cornea (Figs. 9.11 and 9.12). This brings the denuded edges of the eyelids into apposition.

8. Interrupted 7/0 Vicryl sutures are then placed through the anterior lips of the gray line incisions and tied (Fig. 9.13).

9. Topical antibiotic ointment is applied to the eyelids.

There is no requirement for the use of any external bolsters with this surgical technique.

Postoperative Care

Topical antibiotic ointment is applied to the eyelids for 2 weeks. The 7/0 Vicryl sutures are carefully removed after 2 weeks.

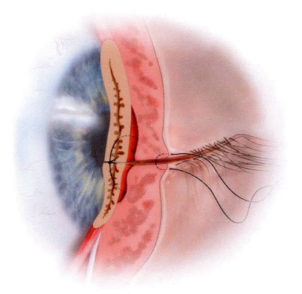

Figure 9.13 Interrupted 7/0 Vicryl sutures are placed through the anterior lips of the gray line incisions.

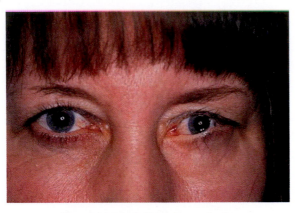

Figure 9.14 A healed lateral tarsorrhaphy.

The eyelids fuse laterally (Fig. 9.14). The tarsorrhaphy can be partially or completely reversed as required by simply dividing the eyelids with straight scissors.

Medial Canthoplasty

In this procedure the eyelids medial to the puncta are fused. This procedure is often used in addition to a lateral tarsorrhaphy to further improve corneal protection in a patient with a facial palsy. It also helps to prevent the development of a medial lower lid ectropion.

Surgical Procedure

1. The upper and lower lids are injected subcutaneously with 2 to 3 ml of 0.5% Bupivacaine with 1:200,000 units of adrenaline mixed 50:50 with 2% lidocaine with 1:80,000 units of adrenaline.
2. The eyelids are split medial to the puncta and anterior to the canaliculi using a Beaver microsharp blade (7530) (Fig. 9.15A). The canaliculi are protected with the placement of 00 Bowman probes.
3. The skin is undermined using blunt-tipped Westcott scissors (Fig. 9.15A).
4. A vertical relieving incision is made inferiorly at the medial aspect of the inferior skin flap (Fig. 9.15A).
5. Two 7/0 Vicryl sutures are passed though the pericanalicular tissue and tied (Fig. 9.15B).
6. The inferior skin flap is drawn medially and the "dog ear" removed (Fig. 9.16A).
7. The skin is closed with interrupted 7/0 Vicryl sutures (Fig. 9.16B).

Postoperative Care

Topical antibiotic ointment is applied to the eyelids for 2 weeks. The 7/0 Vicryl sutures are carefully removed after 2 weeks. The eyelids fuse medially.

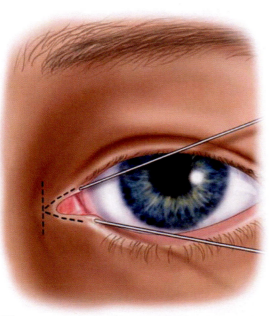

(A)

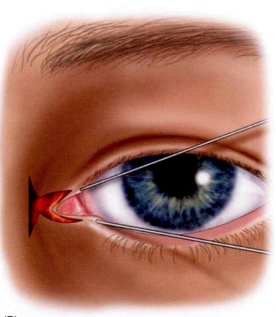

(B)

Figure 9.15 (**A**) A vertical incision is marked just medial to the medial commissure using gentian violet. (**B**) The eyelid skin is incised medial to the puncta and anterior to the canaliculi using a no. 15 Bard Parker blade. The canaliculi are protected by inserting 00 Bowman probes.

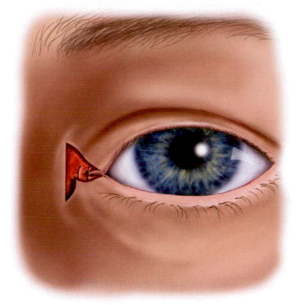

(A)

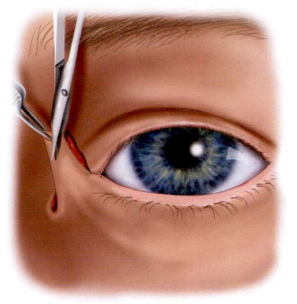

(B)

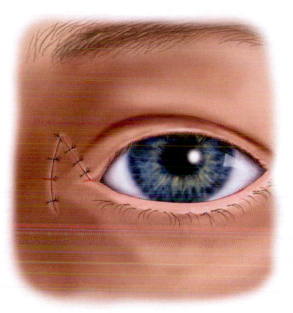

(C)

Figure 9.16 (**A**) Two 7/0 Vicryl sutures are passed though the pericanalicular tissue and tied. (**B**) The inferior skin flap is drawn medially and the dog-ear removed with Westcott scissors. (**C**) The skin is closed with interrupted 7/0 Vicryl sutures.

A patient who has undergone a medial canthoplasty and a small lateral tarsorrhaphy is shown in Figure 9.17. The medial canthoplasty can be partially or completely reversed as required by simply dividing the eyelids with straight scissors.

Müllerectomy and Levator Aponeurosis Recession
A gentle recession of the upper eyelid retractors may benefit the patient with a chronic facial palsy with upper eyelid retraction who has lagophthalmos but a moderate Bell's phenomenon, normal corneal sensation and normal tear production. Such patients may demonstrate exposure signs that affect only the inferior 1/3 of the cornea. The procedure can be performed under local anesthesia, with or without sedation.

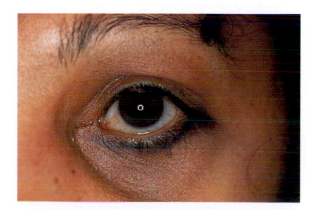

Figure 9.17 A patient who has undergone a medial canthoplasty and a small lateral tarsorrhaphy.

Surgical Procedure

1. The upper eyelid is injected subcutaneously along the skin crease with 1.5 to 2 ml of 0.5% Bupivacaine with 1:200,000 units of adrenaline mixed 50:50 with 2% lidocaine with 1:80,000 units of adrenaline.
2. A 4/0 silk traction suture is placed through the gray line of the upper eyelid.
3. The upper eyelid is everted over a medium Desmarres retractor and a further 1 ml of the same local anesthetic solution is injected subconjunctivally. The retractor is removed.
4. Pressure is applied to the eyelid for 5 minutes.
5. The eyelid is again everted over the Desmarres retractor.
6. A conjunctival incision is made at the superior border of the tarsus with a no. 15 Bard Parker blade.
7. The conjunctiva is grasped centrally with Paufique forceps and pulled forward.
8. Using blunt-tipped Westcott scissors, Müller's muscle is opened along the length of the eyelid exposing the avascular space between Müller's muscle and the levator aponeurosis.
9. A Müllerectomy is performed by peeling Müller's muscle off the conjunctiva using the slightly opened blunt-tipped blades of a pair of Westcott scissors.
10. The retractor is removed and the patient observed in a sitting position.
11. If the eyelid is still retracted, a gentle weakening of the lateral levator aponeurosis is undertaken. The eyelid is everted over the retractor again.
12. The levator aponeurosis is now gently incised vertically with the Westcott scissors in the lateral 2/3 of the eyelid.
13. The Desmarres retractor is removed and the patient is placed into a sitting position again. The eyelid height and contour are inspected. The end point of the procedure is reached when the upper eyelid is 1.5 to 2 mm lower than the fellow upper eyelid.
14. No sutures are required.
15. The traction suture is removed.
16. Antibiotic ointment is instilled into the eye.
17. Cool packs are applied.

Postoperative Care

Topical antibiotic drops are prescribed 4 times a day for 2 weeks. The patient is instructed to apply traction to the eyelid lashes and eyelid margin to maintain the desired eyelid height and contour as soon as the eyelid has risen to this position (Fig. 9.18).

Gold Weight Insertion

Gold weight implantation is a simple and useful procedure for the patient with lagophthalmos but who has a good Bell's phenomenon, normal corneal sensation, and normal tear production. It is particularly useful in the patient who has had a lateral tarsorrhaphy performed and is dissatisfied with the cosmetic appearance, and wishes for the procedure to be reversed. The success of gold weight implantation depends on careful patient selection. It is not advisable to implant a gold weight into patients with very thin pale skin, with a very atrophic orbicularis muscle and an upper lid sulcus defect. The weight is likely to be visible and obtrusive in such individuals. Patients should be carefully counseled preoperatively so that they understand the aims of the procedure and the disadvantages as well as the advantages. The procedure improves eyelid closure but it does not restore a normal reflex blink.

Advantages

1. Simple surgical procedure
2. Reversible
3. Few complications

Disadvantages

1. Eyelid closure may be impeded in the fully recumbent position
2. The gold weight may be visible
3. The gold weight may migrate or extrude
4. The patient may suffer an allergic reaction

Preoperative Evaluation

It is relatively simple to determine the weight required for complete eyelid closure in the case of a patient who has not previously undergone any eyelid surgery. It is more difficult in the case of a patient with a lateral tarsorrhaphy that is to be opened at the time of placement of the weight. A weight is

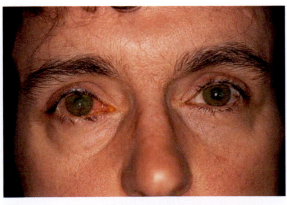

(A)

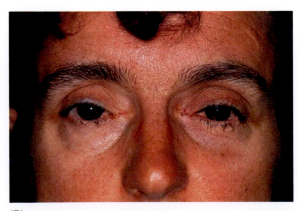

(B)

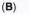

Figure 9.18 (**A**) A patient with a bilateral facial palsy and bilateral exposure keratopathy who has reduced corneal sensation. (**B**) The exposure keratopathy has resolved following a bilateral upper eyelid retractor recession and a bilateral medial canthoplasty.

selected and fixated to the upper eyelid skin just below the skin crease with adhesive tape. The upper eyelid position and degree of closure are assessed (Fig. 9.19).

The optimum weight is that which creates a minimal degree of ptosis but which permits complete eyelid closure. Generally, a 1.0 or 1.2 g weight is used. Although the weights are available commercially, it is preferable to have them shaped to the contour of the patient's individual tarsus. This is a task which can be undertaken by an ocularist.

Surgical Procedure
1. A skin crease incision is marked at the desired level in the upper eyelid using gentian violet and a cocktail stick after cleansing the skin with an alcohol wipe.
2. The upper eyelid is injected subcutaneously along the skin crease with 1.5 to 2 ml of 0.5% Bupivacaine with 1:200,000 units of adrenaline mixed 50:50 with 2% lidocaine with 1:80,000 units of adrenaline.
3. A 4/0 silk traction suture is placed through the gray line of the upper lid and fixated to the face drapes with an artery clip.
4. A 7-mm skin crease incision is made with a no. 15 Bard Parker blade (Fig. 9.20).

5. The orbicularis muscle is grasped and opened with Westcott scissors down to the tarsal plate.
6. The glistening white tarsal plate is identified and a space opened medially, laterally, and also inferiorly, taking care to avoid damaging the lash roots.
7. If the patient has significant eyelid retraction, the eyelid retractors may be gently recessed prior to insertion of the gold weight.
8. The gold weight is inserted into the space created. Some surgeons fixate the weight to the tarsus with nonabsorbable sutures (Fig. 9.21). Care should be taken to avoid passing such sutures through the full thickness of the tarsus and to avoid causing any buckling of the tarsus.
9. The orbicularis muscle is closed over the weight with interrupted 7/0 Vicryl sutures (Fig. 9.22).
10. The skin is closed with interrupted 7/0 Vicryl sutures.

Postoperative Care

Topical antibiotic ointment is applied to the eyelid wound for 2 weeks. The 7/0 Vicryl sutures are carefully removed after 2 weeks. The patient should continue to use preservative-free topical lubricants, although the frequency of instillation can be reduced.

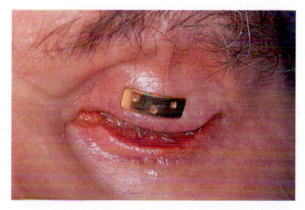

Figure 9.19 A gold eyelid weight fixated to the upper eyelid with a small piece of adhesive tape. The patient is able to effect a passive closure of the eye.

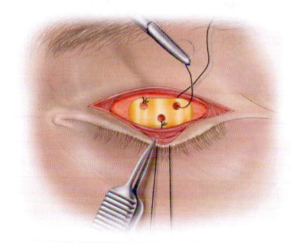

Figure 9.21 The gold weight can be fixated to the tarsus using nonabsorbable sutures passed through holes in the gold weight.

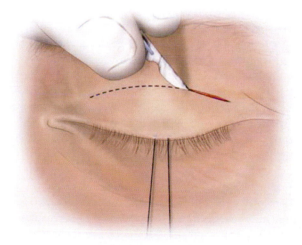

Figure 9.20 A small central incision is made. This reduces the risk of postoperative exposure of the implant. It also reduces the degree and duration of postoperative pretarsal edema and minimizes postoperative sensory loss.

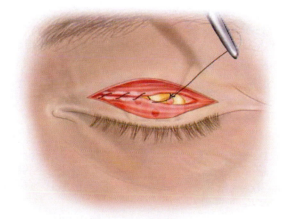

Figure 9.22 The orbicularis muscle is reapproximated before the skin is closed.

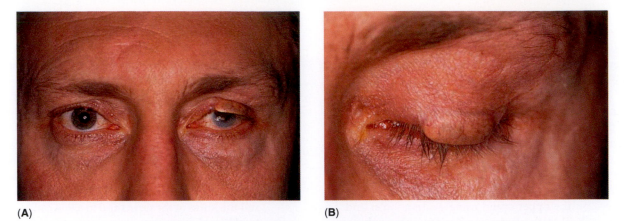

Figure 9.23 (**A**) A patient with a left upper eyelid gold weight which has migrated anteriorly. (**B**) A close-up photograph of the left upper eyelid demonstrating the abnormal position of the gold weight, which is clearly visible through the thinned and stretched upper eyelid skin.

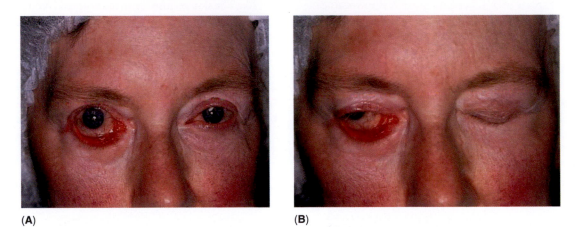

Figure 9.24 (**A**) A patient with a right facial palsy who has a severe lower eyelid ectropion. The ectropion is not only paralytic in etiology but is also cicatricial (due to skin excoriation secondary to chronic epiphora) and mechanical (secondary to a mild mid-face ptosis). (**B**) The patient also has marked lagophthalmos.

Complications

Complications are usually minimal. A patient who is allergic to gold may develop an apparent chronic cellulitis that resolves when the weight is removed. Some upper lid swelling and intermittent redness around the weight does not necessitate removal in the absence of other symptoms or signs. A ptosis of 1 to 1.5 mm is common and usually resolves after removal of the gold weight. If the weight migrates or becomes exposed, elective removal of the weight is undertaken (Fig. 9.23).

Additional Eyelid Closure Procedures

Most patients with lagophthalmos due to a facial palsy can be managed with the procedures described above. A number of other procedures have been described to effect closure of the eyelid:

1. Silicone rod cerclage
2. Palpebral spring implantation
3. Temporalis fascia transfer

The silicone rod cerclage consists of placing a rod of silicone around the upper and lower eyelids. When the upper eyelid opens, tension is placed on the silicone rod cerclage. When the patient relaxes the levator muscle, the stretched cerclage causes closure of the eyelid.

The palpebral spring consists of a piece of orthodontic wire fashioned into a spring and placed laterally in the upper eyelid.

As the eyelid is opened, tension is placed on the wire. Once the levator muscle relaxes, the tension of the spring causes the eyelid to close.

With the temporalis fascia transfer, the force of closure is generated by a cerclage around the eyelid of a strip of temporalis fascia attached to the temporalis muscle. When the patient clenches the jaw, tension is placed on the eyelid, causing it to close.

Both the silicone rod cerclage and the palpebral spring procedures are technically more demanding than gold weight implantation and have a tendency to extrude. For this reason, these procedures are not advocated by the author.

The temporalis fascia transfer relies on a conscious effort being made by the patient to clench the jaw in order to close the eyelid. The patient still experiences lagophthalmos at night as the patient's temporalis muscle relaxes. The temporalis fascia tends to loosen with time. This is not a procedure which is used by the author.

The Correction of Lower Eyelid Ectropion

A patient with a mild degree of paralytic ectropion and lagophthalmos may benefit from a simple lateral tarsorrhaphy alone. The management of greater degrees of ectropion in a patient with a facial palsy depends on an evaluation of the etiology of the ectropion, e.g., chronic epiphora may lead to cicatricial changes that may require a skin graft procedure (Figs. 9.24 and 9.25).

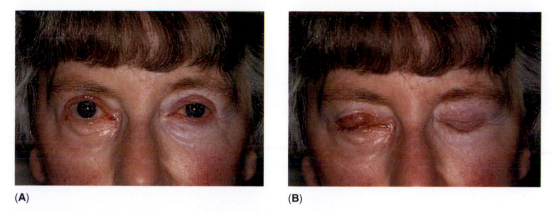

(A)　　　　　　　　**(B)**

Figure 9.25 (**A**) The same patient (as in Fig. 7.23) following a lower eyelid full-thickness skin graft and lateral tarsal strip procedure. (**B**) Her lagophthalmos has also been improved with the placement of an upper eyelid gold weight.

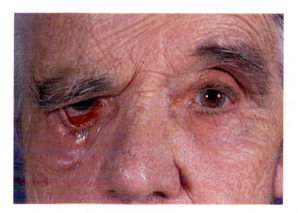

Figure 9.26 A patient with a right lower motor neuron facial palsy. Her right brow ptosis is causing a marked restriction of her visual field.

This is discussed in detail in chapter 6. In patients who are poor candidates for a facial reanimation procedure by a specialist plastic surgeon, the mid-face ptosis may be addressed either with a static sling using autogenous fascia lata to pull the lip and face upward toward the zygomatic arch, or with a sub-orbicularis oculi fat (SOOF) or mid-face lift. These procedures help to eliminate the inferior traction of the sagging face from the lower eyelid.

In a fascia lata facial suspension, the fascial strips must be inserted from the muscles around the mouth and lip subcutaneously using a Wright's fascia lata needle. The strips are then fixated near the zygomatic arch and must be tightened as much as possible.

In an SOOF lift, the inferior orbital margin is approached via a lower eyelid transconjunctival incision combined with a lateral canthotomy and inferior cantholysis. The SOOF lateral to the infraorbital neurovascular bundle is raised down to the lower border of the maxilla. The SOOF is raised and reattached with nonabsorbable sutures to the arcus marginalis and to the superficial temporal fascia. In patients with a more severe mid-face ptosis, a subperiosteal mid-face lift may be performed. In such patients the advanced tissues are fixated using polypropylene sutures passed through drill holes in the bone of the inferior orbital margin, or with the use of a mid-face Endotine implant which is fixated to the lateral orbital margin using titanium or bioabsorbable

screws. These surgical approaches are discussed in more detail in chapter 15.

In spite of the successful correction of a lower eyelid ectropion, and the improvement of lagophthalmos and exposure keratopathy, the patient may still experience chronic epiphora due to a poor lacrimal pump mechanism. In such cases, it may be necessary to resort to an endoscopic conjunctivo-dacryocystorhinostomy (CDCR) with placement of a Lester Jones tube. This is discussed in detail in chapter 20.

The Management of Brow Ptosis
A unilateral brow ptosis may be severe enough to cause impairment of the superior visual field as well as a cosmetic deformity (Fig. 9.26). It can cause a pseudo-blepharoptosis, and may lead to a secondary misdirection of the upper eyelid lashes with constant ocular irritation.

Although a number of different surgical approaches for the management of a brow ptosis complicating a facial palsy have been described, the preferred approaches are:

1. A direct brow lift
2. An endoscopic brow lift

A Direct Brow Lift
A direct brow lift is a simple but effective procedure to correct a unilateral brow ptosis (Fig. 9.27). It can be combined, if necessary, with an upper lid blepharoplasty. If a blepharoplasty is deemed to be necessary, the brow lift should be performed first. The blepharoplasty should be very conservative to avoid aggravating any lagophthalmos. This procedure is discussed in more detail in chapter 16.

Endoscopic Brow Lift
An endoscopic approach to the management of a unilateral brow ptosis has a number of advantages but also some disadvantages.

Advantages
1. Incisional scars which hidden behind the hairline.
2. A reduced risk of postoperative sensory loss in the forehead.
3. A faster postoperative recovery.

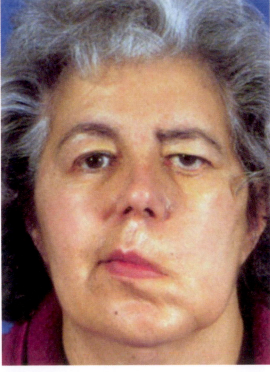

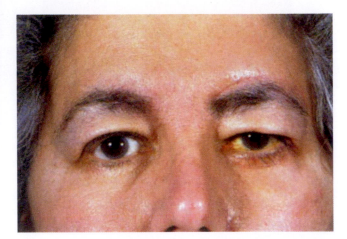

(A)   (B)

Figure 9.27 (**A**) A patient with a left facial palsy and a moderate left brow ptosis. (**B**) The appearance of the eyebrows at rest 2 weeks after a left direct brow lift. A left lateral tarsal strip procedure has also been performed.

Disadvantages
1. Time consuming
2. Expensive
3. A higher recurrence rate

This procedure is described in more detail in chapter 16.

ABERRANT REINNERVATION OF THE FACIAL NERVE

Aberrant reinnervation following recovery from a facial palsy is relatively common and patients should be warned about its possible occurrence. The degree of disability from aberrant reinnervation is variable. Some patients experience complete eyelid closure when using the perioral muscles. Such patients may be treated with botulinum toxin injections to the orbicularis oculi muscle, but such treatment inevitably leaves the patient with lagophthalmos and the need for frequent topical lubricants.

Corneal Neurotization

Direct neurotization of the cornea using the contralateral, supraorbital, and supratrochlear branches of the ophthalmic division of the trigeminal nerve is a procedure that may restore some corneal sensation to selected patients with a unilateral facial palsy and an anesthetic cornea.

FURTHER READING
1. Catalano PJ, Bergstein MJ, Biller HF. Comprehensive management of the eye in facial paralysis. Arch Otolaryngol Head Neck Surg 1995; 121: 81–6.
2. Facial Nerve Disorders Committee. Facial Nerve Grading System 2.0, Otolaryngology-Head and Neck Surgery 2009; 140: 445–50.
3. Leatherbarrow B, Collin JR. Eyelid surgery in facial palsy. Eye 1991; 5: 585–90.
4. Lee V, Currie Z, Collin JRO. Ophthalmic management of facial nerve palsy. Eye 2004; 18: 1225–34.
5. Mavrikakis I, Malhotra R. Techniques for upper eyelid loading. Ophthal Plast Reconstr Surg 2006; 22(5): 325–30.
6. May M. The Facial Nerve. New York: Thieme Stratton, 1986.
7. Olver JM. Raising the sub-orbicularis oculi fat (SOOF): its role in chronic facial palsy. BR J Ophthalmol 2000; 84: 1401–6.
8. Rahman I, Sadiq SA. Ophthalmic management of facial nerve palsy: a review. Surv Ophthalmol 2007; 52(2): 121–44.
9. Reitzen SD, Babb JS, Lalwani AK. Significance and reliability of the House–Brackmann grading system for regional facial nerve function. Otolaryngol-Head Neck Surg 2009; 140: 154–8.
10. Terzis JK, Dryer MM, Bodner BI. Corneal neurotisation: a novel solution to neurotrophic keratopathy. Plast Reconstr Surg 2009; 123(10): 112–20.
11. Wulc AE, Dryden RM, Khatchaturian T. Where is the gray line? Arch Ophthalmol 1987; 105: 1092–8.

10 Eyelid/periocular tumors

INTRODUCTION

Eyelid and periocular skin lesions are very common in patients referred to ophthalmologists. The main goal in the evaluation of these lesions is to differentiate malignant from benign lesions, and to recognize the relevance of some lesions as markers of the potential for systemic malignancies, e.g., Muir–Torre syndrome. In general, the majority of malignant tumors affecting the eyelids and periocular area are slowly enlarging, destructive lesions that distort or frankly destroy eyelid anatomy. There are a number of subtle features that can help to differentiate malignant from benign eyelid tumors (Table 10.1). It can, however, be extremely difficult to make the correct diagnosis of an eyelid lesion without a biopsy. Some malignant lesions may appear relatively innocuous (Fig. 10.1A). Conversely some benign lesions may appear extremely sinister (Fig. 10.2A).

Alternatively, the clinical pattern of some malignant eyelid tumors can simulate other tumor types, e.g., pigmented eyelid tumors are much more frequently basal cell carcinomas than melanomas (Fig. 10.3).

Early diagnosis can significantly reduce morbidity and indeed mortality associated with malignant eyelid tumors. However, malignant eyelid tumors are diagnosed early only if a high degree of clinical suspicion is applied when examining all eyelid lesions. The appropriate management of malignant eyelid tumors requires a thorough understanding of their clinical characteristics and their pathologic behavior.

Slit lamp examination can highlight these various features that help to differentiate benign from malignant tumors (Fig. 10.4). Most benign eyelid tumors can be readily diagnosed on the basis of their typical clinical appearance and behavior. In some cases, however, the diagnosis can only be made with the aid of a biopsy. Changes in the appearance of an eyelid lesion previously thought to be benign, e.g., an increase in size, ulceration, or bleeding, are indications for a biopsy.

KEY POINT

Malignant eyelid tumors are diagnosed early only if a high degree of clinical suspicion is applied when examining all eyelid lesions.

A classification of benign and malignant eyelid tumors is seen in Tables 10.2 and 10.3.

BENIGN EYELID TUMORS

The eyelids have many different components from which a multitude of benign tumors may arise. The majority of benign eyelid tumors arise from structures that comprise the eyelid skin: the epidermis, the dermis, the adnexa (pilosebaceous units, eccrine, and apocrine sweat glands), and pigment cells.

Examples of a number of common and less common benign eyelid tumors are presented.

Benign Lesions of the Epidermis

Achrochordon (papilloma)

The term papilloma is used to describe any lesion that exhibits a papillomatous growth pattern, i.e., a smooth, rounded or pedunculated elevation. The term squamous papilloma is used to describe any papilloma that is non-viral in its etiology. This is the most common benign eyelid lesion seen most commonly in patients over the age of 30 years. Eyelid papillomata present as single or multiple small flesh colored sessile (Fig. 10.5) or pedunculated growths with a central vascular core that bleeds readily on removal of the lesion.

The lesion may also develop on the palpebral or bulbar conjunctiva. Occasionally a malignant lesion can resemble a papilloma (Fig. 10.6). The lesions can be removed surgically. A broad-based lesion affecting the eyelid margin can be shaved and the base cauterized to avoid disruption to the eyelid margin.

Seborrhoeic Keratosis

A seborrhoeic keratosis is the most common benign eyelid tumor. It is most commonly seen in middle-aged and elderly Caucasian patients. It is an epithelial tumor that can occur anywhere on the body. On the eyelids the lesion typically presents with a greasy appearance, and may be sessile, lobulated, papillary, or pedunculated. The surface of the lesion has friable excrescences (Fig. 10.7). The lesion should not usually present difficulties in clinical diagnosis but they can be confused with verruca vulgaris, actinic keratosis, pigmented basal cell carcinoma, and eyelid melanoma.

These lesions are easily removed by simple shave excision leaving a flat surface which re-epithelializes.

Inverted Follicular Keratosis

Inverted follicular keratosis is a benign lesion which occurs in older patients and more commonly affects males (Fig. 10.8). It presents as a small hyperkeratotic or warty mass which may show scaling. It is often mistaken for a malignant lesion, particularly when it is associated with the development of a cutaneous horn. It is treated by complete surgical excision to prevent recurrence.

Cutaneous Horn

Cutaneous horn is the term used to describe a protruberant projection of packed keratin that resembles a horn seen in animals (Fig. 10.9). It is more commonly seen in elderly patients. The horn can be associated with a number of benign, premalignant, and malignant lesions at its base and the underlying diagnosis may be masked. Any such horn should raise the suspicion that the underlying lesion may be a squamous cell carcinoma. A cutaneous horn may also be associated with: verruca vulgaris, actinic keratosis, seborrhoeic keratosis, inverted follicular keratosis, tricholemmoma, and basal cell carcinoma.

In most patients the diagnosis is uncertain until the lesion has been removed and submitted for histopathological examination. As the cutaneous horn may overly a malignant lesion, a complete surgical excision biopsy should be performed.

Epidermoid Cyst

An epidermoid cyst (epidermal inclusion cyst) is a very common lesion which arises from entrapment of surface epithelium. This can occur following surgery or spontaneously. The lesion presents as a slowly growing round, firm, whitish or yellowish lump, which is usually solitary and mobile (Fig. 10.10). A central pore may be seen. Rupture of the cyst wall can result in an inflammatory foreign body reaction or a secondary infection.

The lesion should be completely removed. Incomplete removal results in recurrence of the lesion.

Table 10.1 Clinical signs suggestive of malignancy

- A localized loss of lashes
- Obliteration of the eyelid margin
- Pearly telangiectatic change
- Ulceration
- A new enlarging pigmented lesion
- An area of diffuse induration
- Irregular borders
- A scirrhous retracted area

Dermoid Cyst

A dermoid cyst is a choristoma that results from the sequestration of skin during embryonic development. Continued secretion by sebaceous and sweat glands contained within the lesion cause a gradual increase in size of the cyst. The cyst also contains hairs. The cyst is present at birth but may not become evident until adulthood. The cyst may lie outside the orbit but may have an extension into the orbit. A "dumb-bell" dermoid cyst has an orbital extension and an extraorbital extension, usually positioned over the lateral orbital wall. Rupture of the cyst releases secretions that are highly irritant and cause an acute inflammatory reaction.

Most dermoid cysts are seen in children and are located over the fronto-zygomatic suture (Fig. 10.11). They can occur in the superomedial aspect of the eyelid/orbit where they must be differentiated from a meningocoele or meningo-encephalo-coele by means of a CT scan. Any dermoid cyst with suspected intraorbital extension should be scanned prior to surgical intervention.

Treatment of a dermoid cyst consists of complete surgical excision. Most lesions can be removed via an upper lid skin crease incision, avoiding a visible scar (Fig. 10.12A and B). Care should be taken to ensure that the cyst is removed completely and without rupturing the cyst wall. Great care should also be taken to avoid intraoperative damage to the trochlea when removing a medial canthal dermoid cyst.

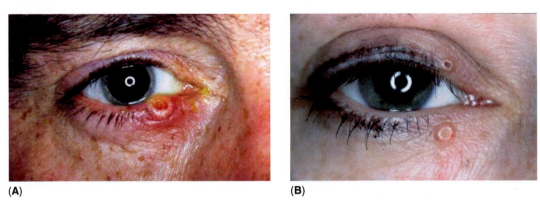

(A)   **(B)**

Figure 10.1 (**A**) A lower eyelid lesion referred to as a suspected molluscum contagiosum. A incisional biopsy proved this lesion to be a squamous cell carcinoma. (**B**) Typical molluscum contagiosum lesions of the eyelid.

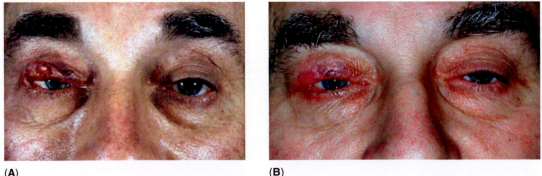

(A)   **(B)**

Figure 10.2 (**A**) This patient was referred with a suspected upper eyelid squamous cell carcinoma. A biopsy proved the lesion to be a cryptococcus infection with no evidence of malignancy. (**B**) The patient following repair of an upper lid wedge incisional biopsy and a 6 week course of Fluconazole.

Any dermoid cyst with suspected intraorbital extension should be scanned prior to surgical intervention. Great care should be taken to avoid intraoperative damage to the trochlea when removing a medial canthal dermoid cyst.

Phakomatous Choristoma

Phakomatous choristoma is a rare congenital lesion that results from surface ectodermal cells destined to form the lens plate and lens vesicle in the embryo, remaining outside the optic vesicle during closure of the embryonic fissure. These cells multiply and form the lesion in the antero-inferior aspect of the lower eyelid (Fig. 10.13). The eye is usually free from any associated developmental anomalies. The lesion is managed by surgical excision.

Milia

Milia are small, raised, round, white, well-circumscribed, superficial, keratin cysts (Fig. 10.14). They are due to occlusion of pilosebaceous units. These are frequently seen in the eyelids. They are particularly common in newborn babies. They may occur spontaneously or can occur following trauma or treatments, e.g., chemical peeling. As in the example above, milia may be seen in young patients with Gorlin's syndrome (basal cell nevus syndrome).

The lesions can be removed for cosmetic reasons by incising them with the cutting edge of a sterile needle.

Molluscum Contagiosum

The skin lesions are usually multiple, dome-shaped, and umbilicated papules (Fig. 10.15). They are self-limiting in immuno-competent patients. An associated follicular conjunctivitis may occur. The lesions can be treated by incision and curettage, surgical excision, electrodessication, and cryotherapy. Severe and aggressive involvement of the periocular region may occur in patients with AIDS or who are otherwise severely immuno-compromised.

Verruca Vulgaris

A verruca vulgaris is a papilloma caused by the human papillomavirus (Fig. 10.16). The lesion may appear as a filiform or flat wart. The lesion begins as a small brown papule that slowly enlarges and develops an elevated irregular hyperkeratotic, papillomatous surface. The filiform type is the most common variety seen on the eyelids. Lesions that involve the eyelid margin may be associated with a papillary conjunctivitis from the shedding of viral particles into the conjunctival sac.

Although the lesion can be treated in a variety of ways, e.g., cryotherapy, chemical cautery, electrodessication, complete surgical excision is preferable.

Benign Lesions of the Dermis

Capillary Hemangioma

A capillary hemangioma represents the most common benign periocular tumor of infancy. It is thought to be a vascular hamartoma. The clinical appearance varies with the depth of the lesion (Fig. 10.17). The lesion may present as a superficial cutaneous lesion (a strawberry hemangioma), a subcutaneous lesion, an orbital lesion or a combination of all three. Initially the hemangioma typically presents as a flat red lesion with overlying telangiectases, and then grows into a red, elevated soft painless compressible mass. A subcutaneous hemangioma presents as a bluish-purple mass. The extent of the lesion may need to be determined by imaging using CT, MRI, or ultrasound scanning.

The tumor tends to grow rapidly during the first few months of life before becoming dormant and then undergoing spontaneous regression. Infants with such a tumor should be kept in regular review and managed conservatively if possible.

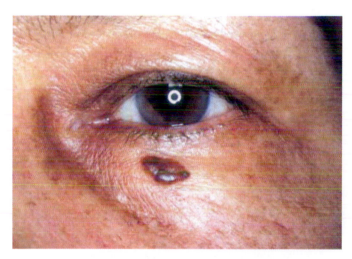

Figure 10.3 A pigmented basal cell carcinoma.

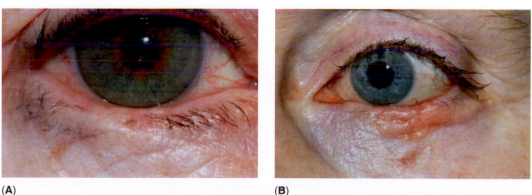

(A)   **(B)**

Figure 10.4 (**A**) An early lower eyelid margin basal cell carcinoma demonstrating a typical localized loss of eyelashes, and pearly telangiectatic changes. (**B**) A more advanced lower eyelid margin basal cell carcinoma demonstrating a typical localized loss of eyelashes, pearly raised edges and distortion of the eyelid margin.

Although benign the lesion may cause amblyopia from occlusion or secondary astigmatism. Lesions that threaten to cause amblyopia have traditionally been treated with intralesional steroid injections (triamcinolone and betamethasone) or with systemic steroids. Such patients should be monitored in conjunction with a pediatrician in view of the risks of growth retardation from the use of steroids. Intralesional steroid injection also carries the small risk of visual loss from emboli affecting the arterial blood flow to the retina and occlusion of the central retinal artery from retrobulbar hemorrhage. An alternative approach to the management of capillary hemangiomas using systemic Propranolol is showing considerable promise and should be considered.

Surgical debulking or a complete surgical excision may be required for those well-defined localized lesions that fail to respond to medical management (Fig. 10.18).

Cavernous Hemangioma

A cavernous hemangioma is rarely seen as an isolated eyelid lesion. It represents a hamartoma and is seen much more frequently in the orbit where it occurs as the most benign orbital tumor in adults. In contrast to the lesion seen in the orbit, an eyelid cavernous hemangioma is not encapsulated and tends to be adherent to the overlying dermis. A subtype termed sinusoidal cavernous hemangioma, involves the eyelid and adjacent brow or cheek and has a more aggressive growth pattern (Fig. 10.19). It is dark blue in appearance through the overlying thinned skin and compressible. As the lesion rarely appears prior to middle childhood, it seldom causes amblyopia. Although the lesion can be treated with intralesional sclerosing agents or cryotherapy, surgical excision is usually preferred.

Plexiform Neurofibroma

Plexiform neurofibromas are pathognomonic for type 1 neurofibromatosis (NF-1). The tumor arises from and grows along peripheral nerves. The lesions typically present during the first decade of childhood and may be responsible for occlusion amblyopia. The lesions typically present with a diffuse infiltration of the eyelid and orbit. Palpation of the lesions gives a sensation that has been likened to that of feeling a "bag of worms" The upper eyelid is involved in approximately 95% of cases. The lower eyelid is involved in approximately 50% of cases and the brow in approximately 15 to 20% of cases. The upper lid becomes ptotic and gradually assumes an S-shape as it thickens and develops horizontal laxity. The lesions are quite vascular and widely and diffusely infiltrative.

Systemic associations:

- CNS hamartomas
- Phaeochromocytoma
- Breast carcinoma
- Medullary thyroid carcinoma
- Gastrointestinal tumours

Ocular associations:

- Iris nodules (Lisch nodules)
- Congenital glaucoma

Table 10.2 Classification of Benign Eyelid Tumors

Benign lesions of the epidermis
- Achrocordon (skin tag, papilloma, fibroepithelial polyp)
- Seborrhoeic keratosis
- Inverted follicular keratosis
- Cutaneous horn
- Epidermoid cyst (epidermal inclusion cyst)
- Dermoid cyst
- Phakomatous choristoma
- Milia
- Molluscum contagiosum
- Verruca vulgaris

Benign lesions of the dermis
- Capillary hemangioma
- Cavernous hemangioma
- Neurofibroma
- Plexiform neurofibroma
- Pyogenic granuloma
- Pyoderma gangrenosum
- Dermatofibroma (fibrous histiocytoma)
- Xanthelasma
- Xanthoma
- Juvenile xanthogranuloma
- Xanthogranuloma
- Varix

Benign lesions of the adnexa
- Chalazion

Benign tumors of sweat gland origin
- Syringoma
- Eccrine spiradenoma

Benign tumors of hair follicle origin
- Trichofolliculoma
- Trichoepithelioma
- Tricholemmoma
- Pilomatrixoma (calcifying epithelioma of Malherbe)
- Sebaceous cyst (tricholemmal cyst)

Benign tumors of sebaceous gland origin
- Sebaceous gland hyperplasia
- Sebaceous adenoma

Benign pigmentary lesions
- Congenital nevus
- Junctional nevus
- Compound nevus
- Intradermal nevus
- Nevus of Ota (oculodermal melanocytosis)
- Lentigo simplex
- Lentigo senilis

Table 10.3 Classification of Malignant Eyelid Tumors

Epithelial
- Basal cell carcinoma
- Sebaceous gland carcinoma
- Squamous cell carcinoma
- Keratoacanthoma

Non-epithelial
- Merkel cell tumor
- Melanoma
- Kaposi's sarcoma
- Lymphoma—mycosis fungoides
- Metastatic tumors
- Angiosarcoma
- Microcystic adnexal carcinoma
- Primary mucinous carcinoma

- Retinal astrocytic hamartoma
- Optic nerve glioma
- Optic nerve meningioma
- Pulsating exophthalmos due to sphenoid wing mal-development (Fig. 10.20)

Plexiform neurofibromas are extremely difficult to manage because of their infiltrative growth pattern and vascularity. Surgical debulking may be undertaken to improve a patient's visual function and cosmetic appearance but this usually has to be repeated at regular intervals.

Pyogenic Granuloma

A pyogenic granuloma is a common benign vascular lesion. The lesion appears as a soft, friable, fleshy, often pedunculated mass. It may show superficial ulceration and may bleed easily (Fig. 10.21). It may occur following surgery or trauma, in relation to foreign bodies e.g., exposed retained sutures, or in association with inflammatory processes. The lesion may also be seen on mucosal surfaces, e.g., adjacent to a motility peg (Fig. 21.33B) to a silicone stent intranasally. An eyelid pyogenic granuloma may be misdiagnosed clinically as a

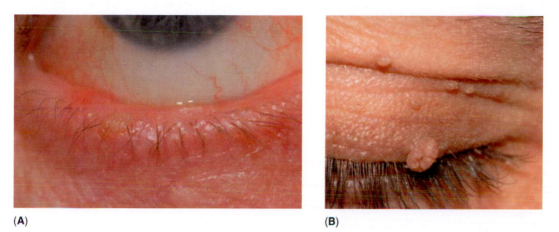

(A)   (B)

Figure 10.5 (**A**) A sessile eyelid margin papilloma. (**B**) Multiple pedunculated eyelid papillomata.

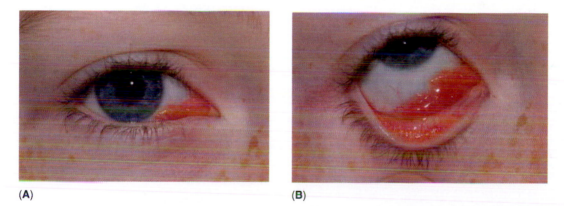

(A)   (B)

Figure 10.6 (**A**) A patient with a lesion initially diagnosed as a conjunctival papilloma. (**B**) The lesion showed multiple finger-like projections but an incisional biopsy proved the lesion to be a rhabdomyosarcoma.

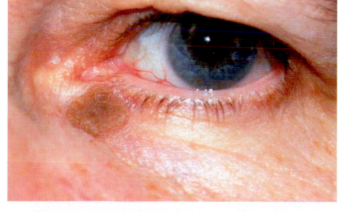

Figure 10.7 A lower lid seborrhoeic keratosis (seborrhoeic wart).

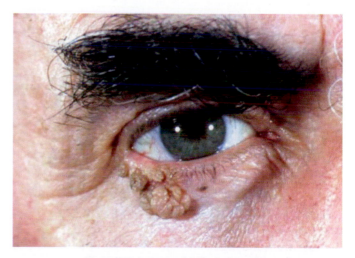

Figure 10.8 An inverted follicular keratosis.

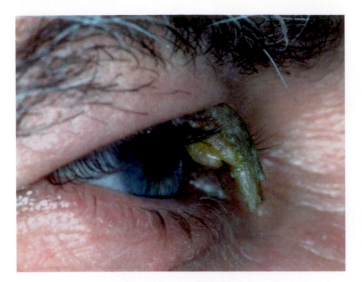

Figure 10.9 A cutaneous horn.

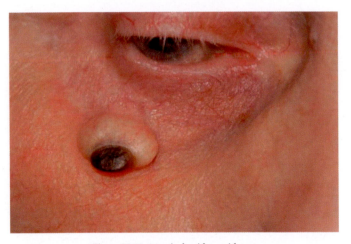

Figure 10.10 A typical epidermoid cyst.

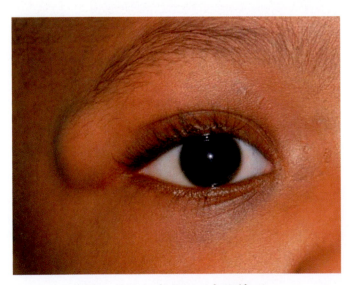

Figure 10.11 A subcutaneous dermoid cyst.

capillary hemangioma, Kaposi's sarcoma, or a basal cell carcinoma.

Treatment is by surgical excision with cautery to the base of the lesion, and by removal or treatment of the inciting factor,

e.g., incision and curettage of an eyelid chalazion. The application of topical steroids to a conjunctival pyogenic granuloma may help the lesion to resolve.

Pyoderma Gangrenosum

Pyoderma gangrenosum is a rare but serious neutrophilic dermatosis. It is commonly misdiagnosed or diagnosed late in the course of the disorder. Typically a deep ulcer with a well-defined border is seen, usually with a violet or blue edge, which is often undermined. The surrounding skin is erythematous and indurated. Lesions may occur at the site of minor trauma. It is most commonly seen on the legs and is very rarely seen in the periocular area. The lesions are usually painful and the pain can be severe. When the lesions begin to heal, the scars are often cribriform (Fig. 10.22). Patients with pyoderma gangrenosum are often systemically unwell with fever and malaise. Fifty percent are associated with systemic disorders, e.g., inflammatory bowel disease, rheumatoid arthritis, and acute myeloid leukemia.

The lesions may require systemic steroid treatment, topical Tacrolimus or systemic treatment with Cyclosporine, Azathioprine, or Infliximab.

Xanthelasma

Xanthelasmata are yellow, plaque-like lipid deposits that initially lie within the superficial dermis but can slowly enlarge and extend beyond the dermis to involve the orbicularis muscle. They typically appear on the medial aspect of the upper and lower eyelids of middle-aged adults, affecting women more frequently than men (Fig. 10.23).

Approximately 50% of patients presenting with xanthelasmata have abnormal serum lipids. Patients should therefore be investigated for serum lipid abnormalities and diabetes as potential underlying causes. Some xanthelasmata have been shown to regress with the use of statins.

The lesions can be treated for cosmetic reasons by surgical excision, CO_2 or argon laser ablation or with the topical application of 90% trichloro-acetic acid. Unfortunately, recurrences of the lesions are common regardless of the treatment modality selected.

Surgical excision is difficult, particularly in younger patients, as the lesions tend to lie medial to the area of skin normally excised in the course of a cosmetic or functional blepharoplasty, leaving visible scarring or the potential for lagophthalmos or cicatricial ectropion. For the more usual lesions confined to the superficial dermis, the topical application of 90% trichloro-acetic acid is simple and quick to perform. The acid is applied, after the administration of local anesthesia, using a cocktail stick dipped into the acid. The moistened cocktail stick is then used to apply the acid to the surface of the lesion which rapidly frosts. As soon as the surface of the lesion frosts the application of acid is stopped. The patient is asked to apply topical antibiotic ointment to the wound for a week. A retreatment is undertaken after a few weeks if the lesion has not fully responded.

Xanthoma

Xanthomata of the eyelids are quite rare and usually associated with hyperlipidemia. The lesions are situated more deeply in the dermis than xanthelasmata (Fig. 10.24).

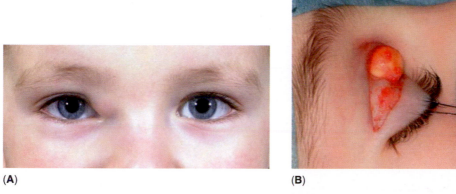

(A)   **(B)**

Figure 10.12 (**A**) A medial canthal dermoid cyst. (**B**) A medial canthal dermoid cyst being removed via an upper lid skin crease incision.

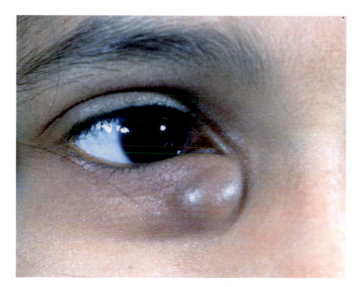

Figure 10.13 A phakomatous choristoma.

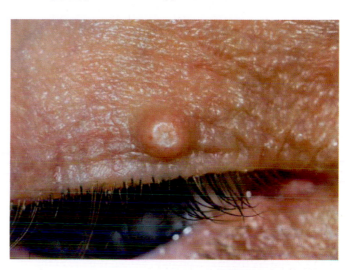

Figure 10.15 A molluscum contagiosum.

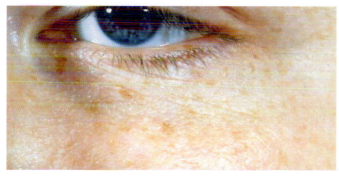

Figure 10.14 Milia.

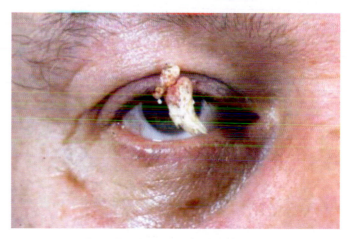

Figure 10.16 A verruca vulgaris (viral wart).

Varix

An eyelid varix consists of a thin-walled venule which appears as an isolated, slightly elevated, dark blue lesion, usually seen in older patients (Fig. 10.25). It is easily compressible. Such a varix is distinct from varices which are forward extensions of orbital varices. An isolated eyelid varix does not communicate with deeper vessels and is not associated with a thrill or bruit. It does not enlarge with a Valsalva manoeuvre. The lesion can easily be removed surgically.

Benign Lesions of the Adnexa

Chalazion

A chalazion develops as a consequence of obstruction to the ducts of the eyelid sebaceous glands (the meibomian glands or the glands of Zeiss). The chalazion is a localized lipogranulomatous reaction to the leaked contents of these glands (Fig. 10.26). Multiple lesions may occur. Large lesions in the upper lid can cause a secondary astigmatism and amblyopia in children. They are often associated with blepharitis and acne rosacea in adults.

Management of chalazia involves treatment of the underlying cause, e.g., daily eyelid scrubs using commercially available eyelid wipes and warm compresses. Chalazia that fail to respond to conservative treatment are usually incised and curetted via a vertical linear incision on the posterior tarsal surface using a chalazion clamp. Smaller chalazia may be injected with steroids

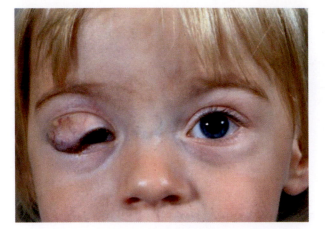

Figure 10.17 A capillary hemangioma of the right upper eyelid.

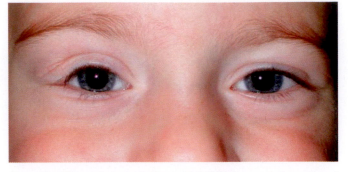

Figure 10.18 The patient seen in Figure 10.17 following surgical resection of the right upper eyelid capillary hemangioma.

but this carries the risk of a central retinal artery occlusion, focal depigmentation of the eyelid skin or even inadvertent ocular perforation.

KEY POINT

It should always be borne in mind that a sebaceous gland carcinoma (SGC) can masquerade as a chronic chalazion. Recurrent chalazia should raise a high index of suspicion and an incisional biopsy should be undertaken.

Benign Tumors of Sweat Gland Origin
Syringoma
Syringomata are the most common benign tumors of the eyelid adnexa. They are benign tumors of sweat gland origin. They most commonly affect young females. They appear as small, flesh-colored, soft, waxy nodules (Fig. 10.27). They may become larger, translucent and cystic. The lower eyelids are predominantly affected.

The lesions can be removed for cosmetic reasons using surgical excision, electrodessication, CO_2 laser ablation, trichloroacetic acid application or cryotherapy. All such treatments, however, carry risks of scarring.

Eccrine Spiradenoma
An eccrine spiradenoma is an uncommon lesion arising from the secretory part of an eccrine gland that tends to occur as a solitary, flesh-colored nodule in early adulthood (Fig. 10.28). The lesion can be tender and occasionally painful. The lesion can be removed surgically.

Apocrine Hidrocystoma
An apocrine hidrocystoma is also known as a sudoriferous cyst of a cyst of Moll. This lesion is often seen near the eyelid margin medially or laterally. The cyst wall is thin and translucent (Fig. 10.29). The cyst is usually filled with clear fluid. The clinical diagnosis is easily made in the vast majority of cases although it can be confused with a cystic basal cell carcinoma. The lesions are easily removed surgically.

Benign Tumors of Hair Follicle Origin
Pilomatrixoma
A pilomatrixoma (also known a calcifying epithelioma of Malherbe) is a tumor that develops from hair matrix cells.

The eyelid and eyebrow are sites of predilection for this tumor. It usually presents as a solitary, slowly growing, subcutaneous solid or cystic nodular mass. The overlying skin may be normal but in some cases it is stretched revealing pale areas and dilated vessels on the surface of the lesion (Fig. 10.30).

The tumor should be removed surgically in its entirety along with the overlying skin in order to prevent a recurrence.

Sebaceous Cyst (Tricholemmal Cyst)
A sebaceous cyst is derived from the outer root sheath of a hair follicle and contains cholesterol-rich debris and keratin, and is surrounded by a well-keratinized epidermal wall. In contrast to an epidermoid cyst, a sebaceous cyst has no central punctum. They are seen on hair-bearing skin and commonly affect the scalp. They appear as single or multiple smooth, painless, round, and mobile cysts (Fig. 10.31).

If the lesion ruptures, it discharges thick, cheesy, and white contents. Spontaneous or traumatic rupture of the cyst can result in an acute inflammatory reaction or secondary infection.

The lesions can be removed surgically and the cyst wall should be maintained intact during the surgical dissection.

Sebaceous Adenoma
A sebaceous adenoma is a relatively rare, usually solitary lesion occurring in patients over the age of 40 years. The lesion typically affects the eyelid and brow. The lesion presents as a slowly enlarging, well defined, firm, smooth, and dome-shaped mass which may have telangiectatic vessels lying within it (Fig. 10.32). The lesion may have a central umbilication and may ulcerate or bleed. The lesion should be excised with clear margins to prevent recurrence.

A sebaceous adenoma may occur in combination with a keratoacanthoma as part of Muir-Torre syndrome (MTS). The defining feature of this syndrome is the combination of sebaceous gland tumors and at least one visceral cancer. The finding of such a tumor is a marker for MTS and should prompt a search for an occult malignancy. The cutaneous lesion may occur as much as 25 years before the internal malignancy. Colorectal cancer is the commonest visceral neoplasm to occur in MTS.

The genetic disorder in MTS is an autosomal dominant inherited germ line mutation in one of the DNA mismatch repair genes, most commonly hMSH2. It is inherited with a high degree of penetrance and variable expression. The male-female ratio is 3:2. Children of an MTS individual, therefore, have a 50% risk of inheriting the cancer predisposition.

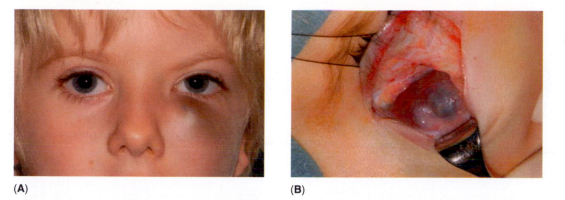

Figure 10.19 (**A**) A sinusoidal cavernous hemangioma of the left lower eyelid extending into the cheek. (**B**) A typical dark blue, lobulated appearance of the cavernous hemangioma seen at surgery.

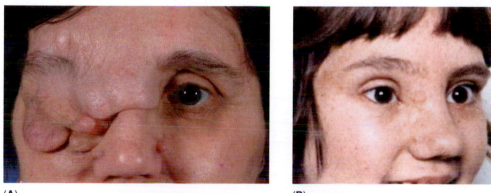

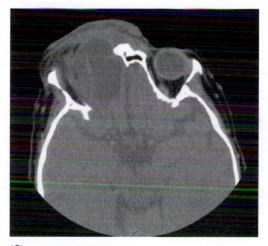

Figure 10.20 (**A**) A patient with an extensive plexiform neurofibroma. (**B**) A photograph of the same patient aged 12 years. (**C**) An axial CT scan of the patient showing a severe sphenoid wing maldevelopment with an encephalocoele.

In families where the germ line mutation can be identified, those individuals who have inherited the mutation should be offered regular screening examinations. Screening for malignancy at all possible sites is impractical in MTS given the wide range of associated malignancies, and screening should probably concentrate on the colorectum, female genital tract, and possibly renal tract.

Families with MTS are probably more common than is recognized, but sebaceous gland tumors are rare and the diagnosis of such a tumor should suggest the possibility of the syndrome and prompt a search for associated malignancies, and for the underlying genetic mutation.

Tricholemmoma

A tricholemmoma arises from a hair sheath as a solitary lesion or in multiple forms. The solitary variety is more commonly seen, usually appearing in older patients, in whom it appears as a flesh-colored verrucous or papillomatous lesion on the face, nose or eyelid. It may be mistaken for a basal cell carcinoma (Fig. 10.33).

Trichoepithelioma

Trichoepithelioma is a lesion which arises from a hair follicle which can occur as a single lesion or which can occur as multiple lesions in an inherited fashion (epithelioma adenoides cysticum

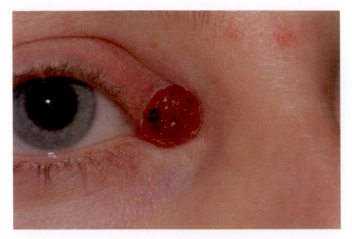

Figure 10.21 A pyogenic granuloma.

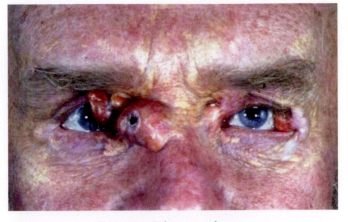

Figure 10.24 Tuberous xanthomata.

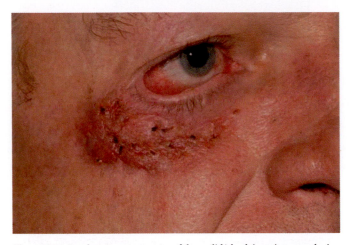

Figure 10.22 Pyoderma gangrenosum of the eyelid/cheek junction seen during the healing phase showing a cribriform appearance. The lesion occurred at the site of very minor trauma.

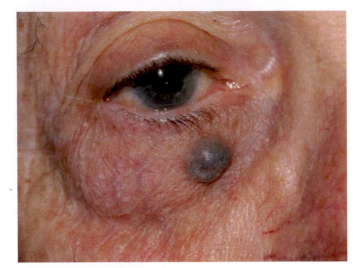

Figure 10.25 An eyelid varix.

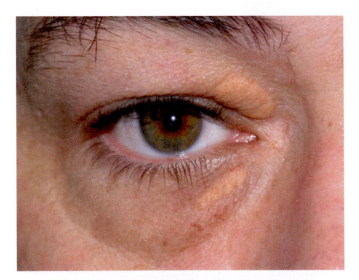

Figure 10.23 Xanthelasmata of the upper and lower eyelids.

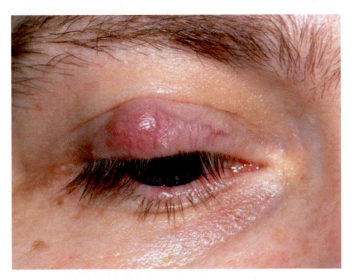

Figure 10.26 An upper eyelid chalazion.

of Brooke). These lesions tend to occur in middle-aged adults and may affect the scalp, neck, and trunk in addition to the eyelids. They appear as small flesh-colored, firm, raised papules ranging from 2 to 6 mm in diameter (Fig. 10.34). Solitary lesions can be removed surgically but multiple lesions require CO_2 laser ablation.

Benign Pigmentary Lesions

Melanocytic Nevus (Nevocellular Nevus)

Melanocytic nevi are collections of melanocytes that may be congenital or acquired. Congenital nevi are thought to be due to errors in the development and migration of cells derived from the neural crest. "Kissing nevi" are the result of such cells

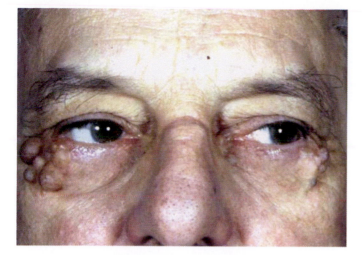

Figure 10.27 Multiple eyelid syringomata.

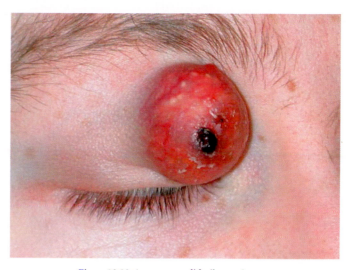

Figure 10.30 An upper eyelid pilomatrixoma.

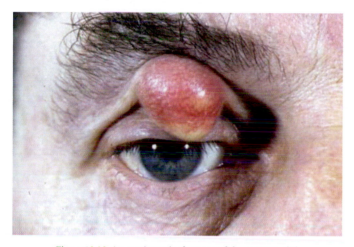

Figure 10.28 An eccrine spiradenoma of the upper eyelid.

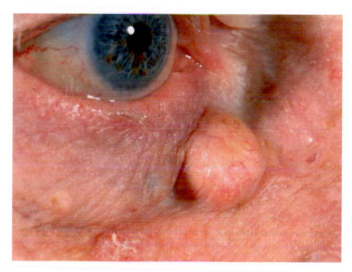

Figure 10.31 A sebaceous cyst.

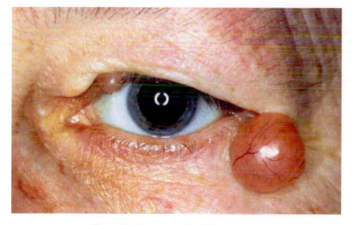

Figure 10.29 An apocrine hidrocystoma.

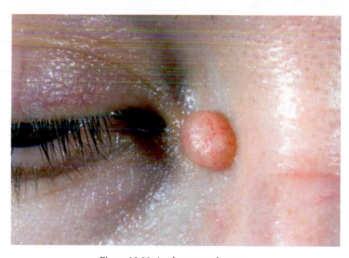

Figure 10.32 A sebaceous adenoma.

becoming sequestered along the palpebral fissure in the embryo prior to separation of the eyelids (Figs. 10.35 and 10.38).

Acquired melanocytic nevi appear during the first 3 to 4 decades of life and are particularly common in fair-skinned individuals. Considerable variation exists in the clinical appearance of melanocytic nevi. Their appearance on the eyelid margin or eyelid skin is quite common. They can be divided into three histological types: junctional. compound, and intradermal.

Junctional nevi arise from the deeper layers of the epidermis and do not involve the dermis. They tend to appear as flat macules which are round or oval in shape. These lesions tend to grow very slowly.

Compound nevi have features of both junctional and intradermal nevi. They are more common than purely

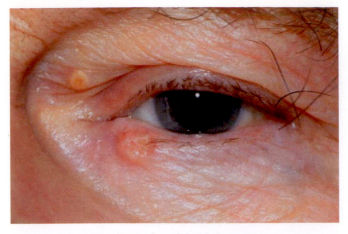

Figure 10.33 A lower lid tricholemmoma.

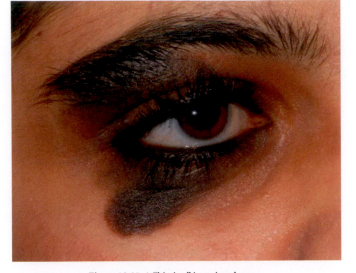

Figure 10.35 A "kissing" junctional nevus.

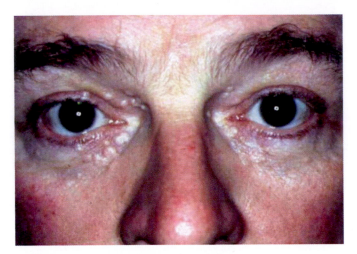

Figure 10.34 Trichoepitheliomata.

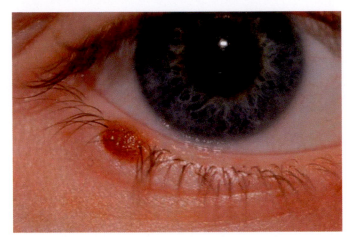

Figure 10.36 A compound nevus.

junctional nevi and tend to affect older children and young adults (Fig. 10.36).

Intradermal nevi are the most common of these three types of nevi and are mostly commonly seen in adults. They tend to present as dome-shaped, sessile, verrucous or even polypoid lesions, which may contain hairs. These lesions are often found on the lid margin (Fig. 10.37). The lesions may vary in color from light brown to flesh-colored.

Both junctional and compound nevi have the potential, albeit very infrequent, for malignant transformation, whereas intradermal nevi very rarely show such transformation.

The surgical management consists of surgical excision for cosmetic reasons but preoperative biopsy is warranted should any lesion show suspicious features e.g., change in size or color, pain, irritation, bleeding or ulceration.

Shave biopsy is preferable for clearly benign eyelid margin lesions (Fig. 10.39).

Nevus of Ota (Oculodermal Melanocytosis)

Nevus of Ota presents as a bluish-gray discoloration of the eyelid and periorbital skin (Fig. 10.40). It is usually unilateral but can occur bilaterally. There is frequently a patchy, bluish discoloration of the sclera of the ipsilateral eye, and occasionally of the conjunctiva, episclera, uveal tract, and optic disc. The oral and nasal mucosa may also be affected. The lesions

can be present at birth or they may begin to appear during the first year of life or later during adolescence. They tend to extend gradually.

Malignant transformation of the skin lesions is extremely rare but there is an increased incidence of uveal melanomas in this condition. No specific treatment is available for nevus of Ota but patients should be kept under regular review with dilated fundoscopy to exclude the development of a uveal melanoma.

Lentigines

Lentigines are acquired macules varying from light to dark brown in appearance. There are three main varieties: *lentigo simplex*, *lentigo senilis*, and *lentigo maligna* (Hutchinson's freckle). *Lentigo simplex* lesions appear as small, well-circumscribed macules which do not darken with exposure to sunlight. They are entirely benign. *Lentigo senilis* lesions appear as regular light to dark brown gradually enlarging macules appearing in patients usually over 50 years of age. They are seen in areas of the skin exposed to sunlight, particularly the face and arms. They are benign. In contrast *lentigo maligna* lesions have malignant potential. These lesions have a variable degree of pigmentation with irregular borders. They tend to occur in the lateral cheek

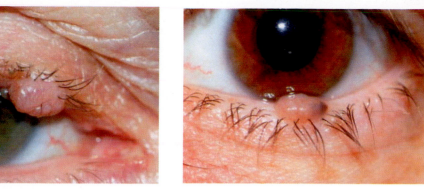

(A)   (B)

Figure 10.37 Eyelid margin intradermal nevi.

and temple regions, affecting patients usually over 50 years of age (Fig. 10.41). As malignant transformation may affect up to 50% of such lesions, surgical excision at an early stage is warranted although some clinicians follow a policy of close observation with biopsy of in the event of a change in size, pigmentation or shape.

A general physical examination should not be overlooked when assessing a patient with a periocular lesion. The purpose of this examination is to gain further clues as to the underlying diagnosis. In some patients, however, more than one pathological abnormality may exist (Fig. 10.42).

BIOPSY OF EYELID AND PERIOCULAR LESIONS
A number of lesions, however, cannot be easily and reliably differentiated from malignant eyelid lesion and require a biopsy. For small lesions an *excisional* biopsy serves two functions: diagnosis and treatment. For larger lesions an *incisional* biopsy is undertaken for diagnostic purposes. Shave biopsies should only be used for lesions in which characteristic histopathological changes are anticipated to be confined to the epidermis or superficial dermis, e.g., seborrhoeic keratosis. Exceptions to this rule include nevi affecting the eyelid margin. Although an intradermal nevus by definition extends into the dermis, it is reasonable to perform a shave biopsy as the visible portion of the lesion is removed without subjecting the patient to a more invasive procedure. This leaves a good cosmetic result with an intact eyelid margin (Fig. 10.37).

BIOPSY TECHNIQUE
It is important that biopsies are performed meticulously or errors in diagnosis will occur. *The tissue must be handled very carefully in order not to induce crush artefact.* The tissue sample should be of adequate size and depth and ideally should include adjacent normal eyelid tissue. This is of particular importance with regard to biopsies of suspected keratoacanthoma. The periphery of the lesion should be selected for incisional biopsy. Material taken from an area of central ulceration may only yield necrotic material.

If an SGC is suspected it is important to alert the pathologist of this suspicion so that appropriate lipid stains are utilized. Some biopsy material may need to be presented on filter paper because of the very small size of the samples e.g., random conjunctival sac biopsies in cases of suspected diffuse SGC.

It is important to orientate tissue for the pathologist where biopsies are attempted excisional biopsies in case one or more edges are not clear of tumor involvement. Sutures of various lengths can be employed as markers for this purpose. A tumor excision map should be enclosed with the pathology form to assist the pathologist.

KEY POINTS

All eyelid lesions that are removed should be submitted for histopathological examination and the patient should be informed of the result.

It is not acceptable to reconstruct an eyelid or periocular tissue defect following the removal of a malignant tumor (except by simple direct closure) before first obtaining histological confirmation that the tumor margins are clear.

MALIGNANT EYELID TUMORS
Basal Cell Carcinoma
A basal cell carcinoma (BCC) is a malignant tumor that is derived from the cells of the basal layer of the epidermis. BCCs are the most common malignant tumor of the eyelids accounting for approximately 90 to 95% of all malignant epithelial eyelid tumors. Ultraviolet light exposure is an important etiological factor in the development of eyelid epithelial malignancies. This tumor is prevalent in fair-skinned individuals. The effects of sun exposure are cumulative, as reflected in the increasing incidence of the tumor with advancing age. BCC may, however, occur in younger patients, particularly those with a tumor diathesis such as the basal cell nevus syndrome (Gorlin's syndrome) (Fig. 10.43).

In descending order of frequency, BCCs involve the following locations (Fig. 10.44):

- Lower eyelid (50–60%)
- Medial canthus (25–30%)
- Upper eyelid (15%)
- Lateral canthus (5%)

Clinical Features
BCCs have a variety of clinical appearances reflecting the various histopathological patterns of the tumor. The tumor arises from undifferentiated cells in the basal layer of the epidermis. As these cells do not produce keratin BCCs are not associated with hyperkeratosis in contrast to squamous cell carcinomas.

The most common presentation is a nodular pattern. The epithelial proliferation produces a solid pearly lesion contiguous with the surface epithelium. The superficial nature of telangiectatic vessels may predispose these lesions to spontaneous bleeding. With prolonged growth, central umbilication and ulceration occurs. The typical presentation is of a chronic, indurated, non-tender, raised, pearly, telangiectatic, well-circumscribed lesion with an elevated surround and depressed crater-like centre (Fig. 10.45).

Clinical Varieties
- Nodular
- Ulcerative
- Cystic
- Pigmented
- Morpheaform

The most commonly encountered morphologic patterns of basal cell carcinoma are the nodular and ulcerative forms. Nodular basal cell carcinomas may assume various clinical presentations such as papilloma (secondary to increased keratin production), a nevus (secondary to pigmentation), and a cyst (due to central tumor necrosis). The variety of clinical presentations of basal cell carcinoma accounts for the high incidence of misdiagnosis. Clinical awareness of the various presentations of the tumor minimizes incorrect clinical diagnoses and management. The pigmented BCC is easily mistaken for an eyelid melanoma, which is in fact very rare (Fig. 10.46).

Occasionally patients present with a lower eyelid ectropion that has occurred as a consequence of the cicatricial effects of a BCC (Fig. 10.47A). The underlying BCC may be missed with a cursory examination (Fig. 10.47B).

The morpheaform lesion has clinically indistinct margins and has a tendency to deep invasion, especially at the medial canthus. Orbital invasion by a BCC is manifested clinically as a fixed, non-mobile tumor and/or a "frozen globe". Although BCCs "never" metastasize, approximately 130 cases of metastases have been described in the literature.

The most difficult BCCs to manage are as follows.

- Morpheaform BCCs (Fig. 10.48A).
- BCCs that are fixed to bone (Fig. 10.48B).
- Medial canthal BCCs (Fig. 10.48C).
- BCCs with orbital invasion (Fig. 10.48D).
- Recurrent BCCs, especially following radiotherapy (Fig. 10.48E).
- BCCs in patients with basal cell nevus syndrome.

Basal Cell Nevus Syndrome (Gorlin's Syndrome)
Basal cell nevus syndrome is an autosomal dominant disorder with a prevalence estimated at 1/56,000. It shows variable expression. It is characterised by specific developmental malformations in addition to a predisposition to characteristic neoplasia. The major associated components include

- Multiple nevoid BCCs
- Odontogenic keratocysts of the jaw

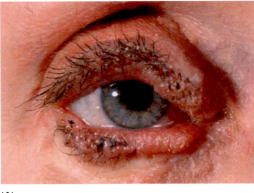

(A)   (B)

Figure 10.38 "Kissing" compound nevi.

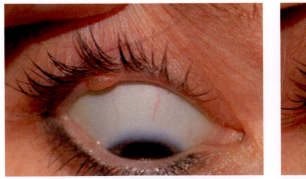
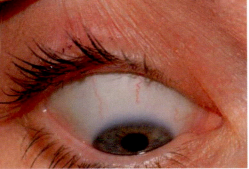

(A)   (B)

Figure 10.39 (**A**) Intradermal nevus of the upper eyelid margin. This is best managed by a simple shave excision with cautery to the base leaving the wound to granulate. This yields the best cosmetic result. (**B**) Postoperative appearance 5 days following simple shave excision.

- Palmar and plantar pits (Fig. 10.49)
- Characteristic ectopic calcifications
- Skeletal developmental anomalies, particularly of the vertebrae and ribs

The predisposition to neoplasia particularly results in multiple basal cell carcinoma at a young age, as well as medulloblastoma in about 3 to 5% of patients, and ovarian fibroma.

Clinical Features
Up to 26% of patients also have ophthalmic manifestations which may include

- Periocular BCC
- Strabismus
- Nystagmus
- Cataract
- Glaucoma
- Eyelid epidermal or dermal cysts
- Periocular milia

Some patients have a typical facies with a broad nasal bridge, hypertelorism, mandibular prognathism, plus frontal and parietal bossing (Fig. 10.50).

Due to the multi-system nature of the disorder, patients with BCNS present at a variety of ages, with considerable variability in clinical features, and to a variety of practitioners. Many undergo a wide variety of medical and surgical treatments, spanning many years. Through a combination of the disease process itself and the effects of repeated surgeries, many patients acquire disfigured features that cause both functional and cosmetic problems (Fig. 10.51).

Following diagnosis, a structured referral plan to all the potentially relevant specialties is important. Multi-disciplinary care is required for these patients from an early age, including referral for genetic counseling.

SQUAMOUS CELL CARCINOMA

Squamous cell carcinoma (SCC) is a malignant tumor that most commonly affects older, fair-skinned individuals. SCCs arise from keratinocytes in the epidermis. In the eyelids they are similar to those occurring elsewhere on the skin, with relatively low overall metastatic potential and low tumor-induced mortality. They tend to arise in areas of skin showing precancerous changes, e.g., actinic or solar keratosis. They may also arise in patients who are immuno-deficient, e.g., organ transplant patients taking long term immunosuppressive

agents, or who have other intrinsic predisposition, e.g., xeroderma pigmentosum (Fig. 10.52).

They represent approximately 2 to 5% of all malignant eyelid lesions. The tumors tend to spread to regional nodes but direct perineural invasion into the CNS is usually the cause of death in this group of patients. A patient with a periocular SCC who develops a cranial nerve palsy has neurotrophic spread until proven otherwise.

Clinical Features
There is no pathognomonic presentation. The lower eyelid is the most common periocular site to be involved. These tumors tend to appear as thick, erythematous, elevated, lesions with indurated borders and with a scaly surface (Fig. 10.53).

Cutaneous horn formation or extensive keratinisation are the most consistent features (Fig. 10.54).

When these tumors occur at the eyelid margin the lashes are destroyed. With chronicity and cicatricial changes of the skin, a secondary ectropion may occur. The lesions have a tendency to ulcerate, become friable, and to bleed easily. The lesion may necrose and develop a secondary infection (Fig. 10.55).

The clinical features of the tumor are an exaggeration of those found with actinic keratosis. The lesions of actinic keratosis occur in areas of actinic damage and appear as flesh-colored, yellow/brown plaques, sometimes with erythema. As these areas have malignant potential such patients should be closely monitored.

Benign tumors such as inverted follicular keratosis, or verruca vulgaris, can simulate features of squamous cell carcinoma.

KERATOACANTHOMA

Keratoacanthoma is a relatively uncommon epithelial tumor usually occurring on the lower eyelid in patients over 50 years of age. The lesion may occur as part of Muir-Torre syndrome.

Clinical Features
Classically the lesion commences as a small, flesh-colored papule, which rapidly develops into a dome-shaped violaceous or brownish nodule with a central keratin-filled crater and elevated, rolled margins (Fig. 10.56). The lesion may increase in size quite rapidly. The lesion then tends to regress spontaneously over the course of 3 to 6 months leaving an atrophic scar. Although this lesion has long been regarded as a benign, self-limiting lesion that mimics a squamous cell carcinoma both clinically and pathologically, it should be regarded as a low grade squamous cell carcinoma and should be completely surgically

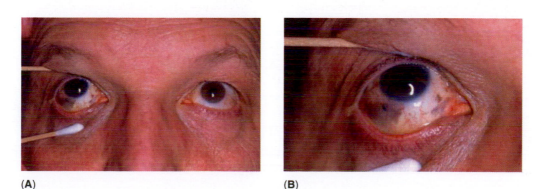

(A) (B)

Figure 10.40 (**A**) A patient with a nevus of Ota. (**B**) A close-up photograph of the eye showing typical slate gray discoloration of the sclera.

excised while still small. Where surgery cannot be undertaken, cryotherapy, radiotherapy, and topical 5-fluorouracil may be used as alternative treatment modalities.

SEBACEOUS GLAND CARCINOMA

SGC is a highly malignant tumor that arises from sebaceous glands. SGCs are very rare, with a predilection for the periocular area. They can arise from the meibomian glands, the glands of Zeiss, and from the adnexal sebaceous glands. SGCs of the eyelids have a tendency to produce widespread metastases, whereas such tumors occurring elsewhere on the skin rarely metastasize. SGC occurs with increasing frequency with advancing age.

Clinical Features

The tumor has a predilection for the upper eyelid, but diffuse upper and lower eyelid involvement may occur in patients presenting with chronic blepharoconjunctivitis. The tumor can mimic a chalazion (Fig. 10.57) and blepharitis/blepharoconjunctivitis (Fig. 10.58). The tumor affects females more commonly than males and is also more common in oriental patients.

KEY POINT

This tumor is well recognized for its ability to masquerade as chronic blepharitis/blepharoconjunctivitis or recurrent chalazion ("masquerade syndrome"). Recurrent chalazion or atypical solid chalazia, or unilateral blepharitis/blepharoconjunctivitis, should alert the ophthalmologist to the possibility of an underlying SGC.

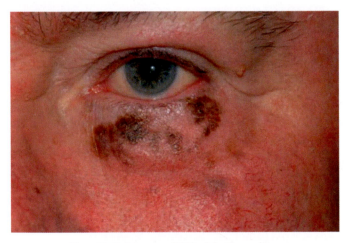

Figure 10.41 A lower eyelid/cheek lentigo maligna.

Histopathological features of SGC are characteristic and may be confirmed by lipid stains (oil red O) on fresh tissue specimens. Multicentric origin is a feature of some SGCs. Clinical presentation of chronic blepharoconjunctivitis has been correlated with the pathologic features of Pagetoid involvement of the surface epithelium. The tumor can show multicentric spread to the conjunctiva, corneal epithelium, and can spread to the nasal cavity via the lacrimal drainage system.

Despite the characteristic features, the tumor is frequently misdiagnosed. The aggressive behavior and significant morbidity and mortality associated with SGCs have traditionally been attributed to the misdiagnosed tumors. It is clear that early diagnosis and appropriate therapy significantly reduce the long-term morbidity and mortality associated with this tumor. An advanced neglected SGC is shown in Figure 10.59.

Poor Prognostic Factors

- Invasion—vascular, lymphatic, or orbital
- Diffuse involvement of both eyelids
- Multicentric origin
- Tumor diameter > 10 mm
- Symptoms present > 6 months

The following points should also be noted:

- In the Pagetoid pattern there is often involvement of both eyelids as well as the conjunctiva.
- Approximately 30% of SGCs recur.
- Systemic extension occurs by contiguous growth, lymphatic spread, and haematogenous seeding.
- The tumor spreads mainly to the orbit, the preauricular/submandibular nodes or parotid gland and less frequently to the cervical nodes, lung, pleura, liver, brain and skull.
- Some patients remain alive and well for long periods with regional node involvement. Radical neck dissection for isolated cervical node disease is therefore often indicated.
- Mortality is approximately 10 to 20%, mainly due to late diagnosis.

Diagnosis

A high index of suspicion is required to make the diagnosis early.

- A shave biopsy may only show inflammation.
- A full thickness eyelid biopsy is required.

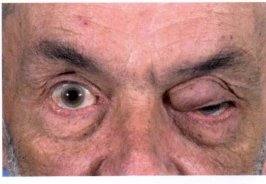

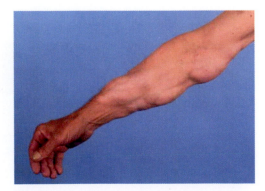

(A)   **(B)**

Figure 10.42 (**A**) A rubbery, painless, mass in the left upper eyelid. (**B**) Multiple subcutaneous lipomata in the same patient. The lesion in the patient's eyelid proved to be a lymphoma.

- Random conjunctival biopsies should be performed.
- Lipid stains are required—alert the pathologist about the suspected diagnosis.

MERKEL CELL TUMOR

Merkel cell tumor is a rare and highly aggressive malignant tumor composed of cells of neural crest origin. Merkel cell

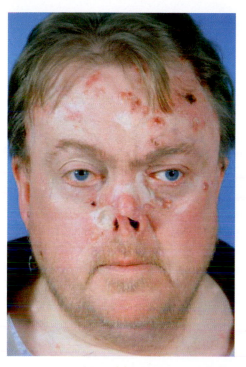

Figure 10.43 A patient with basal cell nevus syndrome.

tumors account for less than 1% of malignant eyelid tumors and tend to affect elderly Caucasian individuals. The tumors metastasize to the regional lymph nodes initially. Metastatic disease is responsible for a 30 to 50% of 2-year mortality.

Clinical Features

The tumor typically presents as a solitary, painless, violaceous or red, dome-shaped nodule with a shiny surface and fine telangiectases (Fig. 10.60). A Merkel cell tumor usually grows very rapidly. It can affect both upper and lower eyelids but is seen more frequently in the upper eyelid.

The tumor should be managed by means of an urgent, aggressive, surgical excision. Unfortunately recurrences following treatment are common.

MELANOMA

Cutaneous melanoma is an invasive proliferation of malignant melanocytes. This tumor is seen rarely in the eyelid and accounts for approximately 1% of all malignant eyelid tumors. Pigmented BCCs are ten times more common than melanoma as a cause of pigmented eyelid tumors. Forty percent of eyelid melanomas are, however, non-pigmented.

Classification

- Lentigo maligna melanoma
- Superficial spreading melanoma
- Nodular melanoma

Nodular melanoma and lentigo maligna melanoma are the most common type affecting the eyelids.

Clinical Features

These tumors tend to have irregular borders, variegated pigmentation often with inflammation, occasional bleeding and ulceration. Occasionally the eyelid may be secondarily involved by a conjunctival melanoma.

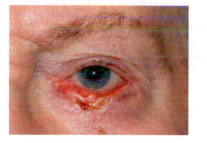
(A)

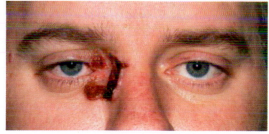
(B)

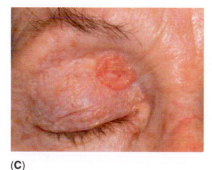
(C)

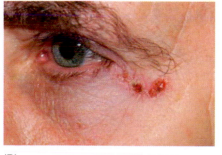
(D)

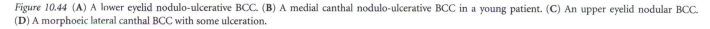

Figure 10.44 (**A**) A lower eyelid nodulo-ulcerative BCC. (**B**) A medial canthal nodulo-ulcerative BCC in a young patient. (**C**) An upper eyelid nodular BCC. (**D**) A morphoeic lateral canthal BCC with some ulceration.

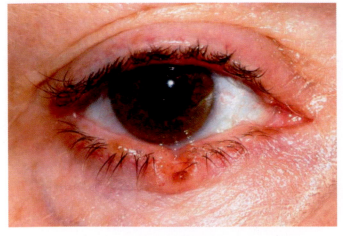

Figure 10.45 A typical lower eyelid nodulo-ulcerative BCC.

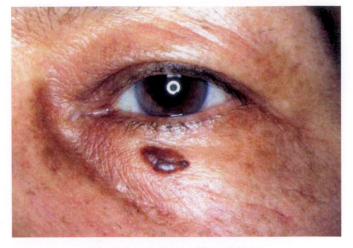

Figure 10.46 A pigmented lower lid BCC.

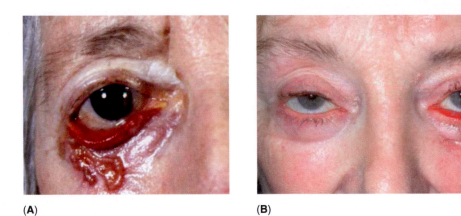

(A)   (B)

Figure 10.47 (**A**) A clinically obvious BCC with a secondary lower eyelid cicatricial ectropion. (**B**) A lower lid ectropion secondary to a BCC adherent to the inferior orbital margin. The presence of the BCC would be easily missed on a cursory examination.

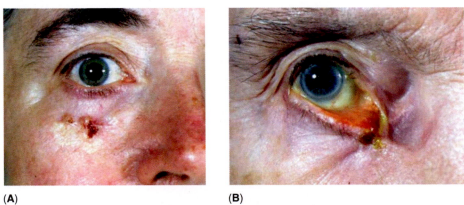

(A)   (B)

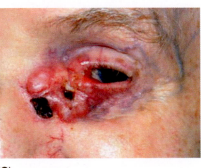

(C)

Figure 10.48 (**A**) An extensive right lower eyelid morpheaform BCC with some nodular change. (**B**) A right lower eyelid nodulo-ulcerative BCC fixed to the inferior orbital margin. (**C**) An extensive left medial canthal BCC with orbital invasion. (*Continued*)

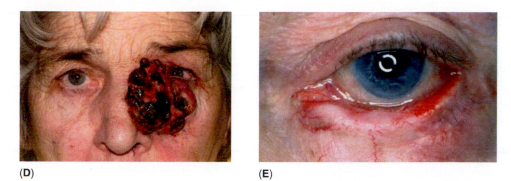

Figure 10.48 (*Continued*) (**D**) A neglected periocular BCC with orbital invasion. (**E**) Recurrence of a lower eyelid BCC after previous radiotherapy.

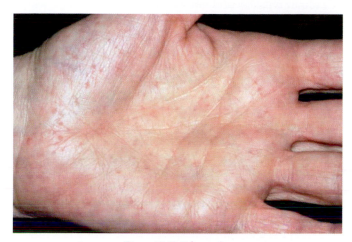

Figure 10.49 Palmar pits.

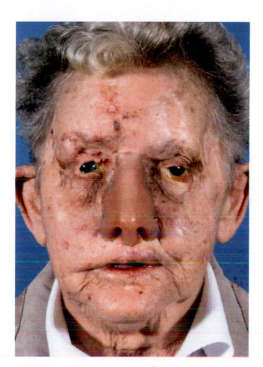

Figure 10.51 A patient with basal cell nevus syndrome and a prosthetic nose showing facial disfigurement following multiple surgical procedures over the course of 40 years.

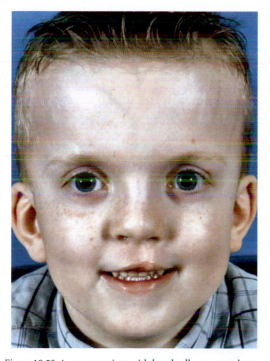

Figure 10.50 A young patient with basal cell nevus syndrome.

Superficial spreading melanoma appears typically as a brown lesion with shades of blue, red, and white. It is initially flat but becomes nodular, indurated, and irregular with an increase in vertical growth (Fig. 10.61). Nodular melanoma typically appears as a nodule or plaque, is dark brown or black in color but can be amelanotic. It shows little radial but extensive and rapid vertical growth (Fig. 10.62). It may ulcerate and bleed.

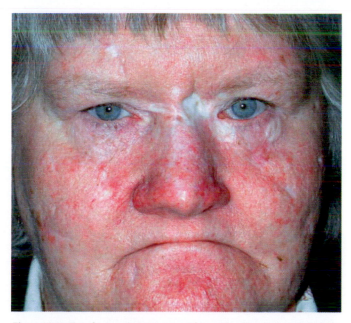

Figure 10.52 Xeroderma pigmentosum. This patient has had several SCCs removed from the eyelids and periocular area with skin graft reconstructions.

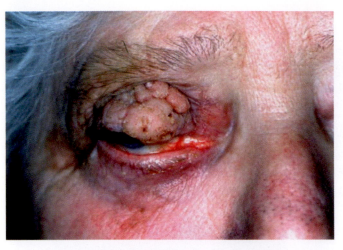

Figure 10.53 An upper eyelid squamous cell carcinoma.

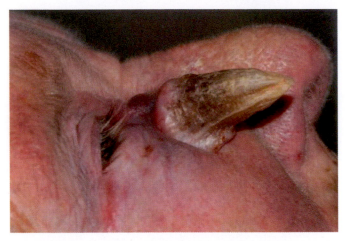

Figure 10.54 A large cutaneous horn in a patient with an underlying lower lid squamous cell carcinoma.

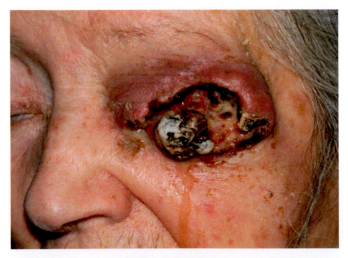

Figure 10.55 A neglected necrotic, ulcerated squamous cell carcinoma.

Two classic histological classifications are based on:

- Anatomic level of involvement (Clark)
- Tumor thickness (Breslow)

Prognosis and metastatic potential are linked to the depth of invasion and thickness of the tumor. Tumor thickness is the most important predictor of prognosis. Lesions which measure less than 0.75 mm in thickness have a 98% 5-year survival, whereas lesions with a thickness greater than 4 mm have a 5-year survival rate which is less than 50%.

KAPOSI'S SARCOMA

Prior to 1981 most cases of Kaposi's sarcoma occurred in elderly Italian/Jewish men or African children. It very rarely involved periocular structures prior to AIDS but is now a relatively common manifestation of AIDS, affecting up to 25% of patients with the disease.

Clinical Features

The tumor typically presents as a red to brown macule which enlarges to become a more elevated, highly vascular, purple or violaceous nodule on the eyelid skin, caruncle or conjunctiva (Fig. 10.63). The conjunctiva may be diffusely involved and simulate inflammation.

MYCOSIS FUNGOIDES

Mycosis fungoides is a cutaneous T-cell lymphoma which typically affected patients over the age of 45 to 50.

Clinical Features

The disease tends to progress through three different phases: a pruritic, eczematous dermatitis phase with erythroderma, followed by a phase characterized by infiltrating plaque-like lesions and scaling, and terminating in a tumor phase (Fig. 10.64). It is the final phase in which eyelid lesions are seen. Full-thickness ulceration of the eyelid can occur and cicatricial ectropion. Other ophthalmic manifestations include conjunctival disease, keratitis, uveitis, and glaucoma. The diagnosis can be difficult because the early phases of the disease often resemble eczema or even psoriasis. Diagnosis is generally made following skin biopsies. Several biopsies are recommended, to be more certain of the diagnosis. The diagnosis is made through a combination of the clinical picture and examination, and is confirmed by biopsy.

METASTATIC TUMORS

Metastatic disease involving the eyelids accounts for less than 1% of all malignant eyelid tumors. The more frequent primary tumor sites are: breast, cutaneous melanoma, bronchus, colon, and prostate gland.

Clinical Features

Eyelid metastases may present with a diffuse, painless, full thickness, firm induration of the eyelid, a subcutaneous nodule, or as a solitary ulcerated lesion. It is rare to see multiple lesions in one or more eyelids.

An incisional biopsy is required to establish the diagnosis.

OTHER RARE EYELID TUMORS

- Angiosarcoma
- Microcystic adnexal carcinoma
- Primary mucinous carcinoma

These highly malignant tumors are extremely rare and require a biopsy to establish the correct diagnosis.

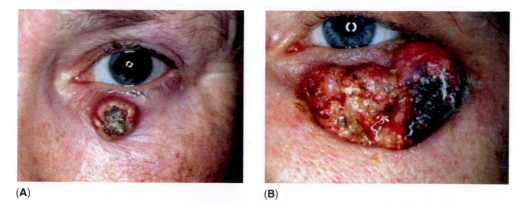

(A)   (B)

Figure 10.56 (**A**) A small keratoacanthoma in a middle-aged patient. (**B**) A large keratoacanthoma in a young patient.

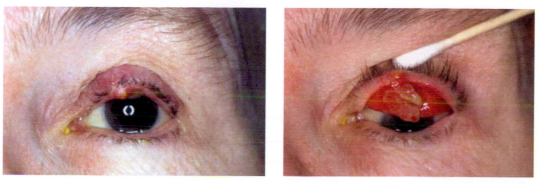

(A)   (B)

Figure 10.57 (**A**) A left upper eyelid sebaceous gland carcinoma (SGC) masquerading as a recurrent chalazion. (**B**) The appearances of the tumor on eversion of the upper eyelid.

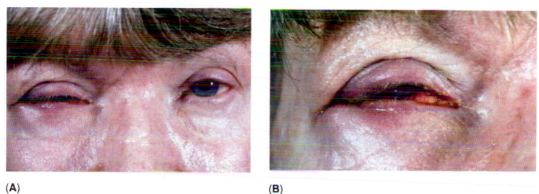

(A)   (B)

Figure 10.58 (**A**) An SGC masquerading as chronic unilateral blepharoconjunctivitis in a patient with acne rosacea. (**B**) A close-up photograph of the same patient.

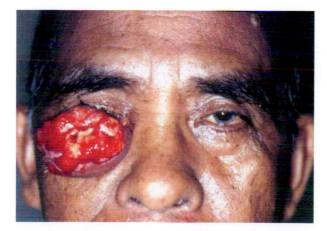

Figure 10.59 An advanced neglected SGC.

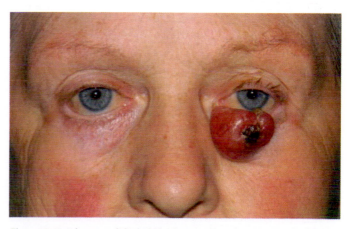

Figure 10.60 A lower eyelid Merkel cell tumor demonstrating typical clinical features.

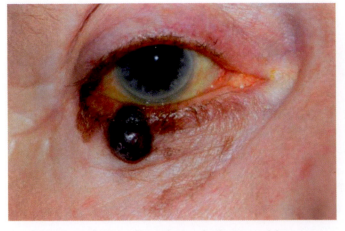

Figure 10.61 A superficial spreading melanoma developing a nodular component.

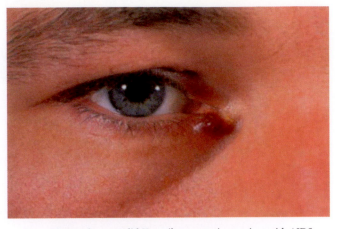

Figure 10.63 A lower eyelid Kaposi's sarcoma in a patient with AIDS.

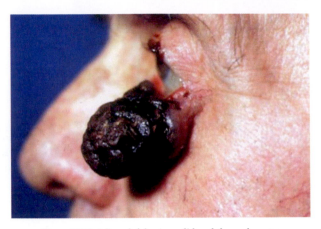

Figure 10.62 A large left lower eyelid nodular melanoma.

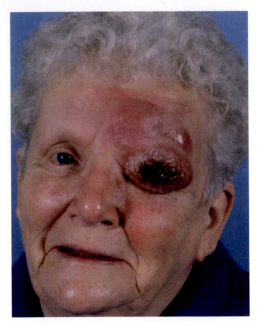

Figure 10.64 A patient with mycosis fungoides.

FURTHER READING

1. American Academy of Ophthalmology. Basic and Clinical Science Course: Orbit, Eyelids, and Lacrimal System, section 7,. San Francisco, CA: The American Academy of Ophthalmology, 2006/7: 201–5.

2. Skalicky SE, Holt PE, Giblin NM, Taylor S, Conway RM. Australian cancer network clinical practice guidelines for the management of ocular and periocular melanoma: an evidence-based literature analysis. (Review). Clin Experiment Ophthalmol 2008; 36(7): 646–58.

3. Conlon MR, Leatherbarrow B, Nerad JA: Benign eyelid tumors. In: Bosniak S, eds,. Principles and Practice of Opbthalmic Plastic and Reconstructive Surgery, chap 31. Philadelphia, PA: WB Saunders, 1996: 323–41.

4. Doxanas MT: Malignant epithelial eyelid tumors. In Bosniak S, ed., Principles and Practice of Opbthalmic Plastic and Reconstructive Surgery, chap 32. Philadelphia, PA: W.B. Saunders, 1996: 342–51.

5. Howard GR, Nerad JA, Carter KD, Whitaker DC. Clinical characteristics associated with orbital invasion of cutaneous basal cell and squamous cell tumors of the eyelid. Am J Opbthalmol 1992; 113: 123–33.

6. Kivela T. Tarkkanen A. The Merkel cell and associated neoplasms in the eyelids and periocular region. Surv Ophthalmol 1990; 35(Suppl 3): 171–87.

7. Margo CE, Waltz K. Basal cell carcinoma of the eyelid and periocular skin. Surv Ophthalmol 1993; 38: 169–92.

8. McCord CD, ed. Management of eyelid neoplastic disease. In: Eyelid Surgery: Principles and Techniques, chap 25. Philadelphia, PA: Lippincott-Raven, 1995: 312–29.

9. Mencia-Gutiérrez E, Gutiérrez-Diaz E, Redondo-Marcos I, et al. Cutaneous horns of the eyelid: A clinicopathological study of 48 cases. J Cutaneous Pathol 2004; 31: 539–43.

10. Missotten GS, de Wolff-Rouendaal D, de Keizer RJW. Merkel cell carcinoma of the eyelid. Am Acad Ophthalmol 2008; 115: 195–201.

11. Nerad JA, Whitaker DC: Periocular basal cell carcinoma in adults 35 years of age and younger. Am J Opbthalmol 1998; 106: 723–9.

12. Özdal PC, Codère F, Callejo S,Caissie AL, Burnier MN. Accuracy of the Clinical Diagnosis of Chalazion, Eye 2004; 18: 135–8.

13. Sacks EH, Lisman RD: Diagnosis and management of seba ceous gland carcinoma. In Bosniak S, ed., Principles and Practice of Ophthalmic Plastic and Reconstructive Surgery, chap 13, vol 13. , Philadelphia, PA: W.B. Saunders, 1996: 190–5.

14. Simon GJB, Huang L, Nakra T, et al. Intralesional triamcinolone acetonide injection for primary and recurrent Chalazia: is it really effective? Am Acad Ophthalmol 2005; 112: 913–7.

15. Snow S, Madjar DD, Hardy S, et al. Microcystic adnexal carcinoma: report of 13 cases and review of the literature. Dermatol Surg 2001; 27(4): 401–8.

16. Song A, Carter KD, Syed NA, Song J, Nerad JA. Sebaceous cell carcinoma of the ocular adnexa: clinical presentations, histopathology and outcomes. Ophthal Plast Reconstr Surg 2008; 24(3): 194–200.

17. Song A, Carter KD, Syed NA. Song J. Nerad JA. Sebaceous cell carcinoma of the ocular adnexa: clinical presentations, histopathology, and outcomes. Ophthal Plast Reconstr Surg 2008; 24(3): 194–200.

18. Tanenbaum M, Grove AS, McCord CD: Eyelid tumors: diagnosis and management. In McCord CD, Tanenhaum M, Nunery WR, eds., Oculoplastic Surgery, 3rd edn, chap 6. New York, NY: Raven Press, 1995; 6145–74.

19. Von Domarus H, Steven PJ. Metastatic basal cell carcinoma. Report of five cases and review of 170 cases in the literature. J Am Acad Dermatol 1984; 10: 1043–60.

11 Management of malignant eyelid/periocular tumors

INTRODUCTION

Many different treatment modalities have been advocated, by a variety of medical practitioners, for the management of malignant tumors in the periocular region. It is essential that the treatment modality best suited to the needs of the individual patient is selected.

The management of all malignant eyelid tumors depends on:

- Correct histological diagnosis
- Assessment of tumor margins
- Assessment of local and systemic tumor spread

The vast majority of malignant periocular tumors are non-melanoma cutaneous malignancies (basal and squamous cell carcinomas). The major considerations in selecting a treatment for these tumors are:

- The selected treatment modality must be capable of totally eradicating all tumor cells to which it is applied.
- A mechanism must exist to ensure that the treatment is applied to all the existing tumor cells.

Tumors of the eyelids and canthi often exhibit slender strands and shoots of cancer cells which can infiltrate the local tissues beyond the clinically apparent borders of the tumor. For this reason appropriate monitoring to ensure that the treatment modality reaches all of the tumor cells is essential. Numerous studies have demonstrated that clinical judgment of tumor margins is inadequate, significantly underestimating the area of microscopic tumor involvement. The introduction of frozen-section control to document adequacy of tumor excision marked a major advancement in the treatment of malignant eyelid tumors and now constitutes the standard of care. Any treatment modality that does not utilize microscopic monitoring of tumor margins must instead encompass a wider area of adjacent normal tissue in the hope that any microscopic extensions of tumor will fall within this area.

The goals in the surgical management of malignant eyelid tumors are:

- Complete eradication of the tumor
- Minimal sacrifice of normal adjacent tissues

These concepts are of the utmost importance in the surgical management of periocular malignancy because of the complex nature of the periocular tissues and the functional importance of the eyelids in ocular protection, in addition to the grave risks that are posed by tumor recurrence in this area.

Mohs' micrographic surgery represents the gold standard in the management of basal cell and squamous cell carcinomas.

In the periocular region, focal malignancy can be treated with:

- Surgery
- Irradiation
- Cryotherapy

- Photodynamic therapy (PDT)
- Topical chemotherapeutic agents

The choice of therapy depends on:

- The size of the tumor
- The location of the tumor
- The type of tumor
- The age and general health of the patient
- The clinician's relative expertise

The choice of treatment is particularly important in:

- Diffuse tumors
- Tumour extension to bone/the orbit
- Patients with a cancer diathesis, e.g., the basal cell nevus syndrome
- Young patients

A comprehensive examination of the patient is important, with palpation of the regional lymph nodes and a whole body skin examination wherever possible. If orbital invasion is suspected from the clinical examination, e.g., restriction of ocular motility, it is appropriate to request thin-section, high-resolution computed tomography (CT) scans with bone windows. In selected cases, chest and abdominal CT is required with liver function tests to evaluate systemic spread. Such patients should be managed with the assistance of an oncologist. If systemic spread is found, palliation only may be preferable.

The follow-up of patients with periocular malignant tumors is very important and depends on a number of variable factors. A protocol for this should be set up by clinicians involved in the management of these patients.

BASAL CELL CARCINOMA

Unfortunately, basal cell carcinomas have traditionally been regarded as relatively benign, rarely invasive tumors by many different clinicians in a variety of specialties and as such have commonly been casually excised. This has been associated with a high incidence of recurrence, unnecessary morbidity, and occasionally avoidable mortality. A dedicated approach to tumor eradication is clearly essential in the management of patients who have a basal cell carcinoma. The main options for the management of these tumors in the periocular area are:

- Surgery in conjunction with histological monitoring of tumor margins
- Irradiation
- Cryotherapy
- PDT
- Topical chemotherapeutic agents

The surgical management of basal cell carcinoma consists of surgical removal of the tumor, with monitoring of the excised margins, either by formalin-fixed, paraffin-embedded or frozen section control. A close working relationship with a specialist pathologist offers a major advantage in the efficient delivery of such care. In the majority of cases the diagnosis is evident on clinical grounds alone. *Where the diagnosis is unclear, a biopsy should be performed before definitive treatment.* For small well-defined tumors an excisional biopsy with a 2 to 3 mm margin serves not only to establish the histological diagnosis but also as a definitive treatment if the excision margins prove to be clear. Mohs' micrographic surgery is now considered by many to represent the *gold standard* in the management of periocular basal cell carcinomas, particularly for poorly defined or critically sited tumors. Unfortunately, this treatment modality is unavailable in many centers in this and other countries. Where Mohs' surgery is not available, so-called "Slow Mohs'" techniques have evolved using formalin-fixed, paraffin-embedded sections with delayed reconstruction of the periocular defect with good outcomes and low recurrence rates. Standard frozen section control may be required for patients who require surgery under general anesthesia e.g., patients with extensive periocular tumors and dementia. It is important to orientate the specimen using sutures of varying length and a tumor map should be recorded for the pathologist, e.g., "the long silk suture marks the lateral aspect of the excision, the short suture the superior aspect and the intermediate suture the medial aspect."

Although it is reasonable to close small defects immediately, no defect should be formally reconstructed without definitive histopathological evidence of complete tumor clearance. Exenteration is reserved for cases where orbital invasion has occurred and aggressive surgical management is appropriate for the individual patient.

Surgery continues to be the main treatment modality for the management of periocular basal cell carcinomas but it should be recognized that new pharmacological agents, such as immunomodulators, topical chemotherapeutic agents, and PDT, have emerged and have shown some promising results. PDT, usually undertaken by a dermatologist, may have a role to play in small superficial basal cell carcinomas in patients with basal cell nevus syndrome (Gorlin's syndrome).

Radiotherapy and cryotherapy also have their own limited role to play in the management of periocular basal cell carcinomas.

KEY POINT

A tumor defect should not be formally reconstructed, except by simple direct closure if appropriate, until definitive histopathological evidence of complete tumor removal has been obtained.

Irradiation

Historically, irradiation as a treatment modality for periocular cutaneous malignancies was very popular in the United Kingdom, and a number of studies reported better than 90% cure rates for periocular basal cell carcinomas. More recently, however, investigators have noted that basal cell carcinomas treated by irradiation recur at a higher rate and behave more aggressively than tumors treated by surgical excision.

The radiation dose used to treat patients varies, depending on the size of the lesion and the estimate of its depth. The treatments are usually fractionated over several weeks, depending on local protocols. The proponents of radiation therapy point to the lack of discomfort with radiation treatment and to the fact that no hospitalization or anesthesia is required.

Although radiation therapy is no longer to be recommended as the treatment of choice for periocular cutaneous malignancies, there are occasionally patients who, for various reasons, cannot undergo surgical excision and reconstruction and for whom radiation may be useful. However, it is important to continue to look closely for evidence of recurrence well beyond the 5-year postoperative period routinely utilized for surgically managed cutaneous malignancies.

Disadvantages
It is now generally accepted that basal cell carcinomas recurring after radiation therapy are more difficult to diagnose, present at a more advanced stage, cause more extensive destruction, and are much more difficult to eradicate. The greater extent of destruction may be explained by the presence of adjacent radio dermatitis, which may mask underlying tumor recurrence and allow the tumor to grow more extensively before it can be clinically detected (Fig. 11.1). The damaging effect of radiation on periocular tissues poses another drawback to its use.

Note the potential complications associated with the use of irradiation for treatment of periocular malignancy:

- Skin necrosis
- Cicatricial ectropion
- Telangiectasia
- Epiphora
- Loss of eyelashes
- Keratitis
- Cataract
- Dry eye
- Keratinization of the palpebral conjunctiva

Note: The most serious complications following radiotherapy occur after treatment of large tumors of the upper eyelid even when the eye is shielded.

Although most surgeons would oppose the use of radiotherapy as the primary modality in treating periocular skin cancers, it is felt to be specifically contraindicated for lesions in the medial canthus, lesions greater than 1 cm and recurrent tumors.

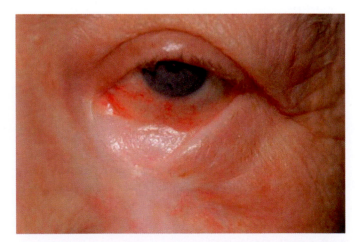

Figure 11.1 Severe lower eyelid scarring with eyelid retraction and conjunctival exposure following radiotherapy treatment for a lower eyelid basal cell carcinoma.

Although a number of studies reported high success rates with radiation for periocular basal cell carcinomas, many of these studies did not include long-term follow-up. Investigators have now determined that it may take longer for a recurrence of a radiation-treated malignancy to become clinically apparent than for a surgically treated tumor. Recent studies with longer follow-up have reported a recurrence rate between 17% and 20%.

The radiation changes induced in surrounding tissue make it more difficult to track recurrent tumors micrographically and render subsequent reconstruction after excision more difficult. It has also been reported that radiation therapy may disturb the protective barrier offered by the periosteum and allow for greater likelihood of bony cancerous involvement with recurrences. A final concern with radiation therapy, which is not shared by other treatment modalities, is that the treatment itself may induce new tumor formation.

Note: Tumors which recur after radiation are often poorly controlled with other modalities

Cryotherapy

Cryotherapy is an effective alternative therapy for small localized basal cell carcinomas, especially those located in the vicinity of the puncta/canaliculi which are relatively resistant to damage by the temperatures required to kill tumor cells. It is useful in debilitated patients who are unfit for surgery. It is a single session treatment (cf. radiotherapy). *A diagnostic biopsy should be performed prior to treatment.* The entire tumor must be frozen to −30°C. Liquid nitrogen is the most effective freezing agent. The globe and adjacent tissue must be adequately protected from the effects of the cryotherapy. A thermocouple should be inserted under the estimated deepest part of the tumor with a second thermocouple placed 5 to 10 mm peripheral to the tumor and a cycle of freeze-thaw, freeze-thaw is utilized, spraying the tumor with liquid nitrogen.

Disadvantages
There is an approximate 10% recurrence rate due to the inadvertent inclusion of morpheaform/diffuse tumors. There is a profound tissue reaction to cryotherapy with exudation and a prolonged period of healing.

Note the potential complications associated with the use of cryotherapy for treatment of periocular malignancy:

- Eyelid notching
- Ectropion
- Hypertrophic scarring
- Pseudoepitheliomatous hyperplasia
- Symblephara

Pseudoepitheliomatous hyperplasia is difficult to manage as it can mimic recurrent tumor.

Mohs' Micrographic Surgery

Mohs' micrographic surgery is a refinement of frozen-section control of tumor margins that, by mapping tumor planes, allows a three-dimensional assessment of tumor margins rather than the two-dimensional analysis provided by routine frozen section. In this technique, the surgical removal of the tumor is performed by a dermatological surgeon with specialized training in tumor excision and mapping of margins.

The unique feature of Mohs' micrographic surgery is that it removes the skin cancer in a sequence of horizontal layers monitored by microscopic examination of horizontal sections through the undersurface of each layer. Careful mapping of residual cancer in each layer is possible, and subsequent horizontal layers are then excised in cancer-bearing areas until cancer-free histological layers are obtained at the base and on all sides of the skin cancer.

Advantages
Mohs' micrographic excision has been shown to give the highest cure rate for most cutaneous malignancies occurring on various body surfaces. In addition to its high cure rate, the technique offers several other advantages. The Mohs' technique obviates the need to remove generous margins of clinically normal adjacent tissue by allowing precise layer-by-layer mapping of tumor cells. This is extremely important in the periocular regions because of the specialized nature of the periocular tissues and the challenges in creating ready substitutes that will obtain a satisfactory functional and cosmetic result.

Because routine frozen-section monitoring of periocular skin cancers in the operating theatre involves a significant loss of time while waiting for turn around of results from the pathologist, Mohs' micrographic excision performed in the dermatologist's minor operating theatre allows for more efficient use of operating theatre time.

Although small wounds may be allowed to granulate, excision in the majority of periocular cases is followed by immediate or next day reconstruction, by a separate oculoplastic surgeon who has expertise in reconstructing periocular defects. Reconstruction can be scheduled immediately following Mohs' micrographic excision or on a subsequent day with better prediction of the operating theatre time required. Taking responsibility for tumor excision out of the hands of the reconstructing surgeon also assures that concern over the difficulties of reconstruction do not limit aggressive tissue removal where it is required.

Mohs' micrographic excision has been shown to provide the most effective treatment for non-melanoma cutaneous malignancies, i.e., basal cell and squamous cell carcinomas. It is not suitable for the management of sebaceous gland carcinomas. However, it is particularly recommended for the following types of periocular cutaneous malignancy:

- Skin tumors arising in the medial canthal region, where, because of natural tissue planes, the risk of deeper invasion is greater and where the borders of involved tissue are more difficult to define
- Recurrent skin tumors
- Large primary skin tumors of long duration
- Morpheaform basal cell carcinomas
- Any tumors whose clinical borders are not obviously demarcated
- Tumors in young patients

Disadvantages
Although Mohs' micrographic surgery allows for the most precise histological monitoring, some cancer cells may rarely be left behind and a 2 to 3% long-term recurrence rate has

been reported for primary periocular skin cancers. Careful follow-up, searching for early signs of recurrence, remains important.

For periocular tumors the surgical excision and surgical reconstruction are usually divided between two surgeons and often at two different physical locations. In addition, Mohs' micrographic surgeons are not available in many centers in this and other countries.

Photodynamic Therapy
PDT can be considered for the management of small periocular basal cell carcinomas in patients with basal cell nevus syndrome (Gorlin's syndrome). Its role in the management of periocular basal cell carcinomas is otherwise very limited. This treatment is usually undertaken by a dermatologist.

Topical Chemotherapeutic Agents
Agents such as topical Imiquimod 5% cream can be considered in the treatment of eyelid basal cell carcinoma for selected patients. Imiquimod *has to be applied* once daily, 5 days per week, for 6 weeks and can be associated with an aggressive tissue reaction. Such treatment is usually undertaken by a dermatologist.

SQUAMOUS CELL CARCINOMA
The following treatment modalities are used for the management of eyelid/periocular squamous cell carcinoma:

- Surgery in conjunction with histological monitoring of tumor margins
- Radiation

The surgical management of squamous cell carcinoma consists of surgical removal of the tumor with monitoring of the excised margins, either by formalin-fixed, paraffin-embedded, or frozen-section control. It is appropriate to obtain a biopsy of a suspicious tumor before undertaking a definitive surgical procedure. *Great care should be taken to obtain a representative section of the tumor.* Shave biopsies do not allow determination of dermal invasion by the epithelial tumor. Benign tumors such as actinic keratosis, inverted follicular keratosis, and pseudoepitheliomatous hyperplasia can be differentiated only by evaluation of dermal extension. As such, the pathologist is frequently forced to give a diagnosis of squamous cell carcinoma because inadequate tissue has been submitted for review. It is not unusual for a tumor that has been reported as squamous cell carcinoma to have resolved by the time definitive surgical resection can be scheduled for this reason.

Biopsy Technique
If the lesion is small, an excisional biopsy with direct closure of the defect should be performed. If the lesion is larger, an incisional biopsy should be performed. The specimen should be handled with care to avoid any crush artifact. If the lesion involves the eyelid margin, the biopsy should be full thickness.

Wherever possible, the base of the lesion and adjacent normal tissue should be included. "Laissez-faire" is useful for healing of many biopsy sites.

As in the management of basal cell carcinoma, Mohs' surgery is the *gold standard*. If this is not available, however, the excised specimen should be removed with a 3 to 4 mm margin, oriented using sutures of varying length and a tumor map recorded for the pathologist, e.g., "the long silk suture marks the lateral aspect of the excision, the short suture the superior aspect and the intermediate suture the medial aspect". The result of formalin-fixed, paraffin-embedded sections should be awaited with delayed reconstruction of the periocular defect. Exenteration is reserved for cases where orbital invasion has occurred and aggressive surgical management is appropriate for the individual patient.

SEBACEOUS GLAND CARCINOMA
The preferred management of sebaceous gland carcinoma consists of complete surgical extirpation of the tumor. With heightened appreciation of the clinical presentation of the tumor, early surgical excision significantly enhances the long-term prognosis. Numerous procedures for incision and drainage of suspected recurrent chalazia delay the appropriate diagnosis of sebaceous gland carcinoma.

Localized sebaceous gland carcinoma is managed by an incisional biopsy and formalin-fixed, paraffin-embedded histological examination to establish the diagnosis. A full-thickness block resection of the eyelid is required to establish the diagnosis in patients with diffuse thickening of the eyelid. An incisional biopsy is appropriate in the patient presenting with a solid mass. The tumor can arise from multifocal non-contiguous tumor origins. It is for this reason that it is not appropriate to subject this tumor to Mohs' micrographic surgery nor is intraoperative frozen-section control of the surgical margins appropriate. The pathologist should be warned about the suspected diagnosis.

Following confirmation of the diagnosis a wide resection of the tumor is performed and the specimen sent for formalin-fixed, paraffin-embedded histopathological analysis. *Because of the possible multicentric origin of sebaceous gland carcinoma, it is important to perform random conjunctival sac biopsies which should be carefully mapped and recorded.* If the pathologist is able to confirm that the margins are clear and that the random biopsies do not contain tumor, the defect can be reconstructed.

Close postoperative observation is always crucial in the management of these patients to exclude recurrent disease. In patients with diffuse eyelid/conjunctival involvement or orbital extension, orbital exenteration is recommended.

Radiation therapy has a limited role in the management of sebaceous gland carcinoma. The tumor is radiosensitive and does respond to radiation therapy, but recurrences are inevitable. In addition, patients develop significant ocular complications such as keratitis, radiation retinopathy, and severe pain. Radiation therapy is therefore considered a palliative procedure to reduce tumor size. It should not be viewed as a curative modality.

MELANOMA
Surgery
The extent of tumor-free margins for eyelid melanoma does not correlate with survival, but the use of very narrow excisions

of 5 mm or less is associated with a greater frequency of local recurrence. It is therefore appropriate to take wide tissue margins of 10 mm from the macroscopic edge of the tumor wherever possible with formalin-fixed, paraffin-embedded sections and delayed reconstruction of the tumor excision defect. Margin control by mapped serial excision or a modified Mohs' micrographic surgery using paraffin sections is a useful technique to ensure complete excision and minimization of local recurrence.

The management of a patient presenting with an eyelid melanoma should be discussed at a skin cancer multidisciplinary team meeting. If the tumor has extended to Clark level IV or V or its Breslow thickness exceeds 1.5 mm, a referral for lymph node dissection should be considered. Clark's level > or = IV or Breslow thickness > or = 1.5 mm are poor prognostic indicators for melanomas of the eyelid skin. Clinicians should have a high level of suspicion for occult regional lymph node metastasis when treating patients with these tumors. Careful postoperative surveillance for local and regional recurrence is indicated.

Radiation

Radiotherapy is rarely used in the primary management of eyelid melanoma, except in patients who are unfit for surgery. Its use is associated with significant ocular morbidity.

Topical Chemotherapeutic Agents

Imiquimod 5% cream appears to be effective in the treatment of lentigo maligna melanoma and can be considered for selected patients. Such treatment is usually undertaken by a specialist dermatologist.

RARER MALIGNANT EYELID TUMORS

The management of a patient presenting with rarer malignant eyelid tumors should be discussed at a skin cancer multidisciplinary team meeting.

Merkel Cell Tumor

Merkel cell tumor is a rare but highly malignant tumor which tends to metastasize early and which has a high local recurrence rate. It should be managed by urgent aggressive surgical resection with wide margins. Postoperative adjuvant radiotherapy should also be considered. Prophylactic regional node dissection may also be required.

Metastatic Eyelid Tumor

The management of metastatic eyelid tumors is the realm of the oncologist and usually involves chemotherapy and/or radiation therapy. Surgical excision can be considered if the tumor is localized and unresponsive to other modalities.

Lymphoma

The management of eyelid lymphoma is also the realm of the oncologist following the establishment of the diagnosis by incisional biopsy.

Kaposi's Sarcoma

Local control is usually achieved with radiotherapy to which the tumor responds very well.

Angiosarcoma

The preferred treatment for angiosarcoma of the eyelid is wide surgical resection with adjuvant radiotherapy.

Microcystic Adnexal Carcinoma

Several treatment modalities have been used for the management of this tumor, including standard excision with wide margins, Mohs' micrographic surgery, irradiation, and chemotherapy. In general, Mohs' micrographic surgery offers the highest likelihood of clear margins and cure with the fewest procedures.

Primary Mucinous Carcinoma

Several treatment modalities have also been used for the management of this tumor, including standard excision with wide margins, Mohs' micrographic surgery, irradiation, and chemotherapy. In general, Mohs' micrographic surgery offers the highest likelihood of clear margins and cure with the fewest procedures.

FURTHER READING

1. Abide JM, Nahai F, Bennett RG. The meaning of surgical margins. Plast Reconstr Surg 1984; 73: 492–6.
2. American Academy of Ophthalmology. Basic and Clinical Science Course: Orbit, eEyelids, and Lacrimal System, section 7. San Francisco, CA: The American Academy of Ophthalmology, 2006/7: 201–5.
3. Anderson RL, Ceilley RI. Multispeciality approach to excision and reconstruction of eyelid tumors. Ophthalmology 1978; 85: 1150–63.
4. Carter KD, Nerad JA, Whitaker DC. Clinical factors influencing periocular surgical defects after Mohs' micrographic surgery. Ophthal Plast Reconstr Surg 1999; 15: 83–91.
5. Chan FM, O'Donnell BA, Whitehead K, Ryman W, Sullivan TJ. Treatment and outcomes of malignant melanoma of the eyelid: a review of 29 cases in Australia. Ophthalmology 2007; 114(1): 187–92,.
6. Choontanom R, Thanos S, Busse H, Stupp T. Treatment of basal cell carcinoma of the eyelids with 5% topical imiquimod: a 3 year follow-up study. Graefe's Arch Clin Exp Ophthalmol 2007; 245:1217–20.
7. Committee on Guidelines of Care. Task force on basal cell carcinoma. Guidelines of care for basal cell carcinoma. J Am Acad Dermatol 1992; 26(1): 117–20.
8. De Potter P, Shields CL, Shields JA. Sebaceous gland carcinoma of the eyelids. Int Ophthalmol Clin 1993; 33: 5–9.
9. Gupta AK, Davey V, McPhail H. Evaluation of the effectiveness of imiquimod and 5-fluorouracil for the treatment of acitinic keratosis: critical review and meta-analysis of efficacy studies. J Cutaneous Med Surg 2005; 9(5): 209–14.
10. Inkster C, Ashworth J, Murdoch JR, et al. Oculoplastic reconstruction following Mohs' surgery. Eye 1998; 12: 214–18.
11. Lee S, Selva D, Huilgol SC, Goldberg RA, Leibovitch I. Pharmacological treatments for basal cell carcinoma. Drugs 2007; 67(6): 915–34.
12. Leshin B, Yeatts P, Anscher M, Montano G, Dutton JJ. Management of periocular basal cell carcinoma: Mohs' micrographic surgery versus radiotherapy. Surv Ophthalmol 1993; 38: 193–212.
13. Mahoney MH, Joseph MG, Temple C. Topical imiquimod therapy for lentigo maligna. Ann Plast Surg 2008; 61: 419–24.
14. Malhotra R, Chen C, Huilgol SC, Hill DC, Selva D. Mapped serial excision for periocular lentigo maligna melanoma. Ophthalmology 2003; 110: 2011–18.
15. Mohs FE. Micrographic surgery for the microscopically controlled excision of eyelid cancers. Arch Ophthalmol 1986; 104: 901–9.
16. Morris DS, Elzaridi E, Clarke L, Dickinson AJ, Lawrence C M. Periocular basal cell carcinoma: 5-year outcome following slow Mohs surgery with formalin-fixed paraffin-embedded sections and delayed closure. Br J Ophthalmol 2009; 93(4): 474–6.
17. Neubert T, Lehmann P. Bowen's disease—a review of newer treatment options. Therap Clin Risk Manage 2008; 4(5): 1085–95.

18. Rivlin D, Moy RL. Mohs' surgery for periorbital malignancies. In: Bosniak S, ed. Principles and Practice of Ophthalmic Plastic and Reconstructive Surgery, vol 2. Philadelphia, PA: W.B. Saunders, 1996: 352–5.

19. Sacks EH, Lisman RD. Diagnosis and management of sebaceous gland carcinoma. In: Bosniak S, ed. Principles and Practice of Ophthalmic Plastic and Reconstructive Surgery. Philadelphia, PA: W.B. Saunders, 1996: 190–5.

20. Shields JA, Demirci H, Marr BP, Eagle RC, Shields CL. Sebaceous carcinoma of the eyelids. Ophthalmology 2004: 111: 2151–7.

21. Shriner DL, McCoy DK, Goldberg DJ, Wagner RF Jr. Mohs' micrographic surgery. J Am Acad Dermatol 1998; 39: 79–97.

22. Shumack S, Robinson J, Kossard S, et al. Effifacy of topical 5% imiquimod cream for the treatment of nodular basal cell carcinoma. Arch Dermatol 2002; 138: 1165–71.

23. Tanenbaum M, Grove AS, McCord CD. Eyelid tumors: diagnosis and management. In: McCord CD, Tanenhaum M, Nunery WR, eds. Oculoplastic Surgery, 3rd edn. New York, NY: Raven Press, 1995: 145–74.

24. Telfer NR, Colver GB, Bowers PW. Guidelines for the management of basal cell carcinoma. British Association of Dermatologists. Br J Dermatol 1999; 141:415–23.

25. Telfer NR, Colver GB, Morton CA. Guidelines for the management of basal cell carcinoma. Br J Dermatol 2008; 159: 35–48.

12 Eyelid and periocular reconstruction

INTRODUCTION

The goals in eyelid and periocular reconstruction following eyelid tumor excision are preservation of normal eyelid function for the protection of the eye and restoration of good cosmesis. Of these goals, preservation of normal function is of the utmost importance and takes priority over the cosmetic result. Failure to maintain normal eyelid function, particularly following upper eyelid reconstruction, will have dire consequences for the comfort and visual performance of the patient. In general, it is technically easier to reconstruct eyelid defects following tumor excision surgery than following trauma.

GENERAL PRINCIPLES

A number of surgical procedures can be utilized to reconstruct eyelid defects. In general, where less than 25% of the eyelid has been sacrificed, direct closure of the eyelid is possible. Where the eyelid tissues are very lax, direct closure may be possible for much larger defects occupying 50% or more of the eyelid. Where direct closure without undue tension on the wound is difficult, a simple lateral canthotomy and cantholysis of the appropriate limb of the lateral canthal tendon can facilitate a simple closure.

To reconstruct eyelid defects involving greater degrees of tissue loss, a number of different surgical procedures have been devised. The choice depends on:

- The extent of the eyelid defect
- The state of the remaining periocular tissues
- The visual status of the fellow eye
- The age and general health of the patient
- The surgeon's own expertise

In deciding which procedure is most suited to the individual patient's needs, one should aim to re-establish the following:

- A smooth mucosal surface to line the eyelid and protect the cornea
- An outer layer of skin and muscle
- Structural support between the two lamellae of skin and mucosa originally provided by the tarsal plate
- A smooth, nonabrasive eyelid margin free from keratin and trichiasis
- In the upper eyelid, normal vertical eyelid movement without significant ptosis or lagophthalmos
- Normal horizontal tension with normal medial and lateral canthal tendon positions
- Normal apposition of the eyelid and lacrimal punctum to the globe
- A normal contour to the eyelid

Large eyelid defects generally require composite reconstruction in layers with a variety of tissues from either adjacent sources or from distant sites being used to replace both the anterior and posterior lamellae. It is essential that only one lamella should be reconstructed as a free graft. The other lamella should be reconstructed as a vascularized flap to provide an adequate blood supply to prevent necrosis of the graft.

Many different techniques have been described for use in periocular reconstruction. The techniques, which are described in this chapter, are those most commonly used by the author. It is wise to master the simpler techniques before attempting more complex reconstructions. A combination of techniques may have to be used for more extensive defects.

LOWER EYELID RECONSTRUCTION

Defects of the lower eyelid can be divided into those that involve the eyelid margin and those that do not.

Eyelid Defects Involving the Eyelid Margin

Small Defects

An eyelid defect of 25% or less may be closed directly in most patients. In patients with marked eyelid laxity, even a defect occupying up to 50% or more of the eyelid may be closed directly. The two edges of the defect should be grasped with toothed forceps and pulled together to judge the facility of closure. If there is no excess tension on the lid, the edges may be approximated directly.

Direct Closure

Surgical Procedure

1. A single-armed 5/0 Vicryl suture on a 1/2-circle needle loaded on a Castroviejo needle holder is passed through the most superior aspect of the tarsus just below the eyelid margin, ensuring that the needle and suture are anterior to the conjunctiva to avoid contact with the cornea (Fig. 12.1A).
2. This suture is tied with a single throw and the eyelid margin approximation checked. If this is unsatisfactory, the suture is replaced and the process repeated. Proper placement of this suture will avoid the complications of eyelid notching and trichiasis, and wound dehiscence. Once the margin approximation is good, the suture is untied and the ends fixated to the head drape with a curved artery clip. This elongates the wound, enabling further single-armed 5/0 Vicryl sutures to be placed in the tarsus inferiorly (Fig. 12.1B).
3. Additional 5/0 sutures are then passed through the orbicularis muscle and tied (Fig. 12.2A).
4. A single armed 6/0 black silk suture on a reverse cutting needle loaded on a Castroviejo needle holder is passed through the eyelid margin along the line of the meibomian glands 2 mm from the wound edge emerging 1 mm from the surface. The needle is remounted and passed similarly through the opposing wound emerging 2 mm from the wound edge.

The suture is cut leaving the ends long. The same suture is passed in a similar fashion along the lash line and cut leaving the ends long (Fig. 12.2B).

5. Next, the 6/0 silk sutures are tied with sufficient tension to cause eversion of the edges of the eyelid margin wound. A small amount of pucker is desirable initially, to avoid late lid notching as the lid heals and the wound contracts. The sutures are left long and incorporated into the skin closure sutures to prevent contact with the cornea (Fig. 12.3).

6. The skin is closed with simple interrupted 6/0 black silk sutures.

7. Topical antibiotic ointment is instilled into the eye and the eye closed.

8. A Jelonet dressing is placed over the eye, followed by two eye pads, and a firm compressive bandage is applied to prevent excessive swelling.

Postoperative Care
The dressing is removed after 48 hours and topical antibiotic ointment applied three times per day to the eyelid wound for 2 weeks. The 6/0 sutures are removed in clinic after 2 weeks.

Moderate Defects
Canthotomy and Cantholysis
Where an eyelid defect cannot be closed directly without undue tension on the wound, a lateral canthotomy and inferior cantholysis can be performed.

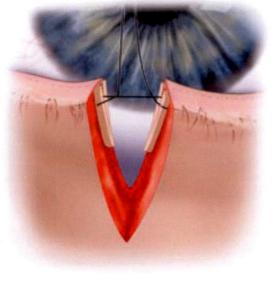
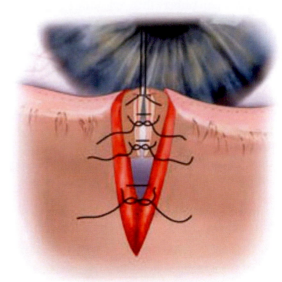

(A)   (B)

Figure 12.1 (**A**) Reapproximation of the eyelid margin is achieved with a single armed 5/0 Vicryl suture passed symmetrically through the superior aspect of the tarsus on each side of the defect. (**B**) Once the eyelid margin is satisfactorily aligned, the initial suture is loosened and used to put the eyelid on gentle traction. The rest of the tarsus is reapproximated with interrupted 5/0 Vicryl sutures.

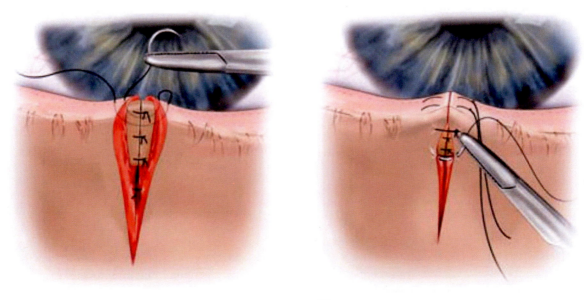

(A)   (B)

Figure 12.2 (**A**) Once the tarsal sutures have been placed, 6/0 silk sutures are placed along the lash line and along the line of the meibomian glands in a vertical mattress fashion. (**B**) The skin is closed with interrupted 6/0 silk sutures.

Surgical Procedure

1. Using a no. 15 Bard Parker blade, a 4 to 5 mm horizontal skin incision is made at the lateral canthus. This is deepened to the periosteum of the lateral orbital margin using curved Westcott scissors.
2. Next, the inferior cantholysis is performed by cutting the tissue between the conjunctiva and the skin using blunt tipped curved Westcott scissors close to the periosteum of the lateral orbital margin with the lateral lid margin drawn up and medially (Fig. 12.4). The eyelid will "give" as the inferior crus of the lateral canthal tendon and the orbital septum are severed.
3. The wound is closed with simple interrupted 6/0 black silk sutures.

Postoperative Care

This is as described above.

Semicircular Rotation Flap

A semicircular rotation flap (Tenzel flap) is useful for the reconstruction of defects up to 70% of the lower eyelid where some tarsus remains on either side of the defect, particularly where the patient's fellow eye has poor vision. Under these circumstances, it is preferable to avoid a procedure, which necessitates closure of the eye for a period of some weeks (e.g., a Hughes tarsoconjunctival flap procedure).

Surgical Procedure

1. A semicircular incision is marked out with gentian violet starting at the lateral canthus, curving superiorly to a level just below the brow and temporally for approximately 2 cm.
2. The skin incision is made using a no. 15 Bard Parker blade.
3. The flap is then widely undermined using blunt-tipped Westcott scissors to the depth of the superficial temporalis fascia, taking care not to damage the temporal branch of the facial nerve that crosses the midportion of the zygomatic arch (Figs. 2.30 and 2.31).
4. A lateral canthotomy and inferior cantholysis are then performed and the eyelid defect is closed as described above.
5. The lateral canthus is suspended with a deep 5/0 Vicryl suture passed through the periosteum of the lateral orbital margin to prevent retraction of the flap (Fig. 12.5).
6. Any residual "dog ear" is removed and the lateral skin wound closed with simple interrupted 6/0 black silk sutures.
7. The conjunctiva of the inferolateral fornix is gently mobilized and sutured to the edge of the flap with interrupted 8/0 Vicryl sutures.

Postoperative Care

This is as described above.

Large Defects

Upper Lid Tarsoconjunctival Pedicle Flap
First stage
The upper lid tarsoconjunctival pedicle flap (Hughes flap) is an excellent technique for the reconstruction of relatively shallow lower eyelid defects involving up to 100% of the eyelid (Fig. 12.6). With defects extending horizontally beyond the eyelids, it can be combined with local periosteal flaps to recreate medial and/or lateral canthal tendons.

> **KEY POINT**
>
> Great care should be taken in the planning and construction of the tarsoconjunctival pedicle flap in order not to compromise the function of the upper eyelid. It is essential that the patient can cope with occlusion of the eye for a period of 3 to 10 weeks.

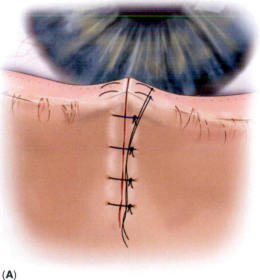

(A)

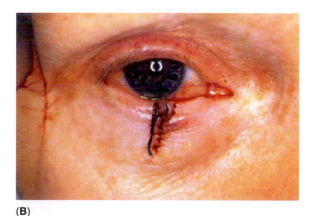

(B)

Figure 12.3 Direct closure of a lower eyelid defect completed with eversion of the eyelid margin wound. The silk sutures have been left along and have been incorporated into the skin closure sutures. The conjunctiva is left to heal spontaneously without suture closure. The skin sutures may be removed in 5 to 7 days but the eyelid margin sutures should be left in place for 14 days.

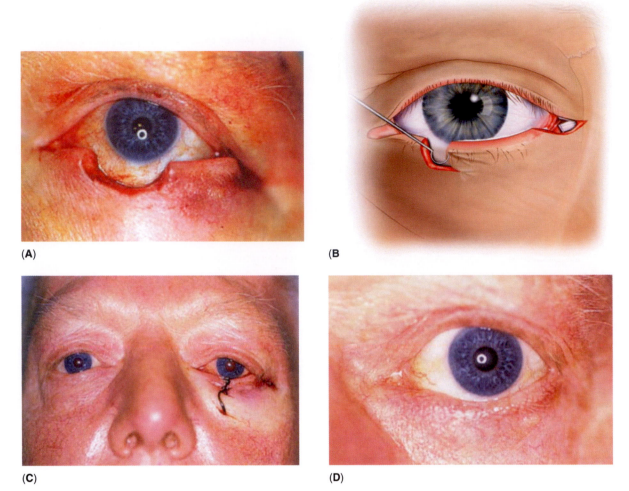

Figure 12.4 (**A**) Lower eyelid defect occupying greater than 30% of the eyelid. (**B**) Reapproximation of the eyelid margins achieved by lateral canthotomy and inferior cantholysis. (**C**) The immediate postoperative appearance. (**D**) The appearance of the eyelid 2 months postoperatively showing some rounding of the lateral canthus and horizontal shortening of the palpebral fissure.

Surgical Procedure

1. The size of the flap to be constructed is ascertained by pulling the edges of the eyelid wound toward each other with a moderate degree of tension using two pairs of Paufique forceps and measuring the residual defect.
2. A 4/0 silk traction suture is passed through the gray line of the upper eyelid, which is everted over a Desmarres retractor.
3. The tarsal conjunctiva is dried with a swab and a series of points, 3.5 mm above the lid margin, are marked with gentian violet. These points are then joined to mark an incision line.
4. A superficial horizontal incision is made centrally along the tarsus 3.5 mm above the lid margin using a no. 15 Bard Parker blade. It is important to leave a tarsal height of 3.5 mm below the incision in order to maintain the structural integrity of the eyelid to prevent an upper eyelid entropion and to prevent any compromise of the blood supply of the eyelid margin.
5. The incision is deepened through the full thickness of the tarsus centrally using the no. 15 blade and the horizontal incision is completed with blunt-tipped Westcott scissors. Vertical relieving cuts are then made at both ends of the tarsal incision.
6. The tarsus and conjunctiva are dissected free from Müller's muscle and the levator aponeurosis up to the superior fornix. The tarsoconjunctival flap is mobilized into the lower lid defect (Fig. 12.7).
7. The tarsus is sutured, edge to edge, to the lower lid tarsus with interrupted 5/0 Vicryl sutures taking great care to ensure that the sutures are passed though the tarsus in a partial thickness fashion. The lower lid conjunctival edge is sutured to the inferior border of the mobilized tarsus with a continuous 7/0 Vicryl suture.
8. Sufficient skin to cover the anterior surface of the flap can often be obtained by advancing a myocutaneous flap from the cheek (Fig. 12.8). This flap can be elevated by bluntly dissecting a skin and muscle flap inferiorly toward the orbital rim.
9. The lid and cheek skin are incised vertically at the medial and lateral borders of the flap using straight iris scissors.

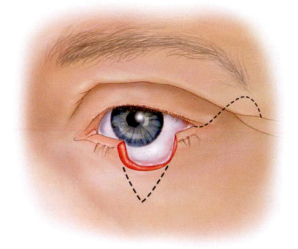

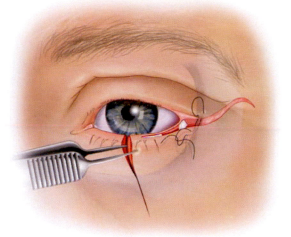

(A)   (B)

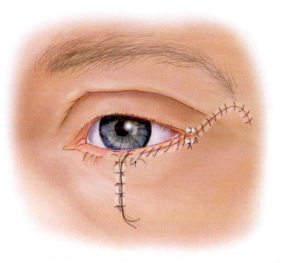

(C)

Figure 12.5 (**A**) A large defect of the lower eyelid. (**B**) A lateral canthotomy and inferior cantholysis with dissection of a semicircular flap. The flap is suspended from the periosteum of the lateral orbital margin with a suture. (**C**) The final appearance following wound closure.

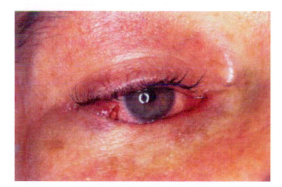

Figure 12.6 A lower eyelid defect suitable for reconstruction using a Hughes procedure.

10. Relaxing triangles (Burow's triangles) may be excised on the inferior medial and lateral edges of the defect to avoid "dog ears" (Fig. 12.8).
11. The skin–muscle is then advanced after sufficient undermining so that it will lie in place without tension.

12. This flap is then sewn into place with its upper border at the appropriate level to produce the new lower lid margin. Two interrupted 5/0 Vicryl sutures are passed through the flap and anchored to the tarsus using a partial thickness pass of the needle (Fig. 12.9).
13. The skin edge is sewn to the superior aspect of the tarsus using interrupted 7/0 Vicryl sutures.
14. Topical antibiotic ointment is instilled into the eye and the eye closed.
15. A Jelonet dressing is placed over the eye, followed by two eye pads and a firm compressive bandage to prevent excessive swelling. If a full-thickness skin graft has been utilized, an additional piece of Jelonet is folded to fit over the skin graft and the same occlusive dressing is applied.

In the patient with relatively tight, non-elastic skin, such an advancement may eventually lead to eyelid retraction or an ectropion when the flap is separated. In such cases, it is wiser

Desmarres retractor
visible through the
levator aponeurosis

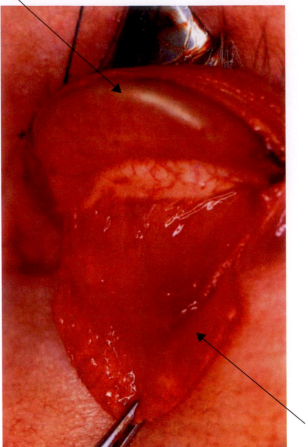

Tarsoconjunctival
flap

Figure 12.7 A tarsoconjunctival flap.

to use a free full-thickness skin graft from the opposite upper lid, preauricular area, retroauricular area, or from the upper inner arm. The graft should not usually be taken from the upper lid of the same eye as the Hughes flap, as the resultant vertical shortening of both the anterior and the posterior lamellae may produce vertical contracture of the donor lid. The skin graft should be thinned meticulously and sutured into place with interrupted 7/0 Vicryl sutures. The graft should fit the defect perfectly and should be sutured under a slight degree of tension (Fig. 12.10).

If possible, a "bucket handle" flap of orbicularis muscle can be advanced after dissecting it free from the overlying skin below the defect. This is then sutured to the superior border of the tarsus with interrupted 7/0 Vicryl sutures. This flap will improve the vascularity of the recipient bed for the skin graft and will help to enhance the resultant cosmetic appearance (Fig. 12.10).

Postoperative Care

The dressing is removed after 48 hours. If a full-thickness skin graft has been utilized, the dressing is not removed for 5 days. The Vicryl sutures are all removed after 2 weeks. The patient is instructed to keep the reconstructed eyelid clean and free of desquamated skin and debris by lifting the upper

lid and by gently cleaning the area with cotton tipped applicators moistened with cool boiled water three times a day. Topical antibiotic is applied to the wounds three times a day for 2 weeks.

If a full-thickness skin graft has been utilized, the patient is instructed to massage the skin graft in an upward and horizontal direction for a few minutes three to four times per day using Lacrilube ointment. A silicone preparation, e.g., Kelocote or Dermatix, can also be applied after a few days to help to prevent undue contracture. The massage is commenced 2 weeks postoperatively. This should be continued for 4 to 6 weeks. If the skin graft thickens, it should be injected with a total of 0.2 to 0.4 ml of Kenalog solution at several different points and the massage continued.

Second Stage

The flap can be opened approximately 3 to 10 weeks (or longer if necessary) after surgery. If a skin graft has been used it is preferable to ensure that the graft is supple and unlikely to contract before the flap is opened to prevent retraction of reconstructed lower eyelid. If the procedure is undertaken under local anesthesia, it is preferable to utilize intravenous sedation, as the administration of local anesthesia can be particularly uncomfortable for such patients.

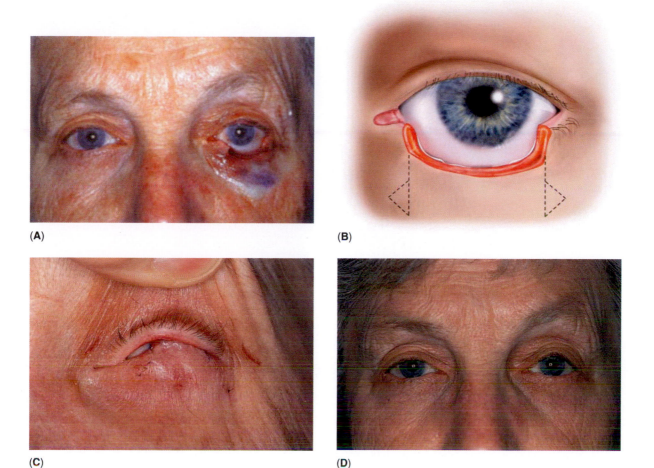

(A)

(B)

(C)

(D)

Figure 12.8 (**A**) A central shallow lower eyelid defect occupying greater than 50% of the eyelid. (**B**) A diagram showing position of Burow's triangles. (**C**) The upper eyelid is being raised showing the typical appearance of a skin-muscle advancement flap. (**D**) The appearance of the reconstructed eyelid 1 month after the second stage division of the flap. The upper eyelid shows some mild retraction.

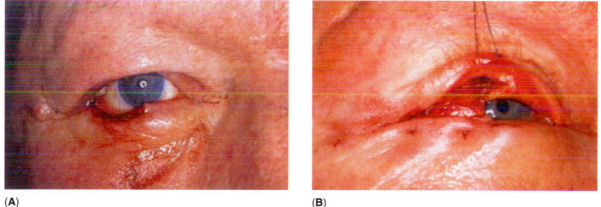

(A)

(B)

Figure 12.9 (**A**) A lateral lower eyelid defect. (**B**) A lateral tarsoconjunctival flap with a skin-muscle advancement flap. The flap is held in the advanced position with two 5/0 Vicryl sutures that are anchored to the tarsus.

Surgical Procedure

1. Two to three milliliters of 0.5% Bupivacaine with 1:200,000 units of adrenaline mixed 50:50 with 2% lidocaine with 1:80,000 units of adrenaline are injected subcutaneously into the upper and lower eyelids. If a skin graft was previously used it is preferable to commence with an infraorbital nerve block.

2. Next, one blade of a pair of blunt-tipped straight Westcott scissors is inserted just above the desired level of the new lid border and the flap is cut open. (It is unnecessary to angle the scissors to leave the conjunctival edge somewhat higher than the anterior skin edge. Traditionally, this provided some conjunctiva posteriorly to be draped forward to create a new mucocutaneous lid margin, but this leaves a reddened lid margin, which is cosmetically poor. It is preferable to allow the lid margin simply to granulate after applying bipolar cautery, as the resultant appearance is far better.)

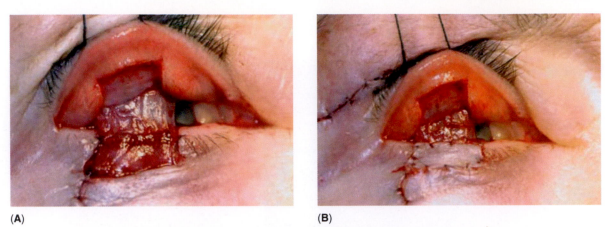

Figure 12.10 (**A**) An upper lid tarsoconjunctival flap with a lower lid orbicularis muscle advancement flap. (**B**) A full-thickness skin graft has been taken from the outer aspect of the upper eyelid just above the skin crease in this patient, as there was plenty of redundant skin. This has been sutured over the orbicularis muscle advancement flap.

3. The upper lid is then everted and the residual flap is excised flush with its attachment to the upper lid tarsus using blunt-tipped Westcott scissors. (If Müller's muscle has been left undisturbed in the original dissection of the flap, eyelid retraction is minimal and no formal attempt is needed to recess the upper lid retractors.)

Postoperative Care
The patient is instructed to keep the eyelid margin meticulously clean and to apply topical antibiotic ointment three times a day for 2 weeks. Topical lubricants should also be prescribed for a few weeks. The Hughes procedure can provide excellent cosmetic and functional results for lower lid reconstruction (Fig. 12.8).

Although the Hughes procedure is traditionally used for the reconstruction of shallow marginal defects of the lower eyelid, it can be used in conjunction with local periosteal flaps for a simplified reconstruction of more extensive defects of the lower lid (Figs. 12.11–12.14). This avoids more invasive procedures and can still be performed under local anesthesia. The term "maximal Hughes procedure" has been coined for this reconstructive technique.

Complications
- Lower eyelid retraction
- Lower eyelid ectropion
- A reddened eyelid margin
- Upper eyelid retraction

These complications following the use of a Hughes procedure can be avoided if the basic principles outlined above are closely adhered to (Fig. 12.15). The lower eyelid will retract if a skin–muscle advancement flap has been used where there is insufficient residual anterior lamella, if the flap has been divided too soon or if the patient has not applied sufficient postoperative massage.

An unsightly eyelid margin is avoided by performing a simple division of the flap without formal overlapping or suturing of the conjunctiva.

Some upper eyelid retraction is inevitable but can be kept to a minimal degree by excluding Müller's muscle from the tarsoconjunctival flap. If an unsatisfactory degree of upper lid retraction does occur, it can be treated using a posterior approach upper lid retractor recession (see chap. 8).

Periosteal Flaps
For the repair of medial or lateral lid defects in which the tarsus and the lateral and/or medial canthal tendons have been completely excised, periosteal flaps provide excellent support for the reconstruction.

Lateral Periosteal Flap
Surgical Procedure
1. A short lateral periosteal flap is created by making two horizontal periosteal incisions over the lateral orbital margin 4 to 5 mm apart with a no. 15 Bard Parker blade. The uppermost incision is made at the level of the insertion of the lateral aspect of the upper eyelid.
2. A vertical relieving incision joining the two horizontal incisions is made over the most lateral aspect of the lateral orbital margin.
3. The flap is then elevated toward the orbit using the sharp-tipped end of a Freer periosteal elevator. The flap is anchored at the junction of the periosteum with the periorbita.
4. The flap is sutured to the lateral margin of the tarsus of the upper lid tarsoconjunctival flap with interrupted 5/0 Vicryl sutures.
5. A longer lateral periosteal flap can be obtained by raising the flap vertically from the lateral orbital margin extending onto the malar eminence. The anchor point, however, remains the same. (Fig. 12.16).
6. Topical antibiotic ointment is instilled into the eye and the eye closed.
7. A Jelonet dressing is placed over the eye, followed by two eye pads and a firm compressive bandage is applied to prevent excessive swelling.

Postoperative Care
This is as described above.

Medial Periosteal Flap
Surgical Procedure
1. A short medial periosteal flap is created by making two horizontal periosteal incisions over the medial orbital margin 4 to 5 mm apart with a no. 15 Bard

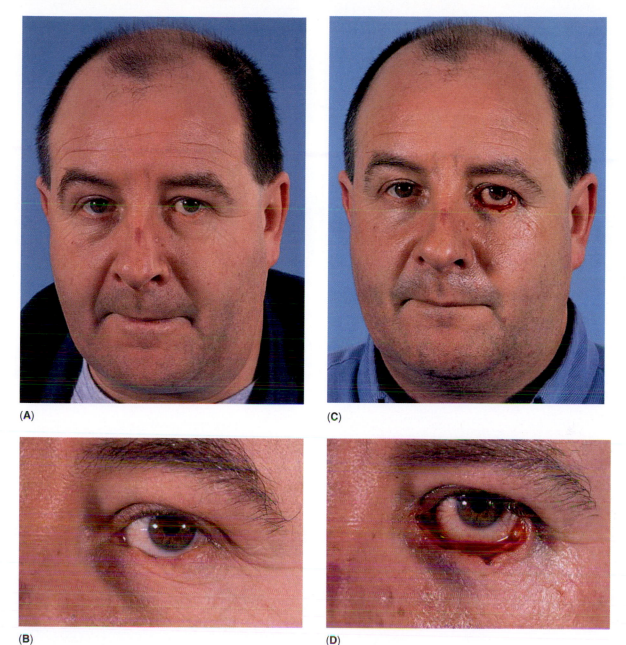

(A)

(C)

(B)

(D)

Figure 12.11 (**A**) A patient presenting with a left lower eyelid morphoeic basal cell carcinoma. (**B**) A close-up of the left lower eyelid morphoeic BCC. (**C**) The same patient following a Mohs' micrographic surgical excision of BCC. (**D**) A close-up of the left lower eyelid Mohs' micrographic surgery defect.

Parker blade. The uppermost incision is made at the level of the insertion of the medial aspect of the upper eyelid. A horizontal skin incision may need to be made extending to the bridge of the nose in order to gain access to an adequate length of periosteum.

2. A vertical relieving incision joining the two horizontal incisions is made over the bridge of the nose.

3. The flap is then elevated toward the orbit using the sharp-tipped end of a Freer periosteal elevator. The flap is anchored at the junction of the periosteum with the periorbita.

4. The flap is sutured to the medial margin of the tarsus of the upper lid tarsoconjunctival flap with interrupted 5/0 Vicryl sutures. Great care needs to be taken as this periosteal flap tends to be thinner and less robust than a lateral periosteal flap.

5. Topical antibiotic ointment is instilled into the eye and the eye closed.

6. A Jelonet dressing is placed over the eye, followed by two eye pads and a firm compressive bandage is applied to prevent excessive swelling.

Postoperative Care
This is as described above.

The Hughes procedure may be combined with other reconstructive techniques, e.g., a Fricke flap, to achieve the best result for an individual patient (Fig. 12.17).

Free Tarsoconjunctival Graft
Adequate tarsal support may be provided by harvesting a free tarsoconjunctival graft from either upper lid. The graft must be covered by a local vascularized myocutaneous advancement, rotation or transposition flap.

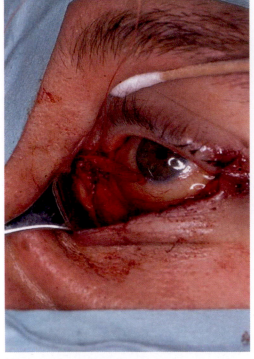

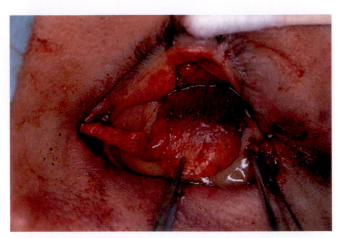

(A)

(B)

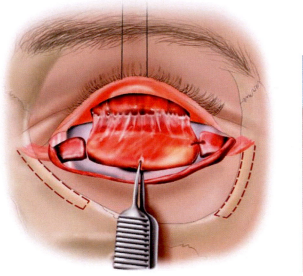

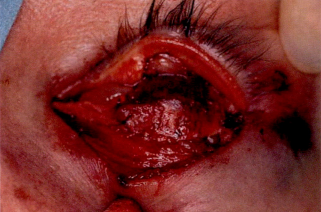

(C)

(D)

Figure 12.12 (**A**) A medial periosteal flap dissected from the frontal process of the maxilla. (**B**) A central tarsoconjunctival flap and medial and lateral periosteal flaps dissected. (**C**) A diagram demonstrating the periosteal flap dissection. (**D**) The flaps sutured into place prior to the skin-muscle advancement flap.

This technique is useful for lower eyelid reconstruction in a monocular patient because it does not occlude the visual axis. If the surgical defect extends to involve the canthal tendons, the free graft should be anchored to periosteal flaps as described above.

Surgical Procedure
1. A 4/0 silk traction suture is passed through the gray line of the upper eyelid, which is everted over a Desmarres retractor.
2. The tarsal conjunctiva is dried with a swab and a series of points 3.5 mm above the lid margin are marked with gentian violet. These points are then joined to mark an incision line.

3. The size of the graft required is determined and marked out.
4. A superficial horizontal incision is made centrally along the tarsus 3.5 mm above the lid margin using a no. 15 Bard Parker blade. It is important to leave a tarsal height of 3.5 mm below the incision in order to maintain the structural integrity of the eyelid to prevent an upper eyelid entropion and to prevent any compromise to the blood supply of the eyelid margin.
5. The incision is deepened through the full thickness of the tarsus centrally using the no. 15 blade and the horizontal incision is completed with blunt-tipped Westcott scissors (Fig. 12.18).

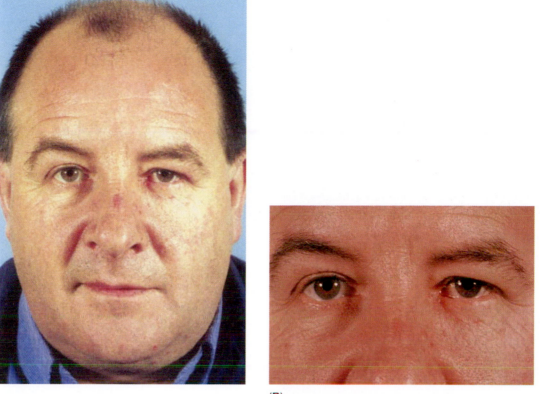

(A)   (B)

Figure 12.13 (**A**) The postoperative appearance of the reconstructed eyelid following a "maximal Hughes procedure". (**B**) A close-up photograph of the same patient.

6. Vertical relieving cuts are then made at both ends of the tarsal incision.
7. The tarsal graft is then dissected from the underlying tissues and amputated at its base.
8. The tarsal graft is sutured into the recipient lower lid defect as described above.
9. A myocutaneous flap (a rotation, transposition, or advancement flap) is then fashioned to lie over the graft.

Postoperative Care
This is as described above.

Mustardé Cheek Rotation Flap
With the development and popularity of other reconstruction techniques and with the tissue-conserving advantages of Mohs' micrographic surgery, the Mustardé cheek rotation flap is utilized far more rarely than in the past. It is reserved for the reconstruction of very extensive deep eyelid defects usually involving more than 75% of the eyelid.

A large myocutaneous cheek flap is dissected and used in conjunction with an adequate mucosal lining posteriorly. The posterior lamellar tarsal substitute is usually a nasal septal cartilage graft or a hard palate graft. The important points in designing a cheek flap are summarized by Mustardé as follows:

A deep inverted triangle must be excised below the defect to allow adequate rotation (Fig. 12.19). The side of the triangle nearest to the nose should be practically vertical. Failure to observe this point will result in a pulling down of the advancing flap because the center of rotation of the leading edge is too far to the lateral side.

The outline of the flap should rise in a curve toward the tail of the eyebrow and hairline and should reach down just in front of the ear as far as the lobule of the ear (Fig. 12.19).

The flap must be adequately undermined from the lowest point of the incision in front of the ear across the whole cheek to within 1 cm below the apex of the excised triangle. Great care must also be exercised to avoid damage to branches of the facial nerve.

Where necessary (in defects of three-quarters or more), a back cut should be made at the lowest point, 1 cm or more below the lobule of the ear. The deep tissue of the flap should be hitched up to the orbital rim, especially at the lateral canthus, to prevent the weight of the flap from pulling on the lid (Fig. 12.20). A typical early result following this reconstructive procedure is shown in Figure 12.21.

KEY POINTS

Cheek flaps can be followed by many complications, including facial-nerve paralysis, hematoma, necrosis of the flap, ectropion, entropion, epiphora, sagging of the reconstructed lower eyelid (Fig. 12.22), and excessive facial scarring. It is very important to plan the design of the flap and to appreciate the plane of dissection to avoid inadvertent injury to the facial nerve branches, which can result in lagophthalmos. Meticulous attention to hemostasis is important, as is placement of a drain and a compressive dressing at the conclusion of surgery.

Surgical Procedure
1. The cheek rotation flap is marked out very carefully with gentian violet. The outline of the flap should

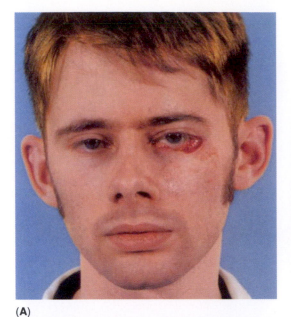
(A)

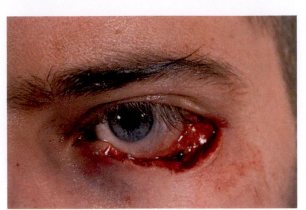
(B)

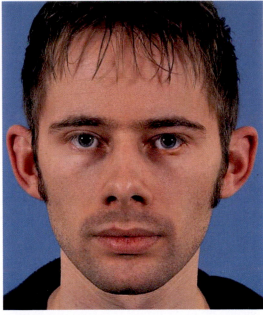
(C)

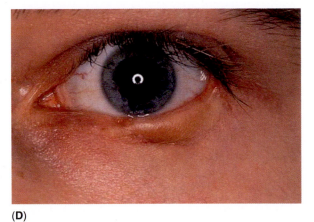
(D)

Figure 12.14 (**A**) A young patient with an extensive lower eyelid Mohs' micrographic surgery defect. (**B**) A close-up of the defect. (**C**) The postoperative appearance following a "maximal Hughes procedure" with a skin graft. (**D**) A close-up photograph of the reconstructed eyelid.

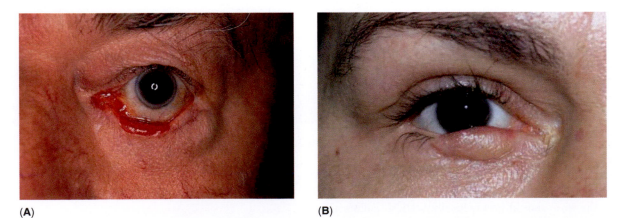
(A)   **(B)**

Figure 12.15 (**A**) An unsatisfactory result from a Hughes procedure with a lower eyelid ectropion, retraction and an unsightly eyelid margin. (**B**) An unsatisfactory result from a poorly divided Hughes flap with a raised irregular eyelid margin and a thickened skin graft. This will require a revision procedure to reshape the eyelid margin and thin the skin graft.

rise in a curve toward the tail of the eyebrow and hairline and should reach down just in front of the ear as far as the lobule of the ear (Fig. 12.19).

2. The midface is then infiltrated with a tumescent solution made up of 500 ml of Ringer's lactate, 25 ml of 0.25% Bupivacaine with 1:200,000 units of adrenaline, 25 ml of 2% lidocaine with 1:80,000

units of adrenaline, 0.5 ml of 1:10,000 adrenaline, 5 ml of triamcinolone 10 mg/ml, and 1500 units of hyaluronidase. The solution is injected using a 20-ml Luer lock syringe and a 21-gauge needle. Approximately 15 to 20 ml of the solution are injected subcutaneously over the central and lateral midface and pressure is then applied to diffuse the solution. The solution is allowed at least 10 minutes to work.

3. The skin is incised along the gentian violet marks using a no. 15 Bard Parker blade.

4. The flap is then undermined in a superficial subcutaneous plane using blunt dissection with blunt-tipped curved Stevens scissors and toothed Adson forceps. The undermining is continued until the flap can be rotated adequately without undue tension.

5. The deep aspect of the flap is sutured to the periosteum of the lateral orbital margin using a 4/0 PDS suture.

6. The medial vertical subcutaneous aspect of the flap is closed with interrupted 5/0 Vicryl sutures.

7. The lateral subcutaneous aspects of the flap are also closed with interrupted 5/0 Vicryl sutures. A vacuum-assisted drain is placed before the wound closure has been completed. This should be sutured to the adjacent skin to prevent the drain from being inadvertently removed (Fig. 12.23).

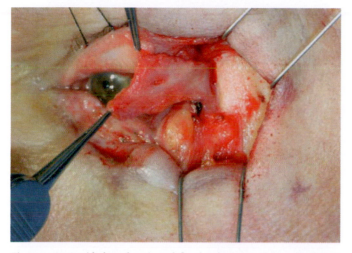

Figure 12.16 A wide lateral periosteal flap has been raised from the lateral orbital margin extending to the zygoma. The anchor point is situated at the internal aspect of the lateral orbital margin at the position of the original lateral canthal tendon. This flap is to be divided into two strips to be used for both upper and lower eyelid reconstruction.

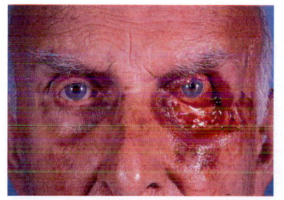

(A)

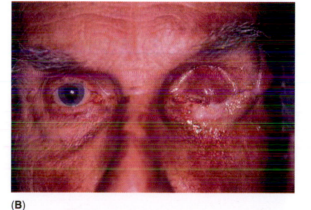

(B)

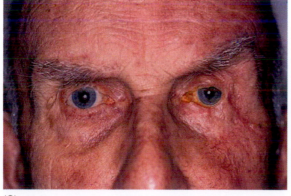

(C)

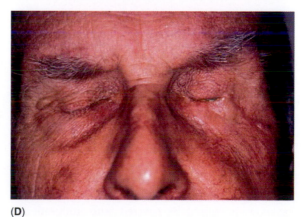

(D)

Figure 12.17 (**A**) An extensive Mohs' micrographic surgery defect of the lower eyelid and lateral part of upper eyelid. (**B**) The defects reconstructed with medial tarsoconjunctival flap, large periosteal flaps and a Fricke flap. (**C**) The postoperative appearance following division of the flaps. (**D**) The adequate closure of the eyelids has been achieved.

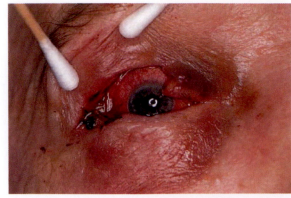

(A)

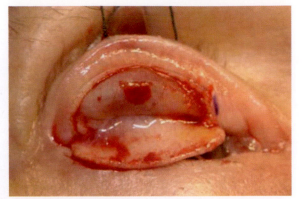

(B)

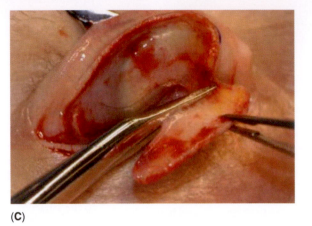

(C)

Figure 12.18 (**A**) An extensive Mohs' micrographic surgery defect of the upper eyelid. (**B, C**) A free tarsoconjunctival graft being harvested.

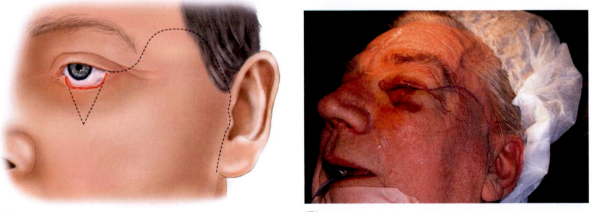

(A)   (B)

Figure 12.19 (**A**) A deep inverted V is excised to permit the flap to rotate adequately. (**B**) The Mustardé cheek rotation flap is marked out.

8. If the lateral preauricular defect cannot be closed directly this can instead be covered with a full thickness skin graft.

9. The medial and lateral skin closure is achieved with interrupted 6/0 Novafil sutures.

10. The skin is sutured to the posterior lamellar flap or graft using interrupted 7/0 Vicryl sutures.

11. The wounds should be covered with antibiotic ointment and Jelonet dressings. Eye pads and gauze swabs should be placed over the wounds and the mid-face and these should be held in place with a bandage that is applied without excessive tension.

Postoperative Care

The patient should keep the head raised postoperatively and avoid any lifting or straining for a week. The dressings are removed after 48 hours and the drain removed postoperatively as soon as the drainage of any blood has ceased. Topical antibiotic ointment is applied to the wounds for 2 weeks. The skin sutures are removed after 2 weeks.

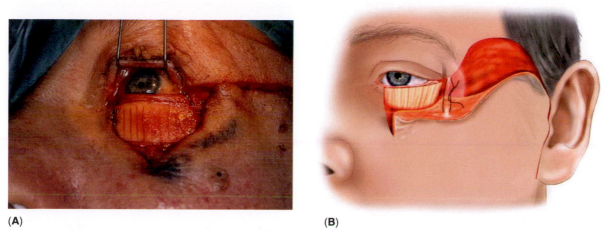

(A) **(B)**

Figure 12.20 (**A**) A nasal septal cartilage graft scored vertically, creating an anterior convexity of the graft. A frill of nasal mucosa is left superiorly to create a muco-cutaneous junction. (**B**) The deep tissue of the flap is hitched to the periosteum of the lateral orbital margin.

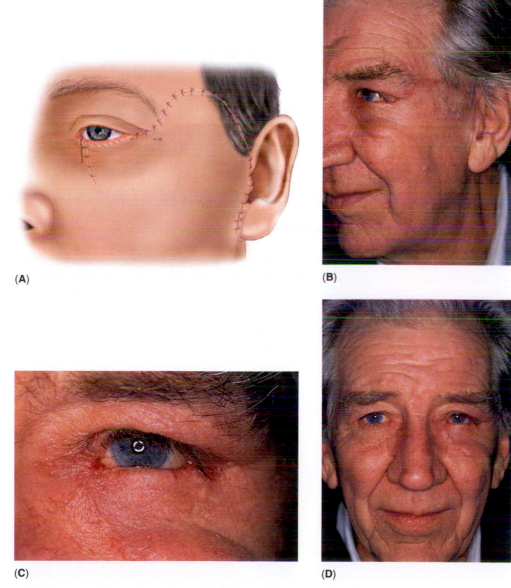

(A) **(B)**

(C) **(D)**

Figure 12.21 (**A**) A check rotation flap and posterior lamellar nasal septal cartilage flap completed. (**B**) A lateral view of a patient 1 week following surgery. (**C**) A close-up view of the reconstructed eyelid. (**D**) A full-face view of the same patient.

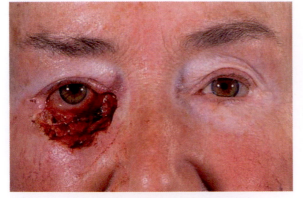

(A)

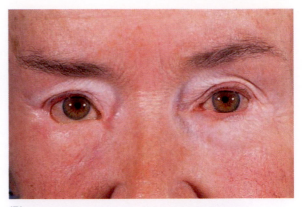

(B)

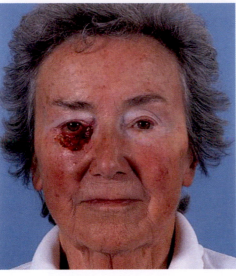

(C)

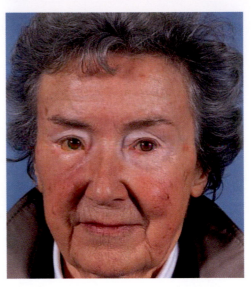

(D)

Figure 12.22 (**A**) An extensive right lower eyelid Mohs' micrographic surgery defect. (**B**) The patient 6 weeks following a Mustard flap reconstruction with nasal septal cartilage graft. The flap was not adequately hitched to the periosteum of the lateral orbital margin, with a resultant sagging of the flap laterally. (**C**) A full-face view of the same patient preoperatively. (**D**) A full-face view of the same patient postoperatively.

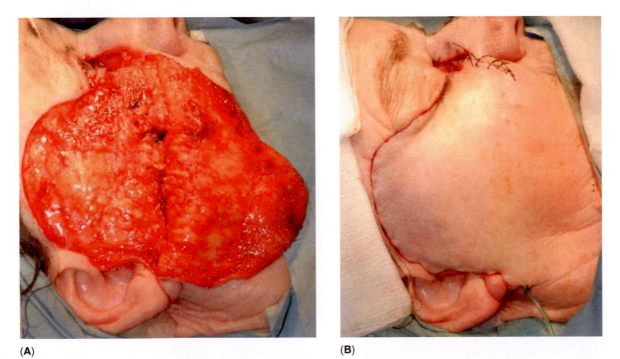

(A)

(B)

Figure 12.23 (**A**) A Mustardé cheek rotation flap dissected. (**B**) The Mustardé cheek flap rotated into position with the initial sutures and drain in place.

The Mustardé cheek rotation flap may be used for the reconstruction of a defect, which extends to involve the medial canthus, and can be used in combination with other local tissue flaps (Fig. 12.24).

The Lower Eyelid Island Flap

The lower eyelid island flap can be used in conjunction with a Mustardé cheek rotation flap for the reconstruction of a medial lower lid defect occupying up to 50% of the eyelid. This is an option for the patient in whom a Hughes flap reconstruction would be inappropriate, or where other options are unsuitable, e.g., a posterior lamellar graft in conjunction with a nasojugal flap (see Fig. 12.33).

Surgical Procedure
1. The Mustardé cheek rotation flap is marked out and prepared as described above.
2. A subciliary incision is made in the temporal remnant of the lower eyelid using a no. 15 Bard Parker blade.
3. The dissection is carried inferiorly in the post-orbicularis oculi muscle plane using blunt-tipped Westcott scissors.
4. A lateral canthotomy and inferior cantholysis are performed keeping the eyelid attached inferiorly by the conjunctiva and the lower eyelid retractors.
5. The lower eyelid remnant is then centered over the pupil and secured in place using medial and lateral periosteal flaps.
6. The subciliary incision is carried temporally to perform a Tenzel semi-circular flap or a full Mustardé cheek rotation flap according to the amount of anterior lamella that is needed to reconstruct the defect. The skin can be displaced all the way nasally to cover the medial canthal area even above the height of the medial canthal tendon as is shown in Figures 12.25, 12.26.
7. It is important to anchor the anterior lamellar flap adequately to minimize the risk of a late postoperative retraction of the lower eyelid.

Postoperative Care

The patient should keep the head raised postoperatively and avoid any lifting or straining for a week. The dressings are removed after 48 hours and the drain removed postoperatively as soon as the drainage of any blood has ceased. Topical antibiotic ointment is applied to the wounds for 2 weeks. The skin sutures are removed after 2 weeks.

OTHER PERIOCULAR FLAPS

There are a number of alternative local periocular flaps, which can be utilized for lower eyelid anterior lamellar reconstruction. A flap can be used from the upper eyelid where there is sufficient redundant tissue. Occasionally, the flap can be created as a "bucket handle" based both temporally and nasally (a Tripier flap). It is essential, however, to ensure that the creation of such flaps does not cause lagophthalmos. It is important to respect a length–width ratio of approximately 4:1 where such flaps are not based on an axial blood supply to avoid necrosis.

A particularly useful flap is the Fricke flap harvested from above the brow and based temporally (Fig. 12.27). It provides good vertical support but requires a second stage revision after approximately 3 to 6 weeks. Other local flaps which are harvested from the lower lateral cheek area or the nasojugal area have the disadvantage of being associated with secondary lymphedema, which can take many months to resolve.

The Fricke Flap
First Stage
Surgical Procedure
1. The length of the flap is marked out using an unfolded swab. One end of the swab is positioned and held at the base of the proposed flap temporally and the other end is drawn to the medial aspect of the lower eyelid defect. The medial aspect of the swab is then moved to the area just above the brow while the lateral end of the swab is maintained in position. This mimics the movement of the Fricke flap and assists the estimation of the length of flap required. The most medial extent of the flap is marked with gentian violet.

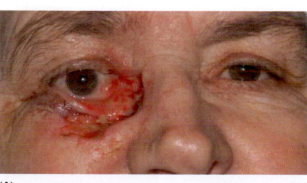
(A)

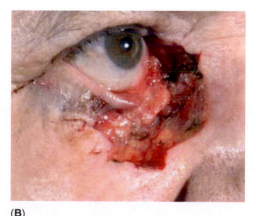
(B)

Figure 12.24 (**A**) An extensive Mohs' surgery defect with loss of skin and orbicularis muscle from the medial half of the lower eyelid and the medial canthus, and loss of the medial aspect of the eyelid and the medial canthal tendon. (**B**) A close-up photograph showing the extent and the depth of the defect.

2. The height of the lower eyelid defect is then measured and the Fricke flap marked out accordingly. The medial aspect of the flap is tapered to mirror the shape of the medial aspect of the lower eyelid defect. The lateral aspect of the flap is kept as wide as possible and should at least respect the ratio of 4:1 for the base to length dimension of the flap.
3. Six to eight milliliters of 0.5% Bupivacaine with 1:200,000 units of adrenaline mixed 50:50 with 2% lidocaine with 1:80,000 units of adrenaline are injected subcutaneously into the flap which has been outlined.
4. A skin incision is made using a no. 15 Bard Parker blade.
5. The flap is dissected with blunt-tipped curved Stevens scissors along the plane between the subcutaneous tissue and the underlying muscles of the brow and lower forehead.
6. Great care should be taken to avoid the excessive use of cautery. Thinning of the flap should also be avoided.

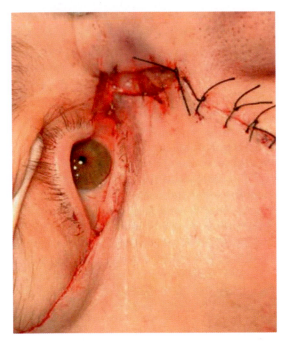

Figure 12.25 A lateral canthotomy and inferior cantholysis have been undertaken and a medial tarsal strip has been sutured to the posterior lacrimal crest. The Mustardé flap has been positioned and the final sutures are to be placed at the medial canthus, taking the tension off the lower eyelid margin.

7. The flap is transposed to lie in the lower eyelid defect. The inferior and medial subcutaneous wound closure is achieved with interrupted 5/0 Vicryl sutures and the skin closure inferiorly and medially is achieved with interrupted 6/0 Novafil sutures. The eyelid margin closure to the posterior lamellar graft or flap is achieved with interrupted 7/0 Vicryl sutures.
8. The forehead wound is closed with interrupted subcutaneous 5/0 Vicryl sutures and interrupted simple 6/0 Novafil sutures are used for the skin closure.
9. The lateral aspect of the flap is left to heal by secondary intention.
10. The wounds should be covered with antibiotic ointment and Jelonet dressings. Eye pads and gauze swabs should be placed over the wounds and these should be held in place with a bandage that is applied without excessive tension.

Postoperative Care
The patient should keep the head raised postoperatively and avoid any lifting or straining for a week. The dressings are removed after 48 hours. Topical antibiotic ointment is applied to the wounds for 2 weeks. The skin sutures are removed after 2 weeks.

Second Stage
Surgical Procedure
1. Three to four milliliters of 0.5% Bupivacaine with 1:200,000 units of adrenaline mixed 50:50 with 2% lidocaine with 1:80,000 units of adrenaline are injected subcutaneously into the lateral aspect of the flap which will have healed to form a tubular tissue flap.
2. The tubular flap is simply excised leaving stumps of tissue medially and laterally. These stumps are gently debulked of subcutaneous fat and the skin closed (Fig. 12.28).

Postoperative Care
This is as described above.

The Fricke flap can be expanded intraoperatively by 10 to 15% with the use of a 14-gauge Foley catheter ("rapid intraoperative tissue expansion"). This is inserted into the forehead subcutaneously via a small incision temporally (Fig. 12.29).

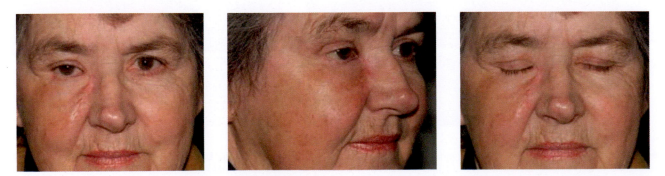

Figure 12.26 The postoperative appearance 2 months following a lower island flap and Mustardé cheek rotation flap reconstruction.

Blunt dissection is used to create a subcutaneous pocket above the eyebrow. The catheter is inflated and deflated at intervals of 10 minutes for approximately 30 minutes.

For the more elective reconstruction of lower eyelid defects a, soft tissue expander can be used and gradually and intermittently inflated over a period of several weeks to recruit additional tissue for a local flap. (An alternative technique is to use an osmotic expander, which gradually self inflates to a predetermined size. This does not require a more extensive dissection to place it but its expansion is less controlled.)

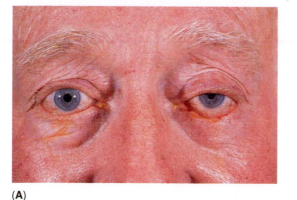

(A)

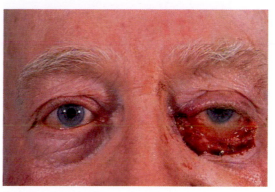

(B)

(C)

(D)

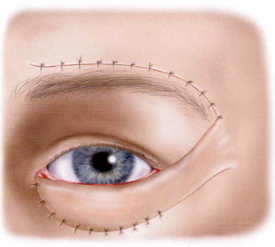

(E)

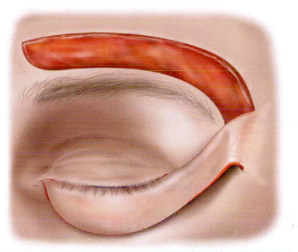

(F)

Figure 12.27 (**A**) A left lower eyelid basal cell carcinoma. (**B**) Extensive left lower eyelid Mohs' micrographic surgery defect. (**C**) A drawing showing a Fricke flap outlined. (**D**) A drawing showing the Fricke flap transposed into the lower eyelid with a 4:1 length-breadth ration. (**E**) A drawing showing the Fricke flap sutured into place leaving the mucocutaneous border of the eyelid margin to heal by secondary intention. (**F**) The final result 2 months postoperatively.

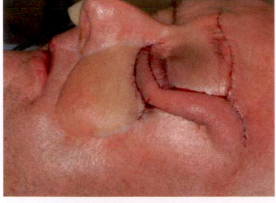
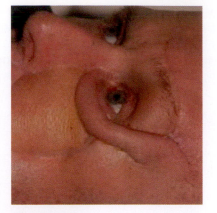

(A)   (B)

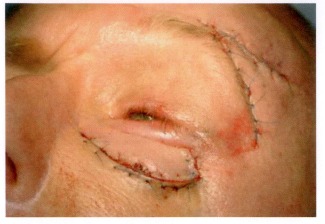

(C)

Figure 12.28 (**A**) The intraoperative appearance of a Fricke flap undertaken for a severe lower eyelid cicatricial ectropion in a patient who had previously undergone a maxillectomy and a free flap reconstruction of the midface. (**B**) The appearance of the Fricke flap 3 weeks postoperatively. (**C**) The intraoperative appearance of the Fricke flap following the second stage debulking of the flap. In this case, part of the flap was returned to the eyebrow to reduce the degree of eyebrow retraction.

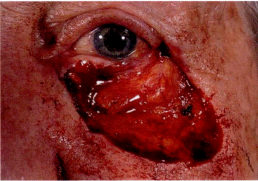
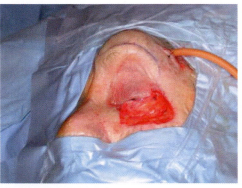

(A)   (B)

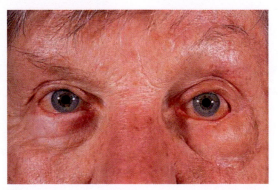

(C)

Figure 12.29 (**A**) An extensive lower eyelid/cheek Mohs' micrographic surgery defect. (**B**) Rapid intraoperative expansion of Fricke flap using Foley catheter. (**C**) The final result after reconstruction with an expanded Fricke flap, a lateral tarsoconjunctival flap, and a skin graft at the inferior aspect of the wound.

Surgical Procedure

1. A "w plasty" incision is marked in the temple avoiding the superficial temporal artery. (Fig. 12.30).
2. Ten to fifteen milliliters of 0.5% Bupivacaine with 1:200,000 units of adrenaline mixed 50:50 with 2% lidocaine with 1:80,000 units of adrenaline are injected subcutaneously into the temple, forehead, and postauricular area.
3. A skin incision is made using a no. 15 Bard Parker blade.
4. The incision is carried through the temporoparietal fascia to the deep temporal fascia using blunt-tipped Stevenss scissors.
5. A tunnel is created leading from the temporal wound anteriorly just above the eyebrow by blunt dissection using Metzenbaum scissors to create a subcutaneous pocket to accommodate the soft tissue expander. The soft tissue expander is shown in Figure 12.30. Blunt dissection is then continued posteriorly to accommodate the injection port.
6. The temple wound is closed with interrupted subcutaneous 5/0 Vicryl sutures and interrupted simple 6/0 Novafil sutures are used for the skin closure.
7. The wounds should be covered with antibiotic ointment and Jelonet dressings. Eye pads and gauze swabs should be placed over the wounds and these should be held in place with a bandage that is applied without excessive tension.
8. The typical postoperative appearance of the position of the soft tissue expander and the injection port is shown in Figure 12.30.

Postoperative Care

The patient should keep the head raised postoperatively and avoid any lifting or straining for a week. The dressings are removed after 48 hours. Topical antibiotic ointment is applied to the wounds for 2 weeks. The skin sutures are removed after 2 weeks.

The expander is gradually inflated at 1 to 2 weekly intervals. The skin overlying the injection port is prepped with an antiseptic agent, e.g., iodine, and 1 to 2ml of sterile saline are injected slowly using a 3 ml Luer lock syringe and a 30-gauge sterile needle. As soon as a satisfactory degree of soft tissue expansion has been achieved, the Fricke flap reconstruction is planned. The soft tissue expander is deflated and removed during the procedure by reopening the temple wound.

The Fricke flap has the disadvantage that it leaves the ipsilateral eyebrow elevated. A regime of firm postoperative massage can help to lower the eyebrow to a satisfactory level. A contralateral direct brow lift can be performed later in order to improve symmetry if necessary.

The Nasojugal Flap

The nasojugal flap is based at the medial aspect of the lower eyelid and extended along the nasojugal fold. The nasojugal flap reconstruction is undertaken as a single stage procedure. A similar flap can be undertaken based as the lateral aspect of the lower eyelid but this flap tends to cause more disruption to lymphatic drainage and can result in persistent edema of the flap. This flap has the advantage of minimizing any potential intraoperative damage to branches of the facial nerve, which could result in lagophthalmos, in contrast to the Mustardé cheek rotation flap.

Surgical Procedure

1. The length of the flap is marked out using an unfolded swab. One end of the swab is positioned and held at the base of the proposed flap medially and the other end is drawn to the lateral aspect of the lower eyelid defect. The lateral aspect of the swab is then moved to the base of the nasojugal fold. This mimics the movement of the nasojugal flap and assists the estimation of the length of flap required. The most inferior extent of the flap is marked with gentian violet.

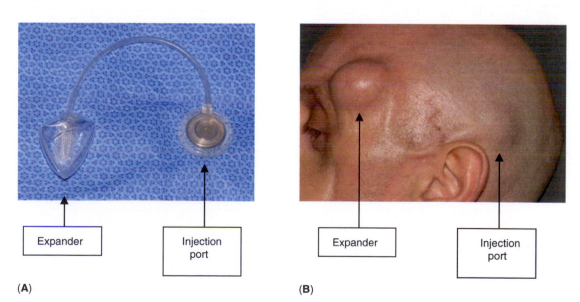

(A)   **(B)**

Figure 12.30 (**A**) A soft tissue expander. (**B**) A soft tissue expander in place in a patient due to undergo a Fricke flap reconstruction of a lower eyelid soft-tissue defect. (This patient is seen in Figure 12.28.)

2. The height of the lower eyelid defect is then measured and the nasojugal flap marked out accordingly. The medial aspect of the flap is kept as wide as possible and should at least respect the ratio of 4:1 for the base to length dimension of the flap.

3. Six to eight millimeters of 0.5% Bupivacaine with 1:200,000 units of adrenaline mixed 50:50 with 2% lidocaine with 1:80,000 units of adrenaline are injected subcutaneously into the flap which has been outlined.

4. A skin incision is made using a no. 15 Bard Parker blade.

5. The flap is dissected with blunt-tipped curved Westcott scissors along the plane between the subcutaneous tissue and the underlying muscle.

6. Great care should be taken to avoid the excessive use of cautery. Thinning of the flap should also be avoided.

7. The flap is transposed to lie in the lower eyelid defect. The inferior and lateral subcutaneous wound closure is achieved with interrupted 5/0 Vicryl sutures and the skin closure inferiorly and laterally is achieved with interrupted 6/0 Novafil sutures. The eyelid margin closure to the posterior lamellar graft or flap is achieved with interrupted 7/0 Vicryl sutures.

8. The nasojugal wound is closed with interrupted subcutaneous 5/0 Vicryl sutures and interrupted simple 6/0 Novafil sutures are used for the skin closure.

9. The wounds should be covered with antibiotic ointment and Jelonet dressings. Eye pads and gauze swabs should be placed over the wounds and these should be held in place with a bandage that is applied without excessive tension.

Postoperative Care

The patient should keep the head raised postoperatively and avoid any lifting or straining for a week. The dressings are removed after 48 hours. Topical antibiotic ointment is applied to the wounds for 2 weeks. The skin sutures are removed after 2 weeks.

Figure 12.31 shows a young patient whose very extensive lower eyelid defect was not reconstructed primarily but was left to granulate initially. A soft tissue expander was inserted subcutaneously into his cheek via a pre-auricular short scar face-lift incision. This was removed after 6 weeks and a nasojugal flap was used, in conjunction with a hard palate graft and medial and lateral periosteal flaps, to reconstruct the lower eyelid (Figs. 12.32 and 12.33).

Eyelid Defects Not Involving the Eyelid Margin

If the lesion is small, the defect may be closed with direct approximation of the skin edges after undermining or with the use of a horizontal skin-muscle advancement flap or a rotation flap (Fig. 12.34). It is important to close the wound horizontally and not vertically to avoid a postoperative ectropion.

Surgical Procedure

1. A subciliary incision is marked out using gentian violet, with the addition of a Tenzel flap if required.

2. Two to three milliliters of 0.5% Bupivacaine with 1:200,000 units of adrenaline mixed 50:50 with 2% lidocaine with 1:80,000 units of adrenaline are injected subcutaneously into the flap which has been outlined.

3. Using a no.15 Bard Parker blade a subciliary skin incision is made extending from the defect to the lateral canthus. This can be extended beyond the lateral canthus as a Tenzel flap if required.

4. Next, the skin–muscle flap is widely undermined using blunt-tipped Westcott scissors.

5. The medial wound is closed with subcutaneous 5/0 Vicryl sutures, commencing at the inferior aspect of the wound. It is essential to anchor the apex of the flap medially so that all tension is removed from the eyelid margin. The skin edges are reapproximated with 6/0 Novafil sutures.

6. The subciliary skin wound is closed with simple interrupted 7/0 Vicryl sutures.

7. Tincture of Benzoin is applied to the skin of the cheek and to the forehead skin and allowed to dry.

8. Topical antibiotic ointment is applied to the wounds, followed by Jelonet. A sterile double eye pad is applied to the eyelids and Micropore tape is applied to the cheek and then fixated to the forehead, drawing the cheek superomedially. This ensures that all tension is taken off the wounds.

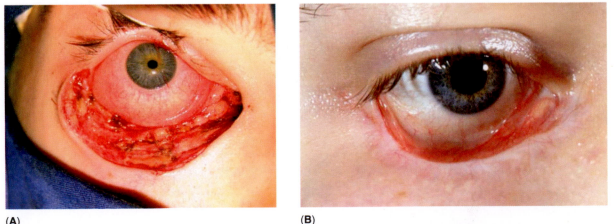

(A)   (B)

Figure 12.31 (**A**) An extensive lower eyelid defect. (**B**) The appearance of the same lower lid defect after allowing healing by "laissez-faire."

Postoperative Care

The patient should keep the head raised postoperatively and avoid any lifting or straining for a week. The dressings are removed after 48 hours. Topical antibiotic ointment is applied to the wounds for 2 weeks. The skin sutures are removed after 2 weeks. The patient should be instructed to massage the eyelid in an upward and inward direction for 3 minutes three times per day after applying Lacrilube ointment to the eyelid skin. The patient should start the massage 2 weeks postoperatively and should continue this for at least 6 weeks.

Full Thickness Skin Graft

With larger superficial lesions or where the adjacent skin is tight, a full-thickness skin graft may be necessary to prevent ectropion of the lower lid (Fig. 12.35). If the defect occupies more than 1/3 of the eyelid or if the eyelid is lax, the skin graft should be combined with a lateral tarsal strip procedure or a lateral eyelid wedge resection in order to prevent a lower eyelid ectropion.

Surgical Procedure

This is described in chapter 13.

Postoperative Care

A compressive dressing should be left in place for 5 to 7 days. The sutures should be removed after 10 to 14 days and postoperative wound massage should be commenced 2 weeks postoperatively to prevent thickening and contracture of the graft. The massage should be undertaken in a horizontal and upward direction for 3 minutes three times a day after applying Lacrilube ointment to the skin graft. The application of a silicone gel, e.g., Dermatix or Kelocote is advantageous but incurs additional expense. If the skin graft shows any tendency to thicken or "pin cushion" (Fig. 12.36), it can be injected at several points with tiny amounts of triamcinolone using a 1 ml Luer lock syringe and a 30-gauge needle. The total dose injected should not need to exceed 0.3 ml.

UPPER EYELID RECONSTRUCTION

Reconstruction of upper eyelid tumor defects must be performed meticulously to avoid ocular surface complications. A number of surgical procedures can be utilized to reconstruct an upper lid defect and it is important to select the procedure best suited to the individual patient's needs.

Lagophthalmos following reconstruction may cause exposure keratopathy, particularly in the absence of a good Bell's phenomenon. The problem is compounded by loss of accessory lacrimal tissue. Lacrimal tissue should be preserved when dissecting in the lateral canthal, lateral levator and lateral anterior orbital areas. Poor eyelid closure is usually due either to adhesions, wound contracture, or to a vertical skin shortage.

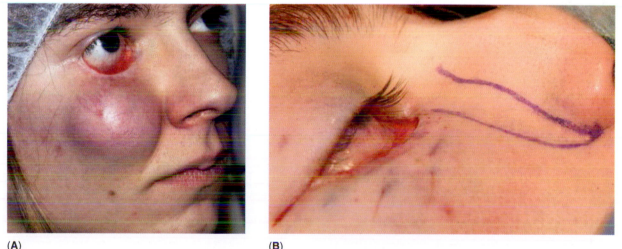

(A) (B)

Figure 12.32 (**A**) A soft tissue expander in situ. (**B**) A nasojugal flap outlined with gentian violet.

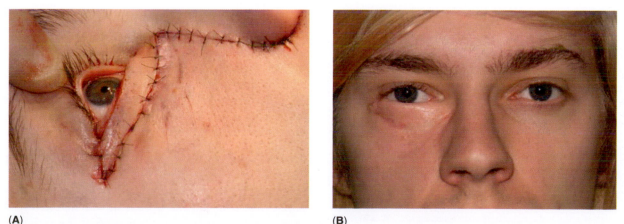

(A) (B)

Figure 12.33 (**A**) The nasojugal flap and hard palate graft sutured into place. (**B**) The postoperative appearance 3 years following the reconstruction.

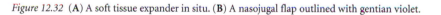

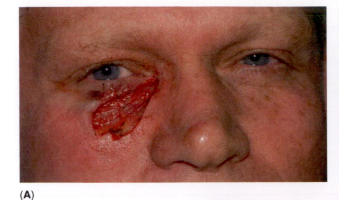
(A)

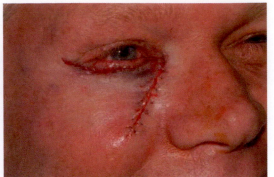
(B)

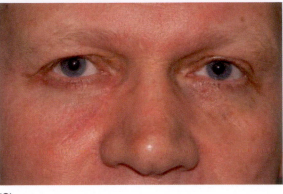
(C)

Figure 12.34 (**A**) A superficial Mohs surgery defect. (**B**) The appearance immediately following a skin advancement flap. (**C**) The postoperative appearance 3 months following surgery.

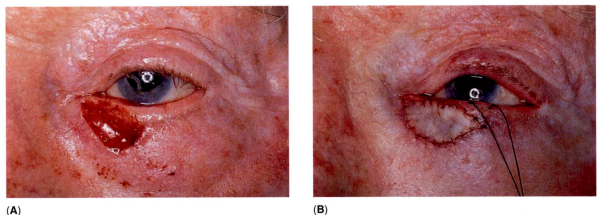
(A)   **(B)**

Figure 12.35 (**A**) Moderate anterior lamellar defect. (**B**) Placement of full-thickness skin graft.

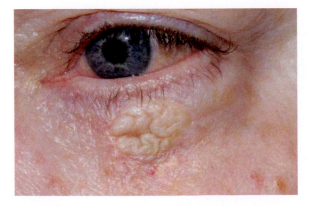

Figure 12.36 A "pin cushioned" full-thickness skin graft.

It may also be caused by over-enthusiastic dissection of lateral periocular flaps, with damage to branches of the facial nerve.

When levator function is preserved following surgical defects of the eyelid, ptosis can usually be avoided or corrected. It is important to carefully identify the cut edges of the levator and to ensure that the levator is reattached to the reconstructed tarsal replacement with a suitable spacer if required.

EYELID DEFECTS INVOLVING THE EYELID MARGIN
Small Defects

As in lower lid reconstruction, an eyelid defect of 25% or less may be closed directly, and in patients with marked eyelid laxity, even a defect occupying up to 50% of the eyelid may be closed directly (Fig. 12.37). The surgical procedure is as

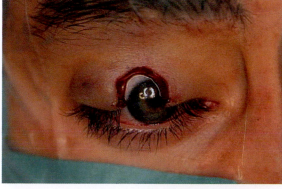
(A)

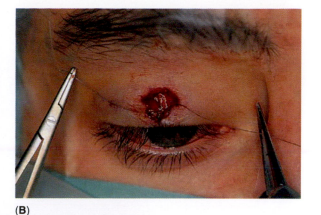
(B)

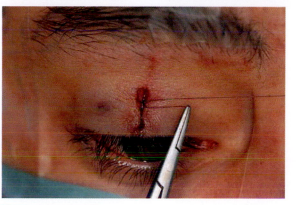
(C)

Figure 12.37 Direct closure of an upper eyelid wedge resection defect.

described above. It is important that the tarsal plate is aligned precisely and closed with 5/0 Vicryl sutures, ensuring that the bites are partial thickness to avoid the possibility of corneal abrasion. After closure of the tarsus, the eyelid margin is closed with interrupted 6/0 silk sutures placed at the gray line and lash margin. All eyelashes should be everted away from the cornea. The ends of the margin sutures are left long and sutured to the external skin tissue to avoid corneal irritation.

MODERATE DEFECTS
Canthotomy and Cantholysis
Where an eyelid defect cannot be closed directly without undue tension on the wound, a lateral canthotomy and superior cantholysis can be performed. *It is very important that the cantholysis is performed meticulously to avoid any inadvertent damage to the levator aponeurosis or to the lacrimal gland.*

KEY POINT

It is essential to keep the blades of the scissors close to the bone of the lateral orbital margin when performing a superior cantholysis to avoid inadvertent trauma to the levator aponeurosis or to the lacrimal gland.

Sliding Tarsoconjunctival Flap
Horizontal advancement of an upper eyelid tarsoconjunctival flap is useful for full-thickness defects of up to 50% of the upper lid margin.

Surgical Procedure

1. Two to three milliliters of 0.5% Bupivacaine with 1:200,000 units of adrenaline mixed 50:50 with 2% lidocaine with 1:80,000 units of adrenaline are injected subcutaneously into the upper eyelid remnant and lateral canthus.
2. The residual upper eyelid tarsus is incised horizontally 3.5 mm above the eyelid margin (Fig. 12.38A).
3. The superior portion of the tarsus is then dissected from the orbicularis muscle and advanced horizontally along with its levator and Müller's muscle attachments (Fig. 12.38B).
4. The tarsoconjunctival advancement flap created is then sutured in a side-to-side fashion to the lower portion of the residual upper lid tarsus using 5/0 Vicryl sutures and to a lateral or medial periosteal flap (Fig. 12.38C and D).
5. The lower portion of the residual upper lid tarsus remains attached to the orbicularis and skin tissue.
6. After the horizontal tarsoconjunctival advancement has been undertaken, the anterior lamellar defect is reconstructed using a full-thickness skin graft or a semicircular cutaneous rotation flap (as described above) (Fig. 12.38E).
7. Topical antibiotic ointment is instilled into the eye and the eye closed.
8. A Jelonet dressing is placed over the eye, followed by two eye pads and a firm compressive bandage to prevent excessive swelling.

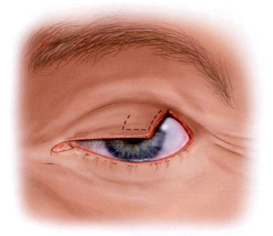

(A)

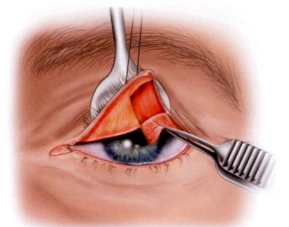

(B)

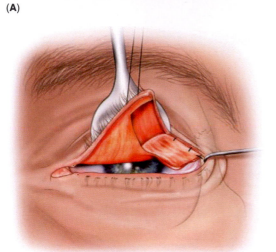

(C)

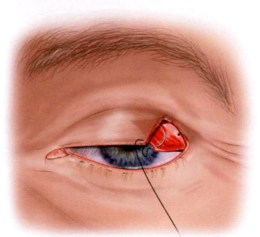

(D)

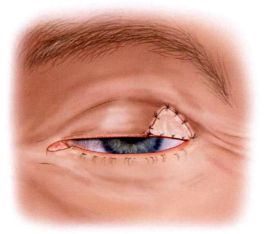

(E)

Figure 12.38 (**A**) The proposed flap is outlined. (**B**) The residual upper eyelid tarsus is incised horizontally 3.5 mm above the eyelid margin and the superior portion of the tarsus is then dissected from the orbicularis muscle. (**C**) The tarsoconjunctival flap is then advanced horizontally along with its levator and Müller's muscle attachments. (**D**) The tarsoconjunctival advancement flap created is then sutured in a side-to-side fashion to the lower portion of the residual upper lid tarsus using 5/0 Vicryl sutures and to a lateral or medial periosteal flap. (**E**) The anterior lamellar defect is reconstructed using a full-thickness skin graft (or a semicircular cutaneous rotation flap).

Postoperative Care

The patient should keep the head raised postoperatively and avoid any lifting or straining for a week. The dressings are removed after 48 hours, or after 5 days if a skin graft has been used. Topical antibiotic ointment is applied to the wounds for 2 weeks. The skin sutures are removed after 2 weeks. The patient should be instructed to massage the eyelid in a horizontal direction for 3 minutes 3 times per day after applying

Lacrilube ointment to the eyelid skin. The patient should start the massage 2 weeks postoperatively and should continue this for at least 6 weeks.

Semicircular Rotation Flap

A lateral, inverted, semicircular rotation flap may be combined with direct closure for full-thickness defects of up to two-thirds of the eyelid margin.

Surgical Procedure

1. An inverted semicircle is marked on the skin surface, beginning at the lateral canthus and extending laterally approximately 3 cm (Fig. 12.39A).
2. Two to three milliliters of 0.5% Bupivacaine with 1:200,000 units of adrenaline mixed 50:50 with 2% lidocaine with 1:80,000 units of adrenaline are injected subcutaneously into the flap which has been outlined.
3. The skin incision is made using a no. 15 Bard Parker blade.
4. The skin and orbicularis muscle are undermined under the entire flap using blunt-tipped Westcott scissors.
5. A lateral canthotomy and a superior cantholysis are then performed, taking care to avoid damage to the levator aponeurosis and to the lacrimal gland.
6. The lateral aspect of the eyelid is then advanced medially to close the defect (Fig. 12.39B).
7. The posterior surface of the advanced semi-circular flap laterally may be covered by a wide lateral periosteal flap or a tarsoconjunctival advancement flap from the lateral aspect of the lower eyelid.
8. If a tarsoconjunctival flap is to be used, the width of the residual upper lid posterior lamellar defect is measured with a caliper and two vertical incisions are marked on the lateral aspect of the lower eyelid the same width apart (Fig. 12.39B).
9. Two vertical, full-thickness incisions are made through the lower eyelid margin using a no. 15 Bard Parker blade and the incisions extended just beyond the inferior border of the tarsal plate using straight iris scissors.
10. The tarsoconjunctival advancement flap is prepared by excising the lower eyelid skin and orbicularis muscle and the eyelash margin from the flap (Fig. 12.39C).
11. The tarsus and conjunctiva are then advanced superiorly into the lateral aspect of the upper eyelid flap and sutured to a small lateral periosteal flap laterally and to the upper eyelid tarsal remnant medially using 5/0 Vicryl sutures, taking great care to ensure that the sutures do not abrade the cornea (Fig. 12.39D).
12. The skin edges of the semicircular flap are carefully sutured to the conjunctival flap with interrupted 8/0 Vicryl sutures, again taking great care to ensure that the sutures do not abrade the cornea (Fig. 12.39E).
13. The lower eyelid defect is then repaired primarily, anterior to the tarsoconjunctival flap.

14. Topical antibiotic ointment is instilled into the eye and the eye closed.
15. A Jelonet dressing is placed over the eye, followed by two eye pads and a firm compressive bandage to prevent excessive swelling.

As an alternative to a semicircular rotation flap, the advanced lower lid tarsoconjunctival flap may be covered with full-thickness skin tissue rather than a rotated, inverted semicircle.

Postoperative Care

The dressing is removed after 48 hours. If a full-thickness skin graft has been utilized, the dressing is not removed for 5 days. The Vicryl sutures are all removed after 2 weeks. Topical antibiotic is applied to the wounds 3 times a day for 2 weeks. Frequent preservative free topical lubricants should be prescribed for a few weeks postoperatively.

If a full-thickness skin graft has been utilized, the aftercare is as described above (see "Hughes flap and skin graft").

The lateral conjunctival flap may be released after 4 to 6 weeks.

LARGE DEFECTS

Free Tarsoconjunctival Graft

Adequate tarsal support may be provided by harvesting a free tarsoconjunctival graft from the opposite upper eyelid, leaving at least 3.5 cm of undisturbed tarsus above the eyelid margin to prevent instability of the eyelid (Fig. 12.18B and C). The graft is sewn edge to edge to the residual tarsus or to the local periosteal flaps with 5/0 Vicryl sutures (Fig. 12.40). The graft must be covered by a local vascularized myocutaneous advancement, rotation, or transposition flap. A skin-muscle advancement flap may be used from the sub-brow area and the secondary defect itself covered with a full-thickness skin graft.

This technique is useful for upper eyelid reconstruction in a monocular patient, because it does not occlude the visual axis. If the surgical defect extends to involve the canthal tendons, the free graft should be anchored to periosteal flaps as described above.

Surgical Procedure

1. Two to three milliliters of 0.5% Bupivacaine with 1:200,000 units of adrenaline mixed 50:50 with 2% lidocaine with 1:80,000 units of adrenaline are injected subcutaneously into the opposite upper eyelid.
2. A 4/0 silk traction suture is passed through the gray line of the opposite upper eyelid, which is everted over a Desmarres retractor.
3. The tarsal conjunctiva is dried with a swab and a series of points 3.5 mm above the lid margin are marked with gentian violet. These points are then joined to mark an incision line.
4. The size of the graft required is determined and marked out.
5. A superficial horizontal incision is made centrally along the tarsus 3.5 mm above the lid margin using a no. 15 Bard Parker blade. It is important to leave a tarsal height of 3.5 mm below the incision in order to maintain the structural integrity of the eyelid to prevent an upper eyelid entropion and to prevent any compromise of the blood supply of the eyelid margin.

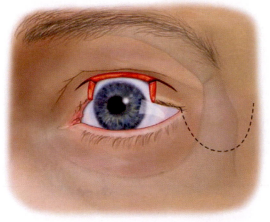

(A)

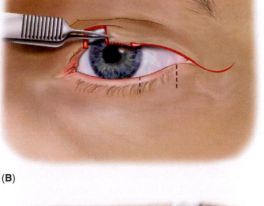

(B)

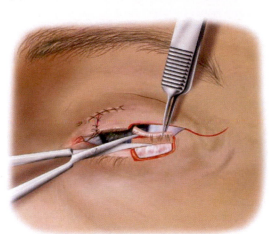

(C)

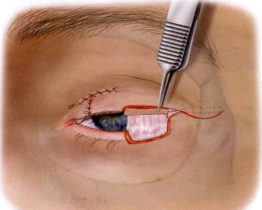

(D)

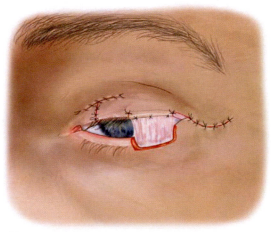

(E)

Figure 12.39 (**A**) An inverted semicircle is marked on the skin surface, beginning at the lateral canthus and extending laterally approximately 3 cm. (**B**) A lateral canthotomy and a superior cantholysis are performed and the lateral aspect of the eyelid is then advanced medially to close the defect in the upper eyelid. The width of the residual upper lid posterior lamellar defect is measured with a caliper and two vertical incisions are marked on the lateral aspect of the lower eyelid the same width apart. (**C**) A lower lid tarsoconjunctival flap is prepared from the lower eyelid and the mucocutaneous junction removed with Westcott scissors. (**D**) The tarsus and conjunctiva from the lower eyelid are advanced superiorly into the lateral aspect of the upper eyelid flap and sutured to a small lateral periosteal flap laterally and to the upper eyelid tarsal remnant medially using 5/0 Vicryl sutures. (**E**) The skin edges are carefully sutured to the conjunctival flap with interrupted 8/0 Vicryl sutures.

6. The incision is deepened through the full thickness of the tarsus centrally using the no. 15 blade and the horizontal incision is completed with blunt-tipped Westcott scissors.

7. Vertical relieving cuts are then made at both ends of the tarsal incision.

8. The tarsal graft is then dissected from the underlying tissues and amputated at its base (Fig. 12.18B and C).

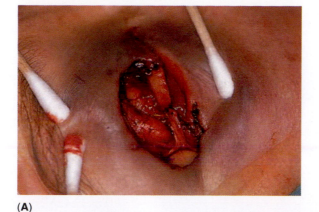

(A)

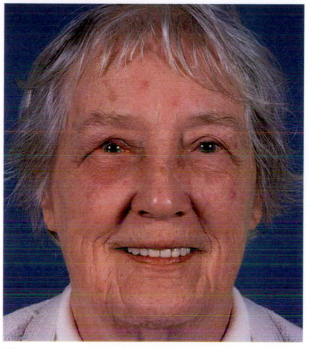

(B)

(C)

Figure 12.40 (**A**) A lateral periosteal flap dissected and attached to a free tarsal graft. (**B**) The preoperative appearance of the patient with a large right upper eyelid squamous cell carcinoma. (**C**) The postoperative appearance after use of an upper eyelid skin-muscle advancement flap.

9. The tarsal graft is sutured into the upper lid edge to edge with the residual tarsus or to periosteal flaps using interrupted 5/0 Vicryl sutures taking care to ensure that the sutures do not pass full thickness with a risk of causing a corneal abrasion.

10. The conjunctiva is sutured to the superior aspect of the graft using interrupted 7/0 Vicryl sutures.

11. The residual eyelid retractors are carefully sutured to the graft using interrupted 5/0 Vicryl sutures. If required, a spacer graft, e.g., a temporalis fascial graft, may need to be used if the levator aponeurosis has been sacrificed.

12. A myocutaneous flap (a rotation, transposition, or advancement flap) is then fashioned to lie over the graft. An advancement flap is quite versatile and the ensuing defect below the brow can in turn be reconstructed using a full thickness skin graft.

13. Topical antibiotic ointment is instilled into the eye and the eye closed.

14. A Jelonet dressing is placed over the eye, followed by two eye pads and a firm compressive bandage to prevent excessive swelling.

Postoperative Care

The dressings are removed after 72 hours. Topical antibiotic ointment is applied to the wounds for 2 weeks and antibiotic drops are prescribed for the fellow eye for a week. The skin sutures are removed after 2 weeks. Preservative free topical lubricants are prescribed for both eyes for a few weeks.

CUTLER BEARD RECONSTRUCTION (MODIFIED)

A Cutler–Beard reconstruction is a two-stage procedure, which is useful for upper eyelid defects covering up to 100% of the eyelid margin.

First Stage

Surgical Procedure

1. Four to five milliliters of 0.5% Bupivacaine with 1:200,000 units of adrenaline mixed 50:50 with

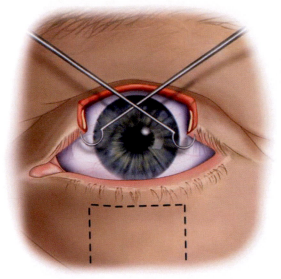

Figure 12.41 The edges of the upper eyelid defect are gently drawn together before the defect is measured.

2% lidocaine with 1:80,000 units of adrenaline are injected subcutaneously into the upper eyelid remnants and into the lower eyelid.

2. The upper lid defect is measured horizontally while gently drawing the edges of the wound together.
3. A three-sided inverted U-shaped incision is marked on the lower eyelid using gentian violet, beginning 4 to 5 mm below the eyelid margin (Fig. 12.41).
4. A 4/0 silk traction suture is passed through the gray line of the lower eyelid, which is everted over a Desmarres retractor.
5. A conjunctival incision is made below the tarsus (Fig. 12.42A).
6. A conjunctival flap is fashioned and dissected into the inferior fornix and onto the globe.
7. The Desmarres retractor is removed.
8. The flap is advanced into the upper eyelid defect and sewn edge to edge to the remaining upper forniceal conjunctiva using 7/0 Vicryl sutures, which are carefully passed through the subconjunctival

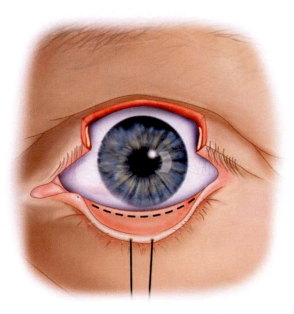

(A)

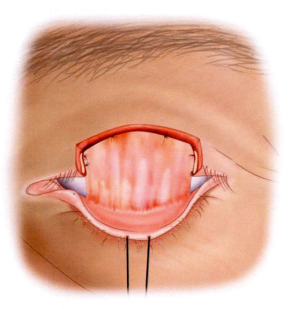

(B)

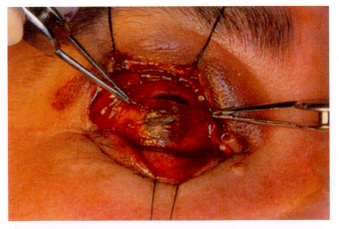

(C)

Figure 12.42 (**A**) A horizontal incision is made through the conjunctiva just below the tarsus. (**B, C**) The conjunctival flap is sutured to the cut edge of the superior forniceal conjunctiva.

tissue with great care being taken to avoid corneal irritation.

9. The cornea is now protected (Fig. 12.42B).
10. Tarsal support to the upper eyelid is replaced by placing an autogenous auricular cartilage graft, which has been suitably shaped, anterior to the conjunctival flap (Fig. 12.43). The technique of harvesting an auricular cartilage graft and the postoperative care is outlined in chapter 13. The alternative is to use an autogenous tarsoconjunctival graft as described above.
11. The edges of the graft are sutured edge to edge to either tarsal remnants or to local periosteal flaps using 5/0 Vicryl sutures.
12. The edge of the levator aponeurosis is sutured to the anterior surface of the superior one-third of the auricular cartilage or tarsoconjunctival graft. If the levator aponeurosis has been resected it may be necessary to interpose a "spacer," e.g., a piece of autogenous temporalis fascia.
13. Next, an incision is made horizontally through the lower eyelid skin and orbicularis muscle just below the tarsus and extended inferiorly to create a skin–muscle advancement flap (Fig. 12.44).
14. The lower lid skin–muscle flap is then advanced posterior to the remaining lower lid tarsal and lid margin bridge to cover the auricular cartilage or tarsoconjunctival graft (Fig. 12.43).
15. The skin-muscle flap is then sutured to the residual upper lid skin using interrupted 7/0 Vicryl sutures (Fig. 12.45).
16. Topical antibiotic ointment is instilled into the eye and the eye closed.
17. A Jelonet dressing is placed over the eye, followed by two eye pads and a firm compressive bandage to prevent excessive swelling.

Postoperative Care

The dressings are removed after 72 hours. Topical antibiotic ointment is applied to the wounds for 2 weeks. The skin sutures are removed after 2 weeks. Preservative free topical lubricants are prescribed for a few weeks.

The bridge flap is left intact for at least 8 weeks prior to separation. Typically, the lower eyelid margin will become ectropic, particularly in an older patient, and the exposed tarsal conjunctiva should be kept protected with the frequent application of Lacrilube ointment. The patient should also use Lacrilube ointment to massage the reconstructed upper eyelid for at least 3 minutes three times per day commencing 2 weeks postoperatively, until the second stage is undertaken.

Second Stage

Surgical Procedure

1. Four to five milliliters of 0.5% Bupivacaine with 1:200,000 units of adrenaline mixed 50:50 with 2% lidocaine with 1:80,000 units of adrenaline are injected subcutaneously into the reconstructed upper eyelid and into the lower eyelid.
2. A very careful skin incision is made through the flap at a position inferior to the lower lid bridge margin using a no. 15 Bard Parker blade.
3. Blunt-tipped Westcott scissors are then used to dissect the bridge flap so that the skin edge is recessed relative to the conjunctiva. Great care is taken to protect the underlying globe from the scissors.
4. The conjunctiva and skin are then sutured together, leaving the edge of the reconstructed eyelid covered by conjunctiva (Fig. 12.46).
5. The inferior margins of the lower lid bridge are freshened with Westcott scissors and the skin edges are sutured to the surrounding lower lid skin.
6. It is common for the lower lid to require a wedge resection at this second stage.

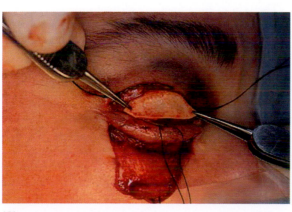

(A)

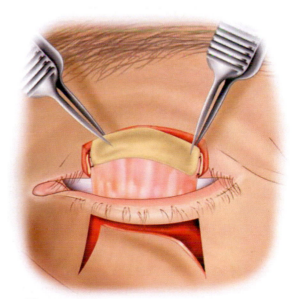

(B)

Figure 12.43 (**A**) An auricular cartilage graft is used to reconstruct the upper eyelid tarsal plate. (**B**) The cartilage graft is sutured to the tarsal remnants or periosteal flaps and to the remaining levator aponeurosis.

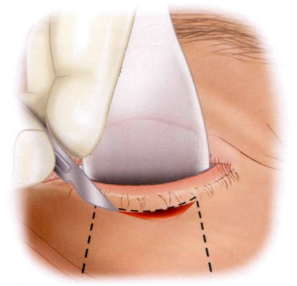

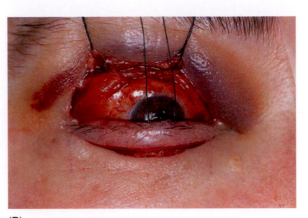

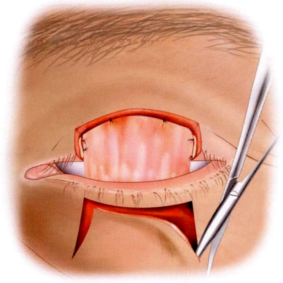

Figure 12.44 (**A**) A horizontal incision is made through the eyelid 4 to 5 mm below the eyelid margin to match the dimension of the upper eyelid defect. (**B**) The incision here is shown before the conjunctival flap has been dissected. (**C**) Two parallel vertical incisions are made to create a skin–muscle advancement flap.

7. Topical antibiotic ointment is instilled into the eye and the eye closed.
8. A Jelonet dressing is placed over the eye, followed by two eye pads and a firm compressive bandage to prevent excessive swelling.

Postoperative Care

The dressings are removed after 24 hours. Topical antibiotic ointment is applied to the wounds for 2 weeks. The skin sutures are removed after 2 weeks. Preservative-free topical lubricants are prescribed and are usually required for the long term.

COMPLICATIONS

It is extremely important to ensure that sutures are kept away from the cornea. It is very difficult to assess a complaint of a foreign body sensation following this reconstruction. Exposed

suture ends abrading the cornea can lead to severe corneal morbidity.

The skin of the upper eyelid may slide anteriorly, bringing fine skin hairs into contact with the cornea. This can be managed either with the application of cryotherapy or with a skin resection at the lid margin, leaving the area to granulate.

A typical result following a Cutler–Beard reconstruction of an upper eyelid defect is shown in Figure 12.47. The use of a large labial mucous membrane graft in conjunction with a Cutler–Beard procedure for the reconstruction of a more extensive upper eyelid and conjunctival defect is demonstrated in Figure 12.48.

Full-thickness Eyelid Composite Graft

A full-thickness en bloc section of tissue from the other upper eyelid may be transplanted into defects of the upper eyelid margin (Fig. 12.49). This technique is useful for upper eyelid

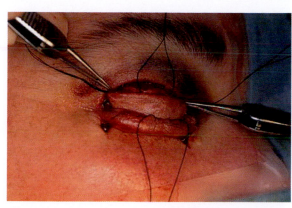

(A)

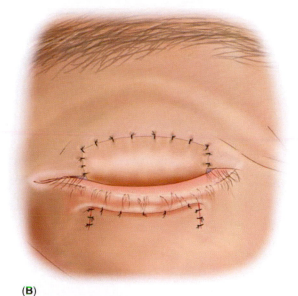

(B)

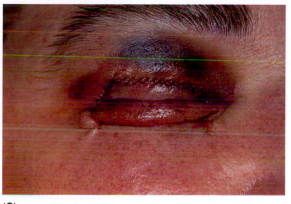

(C)

Figure 12.45 (**A**) The skin–muscle flap is advanced under the lower lid margin. (**B**) The skin edges are closed with interrupted 7/0 Vicryl sutures. (**C**) The appearance of the reconstructed eyelid at the completion of the firs stage of surgery.

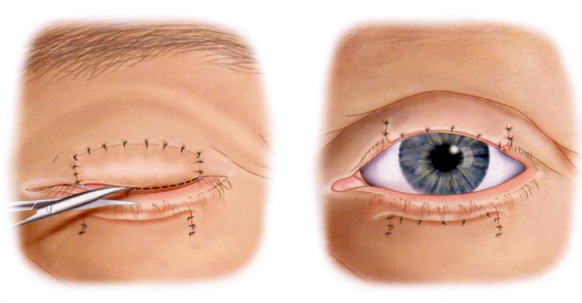

(A)   (B)

Figure 12.46 (**A**) The flap is divided with blunt tipped Westcott scissors, leaving a frill of conjunctiva. (**B**) The lower eyelid defect is refashioned and closed.

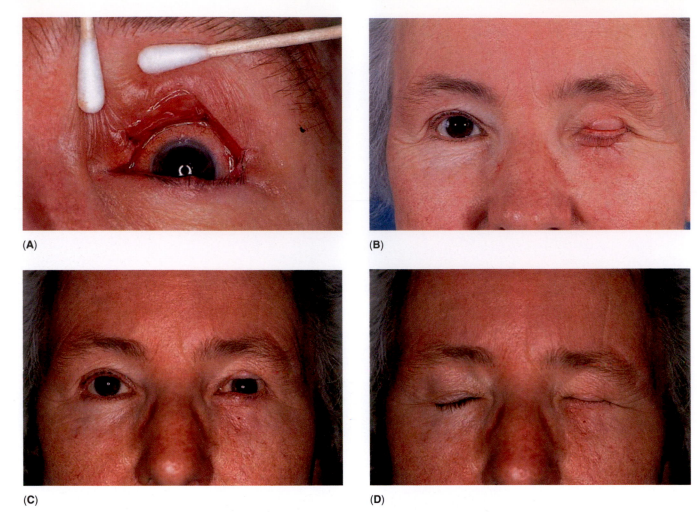

Figure 12.47 (**A**) An extensive upper eyelid defect. (**B**) The postoperative appearance 6 weeks following a Cutler-Beard reconstruction. (**C**) The appearance of the upper eyelid reconstruction 4 weeks following division of flaps and a wedge resection of the lower eyelids. (**D**) A satisfactory passive closure of the reconstructed upper eyelid.

reconstruction in a monocular patient, because it does not occlude the visual axis. The en bloc wedge resection of the normal eyelid should be should be done only when the remaining normal eyelid can be easily repaired by direct closure without risking a mechanical ptosis or a dehiscence from undue tension on the wound. The lashes of the transplanted lid rarely survive but the graft can provide a good eyelid margin. The overlying skin and orbicularis are removed and a rotation/advancement flap fashioned to cover the graft.

Surgical Procedure
The surgical technique and aftercare are outlined in chapter 13.

Rotation of the Lower Lid (The Switch Flap)
Rotation and inversion of the lower lid margin and tarsus into an upper lid defect provides good lid function as well as lashes for the upper eyelid. This procedure is best used, however, for large upper lid defects and it necessitates complete reconstruction of the lower eyelid margin, often utilizing a lateral Mustardé cheek flap reconstruction combined with a hard palate or nasal chondromucosal graft for the reconstruction of the lower eyelid tarsus and conjunctiva. This technique is particularly useful for reconstruction of upper eyelid colobomata.

First Stage
Surgical Procedure
1. The lower eyelid flap is marked to correspond to the upper eyelid defect using gentian violet (Fig. 12.50A).
2. Four to five milliliters of 0.5% Bupivacaine with 1:200,000 units of adrenaline mixed 50:50 with 2% lidocaine with 1:80,000 units of adrenaline are injected subcutaneously into the upper eyelid remnants and into the lower eyelid.
3. The lower eyelid margin is incised vertically with a no. 15 Bard Parker blade just lateral to the inferior punctum. Using sharp-tipped iris scissors, the incision is then continued inferiorly to a position 2 to 3 mm below the tarsus.
4. A horizontal full-thickness incision is made inferiorly in the lower eyelid flap, leaving a 5-mm pedicle intact laterally (Fig. 12.50B).
5. The lower eyelid margin is then inverted and sutured into the upper lid defect in layers using interrupted sutures (Fig. 12.50C). The conjunctiva and skin are reapproximated using 7/0 Vicryl sutures and the levator is sutured to the orbicularis muscle using 5/0 Vicryl sutures.

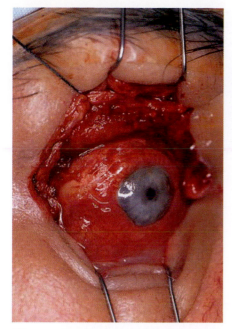

(A)

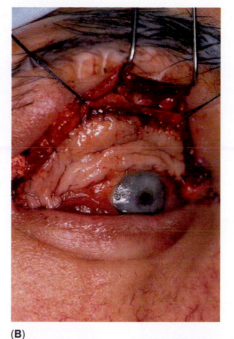

(B)

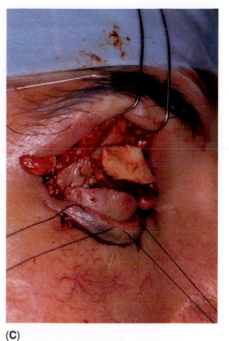

(C)

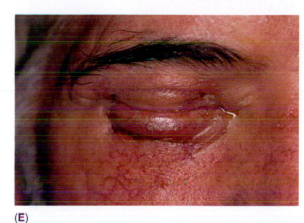

(D)

(E)

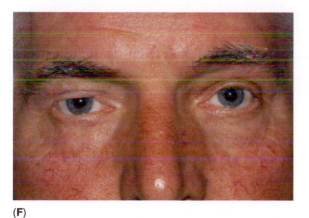

(F)

(G)

Figure 12.48 (**A**) Total loss of the upper eyelid and superior bulbar conjunctiva following tumor resection. (**B**) Reconstruction of the conjunctival defect with a labial mucous membrane graft. (**C**) A Cutler-Beard reconstruction with an autogenous auricular cartilage graft. (**D**) The appearance 2 weeks postoperatively. (**E**) A close-up photograph of the first stage reconstruction. (**F**) The postoperative appearance 5 years following the reconstruction showing a rather flat contour of the eyelid but with a quiet white eye and a clear cornea. (**G**) The patient has good voluntary eyelid closure.

6. Topical antibiotic ointment is instilled into the eye and the eye closed.
7. A Jelonet dressing is placed over the eye, followed by two eye pads and a firm compressive bandage to prevent excessive swelling.

Postoperative Care

The dressings are removed after 48 hours. Topical antibiotic ointment is applied to the wounds for 2 weeks. Arrangements are made to divide the flap 4 to 6 weeks postoperatively.

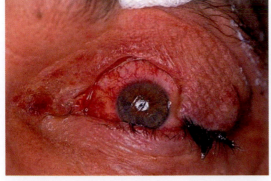

(A)

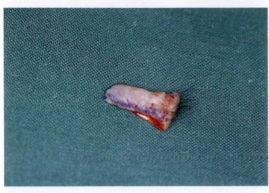

(B)

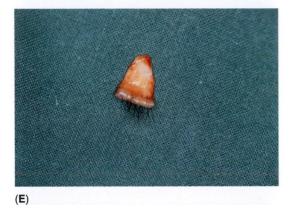

(C)

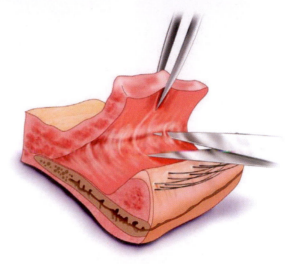

(D)

(E)

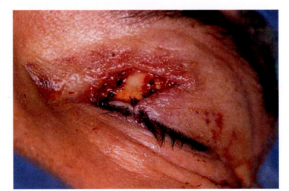

(F)

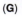

(G)

Figure 12.49 (**A**) An extensive upper eyelid defect. (**B**) A wedge resection marked out on the contralateral upper eyelid. (**C**) The resected eyelid tissue. (**D**) A drawing demonstrating the removal of skin and muscle from the eyelid graft. (**E**) The appearance of the prepared graft. (**F**) The graft sutured into the upper eyelid defect. A lateral canthotomy and superior cantholysis have also been performed. (**G**) The appearance 4 weeks postoperatively.

Second Stage

1. Four to five milliliters of 0.5% Bupivacaine with 1:200,000 units of adrenaline mixed 50:50 with 2% lidocaine with 1:80,000 units of adrenaline are injected subcutaneously into the reconstructed upper eyelid and into the lower eyelid remnants.

2. The pedicle is cut with straight iris scissors taking great care to avoid inadvertent injury to the globe (Fig. 12.50D).

3. The medial aspect of the upper lid wound is opened with blunt-tipped Westcott scissors sufficiently to suture the rotated lower eyelid into position. The medial upper lid wounds are closed in layers (Fig.12.50E).

4. The edges of the lower eyelid remnants are freshened with Westcott scissors and the lower eyelid is reconstructed using a Mustardé cheek rotation flap and posterior lamellar graft or island flap as described above.

Postoperative Care

This is as described above for a Mustardé cheek rotation flap. In addition, preservative free topical lubricants should be prescribed for long term use.

EYELID DEFECTS NOT INVOLVING THE EYELID MARGIN

If a small skin defect can be closed directly, this should be performed horizontally, leaving a vertical scar in order to prevent vertical contracture of the wound and secondary lagophthalmos or eyelid retraction. If horizontal direct closure of the tissue is not possible, a local flap can be used or a full-thickness skin graft may be placed over the defect to prevent lagophthalmos.

FULL-THICKNESS LOSS OF UPPER AND LOWER LIDS

Reconstruction of the upper eyelid becomes much more of a challenge when additional periocular tissue and part of the lower eyelid has been lost. The type of reconstruction will then depend very much on the age and general health of the patient and the visual status of the fellow eye. Frequently, concerns about cosmesis will have to be sacrificed to concerns about adequate corneal protection.

When a full-thickness defect includes the entire upper and lower eyelids, the goal of reconstruction becomes preservation of the globe by complete coverage with mucous membrane and skin tissue. Usually, sufficient conjunctiva is available on the bulbar surface to allow undermining and reflection over the corneal surface. The reflected bulbar conjunctiva inferiorly is sutured to the reflected conjunctiva superiorly. This can then be covered with a full-thickness skin graft or a rotation flap from the lateral face or mid-forehead. After maturation of the tissue, a small opening can be made to permit some central vision. Because the upper and lower eyelids are immobile, only a small palpebral fissure should be created to minimize the risk of lagophthalmos and exposure.

If available bulbar conjunctiva is insufficient to cover the globe, full-thickness buccal mucous membrane may be grafted to the posterior surface of the lateral cheek or midline forehead flap to provide a mucosal lining for the globe.

When ample conjunctiva with a good blood supply is available, the reflected mucosal covering may be adequate to support full-thickness skin grafting externally as an alternative to larger rotation flaps.

MEDIAL CANTHAL RECONSTRUCTION

The medial canthal region is a unique area that represents the convergence of skin units of differing texture, thickness and contour. The unique contour of the medial canthal region is dependent on the interrelationship of the eyelids, brow, cheek, nose, and glabellar regions. This can present difficulties in the reconstruction of surgical defects in this region.

Medial canthal tumor defects can be closed by a variety of methods depending on their size, location, depth, patient age, and patient preference. Spectacle wear by the patient should also be taken into account. The methods include:

1. Laissez-faire
2. Full-thickness skin grafting
3. A variety of local flaps, e.g., a glabellar flap, a bilobed flap, a rhomboid flap, and a median forehead flap
4. A pericranial flap combined with full-thickness skin grafting

If the lacrimal drainage system has been sacrificed, it is not formally reconstructed at the time of reconstruction of a medial canthal tumor defect. The patient may in fact remain symptom-free. If postoperative epiphora is problematic, a conjunctivo-dacryocystorhinostomy with placement of a Lester Jones tube may be undertaken. It is preferable to ensure that the patient has been free from any signs of recurrence of the tumor for a period of at least 3 years before disturbing the local periosteum, an important tumor barrier.

Laissez-faire

Laissez-faire (leaving a wound to heal by secondary intention) can yield excellent results in the medial canthal region, and avoids the need for additional scars in the glabella, medial canthal, and nasal areas. This is particularly useful for small defects in the medial canthus and for defects in elderly or medically unfit patients. It can, however, lead to unsatisfactory scarring and unpredictable results in younger patients. An unsatisfactory result for an elderly patient who declined a formal reconstruction of her extensive medial canthal defect is shown in Figure 12.51.

The term "managed" laissez-faire refers to the active manipulation of a wound before it is allowed to heal by secondary intention. A medial canthal wound can be reduced in size by drawing in the edges of the wound with interrupted 7/0 Vicryl sutures which are fixated to deeper structures within the base of the wound. The patient should be instructed to keep the wound clean and to apply topical antibiotic ointment, but the patient should also be instructed not to remove any surface eschar but to allow this to separate spontaneously.

The main disadvantage of the technique of "managed" laissez-faire is that the wound may take some weeks to heal completely.

Full-thickness Skin Grafting

Full-thickness skin grafting generally yields very good results in the medial canthus, provided the defect is not too deep. Deep defects exposing bone require a local flap. Skin grafting takes longer to perform than a local flap unless an assistant is available to harvest the graft and close the donor site. Patients with thick sebaceous skin are prone to "pin cushioning" of the graft, which will require massage and patience before a satisfactory result is achieved after a period of many months.

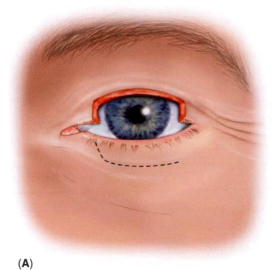

(A)

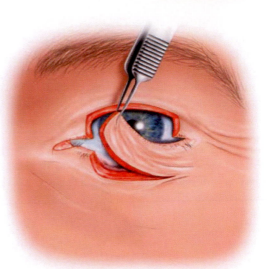

(B)

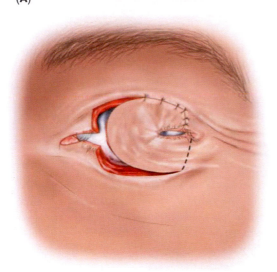

(C)

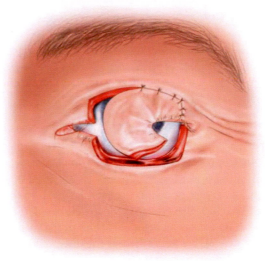

(D)

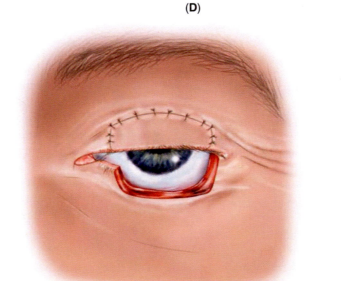

(E)

Figure 12.50 (**A**) The lower eyelid flap is marked to correspond to the upper eyelid defect using gentian violet. (**B**) A horizontal full-thickness incision is made inferiorly in the lower eyelid flap, leaving a 5-mm pedicle intact laterally. (**C**) The lower eyelid margin is then inverted and sutured into the upper lid defect in layers using interrupted sutures. The dotted line shows the position at which the pedicle will be divided at the second stage. (**D**) The pedicle is cut and dissected free of its attachments to the lower eyelid. (**E**) The medial aspect of the upper lid wound is opened with blunt-tipped Westcott scissors, sufficiently to suture the rotated lower eyelid into position. The medial upper lid wounds are then closed in layers. The resulting lower lid defect will need to be reconstructed using a Mustardé cheek rotation flap and a posterior lamellar graft.

Local Flaps

A local flap procedure is relatively quick to perform but such a flap may hide tumor recurrence. As with any formal reconstructive technique other than direct closure, it should only be used after ensuring complete tumor excision by histological monitoring of all the margins of the excised tissue. A number of different flaps can be used including the glabellar flap, the rhomboid flap, and the bilobed flap.

Glabellar Flap

The glabellar flap is a time-honored local flap used for medial canthal reconstruction. The glabellar flap is a V–Y flap which allows the transposition of skin from the glabellar region into a defect. The ideal defect for this flap does not extend laterally below the brow or too far below the medial canthus into the skin of the cheek. It is rounded, so that width and height of the defect are approximately the same.

A number of factors predispose to unsatisfactory results with the glabellar flap, including a large and irregular medial canthal defect; a defect extending across the nose; a defect extending laterally under the brow; young patients; tight facial skin; a very deep medial canthus; a very oval defect oriented vertically and extending well below the lower eyelid; or patients with a continuous brow.

The outline of the flap begins with the location of the apex of the V within the glabellar region. The first arm of the V arises directly from the defect and passes superomedially toward the apex across the medial brow. The second arm arises from the apex at an angle to the first arm and passes inferiorly. The V of the flap thus has two arms, and once the flap has been raised, it has three borders: an inferior, a lateral, and a superior border.

Surgical Procedure

1. Five to seven milliliters of 0.5% Bupivacaine with 1:200,000 units of adrenaline mixed 50:50 with 2% lidocaine with 1:80,000 units of adrenaline are injected subcutaneously into the glabella.
2. The skin is incised along the gentian violet markings using a no. 15 Bard Parker blade.
3. The flap is undermined using Stevens tenotomy scissors. Dissection should be deep to include the

subdermal plexus but should not extend into the procerus or corrugator supercilii muscles. A superficial dissection risks flap necrosis but provides a thinner cosmetically superior flap.

4. Once the flap has been raised, there is a very large defect continuous with the original defect (Fig. 12.52).
5. Closure commences vertically to create a V–Y pattern, and this is facilitated by undermining the tissue margins.
6. Deep 5/0 Vicryl sutures are placed to reduce the tension on the skin closure, which is performed with either 6/0 nylon or 7/0 Vicryl sutures.
7. Once the vertical closure is complete, the original defect is closed with the flap.
8. The deep surface of the flap is anchored to the periosteum with a 5/0 Vicryl suture to reform the concave contour of the medial canthus.
9. Some redundant tissue at the apex of the flap is excised as required.
10. The nasal skin is closed with 6/0 Novafil vertical mattress sutures and the lid skin is closed with 7/0 Vicryl sutures.
11. Antibiotic ointment is applied to the wounds.
12. A dental roll wrapped in Jelonet is applied over the medial canthal flap followed by a further sheet of Jelonet ensuring that the eye is closed and a firm pressure bandage is applied. These measures help prevent the formation of a hematoma and aid in reforming the concave contour of the medial canthus.

Postoperative Care

The dressings are removed after 48 hours. Topical antibiotic ointment is applied to the wounds for 2 weeks. The skin sutures are removed after 2 weeks. Postoperative massage using Lacrilube ointment is commenced after 2 weeks and undertaken for 3 minutes 3 times a day for a minimum period of 6 weeks.

A typical early result of a glabellar flap reconstruction is shown in Figure 12.53.

Rhomboid Flap

The defect is conceptualized as a rhomboid shape with its long axis vertical. The rhomboid consists of two equilateral triangles placed base to base (Fig. 12.54). For medial canthal defects, there are two possible rhomboid flaps. These are constructed as follows. A line of the same length as the bases of the triangles is drawn horizontally across the nose from the base of the triangles. Two vertically oriented lines from the tip of the horizontal line are drawn at an angle of 60° (Fig. 12.54A). These lines are the same length and parallel to the side of the rhomboid. The upper flap is used because of the greater laxity of the upper nasal skin. The resultant scar is also more easily hidden. The flap is oriented parallel to the lines of maximal extensibility (LME), allowing the donor site and defect to be closed with minimal tension (Fig. 12.54B and C). The LME are perpendicular to the horizontally oriented relaxed skin tension lines (RSTL) on the bridge of the nose. The scar from closure of the flap's donor site is hidden in an RSTL. Despite three sections of the scar being oriented almost perpendicular to the RSTL

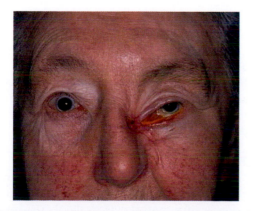

Figure 12.51 A very unsatisfactory result from laissez-faire in an elderly patient who refused medial canthal reconstruction following a Mohs' micrographic surgical excision of a basal cell carcinoma.

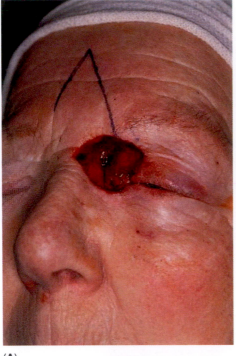

(A)

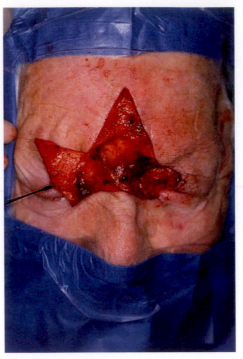

(B)

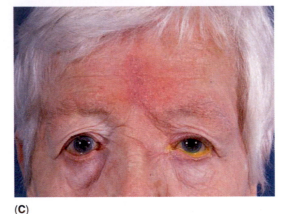

(C)

Figure 12.52 (**A**) A glabellar flap marked out. (**B**) A glabellar flap dissected. (**C**) The postoperative appearance after 2 weeks.

(Fig. 12.54D), this becomes insignificant in most cases after several weeks (Fig. 12.55).

Defects involving the areas above and below the medial palpebral ligament can be closed by rhomboid flaps from the adjoining glabellar and nasal tissues respectively. In closing inferiorly placed defects, the flap can be extended inferiorly by lengthening the vertical incision. In closing defects which extend laterally into the upper or lower lid, the lateral lid skin can be undermined and pulled medially to meet the rhomboid flap. The orientation of the defect parallel to the LME minimizes distortion on surrounding tissues. When the medial palpebral ligament has been excised, periosteal flaps can be used to reattach the cut ends of the tarsal plates (Fig. 12.56). A periosteal flap will pull the lids medially and will help reduce the size of the defect (Fig. 12.57).

The rhomboid flap is extremely versatile. Reconstructing a medial canthal defect with a rhomboid flap enables a close skin match and potentially better cosmesis. A rhomboid flap is quicker to perform than a glabellar flap, is less invasive, and has much shorter suture lines, which heal with less obvious scars in many cases. It can be combined with other medial canthal and periocular reconstructive procedures (Fig. 12.58).

Surgical Procedure
The surgical technique and postoperative care are similar to those described for the glabellar flap above.

Bilobed Flap
The bilobed flap is also a good flap to use for the reconstruction of medial canthal defects. It is described in chapter 1. The surgical technique and postoperative care are similar to those described for the glabellar flap above.

Median Forehead Flap
This flap requires two stages. It is cosmetically disfiguring and very rarely required (Fig. 12.59). For the reconstruction of extensive deep medial canthal defects, the alternative use of a pericranial flap with a full-thickness skin graft is much preferred.

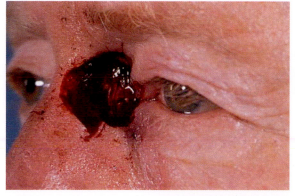

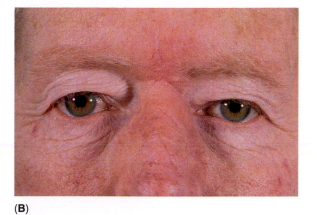

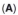

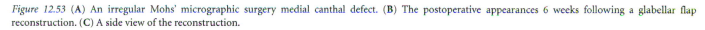

Figure 12.53 (**A**) An irregular Mohs' micrographic surgery medial canthal defect. (**B**) The postoperative appearances 6 weeks following a glabellar flap reconstruction. (**C**) A side view of the reconstruction.

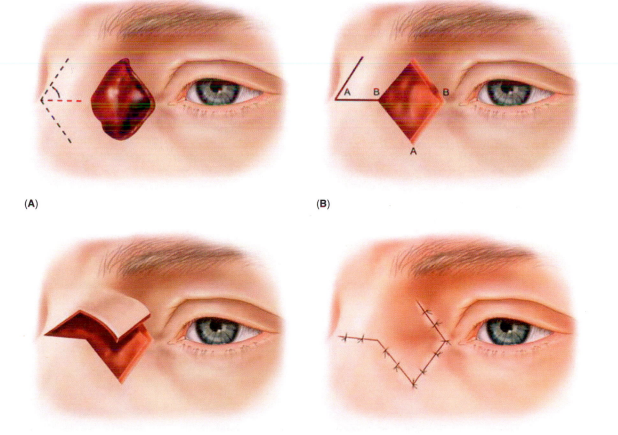

Figure 12.54 (**A**) The rhombhoid flap is marked out, selecting either a superior or inferior flap. (**B**) The incisions are made. (**C**) The flap is undermined and transposed. (**D**) The wounds are closed.

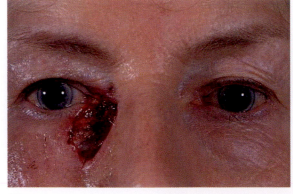

(A)

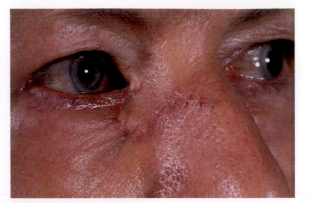

(B)

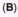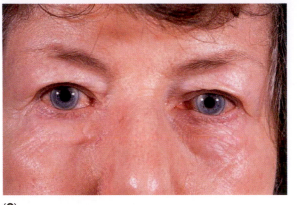

(C)

Figure 12.55 (**A**) A right medial canthal Mohs' micrographic surgery defect. (**B**) The postoperative appearance of medial canthal defect 2 weeks after reconstruction with a rhomboid flap. (**C**) The same patient 6 months after the rhomboid flap reconstruction.

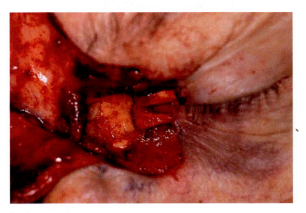

Figure 12.56 Periosteal flaps dissected from the nasal bone can be used to reconstruct a medial canthal tendon.

PERICRANIAL FLAP WITH FULL-THICKNESS SKIN GRAFT

In this procedure, a pericranial flap is dissected from the central forehead regions. The flap is based on the supraorbital vessels on the contralateral side. The flap is sutured into the medial canthal defect to provide some soft tissue volume replacement to the medial canthus and to provide a blood supply to a full-thickness skin graft, which is sutured into place over the flap

This procedure avoids placing a thick tissue flap over a site, which has the potential for tumor recurrence, and it does not affect the position of the eyebrows. The central forehead

wound leaves an unobtrusive scar in patients over the age of 50 years. For younger patients, the flap can be raised with the use of an endoscope, avoiding the need for a forehead incision.

Surgical Procedure

1. Eight to ten milliliters of 0.5% Bupivacaine with 1:200,000 units of adrenaline mixed 50:50 with 2% lidocaine with 1:80,000 units of adrenaline are injected subcutaneously into the glabella and central forehead.
2. A vertical midline incision, approximately 3 to 4 cm long, is made with a no. 15 Bard Parker blade extending superiorly from the glabella leaving a short bridge of skin and deeper tissue between the inferior aspect of the incision and the superior aspect of the medial canthal defect under which the pericranial flap may be tunnelled (Fig. 12.60B).
3. The tissues are dissected down to the pericranium using blunt dissection with Stevens tenotomy scissors, exposing the desired width and length of the pericranial flap while the skin edges are retracted with Desmarres retractors.
4. The required length of the flap is determined by holding a rolled 2 inch × 2 inch gauze swab at the base of the flap's pedicle in the glabella and then extending the swab superiorly toward the hairline. The swab is then rotated to lie in the medial canthal defect. The length of the swab is adjusted until it

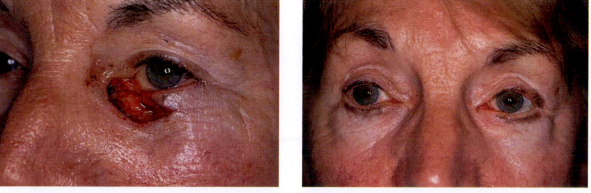

(A)   **(B)**

Figure 12.57 (**A**) A right lower eyelid Mohs' micrographic surgery defect. (**B**) The postoperative result following reconstruction using a medial periosteal flap and a small medial rhomboid flap combined with a small skin graft harvested from the ipsilateral upper eyelid.

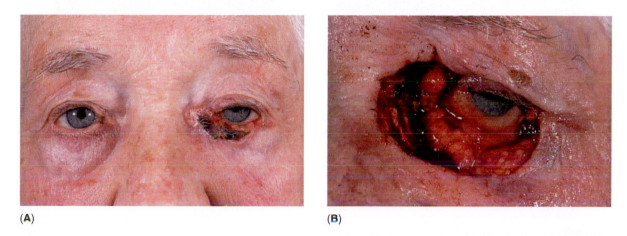

(A)   **(B)**

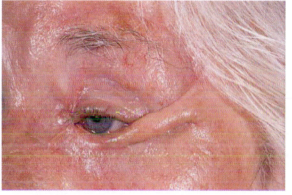

(C)   **(D)**

Figure 12.58 (**A**) A large left lower eyelid and medial canthal basal cell carcinoma. (**B**) An extensive Mohs' micrographic surgery defect. (**C**) The defects reconstructed with a rhomboid flap, hard palate graft, and Fricke flap. Appearance 4 weeks postoperatively. (**D**) The appearance 4 weeks following division of the Fricke flap.

reaches the inferior aspect of the defect without undue tension.

5. The pericranium is dried with a gauze swab and the desired dimensions of the flap outlined with a surgical marker pen.

6. The flap is then cut from pericranium using a no. 15 Bard Parker blade respecting a length to width ration of approximately 4:1 (Fig. 12.60B).

7. The pedicle is based on the supraorbital vessels on the opposite side to that of the medial canthal defect.

8. A subcutaneous dissection of the superior aspect of the medial canthal defect is performed with

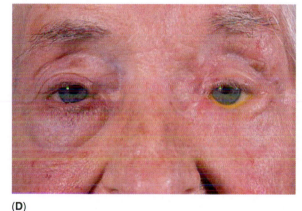

Figure 12.59 A median forehead flap reconstruction of a medial canthal defect.

Stevens scissors and the flap is rotated inferiorly into the defect so that the deep periosteal surface lies on the deep aspect of the medial canthal defect (Fig. 12.60C, D).

9. The flap is then carefully sutured into place with interrupted with 7-0 Vicryl sutures, taking care not to compromise its blood supply by applying undue stretch or tension.

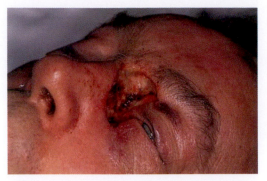

(A)

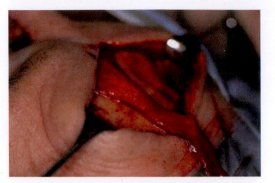

(B)

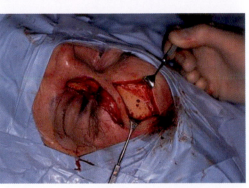

(C)

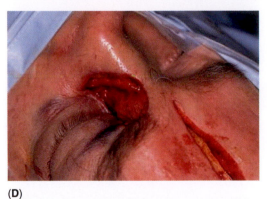

(D)

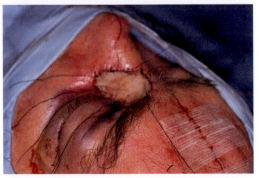

(C)

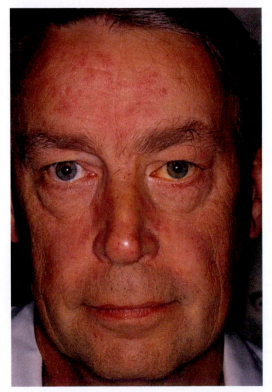

(F)

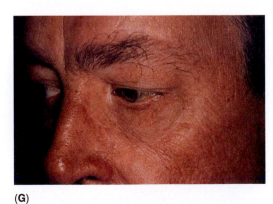

(G)

Figure 12.60 (**A**) An extensive deep medial canthal Mohs' micrographic surgery defect with exposed bone. (**B**) The forehead opened with a vertical incision and a pericranial flap dissected. (**C**) The pericranial flap mobilized beneath the bridge of tissue between the superior aspect of the medial canthal defect and the inferior aspect of the forehead incision. (**D**) The pericranial flap sutured into the medial canthal defect. (**E**) A skin graft placed over the pericranial flap. (**F,G**) The appearance of reconstructed medial canthus 9 months postoperatively.

10. A full-thickness skin graft is then sutured into place over the flap (Fig. 12.60E). Four 4/0 silk bolster sutures are placed and tied over a sponge bolster, which has been covered with a sheet of Jelonet.
11. The forehead wound is closed with interrupted subcutaneous 5/0 Vicryl sutures and then skin approximated with a subcuticular 6/0 Novafil suture. The wound is further supported with the use of Steristrips.
12. Antibiotic ointment is applied to the wounds.
13. A further sheet of Jelonet is applied ensuring that the eye is closed and a bandage is applied lightly in order to prevent undue pressure on the pericranial flap.

Postoperative Care
The dressing is removed after 5 to 7 days and the bolster sutures are carefully removed along with the subcuticular Novafil suture. The remaining skin graft sutures are removed after 2 weeks. Postoperative wound massage should be commenced 2 weeks postoperatively to prevent thickening and contracture of the graft. The massage should be undertaken in a horizontal and upward direction for 3 minutes 3 times a day after applying Lacrilube ointment to the skin graft. The application of a silicone gel, e.g., Dermatix or Kelocote is advantageous but incurs additional expense. If the skin graft shows any tendency to thicken or "pin cushion" (Fig. 13.3), it can be injected at several points with tiny amounts of triamcinolone using a 1-ml Luer lock syringe and a 30-gauge needle. The total dose injected should not need to exceed 0.3 ml.

This procedure avoids placing a thick tissue flap over a site, which has the potential for tumor recurrence, and it does not affect the position of the eyebrows. The central forehead wound leaves an unobtrusive scar in patients over the age of 50 years. For younger patients, the flap can be raised with the use of an endoscope, avoiding the need for a forehead incision.

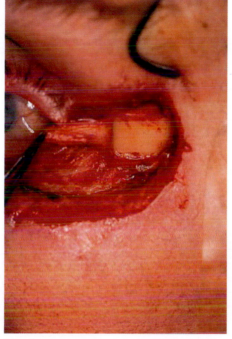

(A)

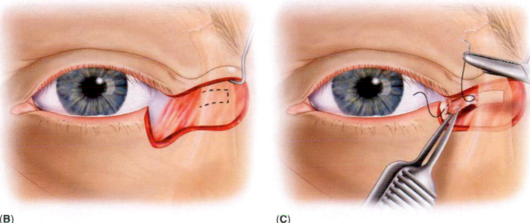

(B)   **(C)**

Figure 12.61 (**A**) A lateral periosteal flap. (**B**) A diagram demonstrating the position of the periosteal flap. (**C**) The flap is mobilized and sutured to the tarsus, recreating a lateral canthal tendon.

LATERAL CANTHAL RECONSTRUCTION

Skin defects at the lateral canthus can be reconstructed with full-thickness skin grafts or with a variety of local flaps. The rhomboid flap is particularly versatile at the lateral canthus. In reconstructing lateral canthal defects, it is important to note that the attachment of the lateral canthal tendon to the lateral orbital tubercle lies posterior to the lateral orbital margin. Attachment of eyelid tissue to the periosteum lying over the lateral orbital rim results in an anteriorly displaced lateral canthal angle.

Periosteal flaps can be raised at the lateral canthus to reconstruct a lateral canthal tendon (Fig. 12.61). A short flap may be raised by incising the periosteum horizontally. If a longer flap is required, this can be raised from the malar eminence and rotated to lie horizontally. The flap should be dissected into the internal aspect of the lateral orbital wall to mimic the anatomical arrangement of the lateral canthal tendon.

The periosteal flap may be split to form both superior and inferior lateral canthal tendon crura. The conjunctiva can be sutured to the edge of the periosteal flaps.

FURTHER READING

1. American Academy of Ophthalmology. Basic and Clinical Science Course: Orbit, Eyelids, and Lacrimal system, section 7. San Francisco, CA: The American Academy of Ophthalmology, 2006/7: 201–5.
2. Anderson RL, Gordy DD. The tarsal strip procedure. Arch Ophthalmol 1979; 97: 2192–6.
3. Bartley GB, Putterman AM. A minor modification of the Hughes' operation for lower eyelid reconstruction. Am J Ophthalmol 1995; 119: 96–7.
4. Bullock JD, Koss N, Flagg SV. Rhomboid flap in ophthalmic plastic surgery. Arch Ophthalmol 1973; 90: 203–5.
5. Cohen MS, Shorr N. Eyelid reconstruction with hard palate mucosa grafts. Ophthal Plast Reconstr Surg 1992; 8: 183–95.
6. Collin JRO. Eyelid reconstruction and tumour management. In: Collin JRO, ed., Manual of Systematic Eyelid Surgery, 2nd edn. London: Churchill Livingstone, 1989: 93.
7. Collin JRO. Eyelid reconstruction and tumour management. In: Manual of Systemic Eyelid Surgery, 3rd edn. Philadelphia, PA: Butterworth-Heinemann Elsevier, 2006: 147–64.
8. Tyers AG, Collin JRO. Colour Atlas of Ophthalmic Plastic Surgery, 3rd edn. Philadelphia, PA:: Butterworth-Heinemann Elsevier, 2008 (ISBN: 978-0-7506-8860-4).
9. Cutler NL, Beard C. A method for partial and total upper lid reconstruction. Am J Ophthalmol 1955; 39: 1.
10. Dailey RA, Habrich D. Medial canthal reconstruction. In: Bosniak S, ed., Principles and Practice of Ophthalmic Plastic and Reconstructive Surgery, vol. 2. Philadelphia, PA: W.B. Saunders, 1996: 387–200.
11. Dryden RM, Wulc AE. The preauricular skin graft in eyelid reconstruction. Arch Ophthalmol 1985; 103: 1579–81.
12. Foster JA, Scheiner AJ, Wulc AE, Wallace IB, Greenbaum SS. Intraoperative tissue expansion in eyelid reconstruction. Ophthalmology 1998; 105: 170–5.
13. Giola VM, Linberg JV, McCormick SA. The anatomy of the lateral canthal tendon. Arch Ophthalmol 1987; 105: 529–32.
14. Hewes EH, Sullivan JH, Beard C. Lower eyelid reconstruction by tarsal transposition. Am J Ophthalmol 1976; 81: 512–14.
15. Hughes WL. Reconstructive Surgery of the Eyelids, 2nd edn. St. Louis,: CV Mosby, 1954.
16. Jackson IT, ed. Local Flaps in Bead and Neck Reconstruction. St Louis, MO: CV Mosby, 1985.
17. Jordan D. Reconstruction of the upper eyelid. In: Bosniak S, ed., Principles and Practice of Ophthalmic Plastic and Reconstructive Surgery, vol. 2. Philadelphia, PA: W.B. Saunders, 1996: 356–86.
18. Leone CR. Periosteal flap for lower eyelid reconstruction. 1992; 114: 513–14.
19. Limberg AA. Mathematical Principles of Local Plastic Procedures on the Surface of the Human Body. Leningrad: Megriz, 1946.
20. Lowry JC, Bartley GB, Garrity JA. The role of second-intention healing in periocular reconstruction. Ophthal Plast Reconstr Surg 1997; 13: 174–88.
21. Maloof AJ, Leatherbarrow B. The glabellar flap dissected. Eye 2000; 14: 597–605.
22. Maloof AJ, Leatherbarrow B. The maximal Hughes procedure. Ophthal Plast Reconstr Surg 2001; 17(2): 96–102.
23. McCord CD, Nunery WR, Tanenbaum M. Reconstruction of the lower eyelid and outer canthus. In: McCord CD, Tanenbaum M, Nunery WR, eds., Oculoplastic Surgery, 3rd edn. New York, NY: Raven Press, 1995: 119–44.
24. McCord CD. System of repair of full-thickness eyelid defects. In: McCord CD, Tanenbaum M, Nunery WR, eds., Oculoplastic Surgery, 3rd edn. New York, NY: Raven Press, 1995: 85–97.
25. Mustard JC. Repair and Reconstruction in the Orbital Region. Edinburgh, UK: Livingstone, 1966.
26. Nerad J. Diagnosis of malignant and benign lid lesions made easy. In: The Requisites-Oculoplastic Surgery. St Louis: Mosby, 2001: 282–311.
27. Ng SG, Inkster CF, Leatherbarrow B. The rhomboid flap in medial canthal reconstruction. Br J Ophthalmol 2001; 85: 556–9.
28. Patrinely JR, Marines HM, Anderson RL. Skin flaps in periorbital reconstruction. Surv Ophthalmol 1987; 31: 249–61.
29. Putterman AM. Viable composite grafting in eyelid reconstruction: a new method of upper and lower lid reconstruction. Am J Ophthalmol 1978; 85: 237–41.
30. Mustardé JC, ed. Repair and Reconstruction in the Orbital Region, 3rd edn. Churchill Livingstone, 1991. (ISBN: 0-443-04023-0).
31. Rohrich RJ, Zbar RI. The evolution of the Hughes tarsoconjunctival flap for the lower eyelid reconstruction. Plast Reconstr Surg 1999; 104: 518–22; quiz 523; discussion 524–6.
32. Shankar J, Nair RG, Sullivan SC. Management of peri-ocular skin tumours by laissez-faire technique: analysis of functional and cosmetic results. Eye 2002; 16(1): 50–3.
33. Shotton FT. Optimal closure of medial canthal defects with rhomboid flaps: "rules of thumb" for flap and rhomboid defect orientations. Ophthal Surg 1983; 14: 46–52.
34. Sullivan TJ, Bray LC. The bilobed flap in medial canthal reconstruction. Aust NZ J Ophthalmol 1995; 23: 42–8.
35. Tenzel RR, Stewart WB. Eyelid reconstruction by the semicircle flap technique. Ophthalmology 1978; 85: 1164–9.
36. Tucker SM, Linberg JV. Vascular anatomy of the eyelids. Ophthalmology 1994; 101: 1118–21.
37. Weinstein GS, Anderson RL, Tse DT, Kersten RC. The use of a periosteal strip for eyelid reconstruction. Arch Ophthalmol 1985; 103: 357–9.
38. Werner MS, Olson JJ, Putterman AM. Composite grafting for eyelid reconstruction. Am J Ophthalmol 1993; 116: 11–6.
39. Wesley RE, McCord CD. Reconstruction of the upper eyelid and medial canthus. In: McCord CD, Tanenbaum M, Nunery WR, eds., Oculoplastic Surgery, 3rd edn. New York, NY: Raven Press, 1995: 99–117.

13   The use of autologous grafts in ophthalmic plastic surgery

INTRODUCTION

Autogenous grafts have widespread application in ophthalmic plastic surgery. By contrast, homologous material such as donor sclera, although very convenient to use, is no longer acceptable to the vast majority of patients because of the small risk of transmissible disease. For this reason, the use of homologous material should be avoided if possible. If the surgeon feels it is in the best interests of the patient to use homologous material, the risks must be explained to the patient and fully informed consent for its use obtained.

SKIN GRAFTS

Skin grafts may be full-thickness or split-thickness grafts. A split-thickness skin graft contains only a portion of the dermis and the graft is harvested using a dermatome (Fig. 13.1), the thickness of the graft being varied by adjustments made on the device. By contrast, a full-thickness skin graft is harvested free hand using a surgical blade. Split-thickness skin grafts contract and have a poor color match with adjacent skin. Full-thickness skin grafts show less of a tendency to contract and are much more commonly utilized in ophthalmic plastic surgery.

Indications

Full-Thickness Skin Graft
- Repair of cicatricial ectropion
- Eyelid/facial reconstruction
- Scar revision surgery

Partial Thickness Skin Graft
- Reconstruction of the exenterated socket
- Skin coverage of large facial skin defects (Fig. 13.2)

Full Thickness Skin Graft

There are a number of potential donor sites for full-thickness skin grafts:

- Upper eyelid
- Postauricular area
- Preauricular area
- Upper inner arm
- Supraclavicular fossa

The choice of donor site is influenced by a number of factors, e.g. the patient's age, the size of graft required, the degree of solar damage of the donor skin.

The upper eyelid skin is easy to harvest, provides an ideal color and texture match for eyelid defects and has no subcutaneous fat. This site does not yield much skin, however, except in older patients with marked dermatochalasis. Removing too much skin may cause lagophthalmos and may exacerbate a brow ptosis. It may also leave the patient with an asymmetrical appearance. The skin above the skin crease is removed in a similar fashion to a blepharoplasty ensuring that the skin to be removed is marked very carefully ensuring that the patient can still close the eyelids passively and ensuring that a minimum of 12 mm of skin is left between the uppermost skin marking and the lowermost part of the eyebrow.

Postauricular skin provides a relatively good color and texture match for eyelid and canthal defects. Its use may be precluded by solar damage in older patients or the use of a hearing aid. The skin to be removed is shared between the ear and the scalp in the mastoid area. The removal of large grafts can leave the ear closer to the skull. Preauricular skin is more readily accessible but may not yield sufficient skin for large defects. It is also a poor site to use in patients who have very greasy skin with prominent sebaceous glands. Such skin is more prone to contracture and a "pin cushion" effect (Fig. 13.3), particularly when used for medial canthal defects.

Surgical Procedure

Meticulous attention to detail is required in order to obtain a good result from a skin graft without complications.

1. The recipient bed must be prepared carefully and all bleeding stopped. The defect should be exaggerated in the eyelids by placing traction sutures through the gray line and placing the eyelid on traction. It must be remembered that it is frequently necessary to tighten the lower eyelid, e.g., with a lateral tarsal strip procedure before placing a skin graft.
2. A piece of Steri-Drape is placed over the defect and outlined with a marker pen (Fig. 13.4). This is cut to the exact size and shape of the defect and used as a template.
3. The template is then transferred to the donor site, where it is outlined with the marker pen (Fig. 13.5A).
4. The donor site is then injected subcutaneously with 0.5% Bupivacaine with 1:200,000 units of adrenaline.
5. The marked incision line is incised with a no. 15 scalpel blade and the graft removed using forceps and the scalpel blade (Fig. 13.5B). The skin should be held under tension as the blade is used to stroke across the skin maintaining a constant depth which should be as shallow as possible, alternatively, Westcott scissors may be used. The defect may need to be converted to an ellipse to effect adequate closure of the wound or to the typical shape of a blepharoplasty incision when the upper eyelid is used.
6. The graft is protected in a gauze swab moistened with saline. This must be stored carefully to avoid inadvertent loss of the graft.

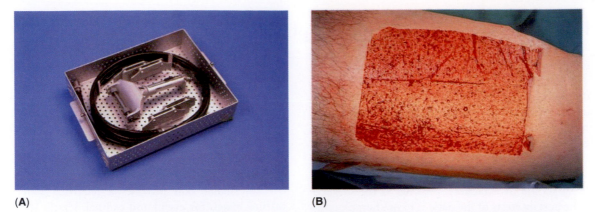

Figure 13.1 (**A**) A Zimmer dermatome. (**B**) The appearance of the donor site after removal of a split-thickness skin graft.

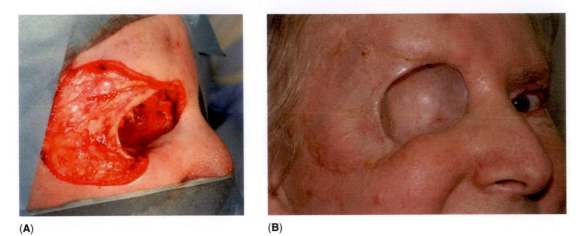

Figure 13.2 (**A**) An intraoperative photograph of a patient who has undergone a total orbital exenteration and the removal of an extensive temporal basal cell carcinoma. (**B**) The appearance of the patient 6 weeks postoperatively following the use of a split-thickness skin graft over the temple defect and in the exenterated socket.

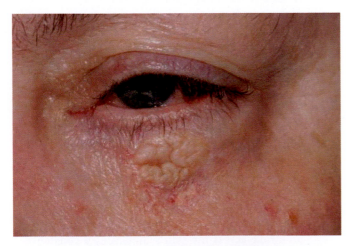

Figure 13.3 A "pin-cushioned" skin graft.

7. The donor site is closed with a 4/0 Nylon suture, either as a continuous simple or blanket suture when the pre- or post-auricular area is used as a donor site. An upper lid defect should be closed with interrupted 7/0 Vicryl sutures. An upper inner arm wound should be closed with interrupted subcutaneous 4/0 Vicryl sutures followed by interrupted 4/0 Nylon sutures for the skin placed in a vertical mattress fashion. A supraclavicular fossa donor site wound can be closed with a subcuticular 6/0 Novafil suture or with interrupted 4/0 Nylon sutures if the wound is under tension.

8. All subcutaneous tissue is completely removed with blunt-tipped Westcott scissors while holding the graft over the index finger of the non-dominant hand (Fig. 13.6). It is important to spend time meticulously thinning the graft in this way until no more tissue can be removed. Large skin grafts are perforated at several points with the tip of the scalpel blade.

9. The graft is then placed on the recipient bed and four interrupted 6/0 silk sutures are placed. The sutures are passed from graft to recipient skin edge. Interrupted 7/0 Vicryl sutures are placed between the silk sutures (Fig. 13.7). The graft should fit snugly into the recipient bed with a slight degree of tension.

10. A piece of sterile sponge is then cut to the size and shape of the graft using the original template. This is covered with Vaseline gauze and placed onto the graft. The silk sutures are tied to each other over the sponge to act as a bolster (Fig. 13.8). This prevents the accumulation of serous fluid or blood under the graft, which will act as a barrier to vascularization. This sponge can be omitted in the case of small lower lid or upper lid grafts which can be covered with Vaseline gauze alone.

11. In the case of an eyelid skin graft, the gray line silk suture is left in place and used to keep the graft stretched and the globe protected. The skin of the cheek or forehead is treated with a small amount

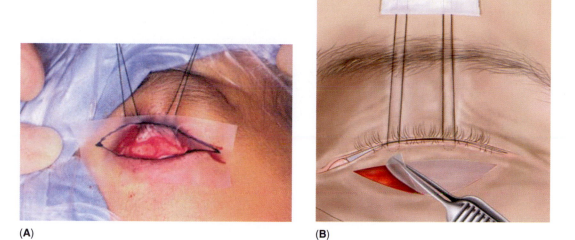

(A)   **(B)**

Figure 13.4 (**A**) A piece of Steri-Drape is used to mark a template. (**B**) The template is cut to size and placed into the defect to ensure the fit is exact.

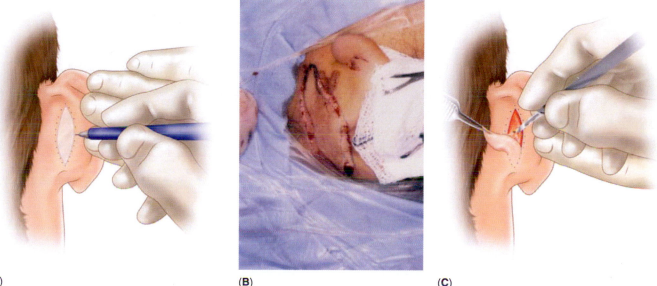

(**A**)   (**B**)   (**C**)

Figure 13.5 (**A**) The template has been placed behind the ear. The template is marked to share the skin equally between the mastoid area and the ear. (**B**) The ear is held forward with Babcock's clamps and an incision made with a no. 15 Bard Parker blade. (**C**) The skin graft is removed using a sweeping action with the blade.

of tincture of benzoin applied with a swab to dry the skin. The silk suture is taped to the cheek in the case of an upper lid graft or to the forehead in the case of a lower lid graft using Steri strips.

12. A pressure dressing consisting of a sheet of Jelonet covering the orbital area and two eye pads is applied and taped into place with Micropore® tape and this is reinforced with a head bandage.

Postoperative Care

The bandage is removed by the patient after 48 hours but the underlying dressing is maintained in place for 5 days. The dressing is then removed along with the silk sutures. The Vicryl sutures are left in place and removed no later than 2 weeks postoperatively. The sutures are also removed from the donor site at this time.

Aftercare of the skin graft is very important. The patient should avoid sun exposure for a period of a few weeks to minimize color changes in the graft. Antibiotic ointment should be applied to the graft three times per day for 2 weeks

and massage of the graft commenced after 2 weeks. Massage should be performed in several directions over the graft for a minimum period of 3 to 4 min three times per day Massage prevents contracture and thickening of the graft and should be continued for 2 to 3 months. Lacrilube (liquid paraffin) ointment is applied to the graft prior to massage. The application of silicone gel, e.g., Kelocote or Dermatix, may also help to prevent contracture and thickening of the graft, but this adds expense. If the graft does thicken, it can be injected with tiny quantities of Triamcinolone (Kenalog®) at several different sites in the graft.

Split-Thickness Skin Graft

The usual donor site for a split-thickness skin graft is the thigh.

Surgical Procedure

1. The thigh is prepared with undiluted iodine solution and the area prepped and draped. The area is injected subcutaneously at several sites using

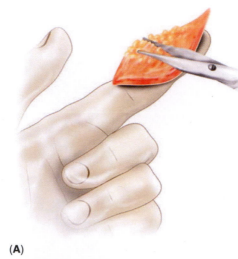

(A)

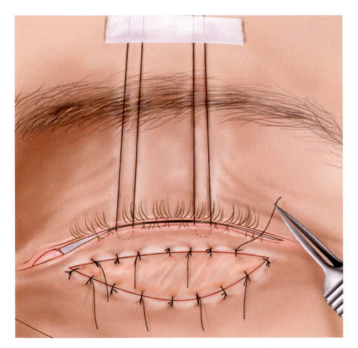

(B)

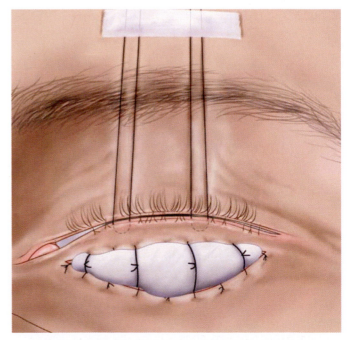

(C)

Figure 13.6 (**A**) The skin graft is draped over the index finger and Westcott scissors are used to thin the graft. (**B**) The subcutaneous fat is meticulously trimmed away. (**C**) The Westcott scissors are used to thin the graft as much as possible.

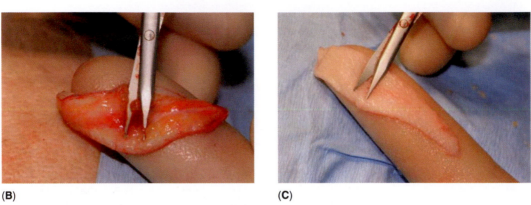

Figure 13.7 The skin graft is sutured to the recipient skin using 7/0 Vicryl sutures; 6/0 Silk sutures are used as bolster sutures.

Figure 13.8 The 6/0 silk sutures are tied over a sponge bolster.

15 to 20 ml of 0.25% Bupivacaine with 1:200,000 units of adrenaline.

2. A light coating of glycerine is applied to the thigh for lubrication.

3. The dermatome is prepared with a blade of an appropriate size and the desired thickness of the graft set on the dermatome (usually 1/16 inch). The dermatome is checked to ensure that it is working correctly.

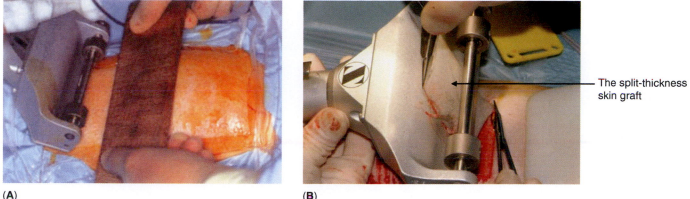

(A)   **(B)**

The split-thickness skin graft

Figure 13.9 (**A**) An assistant is flattening the skin of the thigh ahead of the dermatome. (**B**) The split-thickness skin graft is held with forceps by an assistant as the dermatome is advanced and then the attachment of the skin to the thigh is cut with scissors.

4. The assistant places a small wooden board across the thigh in front of the dermatome in order to flatten the contour of the thigh (Fig. 13.9).
5. The dermatome is applied to the thigh at a shallow angle and slowly advanced while counter traction is applied to the skin of the thigh in the opposite direction.
6. An assistant holds the skin as it emerges from the dermatome. Once the desired amount of skin has been harvested, the dermatome is stopped and the skin attachment to the thigh is cut with Stevens tenotomy scissors.
7. The skin graft is then cut and shaped according to the defect and sutured into place as described for a full-thickness skin graft.
8. The patient should be prescribed appropriate postoperative analgesia to be administered as soon as the effects of the local anesthetic agent begin to wear off.
9. Most split-thickness skin grafts in oculoplastic surgery are used to line an exenterated socket (Fig. 13.10).
10. Such grafts are first placed in a skin graft mesher and enlarged 1:2 (Fig. 13.11).

This effectively enlarges the area of the graft, reducing the size of the donor site. It also ensures egress of serosanguinous fluid. Any remaining skin is returned to the donor site, which aids the rapid healing of the donor site.

Postoperative Care
The thigh wound is covered with an Allevyn Non-Adhesive® (Smith and Nephew) foam dressing and attached using adhesive Opsite Flexifix®(Smith and Nephew) transparent film covering. A piece of Gamgee® (3M), a highly absorbent cotton roll padding with a non-woven cover, and a bandage are also applied to aid hemostasis and to reduce the amount of exudate. This dressing should be changed if any exudate leaks from it. As the wound continues to heal a less absorbent dressing may be considered and an Allevyn Thin® or Compression® (Smith and Nephew) dressing can be used to protect the area from clothing and allow the wound to completely heal. Once healed the area should be then be massaged with Vaseline.

MUCOUS MEMBRANE GRAFT
A mucous membrane graft can be removed free-hand or with the aid of a mucotome. It is generally easier and safer to remove such a graft free hand. The donor sites are the lower lip, upper lip, and the buccal mucosa. The lower lip is preferred. The access is easier and no sutures are required to close the wound which epithelialises spontaneously over the course of 2 to 3 weeks. The buccal mucosa yields more graft material but normally has to be sutured and is not as accessible. Great care must be taken to avoid damage to the parotid duct, whose opening is opposite the upper second molar tooth, when harvesting a buccal graft.

Indications
- Conjunctival replacement following an enucleation
- Fornix reconstruction
- Severe upper eyelid entropion
- Symblepharon division and reconstruction

Any patient who is to undergo an enucleation and who has conjunctival scarring from previous surgery or trauma may require a mucous membrane graft. The patient should be counseled about this possibility prior to surgery and the anesthetist should be informed. The anesthetist should place a throat pack after induction of anesthesia and should place the endotracheal tube to one side of the mouth. The donor site is injected with 0.5% Bupivacaine with 1:200,000 units of adrenaline before the patient is prepared and draped for surgery.

Surgical Procedure
1. The recipient bed must be prepared carefully and all bleeding stopped.
2. A piece of Steri-Drape is placed over the defect and outlined with a marker pen. This is cut to the exact size and shape of the defect and used as a template much in the same way as for a full thickness skin graft.
3. Two Babcock's bowel clamps are placed over the edge of the lower lip, which is protected with gauze swabs moistened with saline. The vermillion border of the lip is included in the clamps, ensuring

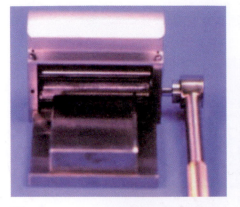
(A)

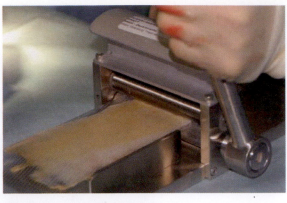
(B)

The split-thickness
skin graft

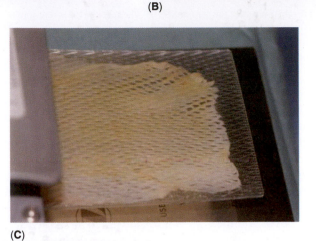
(C)

Figure 13.10 (**A**) A skin graft mesher. (**B**) The split-thickness skin graft is placed on a special plastic sheet guide and passed through the mesher device. (**C**) The appearance of the meshed graft as it passes from the mesher device.

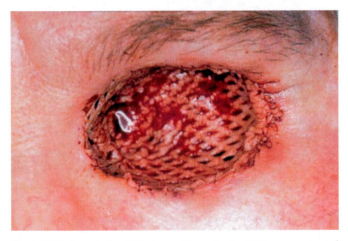

Figure 13.11 A meshed split-thickness skin graft placed into an exenterated socket.

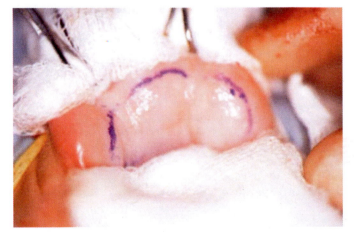

Figure 13.12 The lower lip has been marked and injected with local anaesthetic and then saline in preparation for the removal of a mucous membrane graft. The vermillion border has been protected with a saline-soaked swab and the lip is being retracted with the use of atraumatic Babcock's bowel clamps. A further swab has been placed over the tongue to soak up any blood.

that this area cannot be included in the area used to harvest the graft.

4. The template is then transferred to the donor site, where it is outlined with the marker pen after the mucosa has been dried with a dry swab.
5. The donor site is then injected with saline (Fig. 13.12). This is repeated at intervals, as it aids the dissection of the graft.
6. The marked incision line is gently incised with a no. 15 scalpel blade and the graft removed very carefully using blunt-tipped Westcott scissors and small-toothed forceps (Fig. 13.13). The Westcott

scissors should be kept just under the surface of the graft with the edge of the graft drawn horizontally to ensure that the graft is not inadvertently perforated and that the dissection is not taken too deep. Dissection in a deeper plane risks leaving areas of the lip with sensory loss. Alternatively, a mucotome may be used.

7. The graft is protected in a gauze swab moistened with saline. This must be stored carefully to avoid inadvertent loss of the graft.

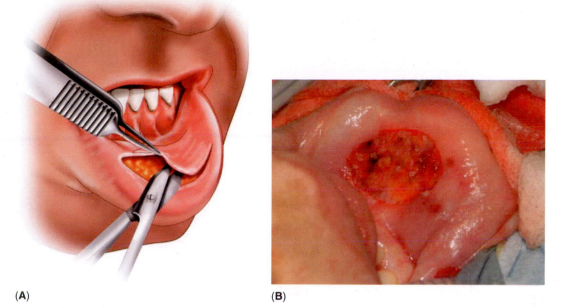

(A)

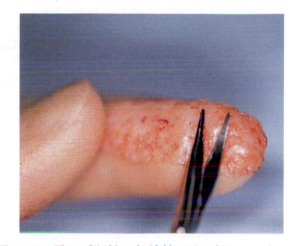

Figure 13.13 (**A**) The mucous membrane graft is harvested with blunt-tipped westcott scissors. (**B**) The appearance of the donor site after the use of bipolar cautery to secure hemostasis.

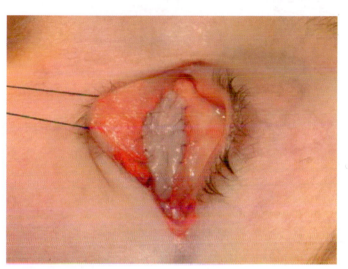

Figure 13.14 The graft is thinned with blunt-tipped Westcott scissors.

Figure 13.15 The mucous membrane graft has been sutured into the inferior fornix of an anophthalmic socket.

8. A swab gently moistened with 1:1000 units of adrenaline is held over the donor site for 5 min and then any bleeding vessels are cauterized using bipolar cautery.
9. The graft is carefully thinned with Westcott scissors removing any fibro-fatty tissue while holding the graft over the index finger of the non-dominant hand (Fig. 13.14).
10. The graft is then placed ensuring that the original graft surface faces upward, on the recipient bed and interrupted 7/0 Vicryl sutures are placed from the graft edge to the recipient conjunctival edge (Fig. 13.15).
11. The graft must be maintained in position with the use of a symblepharon ring when the graft is placed onto the globe or a conformer of an appropriate size and shape when the graft is placed centrally in an anophthalmic socket. If the graft is used to reconstruct a conjunctival fornix it should be held in place with a 240 silicone retinal band and 4/0 Nylon fornix-deepening sutures (see chap. 22).

Postoperative Care

The patient should be prescribed an antiseptic mouthwash for 7 to 10 days and should have a soft bland diet until the donor site has healed. The donor site usually re-epithelializes within 2 to 3 weeks.

HARD PALATE GRAFT

Hard palate mucosa is more rigid than lip or buccal mucosa but has a rougher surface. It does not tend to shrink more than 10% postoperatively. As a general rule it should not be used in the upper eyelid where it may abrade the cornea except in the anophthalmic patient. The anesthetist should place a throat pack after induction of anesthesia. The donor site is injected with 3 to 5 ml of 0.5% Bupivacaine with 1:200,000 units of adrenaline before the patient is prepared and draped for surgery.

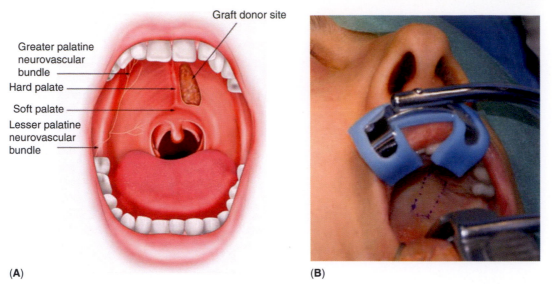

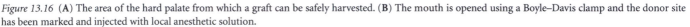

Figure 13.16 (**A**) The area of the hard palate from which a graft can be safely harvested. (**B**) The mouth is opened using a Boyle–Davis clamp and the donor site has been marked and injected with local anesthetic solution.

Indications

- A spacer in lower lid retractor recession
- A posterior lamellar graft in lower eyelid reconstruction
- A graft in severe lower eyelid cicatricial entropion surgery
- A graft for the reconstruction of a contracted socket

Surgical Technique

1. A Boyle–Davis (or similar) retractor is carefully placed, ensuring that the endotracheal tube is not displaced. The patient should be placed in a reverse Trendelenburg position. The surgeon should stand at the side of the patient and should wear a headlight. The anesthetist should tilt the head posteriorly to improve access to the hard palate.
2. The hard palate is dried with a dry swab.
3. The graft size to be harvested is measured and the margins marked on the hard palate, avoiding the gingival border, the midline and the soft palate (Fig. 13.16A).
4. An incision is made with a no. 15 Bard Parker blade through the surface epithelium and into the adipose layer beneath. The periosteum should not be disturbed.
5. The graft is then removed using a no. 66 Beaver blade keeping the dissection plane within the firm adipose layer (Figs. 13.16B and 13.17). Westcott scissors may aid the dissection once the plane has been established with the no. 66 blade.
6. The graft is protected in a gauze swab moistened with saline. This must be stored carefully to avoid inadvertent loss of the graft.
7. A patty gently moistened with 1:1000 units of adrenaline is held over the donor site for 5 min and any bleeding vessels are cauterized using bipolar cautery. The wound is left to heal by secondary intention.
8. Excess adipose tissue is removed with blunt-tipped Westcott scissors while holding the graft over the index finger of the non-dominant hand.

9. The graft is then placed on the recipient bed and interrupted 7/0 Vicryl sutures are placed from the graft edge to the recipient conjunctival edge, ensuring that the sutures are buried.

Postoperative Care

The patient should be prescribed an antiseptic mouthwash for 7 to 10 days and should have a soft bland diet until the donor site has healed. Edentulous patients may replace clean dentures after 2 days. This increases patient comfort and provides a mechanical barrier for the healing area. The donor site usually granulates and re-epithelializes within 2 to 3 weeks.

UPPER EYELID TARSAL GRAFT

A free tarsal graft is harvested from the upper eyelid. Caution should be exercised, however, in the use of such a graft as the tarsus provides structural support for the upper eyelid and the adjacent conjunctiva contains accessory lacrimal tissue. It is important to evert the upper eyelid preoperatively to ensure that the height of the tarsus is adequate. A minimum of 3.5 mm of tarsus from the eyelid margin should be left undisturbed.

Indications

- A posterior lamellar graft in eyelid reconstruction
- A graft in severe upper or lower eyelid cicatricial entropion surgery
- A spacer in lower lid retractor recession

Surgical Procedure

1. One to two ml of 0.5% Bupivacaine with 1:200,000 units of adrenaline mixed 50:50 with Lidocaine with 1:80,000 units of adrenaline are injected subcutaneously into the central aspect of the upper eyelid. A 4/0 Silk traction suture is then passed through the gray line of the upper eyelid and the eyelid is everted over a medium Desmarres retractor and a further 1 ml of 0.5% Bupivacaine with 1:200,000 units of adrenaline is injected subconjunctivally at the superior border of the tarsus.

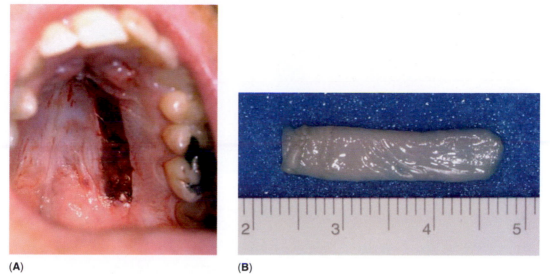

(A)   **(B)**

Figure 13.17 (**A**) The immediate appearance of the donor site following removal of the graft and the use of bipolar cautery. (**B**) The appearance of a hard palate graft with the mucosal surface uppermost.

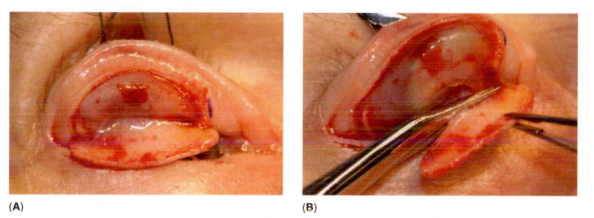

(A)   **(B)**

Figure 13.18 (**A**) The upper eyelid is reverted over a Desmarres retractor and the initial incision is made 3.5 mm above the eyelid margin. (**B**) The tarsal graft is then removed using blunt tipped Westcott scissors.

2. The tarsus is dried and a horizontal incision marked 3.5 mm from the eyelid margin with a sterile gentian violet marker pen.
3. The required width of the graft is also marked on the tarsus (Fig. 13.18A).
4. The tarsus is incised centrally along the horizontal mark with a no. 15 Bard Parker blade and the remainder of the incision is made with blunt-tipped Westcott scissors.
5. Vertical relieving incisions are made and the tarsus dissected from the underlying orbicularis muscle with blunt-tipped Westcott scissors. The graft is then cut free and removed (Fig. 13.18B).
6. The donor area is left to heal by secondary intention.
7. The graft requires no thinning or other preparation prior to its use (Fig. 13.19).

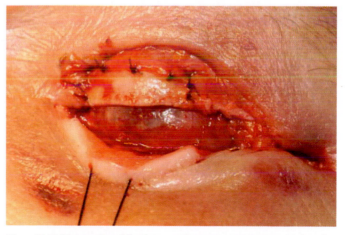

Figure 13.19 The tarsal graft has been used to reconstruct a posterior lamellar defect in the opposite upper eyelid.

Postoperative Care
Antibiotic ointment is instilled in the eye for a week.

AURICULAR CARTILAGE GRAFT
The auricular cartilage graft has a number of indications but its use is limited by the anatomical size and shape of an individual patient's pinna. In contrast to the hard palate graft, the auricular cartilage graft has the disadvantage of lacking a mucosal surface.

Indications
- A tarsal replacement in upper eyelid reconstruction, e.g., as part of a Cutler–Beard procedure (Fig. 13.19).
- A tarsal replacement in upper eyelid entropion surgery, e.g., following an overly aggressive tarsal excision during a Fasanella–Servat procedure.
- A tarsal replacement in lower eyelid reconstruction.

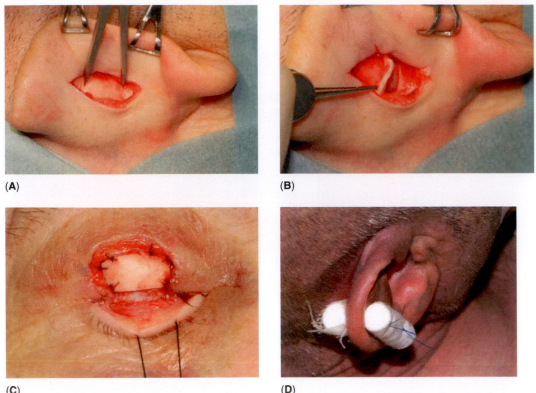

Figure 13.20 (**A**) The auricular cartilage has been exposed via an incision on the posterior surface of the pinna and the required graft is being measured. (**B**) The graft is dissected from the surrounding tissues. (**C**) The graft has been used as part of a Cutler-Beard reconstruction of the upper eyelid. (**D**) Two dental rolls covered in Vaseline gauze are tied together with Nylon sutures passed through the ear. This is done in order to prevent a postoperative hematoma.

Surgical Procedure

1. The pinna is injected subcutaneously with 0.5% Bupivacaine with 1:200,000 units of adrenaline mixed 50:50 with Lidocaine with 1:80,000 units of adrenaline, both anteriorly and posteriorly.
2. Babcock's bowel clamps are placed on the edge of the pinna (Fig. 13.20A).
3. A skin incision is made with a no. 15 Bard Parker blade over the posterior aspect of the pinna centrally. This is deepened to the auricular cartilage with blunt-tipped Westcott scissors.
4. The overlying tissues are dissected from the cartilage until sufficient cartilage has been exposed to enable a graft of sufficient size to be harvested.
5. Next, the graft size is measured and marked out with a gentian violet marker (Fig. 13.20A).
6. An incision is made with a no. 15 Bard Parker blade through the cartilage and the rest of the excision is completed with blunt-tipped Westcott scissors (Fig. 13.20B).
7. The graft is stored carefully in a moistened swab to prevent inadvertent loss.
8. The skin incision is closed with a continuous 6/0 Nylon suture.
9. Two 4/0 Nylon sutures are then passed through the pinna and tied over two dental rolls covered in Jelonet to prevent a hematoma (Fig. 13.21).
10. The graft is then cleaned of any overlying soft tissue and sutured into its recipient bed with interrupted

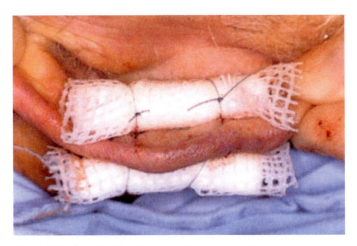

Figure 13.21 Two dental rolls are used to compress the ear to prevent a haematoma.

5/0 Vicryl sutures. Any undulations in the graft can be improved by gentle partial-thickness vertical scoring of the graft with a no. 15 Bard Parker blade.

Postoperative Care
The Nylon sutures are removed after 1 week. Antibiotic ointment is applied to the wounds for 2 weeks.

NASAL SEPTAL CARTILAGE GRAFT
A nasal septal cartilage graft makes an ideal posterior lamellar replacement for lower eyelid reconstruction where the whole of the lower eyelid has been resected. It is usually used in conjunction with a Mustardé cheek rotation flap.

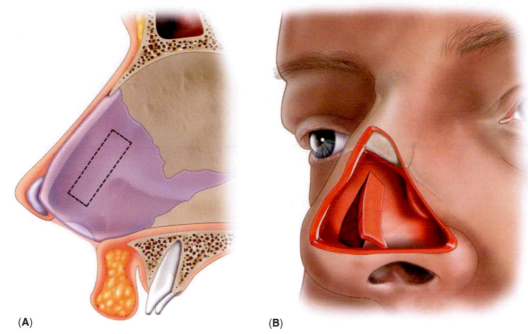

(A) (B)

Figure 13.22 (**A**) A diagram showing the position of the nasal septal cartilage to be removed. (**B**) A diagram showing the nasal septal cartilage being removed.

Surgical Procedure

1. An injection of 0.5% Bupivacaine with 1:200,000 units of adrenaline is given submucosally on one side of the nasal septum to aid separation of the mucosa from the perichondrium. This facilitates removal of the graft without the risk of perforation of the mucosa. Perforation should be avoided as this can lead to whistling and nasal crusting. The same solution is injected submucosally just above the base of the nasal septum on the opposite side in the region of the planned incision.

2. A nasal epistaxis tampon is placed into each nostril and moistened with 5% cocaine solution. This is removed after 5 min.

3. The aim is to harvest a graft measuring approximately 10 to 15 mm × 5 to 8 mm. It is important to leave approximately 0.8mm of cartilage anteriorly to avoid collapse of the nasal strut (Fig. 13.22).

4. Using a 0.4 mm nasal endoscope and a crescent blade, a superficial incision is made through the nasal mucosa at the inferior aspect of the nasal septum, leaving a strut measuring approximately 5 mm above the columella. This incision is then extended through the nasal septum using the sharp end of a Freer periosteal elevator, taking care not to perforate the mucosa on the opposite side.

5. The blunt end of the Freer elevator is then slipped between the nasal septal cartilage and the overlying mucoperichondrium on the opposite side. The elevator is kept against the cartilage and used to sweep the mucosa away. This maneuver is greatly assisted with the use of the nasal endoscope.

6. Vertical cuts are then made with straight blunt-tipped scissors and the most superior attachment of the mucosa and cartilage is severed with a no. 66 Beaver blade.

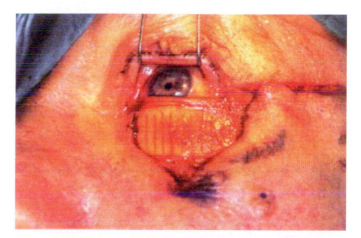

Figure 13.23 A nasal septal cartilage graft. A frill of mucosa has been left proud on the superior surface of the graft and the cartilage has been scored vertically with a blade.

7. The graft is stored carefully in a moistened swab.

8. If an endoscope is not available, the procedure can be undertaken using a nasal speculum and a headlight. If access to the nasal septum is restricted, a nasal alar incision can be made to improve the exposure. The nasal alar incision is then sutured internally with 5/0 Vicryl and the skin closed with interrupted 6/0 Nylon sutures.

9. A fresh nasal epistaxis tampon, lightly coated with antibiotic ointment is inserted into each nostril and left overnight.

10. The graft is very carefully prepared. The nasal cartilage is gently thinned by shaving excess cartilage away using a no. 15 Bard Parker blade. A small strip of cartilage is removed from the border, which will lie against the globe, enabling a strip of mucoperichondrium to be carried over the edge of the cartilage, thereby creating a new eyelid margin (Fig. 13.23).

11. The cartilage may be gently scored vertically to enable the graft to bend towards the globe.

Postoperative Care

The nasal epistaxis tampon is soaked with saline before being gently removed the following day. The nose is gently irrigated with a nasal saline douche or Sinurinse® twice a day for 2 weeks.

DERMIS FAT GRAFT

Fat can be used to replace volume and to prevent/manage subcutaneous adhesions. Dermis is left attached to the fat to provide a blood supply, but postoperative fat atrophy is very variable and unpredictable. Dermis fats in infants, used in the management of the congenital anophthalmic socket, can be seen to grow and may even need to be debulked. This is not seen in adults. Hair follicles and sebaceous units which may be left within the graft usually atrophy but may rarely be responsible for the formation of cysts and the growth of hair. The graft is usually harvested from the upper outer quadrant of the buttock but it is easier and more comfortable for adult patients for the graft to be taken from the lower lateral abdominal wall. In anophthalmic socket reconstruction, the graft may be completely buried but the surface can be left partially exposed when it is used in a volume-deficient socket, which also lacks conjunctival lining. The exposed dermis epithelializes spontaneously over a period of 3 to 4 weeks.

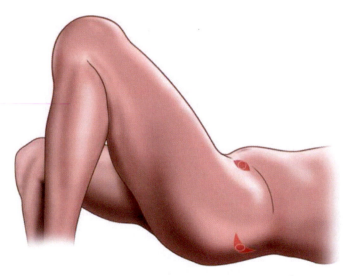

Figure 13.24 The typical donor sites for a dermis fat graft.

Indications

- A primary or secondary orbital implant
- A primary or secondary orbital implant when socket lining is also required
- A replacement orbital implant in the management of an extruding orbital implant
- Prevention/management of subcutaneous adhesions following periorbital surgery/trauma/infection
- Camouflage of upper eyelid sulcus deformity in post-enucleation socket syndrome

Surgical Procedure

1. The size of graft required is outlined on the skin with a gentian violet skin marker pen (Fig. 13.24). A graft to be used as an orbital implant is taken as a circular graft, whereas one to be used within the eyelid is taken as an ellipse (Fig. 13.25).
2. Ten to fifteen milliliters of 0.5% Bupivacaine with 1:200,000 units of adrenaline are injected subcutaneously in the marked area.
3. Saline is injected into the epidermis under pressure using a 10 ml syringe and a fine-gauge needle to create a "peau d'orange" appearance (Fig. 13.26). This is repeated at intervals as required.
4. An incision is made through the epidermis with a no. 15 Bard Parker blade. The edge of the epidermis is grasped with toothed Adson forceps and drawn away as the blade is used to sweep under the epidermis, separating it from the dermis (Fig. 13.27A). The dermis should appear quite pale with multiple bleeding points (Fig. 13.27B). No fat should be visible. The epidermis should ideally be removed in a single sheet.
5. A small incision is made through one edge of the dermis with the blade and the rest of the incision completed with Stevens tenotomy scissors (Fig. 13.28A). The fat is dissected to an approximate depth of 2 to 3 cm and removed with the overlying dermis (Fig. 13.28B). The graft is stored safely in a moistened swab.
6. The donor site is closed with interrupted subcutaneous 4/0 Vicryl sutures and interrupted 4/0 Nylon sutures passed in a vertical mattress fashion for the skin closure.
7. The graft is compressed in a dry swab before it is sutured into the recipient site. In the socket the extraocular muscles are sutured to the edges of the graft and the

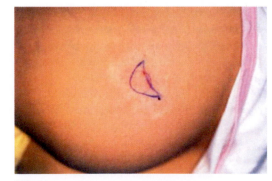

(A)   (B)

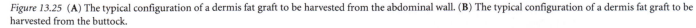

Figure 13.25 (**A**) The typical configuration of a dermis fat graft to be harvested from the abdominal wall. (**B**) The typical configuration of a dermis fat graft to be harvested from the buttock.

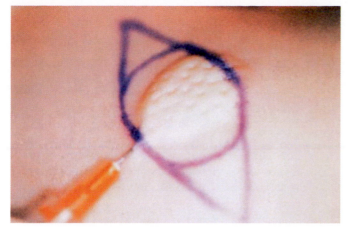

Figure 13.26 Saline is injected into the skin to create a 'peau d' orange' appearance.

conjunctiva either closed over the graft or sutured to its surface, leaving part of the dermis exposed. In the eyelid the dermis is positioned against the periosteum to which it is sutured with interrupted 5/0 Vicryl sutures. The fat is positioned to mimic the anatomical location of the preaponeurotic fat (Figs. 13.29 and 13.30).

Postoperative Care
The skin sutures are removed after 10 to 14 days.

STRUCTURAL FAT GRAFTING
Structural fat grafting is a procedure in which fat cells are harvested from the patient and re-injected into his/her facial subcutaneous tissues. In this procedure fat is harvested by syringe liposuction and the aspirated material centrifuged. This

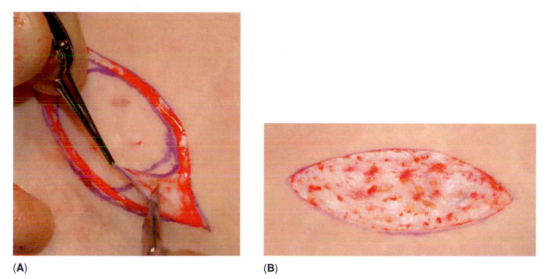

(A)   (B)

Figure 13.27 (A) The epidermis is separated from the dermis using a no.15 blade. (B) The white appearance of the dermis with the epidermis removed. There should be fine bleeding points with little if any fat exposed.

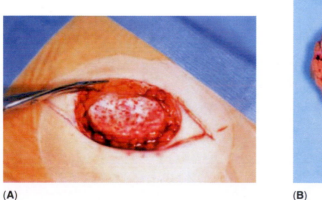

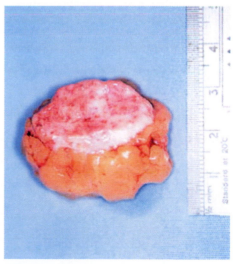

(A)   (B)

Figure 13.28 (A) The dermis fat graft is removed with Stevens scissors. (B) The typical appearance of a dermis fat graft to be used for an orbital implant in an anophthalmic socket reconstruction.

separates into three layers: the uppermost layer is composed primarily of oil, the middle layer is composed of fat, and the bottom layer is composed of blood, serum, and local anesthetic solution. The oil, blood, serum, and local anesthetic solution are removed and the separated fat cells are used for injection.

Indications

Structural fat grafting is used primarily for the cosmetic improvement of facial lines, depressions, and fat atrophy, although it is also used for the cosmetic improvement of depressions and volume loss that are seen following trauma or tumor resections, or following the development of disease states, e.g., Romberg's hemifacial atrophy. It can also be used to treat the post enucleation socket syndrome. In facial rejuvenation, it has the following indications:

- Augmentation of nasolabial folds
- Augmentation of temple hollowing
- Augmentation of the mid-face
- Cosmetic improvement of lower lid tear trough defects
- Volume enhancement of the upper eyelid
- Volume enhancement of the lateral eyebrow

Selection of the Donor Site

Although the lower abdominal wall can be used as a donor site, it is safer to use the "love handle" area, the upper outer quadrant of the buttock or the lateral aspect of the upper thigh.

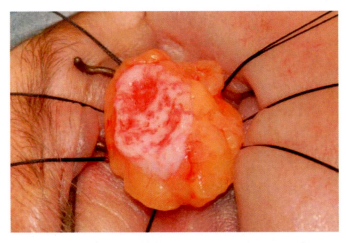

Figure 13.29 A dermis fat graft prepared and ready to be implanted into an anophthalmic socket.

Surgical Procedure

1. The areas of the face to be injected are meticulously marked out using gentian violet marker pen with the patient sitting upright.
2. The donor site area is marked out with gentian violet.
3. The areas of the face to be injected are anesthetized using regional nerve blocks. A mixture of 0.5% Bupivacaine with 1 in 200,000 adrenaline mixed 50:50 with 2% Lidocaine with 1:80,000 units of adrenaline is used. Care should be taken not to exceed the maximum safe limit of local anesthetic solution taking into account the weight of the patient.
4. Five milliliters of the same solution are injected subcutaneously into the inferior aspect of the donor site.
5. A local anesthetic solution for the donor site is prepared using a 50 ml syringe. The following are used:
   - 30 ml of saline for injection
   - 10 ml of 0.5% Bupivacaine
   - 10 ml of 2% Lidocaine
   - 0.25 ml of 1:1000 adrenaline
6. The patient is prepared and draped to allow a meticulous sterile technique.
7. A single stab incision is made through the skin at the inferior aspect of the donor site using a no. 15 Bard Parker blade in a crease, stretch mark or hair bearing area if possible to camouflage the small resulting scar.
8. Using a long blunt-tipped injection cannula attached to a 20 ml Luer lock syringe containing the anesthetic solution transferred from the 50 ml syringe, the cannula is inserted through the stab incision and advanced into the subcutaneous fat, gradually injecting the solution. A further 10 to 20 mls are injected. Ten minutes are allowed for this anesthetic solution to take effect.
9. A few tiny stab incisions are then made in preparation for the fat injections, using a no. 15 Bard Parker blade within skin creases or behind the hairline in the face or temple, depending on the sites of injection. Pressure is applied to these incisions to prevent bleeding.
10. A blunt tipped harvesting cannula is attached to a 10 cm³ Luer lock syringe.
11. The cannula is inserted through the donor site stab incision.
12. The plunger of the syringe is gently manipulated with the thumb and forefinger to provide approximately

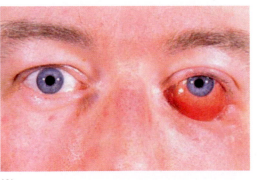

(A)

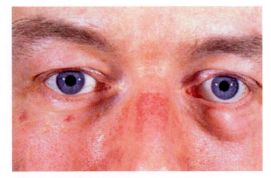

(B)

Figure 13.30 (**A**) A patient referred with an extruding silicone orbital floor implant, scarring and retraction of the lower eyelid into the orbit and chemosis. (**B**) The patient following removal of the implant, release of eyelid adhesions and placement of a dermis fat graft visible as a residual bulge in the lower eyelid.

1 to 2 cm³ of negative pressure space in the barrel of the syringe while the cannula is pushed forward through the subcutaneous fat plane.

13. The cannula is quickly moved back and forth through the fat plane while maintaining the negative pressure on the plunger.

14. After the fat has been harvested, the cannula is removed from the syringe and replaced with a cap.

15. The Luer lock cap is secured to create a seal to prevent any spillage of contents of the syringe during the centrifuging process.

16. The plunger is then removed from the proximal end of the syringe.

17. The syringe is then placed into the sterilized central rotor of a centrifuge.

18. More fat is then harvested in the same way.

19. Each 10 cm³ syringe is placed into an individual sleeve of the centrifuge. The syringes are placed evenly so that each syringe is balanced on the opposite side (Fig. 13.31).

20. The lid on the centrifuge is then closed and locked.

21. The timer is set to 3 min. The recommended centrifugation is 3000 rpm for 3 min. Some surgeons have expressed concern about the possibility of the centrifugation causing damage to the fat cells and some surgeons undertake the centrifugation for as little as 15 secs.

22. The donor site incision is closed with a 6/0 Nylon suture.

23. The cover of the centrifuge is opened only after the rotor has stopped completely.

24. The scrub nurse then removes the centrifuged syringes, taking care to avoid touching the cover or any other non-sterilized parts of the centrifuge.

25. The appearance of the syringe with the separated layers is shown in Figure 13.32.

26. The top oily layer is poured into a sterile glass container and can be used to lubricate the insertion site incisions.

27. The plug is then removed from the Luer lock connection and the blood and fluid is allowed to pour out into a kidney dish or gallipot (Fig. 13.33).

28. The syringes are placed into a sterile rack and a neurosurgical patty is gently inserted into the top of the syringe and used to soak any remaining oil.

29. Any fat, which adheres to the neuropatties or becomes exposed to air, should be discarded.

30. The plunger is replaced and advanced to remove air.

31. A metal Luer lock connector is attached to the 10-ml syringe and a 1 cm³ Luer lock syringe is attached to the other end of the metal connector (Fig. 13.34).

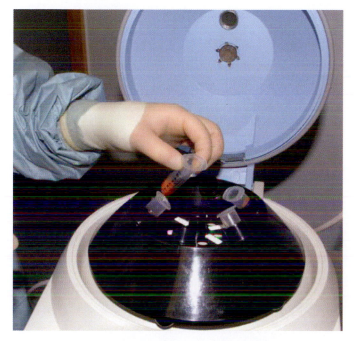

Figure 13.31 The syringes are placed in a centrifuge.

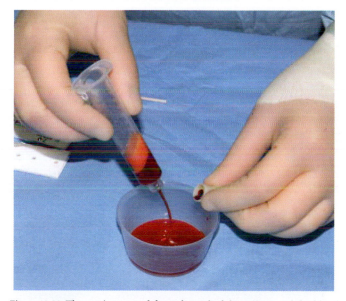

Figure 13.33 The cap is removed from the end of the syringe and the blood and local anesthetic solution is allowed to pour away.

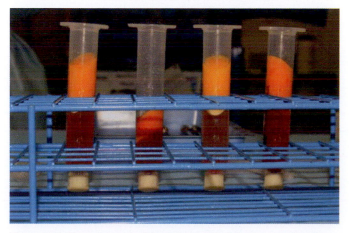

Figure 13.32 The appearance of the syringes of fat following centrifugation.

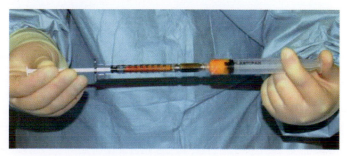

Figure 13.34 The fat is transferred to a series of 1 ml syringes.

32. By gently depressing the plunger on the 10 cc syringe and withdrawing the plunger on the 1 cm³ syringe, the fat is carefully transferred from the 10 cm³ to the 1 cm³ syringe.

33. The 1 cm³ syringe is filled to the 0.8 cm³ mark and any air is expelled before an injection cannula is attached.

34. The fat is now ready for injection into the face, eyelids, temples (or anophthalmic socket) (Fig. 13.35).

The fat should be used as soon as possible after it has been centrifuged. It should be injected using a variety of cannulae, whose tips are especially tailored to the different demands of the tissues to be injected. The tips of the cannulae are blunt to minimize the risk of intravascular injection. The cannula should be inserted while stabilizing the tissues with the opposite hand and 0.1 cm³ of fat only should be injected slowly as the cannula is withdrawn. The process is somewhat tedious, as the fat should be injected gradually and meticulously with multiple passes in different directions. The aim is to place the fat cells in contact with vascularized tissue and not to inject large quantities of fat, most of which will be sequestered and will inevitably atrophy.

In the upper eyelid, if the patient is undergoing an upper lid blepharoplasty or a levator aponeurosis advancement, the fat can be injected directly into the preaponeurotic space before the skin sutures are placed.

The temple is a relatively easy area to begin injections. As experience is gained, the surgeon can then move to the more challenging areas of the face (Fig. 13.36).

The eyelids require meticulous attention to detail and this area should not be overcorrected. The results of mid-face injections, which can be placed at a deeper level than elsewhere in the face, are particularly pleasing in patients who have mid-face fat atrophy with little mid-face ptosis. In the patient with a significant mid-face ptosis, the injections can be combined with mid-face lift surgery.

The tiny stab incisions are closed with interrupted 7/0 Vicryl sutures. No dressings are required. Topical antibiotic ointment is applied to the wounds.

Postoperative Care
The patient should sleep with the head raised at least 30° for the first few days following surgery. Sufficient analgesia should be provided to control pain at the donor site, which can be significant. Clean cool packs should be applied to the recipient sites intermittently for 48 hours. Topical antibiotic ointment to the wounds is continued for a week. Gentle massage to any

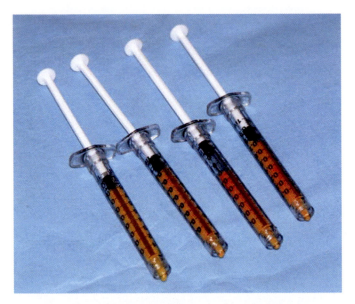

Figure 13.35 Syringes of fat prepared for injection.

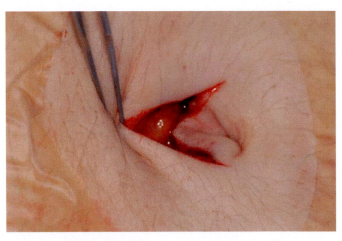

Figure 13.37 A skin incision has been made just below the umbilicus to access subcutaneous fat.

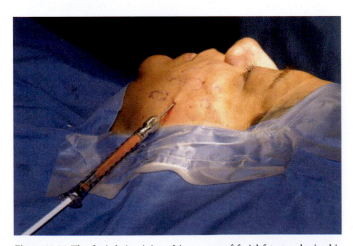

Figure 13.36 The fat is being injected into areas of facial fat atrophy in this patient via a small stab incision.

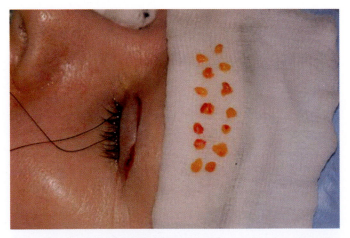

Figure 13.38 Very small "pearls" of fat have been prepared ready to insert into the preaponeurotic space of the upper eyelid.

irregular areas of fat can be commenced after a few days. The patient is advised to avoid vigorous exercise for 3 to 4 weeks.

FAT PEARL GRAFT

Fat can be harvested via a small semicircular incision just below the umbilicus (Fig. 13.37). The fat can be divided into very small fat "pearls" and placed into the eyelids e.g., following an over-resection of upper eyelid fat during a previous blepharoplasty (Fig. 13.38). The fat should not be harvested until the recipient site has been prepared. The fat should be handled meticulously and placed into the recipient site without any delay to reduce the risk of postoperative fat atrophy.

FASCIA LATA GRAFT

Fascia lata is harvested from the lateral aspect of the thigh. Its use can lead to some herniation of the vastus lateralis muscle and an obtrusive scar. It is usually harvested via an incision in the lower aspect of the thigh, although it may be removed via an incision in the superior aspect of the thigh.

Indications

- Frontalis suspension surgery
- Lower eyelid suspension
- Mid-face fascial sling in facial palsy
- Patch grafting of an exposed orbital implant
- Wrapping of an orbital implant

Surgical Technique

1. A 4 to 5 cm incision is marked approximately 10 cm above the knee joint along a line drawn from

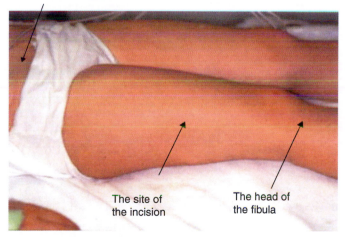

The anterior superior iliac spine

The site of the incision

The head of the fibula

Figure 13.39 The incision for the removal of fascia lata lies on a line running between the anterior superior iliac spine and the head of the fibula.

the head of the fibula to the anterior–superior iliac spine (ASIS) (Fig. 13.39).

2. The incision site and the lateral thigh at several sites along the line extending from the incision site towards the ASIS are injected subcutaneously with 10 to 15 ml of 0.25% Bupivacaine with 1:200,000 units of adrenaline. The volume used depends on the age and the weight of the patient. This is particularly important in children.

3. A skin incision is made with a no. 15 Bard Parker blade. The subcutaneous fat is bluntly dissected using Stevens scissors with a horizontal spreading action until the fascia is exposed. A dry swab is used to clean the surface of the fascia.

4. The fascia first encountered runs circumferentially in contrast to the fascia lata which runs in a vertical direction. The horizontal investing fascia is grasped with Paufique forceps and bluntly stripped in a vertical direction revealing the glistening vertical fibers of the underlying fascia lata.

5. Next a long straight Nelson scissor is inserted between the edge of the horizontal fascia and the fascia lata and pushed up the thigh for a distance of 12 to 15 cm.

6. Two small vertical incisions are made 1 cm apart in the fascia lata with a no. 15 blade. The incisions are continued along fascia up into the thigh using the long straight Nelson scissors. Small blunt-tipped straight scissors are then passed beneath the fascia and the fascia is separated from the underlying muscle along the length of the skin incision.

7. The inferior aspect of the fascia is then cut and the cut end is introduced into a Crawford fascia lata stripper (Figs. 13.40 and 13.41).

8. The stripper is passed along the line of the fascia lata, ensuring that the end of the stripper is passed under the horizontal investing fascia. It is imperative to ensure that the cutting mechanism is locked before the stripper is passed along the fascia.

9. Once the stripper has been passed along the fascia lata to the desired length, as measured on the stripper, the cutting mechanism is unlocked and activated to cut the superior aspect of the fascia.

10. The fascia and the stripper are removed and external pressure applied to the thigh for a few minutes (Fig. 13.42).

11. The fascia is carefully stored in a moistened swab.

12. The thigh wound is closed with interrupted subcutaneous 4/0 Vicryl sutures and the skin is closed

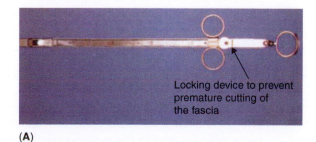

Locking device to prevent premature cutting of the fascia

(A)

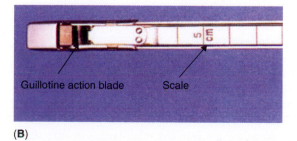

Guillotine action blade   Scale

(B)

Figure 13.40 (**A**) Crawford fascia lata stripper. (**B**) A close-up photograph of the Crawford fascia lata stripper demonstrating the guillotine action blade.

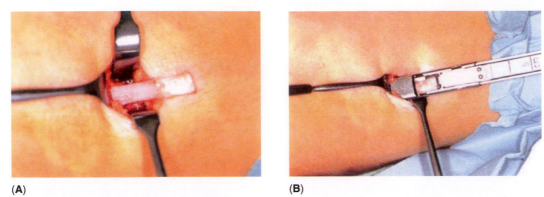

(A)   **(B)**

Figure 13.41 (**A**) The leading strip of fascia lata is dissected free. (**B**) The inferior end of the fascia lata is inserted into the stripper.

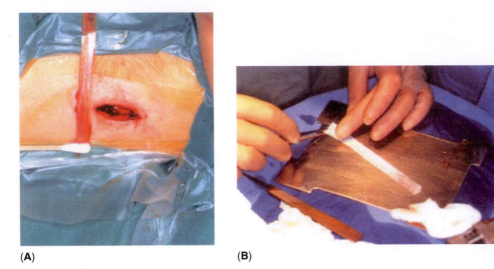

(A)   **(B)**

Figure 13.42 (**A**) The appearance of the fascia lata removed with the stripper. (**B**) The fascia is cleaned of any attached muscle and fat.

with interrupted 4/0 Nylon sutures passed in a vertical mattress fashion.

13. A pressure dressing and bandage are applied.
14. The fascia is then cleaned of any attached fat or fibrous tissue by bluntly rubbing a wet gauze swab along the length of the fascia in a vertical direction.

TEMPORALIS FASCIA GRAFT

Temporalis fascia is readily accessible and its removal leaves a scar hidden behind the hair. This site does not, however, yield the quantity of fascia which is obtainable from the thigh. It does, however, yield more than enough tissue for use in patch grafting of an exposed orbital implant.

Indications
- Patch grafting of an exposed orbital implant
- Lower eyelid suspension
- Surface wrapping of an orbital implant

Surgical Technique
1. The patient's hair is thoroughly cleaned over the temporal fossa with Chlorhexidine (Hibiscrub®) and parted with a comb posterior to the superficial temporal artery.
2. 5 to 10 ml of 0.5% Bupivacaine with 1:200,000 units of adrenaline are injected subcutaneously into the area of the proposed incision.

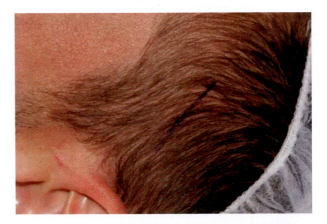

Figure 13.43 The placement of the incision for a temporalis fascia harvest.

3. A 3 to 4 cm incision is made with a No. 15 Bard Parker blade through the skin (Fig. 13.43).
4. The incision is deepened with Stevens tenotomy scissors using a spreading action until the glistening fibres of the deep temporal fascia are visible (Fig. 13.44).
5. The fascia is widely exposed with blunt dissection.
6. Desmarres retractors are inserted and the wound edges moved around to expose the fascia as required.
7. The fascia is incised with a no. 15 Bard Parker blade. The fascia is then dissected from the underlying temporalis muscle with Stevens tenotomy or blunt-tipped Westcott scissors (Fig. 13.45).

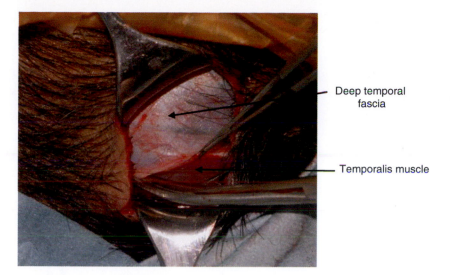

Deep temporal
fascia

Temporalis muscle

Figure 13.44 A temporalis fascial graft being removed with Westcott scissors.

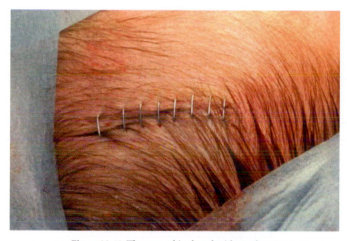

Figure 13.45 The wound is closed with staples.

8. The fascia is stored carefully in a moistened swab.
9. The wound is closed with subcutaneous 5/0 Vicryl sutures and the skin is closed with staples. These are removed after 7 to 10 days.

EYELID COMPOSITE GRAFT

Approximately one-third of the upper eyelid in an older patient may be resected without altering the appearance and function of the eyelid. In patients with marked eyelid laxity an even greater proportion may be removed. The tissue can be used for the reconstruction of a contralateral upper eyelid defect which cannot be closed directly with a lateral canthotomy and cantholysis. The same technique can be used for the lower eyelid. The technique can yield very good cosmetic and functional results but the eyelashes rarely survive (Fig. 13.49).

Surgical Technique

1. The eyelids are injected with 1 to 2 ml of 0.5% Bupivacaine with 1:200,000 units of adrenaline.
2. A full-thickness wedge resection of the upper eyelid is performed (Fig. 13.46). The defect is closed directly.
3. The skin and orbicularis muscle are removed from the tarsus with Westcott scissors (Fig. 13.47).

4. The remaining tarsus with its lid margin and eyelashes are transplanted into the opposite upper eyelid defect. The tarsus is sutured edge to edge with 5/0 Vicryl sutures (Fig. 13.48).
5. The lid margin is sutured with 6/0 Silk sutures placed in a vertical mattress fashion.
6. A local skin–muscle flap is fashioned to advance or rotate over the graft to provide a blood supply.

BONE GRAFT

With the improvement of alloplastic materials now available for the reconstruction of orbital bony defects there is rarely an indication to use bone grafts. The following sites may be used for harvesting bone:

- Calvarium
- Rib
- Iliac crest
- Anterior face of the maxilla

The outer table of the skull yields bone that does not tend to show much resorption. It has the disadvantage, however, of being rigid and brittle. It is very difficult to contour when used for orbital wall defects. It can, however, be stacked piecemeal for simple orbital volume augmentation. The bone can be split from the outer table of the skull in the parietal area using a burr and a curved osteotome. Alternatively, the inner table can be split from a full-thickness piece of calvarium, e.g., following a frontal craniotomy, and used to reconstruct the orbital roof following its removal to gain access to the orbital apex.

Rib grafts can be split, curved, and contoured but show more resorption. The potential donor site morbidity must be considered.

The iliac crest can yield relatively large quantities of corticocancellous bone. The bone does not contour well, however, and also may show resorption. The patient may also experience considerable postoperative pain at the donor site.

The anterior face of the maxilla can yield a small quantity of bone which can be used in the repair of modest-sized orbital floor fractures but this is very rarely justified.

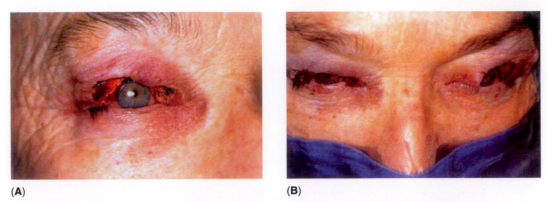

Figure 13.46 (**A**) A large right upper eyelid defect following a Mohs' micrographic surgery resection of a squamous cell carcinoma. (**B**) A wedge resection has been performed on the contralateral upper eyelid.

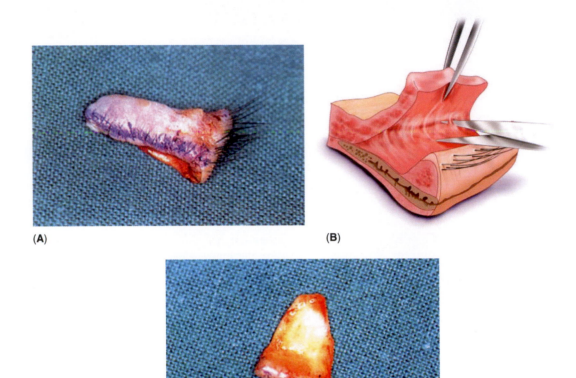

Figure 13.47 (**A**) The wedge resection of upper eyelid. (**B**) The skin and orbicularis muscle are removed. (**C**) The appearance of the composite graft.

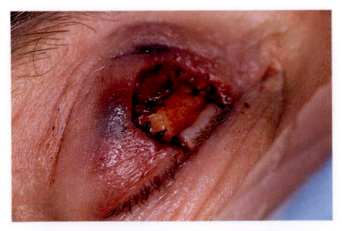

Figure 13.48 The eyelid composite graft sutured into place.

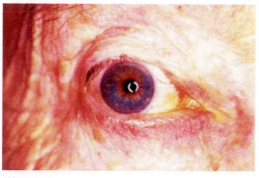

(A)

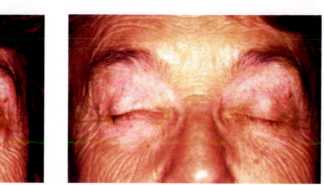

(B)

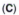

(C)

(D)

Figure 13.49 (**A**) The appearance of the reconstructed eyelid 5 years following the use of a composite graft. (**B**) The appearance of the donor eyelid. (**C**) The patient has a symmetrical appearance. (**D**) There is no lagopthalmos.

FURTHER READING

1. Bartley GB, Kay PP. Posterior lamellar eyelid reconstruction with a hard palate mucosal graft. Am J Ophthalmol 1989; 107: 609–12.
2. Geary PM, Tiernan E. Management of split skin graft donor sites-results of a national survey. J PlastReconstr Aesthetic Surg 2008; 62(12): 1677–83.
3. Hawes MJ. Free autogenous grafts in eyelid tarsoconjunctival reconstruction. Ophthal Surg 1897; 18: 37–41.
4. Henderson HW, Collin JR. Mucous membrane grafting. Dev Ophthalmol 2008; 41: 230–42.

5. Leone CR Jr. Nasal septal cartilage for eyelid reconstruction. Ophthal Surg 1973; 4: 68–71.
6. Levin PS, Stewart WB, Toth BA. The technique of cranial bone grafts in the correction of posttraumatic orbital deformities. Ophthal Plast Reconstr Surg 1987; 3: 77–82.
7. Lisman RD, Smith BC. Dermis-fat grafting. In: Smith BC, ed., Ophthalmic plastic and reconstructive surgery. St. Louis: CV Mosby Co, 1987; 1308–20.
8. Putterman AM. Viable composite grafting in eyelid reconstruction: a new method of upper and lower eyelid reconstruction. Am J Ophthal 1978; 85: 237–41.

14   The evaluation and management of the cosmetic patient

INTRODUCTION

The patient seeking periocular and facial rejuvenation presents many challenges and the inexperienced surgeon should approach such patients with great caution. The surgeon should be very adept at undertaking functional oculoplastic surgery before embarking upon the demands of cosmetic oculoplastic surgery. A good working knowledge of the myriad of non-surgical approaches to the management of such patients should also be acquired to supplement, or indeed, replace surgical interventions where appropriate, as surgery only constitutes one strategy for facial and periocular rejuvenation. The majority of patients who are referred to or who present to an oculoplastic surgeon seek options, which afford good results but involve a minimally invasive approach, minimal risk, and minimal "downtime".

PATIENT CONSULTATION

Consultation Facility

The surgeon embarking upon cosmetic surgery should evaluate his/her consulting facility set-up and staff and ensure that these are tailored to the demands of the cosmetic patient. This can be a major commitment. The initial contact made by a prospective patient may be made with a receptionist, patient-care coordinator, secretary, office administrator, or a nurse. The surgeon should ensure that every member of staff is trained to respond to the initial contact in a professional and knowledgeable manner. The staff should aim to establish a rapport with the patient, which should be reinforced when the patient arrives for a consultation. The staff should be fully conversant with the range of surgical and non-surgical treatments offered by the surgeon and by his/her nurse assistants, and with his/her costs.

The Pre-consultation

The pre-consultation, preferably with an aesthetics nurse practitioner, should begin with a detailed confidential health questionnaire which is very comprehensive and which requests detailed information about the patient's previous facial cosmetic surgical and non-surgical treatments, his/her past ophthalmic history including details of contact lens wear or previous refractive surgery, his/her past medical and surgical history including any tendency to excessive bruising or bleeding, a drug and allergy history, a social history including smoking and alcohol consumption, and a family history. It is extremely important, for example, that information about the prior use of periocular botulinum toxin injections is provided, as such injections can significantly affect the assessment and management of a patient with an eyebrow ptosis and/or blepharoptosis. The questionnaire should be signed by the patient declaring the information to be accurate. The patient should be photographed from a variety of angles, with and without the use of a flash. Ideally, the photography should be standardized. Informed consent should be obtained for the use of the photographs. The precise purpose and intended use of the photographs should be explained to the patient.

A pre-consultation with an aesthetics nurse practitioner is far less intimidating for the patient and an initial rapport can be readily established, which can be continued throughout the various phases of the patient's care. The nurse can help to establish what the patient's main concerns, goals, and expectations are, and can discuss issues such as the timing of the use of postoperative make-up. The patient may reveal concerns about the outcome of treatments undertaken elsewhere and the nurse can then pre-warn the surgeon about these. The nurse can often identify the "difficult" patient and can express reservations about the patient to the surgeon. The patient is far more likely to divulge relevant information about the traumas of a recent separation, divorce, or bereavement, for example, to a nurse. These may prove to be major factors motivating the patient to seek cosmetic surgery for which they are psychologically ill-prepared.

The Surgeon Consultation

The pre-consultation can save a lot of time, allowing the surgeon to concentrate on a comprehensive assessment and examination of the patient, and time to counsel the patient about the pros, cons, risks, and potential complications of the treatments discussed, as well as provide the patient with information about "downtime," aftercare instructions, activity or driving restrictions, and time off work. The surgeon should allow sufficient time for the consultation, and should encourage the patient to go away and consider the options presented. The surgeon should follow-up the consultation with a letter to the patient summarizing the patient's complaints, past history, examination findings, the management options discussed, any preoperative recommendations, e.g., the avoidance of the use of aspirin or anti-inflammatory medications, the expected duration of bruising and swelling, the timing of postoperative clinic visits and the anticipated timing of the removal of sutures, the risks, and potential complications. A separate document which outlines the risks and the potential complications of cosmetic surgery, along with their management, should they occur. It is always helpful to be able to direct the patient to the surgeon's website which should provide great detail about the procedure(s). This letter should also be accompanied by a separate letter from the clinic administrator detailing all the costs of the treatment. Wherever possible, the patient should be encouraged to schedule another, shorter follow-up appointment to go over any outstanding issues and to sign a consent form. It can be difficult to remain focused in an initial consultation and the patient can feel rather overloaded with information, particularly if the patient has not researched the subject in detail prior to the consultation.

The consent form should be type written and standardized, and should never be completed on the day of surgery. It should contain a comprehensive list of all serious or frequently occurring risks, which should be explained in detail to the patient in a manner that neither frightens nor offends. The surgeon should also make it clear how any potential complications would be managed and at what, if any, cost to the patient.

KEY POINT

A consent form for cosmetic surgery should never be completed on the day of surgery.

The dynamics of an effective cosmetic consultation are also very important. The surgeon should listen to the patient's concerns without prematurely interjecting to provide an opinion. The patient who is non-specific about his/her concerns and merely asks for recommendations, should be encouraged to provide more detail so that the surgeon does not make inappropriate recommendations having misunderstood the nature of the patient's concerns. As a general rule, the surgeon should try to remain within the sphere of the patient's complaint and not draw attention to other problems perceived by the surgeon, as this may cause offense. Constant interaction and adjustment of the discussion should occur to ensure that the conversation is progressing in line with the patient's expectations. The surgeon can then determine how receptive the patient will be to alternative options, which may not have been considered by the patient, e.g., many patients who request an upper lid blepharoplasty are surprised to be told that they may benefit from a brow lift.

KEY POINT

The astute patient will appreciate the surgeon whose clear objective is to provide good professional advice and recommendations, which are in the best interests of the patient, rather than one whose main objective is to convert a clinic visit into a surgical case. Such a patient is far more likely to recommend the surgeon to others.

Patient Selection for Surgery

The selection of an appropriate patient for a particular surgical procedure is an acquired skill and is critical to success in cosmetic surgery. It is preferable to decline to operate on patients whose expectations are unrealistic, whose demands are unreasonable, or whose psychological preparedness is in doubt. It is also preferable to decline to operate on the patient who is unduly critical of previous surgery undertaken by a colleague but whose complaint is not legitimate. The surgeon should also beware of the manipulative patient who is impolite to members of staff in the clinic but respectful towards the surgeon.

NON-SURGICAL TREATMENT OPTIONS

There are a wide variety of non-surgical options to select from to help to achieve facial and periocular rejuvenation. These include:

- Botulinum toxin injections
- Dermal filler injections
- Intense pulsed light treatment
- Cutaneous laser resurfacing
- Chemical peels

All non-surgical treatments are associated with small risks of adverse reactions and unwanted side effects. The patient should be provided with detailed information about the treatments and the associated risks and potential complications. Informed consent should be obtained before undertaking any of these treatments.

Botulinum Toxin Injections

Botulinum toxin injections for periocular and facial rejuvenation can be used alone, in combination with other non-surgical treatment modalities, e.g., dermal fillers, and can be used to improve the outcome of some surgical procedures. The injections have an excellent safety record, having long been used in ophthalmic practice for the treatment of essential blepharospasm and strabismus. Their safe and successful use in aesthetic treatments requires an understanding of the anatomy of the muscles of facial expression and a meticulous injection technique, particularly in the periocular area. The major advantage of the use of botulinum toxin injections is the fact that any unwanted effects eventually wear off spontaneously, usually with no long term sequelae.

It is always preferable to be conservative when treating a patient for the first time, as the effects cannot be reversed. It is preferable to offer the patient "top-up" injections after 10 to 14 days to achieve the best results. A clear record should be made of the site and number of injections given, and the dose of each. Once the dose for that individual patient has been established, repeat injections are very simple to undertake, referring back to the previous treatment record.

The author has used Dysport in his practice for over 18 years. Dysport has a relatively long duration of action (approximately 4 months) and is very effective. Its onset of action is usually seen at 3 days following injection, with the maximum effect seen approximately 7 to 10 days following injection.

KEY POINT

It is always preferable to be conservative when treating a patient for the first time, as the effects cannot be reversed. It is preferable to offer the patient "top-up" injections after 10 to 14 days to achieve the best results.

Procedure

A vial of Dysport contains a dry powder and is reconstituted by injecting 2.5 ml of sterile saline using a 3-ml syringe and a 21-gauge needle. The vial and the saline should be checked carefully and the expiry date confirmed with an assistant. The vial is repeatedly inverted and the solution is then withdrawn into a 1-ml Luer lock syringe using a 21-gauge needle. It is preferable not to withdraw more than 0.7 ml of Dysport into the syringe as this makes it more difficult to control the injection. The needle is then removed and exchanged for a 30-gauge needle. Each 0.1 ml gradation on the syringe contains 20 units of Dysport, making it very easy to calculate the dose to be injected.

If the patient prefers, the areas to be injected can be prepared with a topical anesthetic gel to reduce the discomfort of

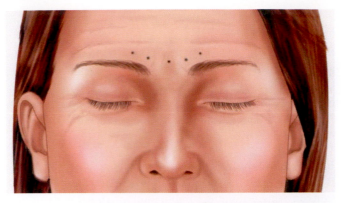

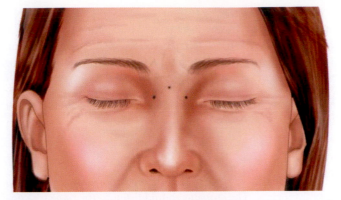

Figure 14.1 The typical sites of injection in the glabella.

Figure 14.2 The typical sites of injection for the treatment of "bunny lines."

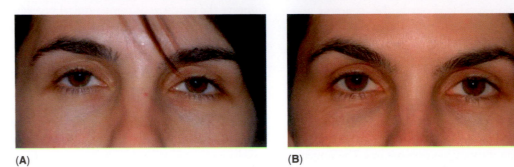

(A)   **(B)**

Figure 14.3 (**A**) Pre-treatment photograph of young female patient. (**B**) Post-treatment photograph of the same patient. A temporal brow lift has been achieved following the injection of Dysport 4 × 20 units to the glabella, and 4 × 10 units to the lateral canthus, and a single 10 unit injection just above and lateral to the tail of the brow.

injection. The patient should refrain from the use of aspirin or anti-inflammatory agents for 10 to 14 days prior to injection to minimize the risk of bruising. The patient is instructed to keep his/her arms by the side during the injections. The practitioner should wear gloves. The injections are given perpendicular to the skin and directly into the underlying muscle. The injections should be given quickly and immediate firm pressure should be applied to the injection sites for 2 to 3 min. The patient should avoid vigorous exercise for a few days following the injections.

The injections can be given at a number of different sites:

- The glabella
- The lateral canthi
- The forehead
- The lower eyelid
- The chin
- The neck
- The upper lip

The Glabella
The most common site for injection is the glabella, targeting the corrugator and depressor supercilii muscles and the medial aspect of the orbital part of the orbicularis oculi muscle. This softens or removes glabellar frown lines. The injections are typically given as four to five separate injections with a total dose of 80 to 120 units. The patient is asked to frown to establish the degree of muscle contraction and then the injections are given quickly into the muscles, injecting at 90° to the surface of the skin, moving from the right to the left sides. Care should be taken not to extend the injections to the adjacent frontalis muscle unless this is intended.

A typical treatment record for a patient is shown in Figure 14.1.

For horizontal lines at the root of the nose, the injections should target the procerus muscle. Some patients develop "bunny lines" when smiling, from overaction of the nasalis muscles. These can be easily treated. This typically requires a single injection on each side of the nose, each containing 5 to 10 units of Dysport (Fig. 14.2).

Patients treated with injections of botulinum toxin given into the glabella, who also suffer from migraine, often notice a significant improvement in their migraine.

The Lateral Canthus
The muscle which is targeted at the lateral canthus is the orbicularis oculi muscle. A series of four to five injections are given after asking the patient to screw the eye up tightly and then relax. The visible veins at the tail of the brow are carefully avoided. The total dose used varies from 30 to 60 units. This treatment softens or removes lateral canthal rhytids. It can also effect a mild to moderate brow lift, particularly when used in conjunction with glabellar injections, due to the unopposed action of the frontalis muscle (Fig. 14.3). If more of a brow lift is also desired, an additional injection is given at the tail of the eyebrow temporally. The dose and injection sites can be modified to take into account any pre-existing brow asymmetry.

A typical treatment record for a patient is shown in Figure 14.4.

The Forehead
Great care should be exercised when injecting into the forehead. The muscle which is targeted in the forehead is the frontalis muscle. The treatment softens horizontal forehead lines very successfully, but the treatment can also result in a very unsatisfactory bilateral brow ptosis, particularly in patients who already have low

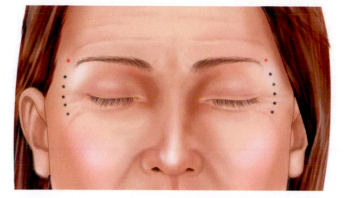

Figure 14.4 The typical sites of injection for the treatment of lateral canthal rhytids (black dots). The red dots depict the additional injection which is used to effect more of a temporal brow lift.

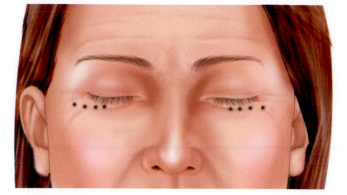

Figure 14.6 The typical sites of injection for the treatment of lateral lower eyelid rhytids.

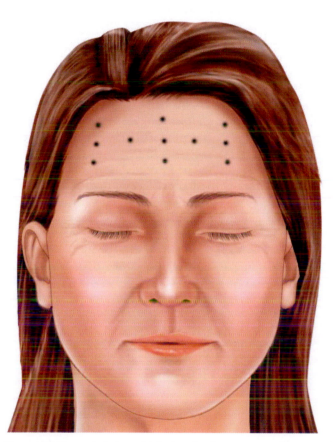

Figure 14.5 The typical sites of injection for the treatment of horizontal forehead lines.

brows. The patient should be counseled on this possibility and, again, an undercorrection should be the initial aim of treatment. Typically, a series of 9 to 12 injections, each at a dose of 10 units, are given across the forehead after asking the patient to raise the eyebrows. The dose and location of each injection may be amended taking into account any asymmetries of the brows.

A typical treatment record for a patient is shown in Figure 14.5.

The Lower Eyelid

Injections in the lower eyelid should be confined to the lateral half to lateral third of the eyelid and should be very conservative. The muscle which is targeted in the lower eyelid is the preseptal orbicularis oculi muscle. The medial aspect of the lower eyelid is avoided to prevent any risk of spread of the toxin to the inferior

oblique muscle, which could result in diplopia. Typically two to three injections are given at a total dose of four to six units. Higher doses can result in a retraction of the lower eyelid or the appearance of a malar "bag" in a predisposed individual due to loss of support of the lateral cheek by the weakened orbicularis muscle.

A typical treatment record for a patient is shown in Figure 14.6.

The Chin

Injections into the chin can help to improve a horizontal line. The mentalis muscle is the target muscle. Typically, two separate injections are given at a total dose of 10 to 15 units. Injections given more laterally over the mandible target the depressor anguli oris, which can help to lift the outer aspect of the lips. Typically, a single injection is given into each muscle at a dose of 10 units. A conservative approach should be adopted to avoid any problems with speech, eating, or drinking.

A typical treatment record for a patient is shown in Figure 14.7.

The Upper Lip

Injections given just above the upper lip can soften vertical upper lip lines ("smoker's lines"), but great caution should be exercised as such injections can cause problems with speech and with eating and drinking. The muscle which is targeted is the orbicularis oris muscle. Two to three injections are given on each side of the philtrum at a total dose not exceeding 10 units.

The Neck

Injections in the neck can help to reduce platysmal bands but such injections are not advised because of the risk of spread of the toxin to involve the muscles of deglutition.

Contraindications

The following are contraindications to the use of botulinum toxin injections:

- A history of myasthenia
- The use of aminoglycoside antibiotics
- Pregnancy or lactation
- An allergy to any known constituent

If patients are to undergo injections prior to surgery, the injections should be given 10 to 14 days prior to the operation. Likewise, injections should not be given following surgery until the postoperative edema has completely resolved. In the presence of edema, the toxin can be carried from the site of injections to other muscles creating secondary problems, e.g., a blepharoptosis.

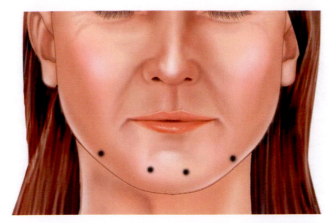

Figure 14.7 The typical sites of injection for the treatment of a horizontal fold in the chin (central injections) and to achieve a lift to the smile (lateral injections).

Side Effects
The patient should be warned about the possible side effects and unwanted effects of botulinum toxin injections.

- Ptosis
- Diplopia
- Lagophthalmos
- Headache

A blepharoptosis can occur from spread of the toxin to involve the levator muscle in the upper eyelid. This is seen when too great a dose of the toxin has been used, too deep an injection has been given, or when there has been bruising and swelling following the injections. Patients should be advised to avoid rubbing the area of injection and vigorous exercise for 3 to 4 days following the injections.

The ptosis can be treated by instilling Iopidine drops, an α-agonist, into the eye. These stimulate Müller's muscle, but the patient must be informed of the additional potential side effects of this topical glaucoma medication.

Diplopia is a very rare occurrence and is usually seen when injections are given inappropriately along the medial aspect of the lower eyelid. There is no specific treatment for this other than occlusion of one eye until the effects of the botulinum toxin have worn off.

Lagophthalmos can occur but this is also a very rare occurrence, and is usually only seen in patients treated for blepharospasm where injections have been given into the pretarsal orbicularis muscle in the upper eyelid.

Some patients experience a headache for 2 to 3 days following injections of botulinum toxin in the glabella, although paradoxically migraine sufferers often notice a marked improvement in their symptoms.

Botulinum toxin reduces sweating and is used for the management of hyperhidrosis. As a consequence of this effect, some patients experience marked dryness of the skin in the glabella and forehead following injections of the toxin.

Other unwanted effects are seen with the inappropriate or excessive use of botulinum toxin, e.g., a brow ptosis, temporal peaking of the eyebrows, and a loss of facial expression. A temporal peaking of one or both eyebrows can be treated with additional injections of botulinum toxin just above the eyebrow but the dose should be very conservative, rarely exceeding 10 units.

Botulinum toxin injections, given appropriately, can yield very good aesthetic results. Patients should be encouraged to maintain the effect of the injections by undergoing repeat injections before the effects wear off spontaneously. The injections can help to maintain the long-term effects of brow lift surgery by weakening the brow depressors. It is also advantageous to inject the brow depressors 2 weeks before undertaking a brow lift procedure.

Dermal Filler Injections
There is a huge demand for dermal filler injections and many companies compete in the ever increasing market for these injections. A surgeon who wishes to embark upon their use needs to decide which fillers to use and needs to be very well informed about the efficacy and safety profile of such fillers. The author does not utilize any permanent synthetic fillers. These are associated with a risk of adverse reactions, e.g., granulomas, and cannot be removed. At the time of writing this text, the author uses only the Restylane® range of fillers and Juvéderm®, which, in his opinion, are relatively safe, versatile and very effective. This is a personal preference but many other such dermal fillers are available to select from. Adverse reactions are very rare. These hyaluronic acid fillers are tailored to the different requirements of different areas of the face, and complications associated with their use are extremely rare. Some of these fillers are also contain Lidocaine, reducing the discomfort associated with their injection.

Restylane® lasts approximately 6 to 12 months, depending on the area of injection, before repeat injections are required to maintain the effects. Restylane offers the advantage that the product can be dissolved away with the use of a very small dose of Hyalase (hyaluronidase) if necessary.

The following Restylane® fillers are used in the face:

Product	Indications
Restylane	Tear trough rejuvenation
	Inflation of the eyebrow
	Improvement of moderate facial lines
Perlane	Nasolabial fold correction
	Augmentation of the hollow temple
Restylane Touch	Improvement of lateral canthal rhytids
Restylane Sub-Q	Cheek enhancement/mid-face lift
Restylane Vital	Skin hydration and rejuvenation
Restylane Lipp	Lip enhancement

With the exception of tear trough injections, most other dermal filler injections can be delegated to a trained aesthetics nurse. Most of the Restylane® products are injected at a single sitting, with the exception of Restylane Vital, which is typically injected as a course of three sessions, each separated by approximately 2 weeks. The injections are relatively simple to perform and are associated with a high level of patient satisfaction. Great care should, however, be taken when injecting in the glabellar area because of the risk of inadvertent

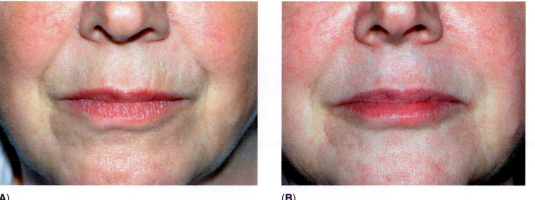

(A)   (B)

Figure 14.8 (**A**) A patient with moderate nasolabial folds before treatment. (**B**) The same patient 1 week following the injection of 1 ml of Perlane along each nasolabial fold.

intravascular injection with embolization of the ophthalmic artery circulation and visual loss.

For the novice practitioner, the nasolabial folds are the simplest areas to treat with a high degree of patient satisfaction.

Procedure

The patient is seated comfortably on a treatment couch in a semi-recumbent position and instructed to keep his/her hands by their side. The practitioner should wear gloves and should use magnification, e.g., surgical loupes. The surgeon stands on the right side of the patient to inject into the right nasolabial fold and vice versa. The nasolabial fold is stretched inferiorly with the non-dominant hand and the needle inserted through the skin at an angle of approximately 30° and passed into the subcutaneous tissue just below the level of the dermis. The filler is injected slowly and the needle then withdrawn. More superficial injections in the area of the nasolabial folds should be avoided. This is repeated at intervals. A topical cream, e.g., Auriderm, is applied to the skin and the nasolabial fold is firmly massaged between thumb and forefinger with the forefinger inside the patient's mouth. This should be continued for 1 to 2 min. Further serial injections can be given at 90° to the initial injections to "cross hatch" the product. More injections, however, increase the risk of bruising. Typically, 1 to 2 ml of Perlane are required for each nasolabial fold.

The massage should be undertaken immediately following the completion of the injections to disperse the filler, avoiding an uneven distribution or lumps. The patient can continue to massage the area for 24 to 48 hours using Auriderm cream following treatment. A result of such treatment is shown in Figure 14.8.

The technique for the injection of the other Restylane products differs, with the filler being injected at different depths. It is wise to undergo formal training in the use of these fillers by an experienced practitioner before undertaking these treatments.

Tear Trough Injections

Perlane or Restylane can be used for tear trough rejuvenation. The author prefers Restylane as this product is injected with a smaller gauge needle, which causes very little discomfort and is less likely to cause bleeding, and Restylane is easier to manipulate with massage.

Tear trough Restylane injections should only be undertaken by a suitably trained and experienced ophthalmic surgeon. The patient should be very carefully selected for this treatment.

In general, the best candidates for this treatment are male or female patients in the age range of 21 to 50 years, who complain of lower eyelid dark circles, which are due to a tear trough defect and not due to pigmentary changes in the skin, and who have no significant lower eyelid or skin laxity. This treatment is suitable for many patients who do not wish to contemplate lower eyelid blepharoplasty surgery, or the ones who are not suitable candidates for such a surgery (Fig. 14.9).

It does not prevent a suitable patient from undergoing such surgery at a later stage. Restylane tear trough injections can also be used for some patients who have developed a "post-blepharoplasty lower eyelid syndrome" with an over-resection of lower eyelid fat.

Contraindications

The following are contraindications to the use of Restylane tear trough injections:

- Inappropriate/unrealistic expectations
- Gross eyelid fat herniation
- The use of anti-coagulants
- Very thin eyelid skin
- Moderate to severe skin laxity
- The use of cutaneous laser treatment

The patient should be counseled appropriately about the pros, cons, risks, and potential complications of treatment and informed consent should be obtained for this. The patient should refrain from the use of aspirin or anti-inflammatory agents for 10 to 14 days prior to the injections. The patient should have realistic expectations of what the treatment can achieve.

Patients who have moderate to severe lower eyelid fat herniation are not suitable candidates for these injections. Patients with very thin lower eyelid skin are more likely to develop problems with an exacerbation of the dark circle appearance as the underlying orbicularis muscle may become more visible or a bluish discoloration may be evident if there is excessive bruising, with staining of the Restylane gel. Patients with a pseudo-proptosis from high axial myopia, or proptosis from thyroid eye disease, are not good candidates for this treatment. Patients who are due to undergo lower eyelid cutaneous laser treatments should not undergo tear trough injections.

The overall satisfaction rate from this treatment in appropriately selected patients is very high (Figs. 14.9 and 14.10).

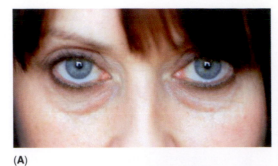
(A)

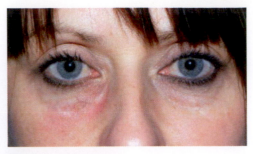
(B)

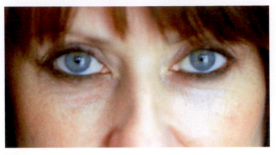
(C)

Figure 14.9 (**A**) The pre-treatment photograph of a patient complaining of lower lid dark circles who wanted to avoid surgical intervention. (**B**) The same patient immediately following tear trough Restylane injections on the right side. (**C**) The post-treatment photograph of the same patient 2 weeks following tear trough Restylane injections.

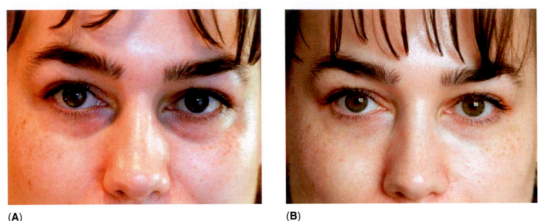
(A)   (B)

Figure 14.10 (**A**) The pre-treatment photograph of a young patient complaining of lower lid dark circles. (**B**) The post-treatment photograph of the same patient 2 weeks following tear trough Restylane injections.

Procedure

The lower eyelid skin is first anesthetized with a topical anesthetic gel for 10 to 15 min, although many patients tolerate the injections very well without this. The injections are given with the patient sitting at an angle of 60° with their arms at their side. Contact lenses should be removed. A drop of proxymethacaine is instilled into each eye.

The surgeon stands on the right side of the patient to inject into the right tear trough and vice versa. The patient is asked to look up during the injections. The surgeon palpates the inferior orbital margin to ensure that the injections are given over the bony margin and not into the orbit. The 30-gauge needle is attached to a 0.5 or 1.0 ml syringe of Restylane. The needle is inserted through the skin of the lower eyelid, starting just nasal to the mid-pupillary line, at an angle of approximately 30° to the skin surface. The needle is inserted into the preperiosteal plane and 0.1 to 0.2 ml of Restylane is injected slowly. The needle is withdrawn and the Restylane is pressed against the inferior orbital rim with the surgeon's forefinger,

using a moderate degree of pressure. If any bleeding is encountered, immediate pressure is applied with a sterile swab. The needle is reinserted and further injections are given along the course of the tear trough, with digital pressure applied to the Restylane after each injection. The injections can be continued in the temporal aspect of the eyelid if required.

The total volume required per eyelid varies from 0.4 to 1.5 ml. Once the injections have been completed, a topical cream, e.g., Auriderm, is applied and the eyelid is gently massaged for a few minutes. The patient continues this gentle massage intermittently at home for 1 to 2 days. No other specific aftercare is required. The patient will experience some swelling and erythema which usually subsides within 3 to 4 days.

Complications

The treatment carries the potential risks of inadvertent injury to the globe or embolization of the retinal vasculature with visual loss, although such a risk is extremely small. The main problems seen after tear trough injections are over-correction

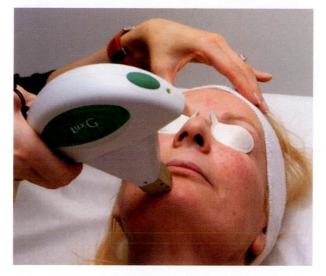

Figure 14.11 A patient undergoing intense pulsed light treatment.

and excessive bruising with a secondary bluish discoloration of the lower eyelids due to blood staining of the gel. For this reason, the injections should not be undertaken on anyone with a tendency to bruise or bleed easily, or who is taking aspirin, anticoagulants, or anti-inflammatory agents. A bluish discoloration is particularly troublesome in male patients, if it occurs, as the use of make-up to camouflage the discoloration is not an option for most male patients. The injections should be very conservative, with a "top-up" injection offered after 1 to 2 weeks, as required. An over-correction can result in "bunching" of the product when smiling with an unnatural appearance. An over-correction can be treated with Hyalase injections.

> **KEY POINT**
>
> The key to success in the use of tear tough rejuvenation injections is good patient selection and a conservative approach.

Intense Pulsed Light Treatment

Intense pulsed light (IPL) can be used to improve the appearance of facial thread veins and melasma, and can help to improve the appearance of facial skin, which shows the effects of age and photo damage. It involves the application of IPL through a small cooled rectangular head on a hand piece (Fig. 14.11). The treatment, which can be undertaken by an aesthetics nurse practitioner, requires the repeated application of the treatment over the course of a few weeks. The patient's skin has to be protected from the sun following the treatment. A result of treatment using IPL is shown in Figure 14.12. The treatment can be alternated with the use of fractional laser skin resurfacing for a greater degree of general skin rejuvenation. A more detailed discussion of this treatment is beyond the scope of this textbook.

Laser Resurfacing

Cutaneous laser resurfacing is a technique mainly used for the treatment of deep skin wrinkles, photo damage, and acne scars. It is usually undertaken with an Erbium YAG 2940 nm wavelength or a CO_2 10,600 nm wavelength laser. The results of treatment with these lasers can be very impressive, particularly for severely photo damaged skin, but the complete surface

ablation achieved is associated with a very disconcerting early postoperative appearance with marked facial edema and erythema, and a long recovery period. It is also associated with the risk of bacterial, viral, or fungal infection, and requires a great deal of aftercare. It is also associated with the risks of hyperpigmentation, hypopigmentation, prolonged erythema, and scarring. As a consequence, the majority of patients now seek less invasive laser resurfacing provided by a fractional laser. The term fractional pertains to the method in which the laser light is transferred. Tiny pinpoints of laser light are used to deliver the laser to the surface of the skin in only a fraction of the area. Several hundred or thousands of pinpoints may be used per square inch, leaving healthy skin in between the ablated areas. This is intended to allow more rapid healing with less risk. The treatment requires 3 to 5 sessions undertaken over a period of weeks and can be alternated with IPL treatment. Through the heating of the deep dermis, fibroblasts are stimulated to form new collagen and elastin helping to bring increased turgor and thickness to the skin. The results of this treatment are far less dramatic than those seen with other ablative lasers but are more acceptable to the patient who seeks minimal "downtime." This treatment requires a commitment on the part of the patient to protect the skin from the adverse effects of the sun, and a commitment to basic post-treatment skin care. This aspect of a patient's care is usually delegated to an aesthetics nurse practitioner.

Laser resurfacing can be used to tighten the lower eyelid skin of a patient who has undergone a transconjunctival blepharoplasty, and who has skin wrinkling, but insufficient skin laxity to justify a "pinch" excision of lower eyelid skin.

A more detailed discussion of laser skin resurfacing is beyond the scope of this textbook.

Chemical Peels

Chemical exfoliation using a combination of Jessner's solution and 35% trichloroacetic acid is a good treatment for patients aged 35 to 45 with mild to moderate skin wrinkling (Fig. 14.13). Like laser resurfacing, it can be used to tighten the lower eyelid skin of a patient who has undergone a transconjunctival blepharoplasty.

A more detailed discussion of chemical exfoliation is beyond the scope of this textbook.

SURGICAL TREATMENT OPTIONS

The surgical options which can be considered for facial rejuvenation are:

- Upper eyelid blepharoplasty
- Lower eyelid blepharoplasty
- Brow lift surgery
- Mid-face lift surgery
- Lower face lift surgery
- Structural fat grafting

Cosmetic upper and lower eyelid blepharoplasty, and mid-face and brow lift surgery are outlined in detail in the next two chapters. A discussion of the surgical techniques involved in lower face-lift and neck rejuvenation surgery is beyond the scope of this textbook and patients requiring such surgical intervention are better served by being referred to an expert facial plastic surgeon.

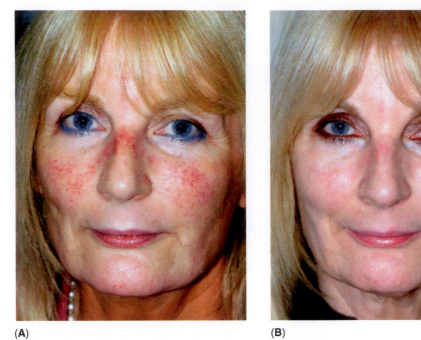

(A)   **(B)**

Figure 14.12 (**A**) A patient with marked facial thread veins. (**B**) The same patient following a course of intense pulsed light treatment.

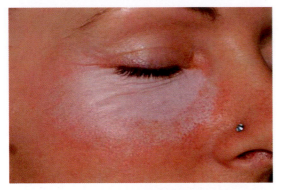   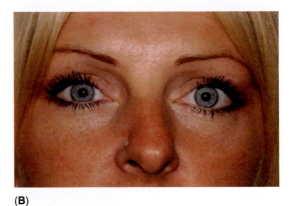

(A)   **(B)**

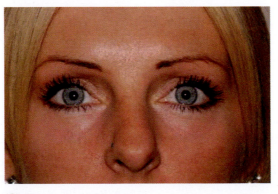

(C)

Figure 14.13 (**A**) A patient undergoing a 35% TCA peel. (**B**) The same patient before treatment. (**C**) The same patient 6 weeks following treatment.

Structural fat Grafting

Structural fat grafting is a procedure in which fat cells are harvested from the patient and re-injected into his/her facial subcutaneous tissues. This can be undertaken alone for facial rejuvenation or it can be used in combination with other surgical procedures, e.g., a lower eyelid blepharoplasty (Fig. 14.14). As with any other facial surgery, the patient must avoid the use of aspirin or anti-inflammatory agents for 10 to 14 days prior to undergoing structural fat grafting.

In this procedure, fat is harvested by syringe liposuction and the aspirated material centrifuged. This separates into three layers: the uppermost layer is composed primarily of oil, the middle layer is composed of fat, and the bottom layer is composed of blood, serum, and local anesthetic solution. The

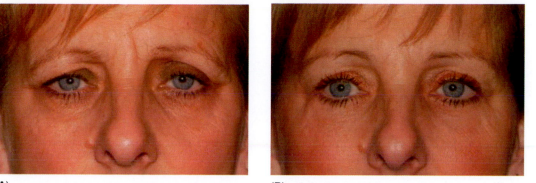

(A)   **(B)**

Figure 14.14 (**A**) Preoperative appearance. (**B**) Appearance of the same patient 4 months after undergoing preoperative botulinum toxin injections to the glabella, a bilateral temporal direct brow lift, bilateral upper and lower eyelid blepharoplasties, and structural fat grafting to the medial aspect of the left upper eyelid and to the upper cheeks.

oil, blood, serum, and local anesthetic solution are removed and the separated fat cells are used for injection.

Indications

Structural fat grafting is used primarily for the cosmetic improvement of facial lines, depressions, and fat atrophy, although it is also used for the cosmetic improvement of depressions and volume loss that are seen following trauma or tumor resections, or following the development of disease states, e.g., Romberg's hemifacial atrophy. It can also be used to treat the post enucleation socket syndrome. In facial rejuvenation, it has the following indications:

- Augmentation of nasolabial folds
- Augmentation of temple hollowing
- Augmentation of the mid-face
- Cosmetic improvement of lower lid tear trough defects
- Volume enhancement of the upper eyelid
- Volume enhancement of the lateral eyebrow

Structural fat grafting can yield very good, long-lasting results but it can also be unpredictable with the development of fat atrophy and the need for further injections. It has also been noted that the technique can provide some skin rejuvenation, which is thought to occur as a consequence of the activity of stem cells in the injected fat.

Selection of the Donor Site

Although the lower abdominal wall can be used as a donor site, it is safer to use the "love handle" area, the upper outer quadrant of the buttock, or the lateral aspect of the upper thigh.

Surgical Technique

The surgical technique is outlined in detail in chapter 13.

Complications

Structural fat grafting is associated with a number of potential complications:

- Fat embolism
- Contour irregularities
- Fat atrophy
- Swelling
- Over-correction

It is preferable to avoid using structural fat injections in the glabella area to avoid the risk of intravascular injection and fat embolism. Contour irregularities can occur and these are more likely to be seen in the tear trough areas. These can respond to massage, although formal surgical debulking or the removal of small pockets of fat using a small cannula is occasionally required. An overcorrection should be avoided by meticulous attention to detail during the injection process. Atrophy of fat requires a repeated injection procedure. Unfortunately, storage of harvested fat is not recommended and further harvesting of fat is required under these circumstances.

FURTHER READING

1. Bozniak S, Cantisano-Zikha M, Purewal BK, Zdinak LA. Combination therapies in oculofacial rejuvenation. Orbit 2006; 25: 4319–26.
2. Deprez P. Textbook of Chemical Peels Superficial, Medium and Deep Peels in Cosmetic Practice. London: Informa Healthcare, 2007 (ISBN-10: 1 84184 495 0).
3. Carruthers A, Carruthers J, eds. Procedures in Cosmetic Dermatology: Botulinum Toxin. Philadelphia, PA: Elsevier Saunders, 2005 (ISBN: 978-1-4160-2470-5).
4. Carruthers A, Carruthers J, eds. Procedures in Cosmetic Dermatology: Soft Tissue Augmentation. Philadelphia, PA: Elsevier Saunders, 2005 (ISBN: 1-4160-2469-7).
5. Goldberg DJ, ed. Procedures in Cosmetic Dermatology: Laser and Lights, vol 2. Philadelphia, PA: Elsevier Saunders, 2005 (ISBN: 1-4160-2387-9).
6. Thomas C. Facial Rejuvenation: Creams, Toxins, Lasers and Surgery. Spoor Informa Healthcare, 2001 (ISBN: 1853177741/9781853177743).
7. Flynn TC. Periocular botulinum toxin. Clin Dermatol 2003; 21: 498–504.
8. Foster JA, Huang W, Perry JD, Holck DL, Wulc AE. Cosmetic uses of botulinum toxin. In: Levine MR, ed. Manual of Oculoplastic Surgery, 3rd edn. Boston, MA: Butterworth-Heinemann, 2003: 93–7.
9. Johnson CM, Alsarraf R. Surgical anatomy of the ageing face. In: The Ageing Face a Systematic Approach. Philadelphia, PA: Saunders Elsevier, 2002: 27–36.
10. Johnson CM, Jr, Alsarraf R. The Ageing Face: A Systematic Approach. Philadelphia, PL: Saunders, 2002.
11. Morris CL, Stinnett SS, Woodward JA. Patient-preferred sites of Restylane injection in periocular and facial soft-tissue augmentation. Ophthal Plast Reconstr Surg 2008; 24(2): 117–21.
12. Romagnoli M, Belmontesi M. Hyaluronic Acid-based Fillers: theory and practice. Clin Dermatol 2008; 26: 123–59.
13. Schanz S, Schippert W, Umler A, et al. Arterial embolisation caused by injection of hyaluronic acid (Restylane). Br J Dermatol 2002; 146:928–9.
14. Taub AF. Treatment of rosacea with intense pulsed light. J Drugs Dermatol 2003; 2:254–9.
15. Teimourian B. Blindness following fat injections. Plast Reconstr Surg 1988; 82: 361.
16. Weiss DD, Carraway JH. Eyelid rejuvenation: a marriage of old and new. Curr Opin Otolaryngol Head Neck Surg 2005; 13: 248–54.

15 Blepharoplasty

INTRODUCTION

The term blepharoplasty is used to refer to an operation in which redundant tissues including skin, or skin and muscle, are excised from the eyelid, and in which fat may be excised, sculpted, or repositioned. The appearance of the eyelids, and the periorbital region, plays a pivotal role in maintaining facial harmony through expression of human character, mood, and emotions, and a successful outcome from this surgery requires great attention to detail.

A blepharoplasty can be performed for both functional and aesthetic reasons. A functional blepharoplasty aims to restore normal function and appearance to an eyelid that has been altered by trauma, infection, inflammation, degeneration, neoplasia, or by a developmental anomaly. A cosmetic blepharoplasty aims to improve the appearance of eyelid tissues that are histologically and functionally normal.

Patients who enquire about, or who are referred for, upper and lower eyelid blepharoplasty tend to present with a variety of aesthetic and functional complaints. These include:

- A tired look
- Hooding of the upper eyelids
- "Drooping" of the upper eyelids
- "Eye bags"
- Skin wrinkling
- Skin folds
- A visual field defect
- Headaches
- Irritation of the upper eyelids
- Lower lid "dark circles" (Fig. 15.1).

Female patients often complain of the inability to place make-up on the upper eyelid.

An upper eyelid blepharoplasty may involve the removal of skin alone, skin and orbicularis muscle, or this may be combined with the removal or sculpting of herniated orbital fat. Occasionally an upper eyelid blepharoplasty will only involve the removal, sculpting, or redraping of fat. The procedure may be combined with an eyebrow lifting or blepharoptosis procedure. The procedure may be performed for functional reasons to improve a patient's visual field restricted by dermatochalasis, or to improve symptoms of irritation from redundant skin hanging over the upper eyelid lashes, and/or for cosmetic reasons.

A lower eyelid blepharoplasty is more frequently performed for cosmetic reasons alone and may also involve the removal of skin and muscle alone or this may be combined with the removal and/or repositioning of herniated orbital fat, the re-suspension of a ptotic orbicularis oculi muscle, a lateral canthal suspension, an orbital decompression procedure for thyroid eye disease, or a mid-face or sub-orbicularis oculi muscle fat (SOOF) lift.

Blepharoplasty is one of the most commonly performed cosmetic operations.

APPLIED ANATOMY

A thorough understanding of the surgical anatomy of the eyebrows, eyelids, and mid-face is essential prior to performing a blepharoplasty. The applied anatomy of the eyebrow, eyelids, and mid-face is presented in detail in chapter 2—"Applied anatomy." This anatomy should be carefully reviewed. Additional aspects of surgically relevant anatomy are presented below.

The Upper Eyelids

The palpebral aperture is almond shaped, with the lateral canthal angle lying slightly higher than the medial canthal angle. The lateral canthal angle is generally slightly higher in females than males and lies approximately 5 mm from the lateral orbital margin (Fig. 15.2). The upper eyelid skin crease is usually approximately 5 to 6 mm above the lash line in males and 7 to 8 mm in females.

The distance between the inferior aspect of the eyebrow and the upper lid skin crease on down gaze should be approximately two-thirds of the distance from the inferior aspect of the eyebrow to the eyelid margin. Likewise, the distance from the skin crease to the eyelid margin in down gaze should be one-third of the distance from the inferior aspect of the eyebrow to the eyelid margin (Fig. 15.2). In general, a minimum distance of 10 to 12 mm should be left between the inferior aspect of the eyebrow and the upper eyelid skin excision marking when performing an upper lid blepharoplasty, and again, in general, approximately 20 mm of skin should be left between the inferior aspect of the eyebrow and the eyelid margin.

It is important to maintain these dimensions. If an excessive amount of upper eyelid skin is removed, reducing the distance from the skin crease to the brow in the presence of a brow ptosis, an unsatisfactory result will occur, with the appearance of the brow being attached to the eyelashes (Fig. 15.3). This may also cause lagophthalmos (Fig. 15.4).

It is important to differentiate prolapsed pre-aponeurotic fat from retro-orbicularis oculi fat (ROOF) that has descended into the upper eyelid (Fig. 15.5).

This may give rise to the appearance of upper eyelid "fullness" (Fig. 15.6).

KEY POINT

The distance between the inferior aspect of the eyebrow and the upper lid skin crease on down gaze should be approximately two-thirds of the distance from the inferior aspect of the eyebrow to the eyelid margin. It is important to maintain these dimensions. In general, a minimum distance of 10 to 12 mm should be left between the inferior aspect of the eyebrow and the upper eyelid skin excision marking when performing an upper lid blepharoplasty.

Although this descended fat can be debulked, it is preferable to reposition this as part of a brow lift procedure.

Some patients have very prominent superolateral bony margins that can also contribute to upper eyelid "fullness." This can be exposed and reduced with the use of a diamond burr during the course of an upper eyelid blepharoplasty (Fig. 15.7).

Subcutaneous thickening of this area in the dysthyroid patient must be recognized. This may not be amenable to improvement by standard blepharoplasty surgery. An overly aggressive upper eyelid blepharoplasty in a patient with thyroid eye disease can markedly worsen symptoms of corneal exposure.

It is important to recognize a prolapsed lacrimal gland that may be responsible for lateral upper eyelid "fullness" or swelling (Fig. 15.8). Prolapsed glands can be repositioned during the course of an upper eyelid blepharoplasty by suturing the gland to the periorbita of the lacrimal gland fossa (Figs. 15.9–15.11).

KEY POINT

It is very important to be able to distinguish the lacrimal gland from orbital fat.

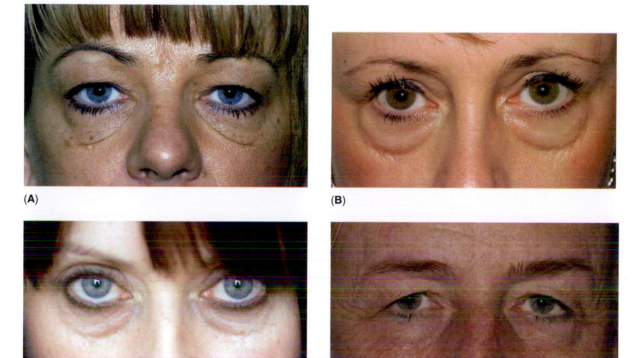

(A)   (B)

(C)   (D)

Figure 15.1 (**A**) A patient complaining of hooded upper lids with an inability to place makeup, and loose folds of skin in the lower eyelids. She was a heavy smoker. (**B**) A patient complaining of unsightly lower eyelid "bags". (**C**) A patient complaining of lower eyelid "dark circles" creating a "tired look." (**D**) A patient complaining of a "blinkered feeling" with a restriction to her visual fields.

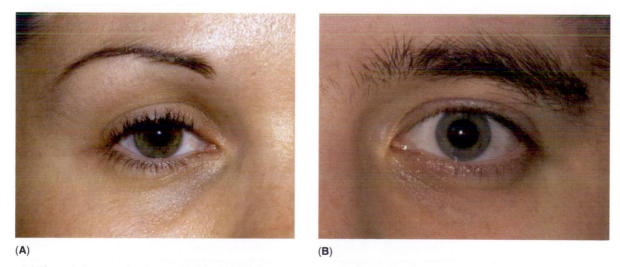

(A)   (B)

Figure 15.2 (**A**) The typical topographical anatomy of the periorbital region of a young female showing a skin crease at 6 to 7 mm above the eyelid margin and an arched eyebrow with the temporal aspect of the eyebrow lying at a higher position than the medial aspect. Note that the eyebrow has been plucked. It is important to take this into consideration when making measurements for skin resection. (**B**) The typical topographical anatomy of the periorbital region of a young male showing a skin crease at 5 to 6 mm above the eyelid margin and a flatter eyebrow contour.

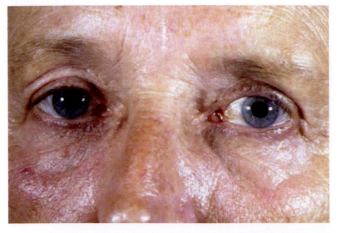

Figure 15.3 A patient following an excessive resection of her left upper eyelid skin with worsening of her brow ptosis. She also has asymmetry of the upper eyelids and brows postoperatively.

Some patients develop orbital fat atrophy creating an upper eyelid sulcus defect. The removal of pre-aponeurotic fat in such patients should be avoided to prevent a postoperative "cadaveric" appearance. A prolapsed medial fat pad in such a patient can be debulked and the fat transplanted to lie evenly in the pre-aponeurotic space. In general, the removal of fat from the upper eyelid should be avoided in the majority of patients.

> **KEY POINT**
>
> In general, the removal of fat from the upper eyelid should be avoided in the majority of patients.

"Fullness" in the medial aspect of the upper eyelid may be caused by a medial eyebrow ptosis. Elevation of the brow, or the use of botulinum toxin injections in the glabella, can be

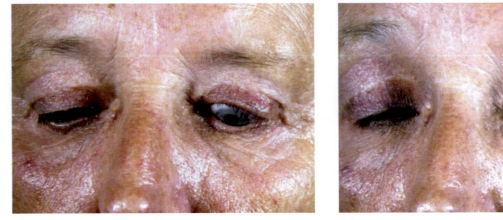

(A)   **(B)**

Figure 15.4 (**A**) The same patient demonstrating severe lag on down gaze. (**B**) The same patient demonstrating lagophthalmos on attempted passive eyelid closure. She also shows very poor placement of the upper lid skin incisions and only 5 to 6 mm of skin between the left upper lid incision and the lowermost position of the eyebrow centrally.

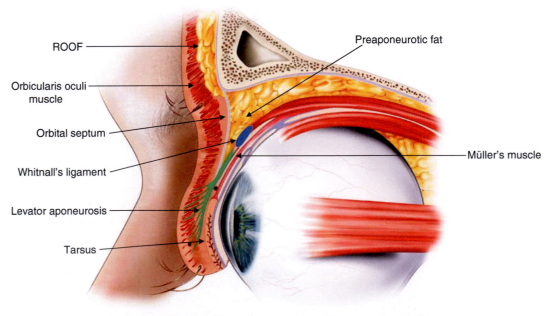

Figure 15.5 Diagram illustrating the position of the pre-aponeurotic fat.

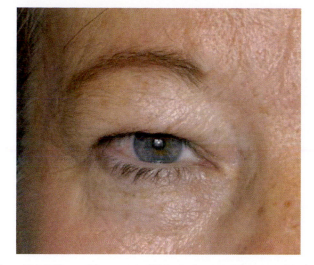

Figure 15.6 Fullness of the upper eyelid due to descent of the retro-orbicularis oculi fat (ROOF).

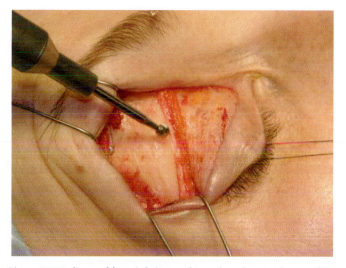

Figure 15.7 A diamond burr is being used to reduce the prominence of the supraorbital margin in this patient.

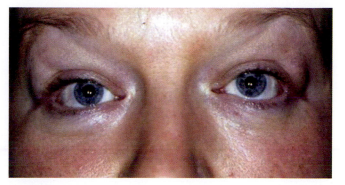

Figure 15.8 A patient with bilateral lateral upper eyelid swellings due to spontaneous lacrimal gland prolapses.

more successful at addressing this problem. Incisions in this area can leave unsatisfactory scarring. It is important to avoid the temptation to "chase a dog-ear" into this area beyond the medial limit of the skin crease during an upper eyelid blepharoplasty as the subsequent scarring can be very unsatisfactory. In such patients, a gentle debulking of the medial fat pad can allow the skin to re-drape with a more satisfactory aesthetic result, but over-resection of fat should be avoided. The fat should not be discarded as it may be required for use in the central aspect of the upper lid or may be of use to help to treat a medial tear trough defect in the lower eyelid.

The upper eyelid skin crease represents the most superior point of attachment between the skin and the levator aponeurosis. This position is just inferior to the insertion of the orbital septum onto the levator aponeurosis. The skin crease lies at a higher level in females, approximately 7 to 8 mm from the lash line, compared to 5 to 6 mm in males. It is important not to raise the skin crease in males to avoid a "feminization" of the eyelid appearance.

The skin crease shows racial differences. In the Oriental eyelid the orbital septum attaches to the levator aponeurosis at a lower level, allowing the preaponeurotic fat to descend into the lower reaches of the eyelid, preventing the levator aponeurosis from forming a high skin crease. A great deal has been written about the oriental eyelid and the oriental blepharoplasty. However, this extends beyond the scope of this textbook.

The skin of the upper eyelid is very thin without any subcutaneous fat. Beneath the skin lies the very vascular orbicularis muscle. Local anesthetic injections should be placed immediately beneath the skin, avoiding the orbicularis muscle, to prevent the occurrence of a hematoma. Deep to the orbicularis muscle above the skin crease lies the orbital septum. This originates from the arcus marginalis along the superior orbital margin. This firm attachment can be utilized to differentiate it from the levator aponeurosis. The orbital septum is a multi-layered structure with a very variable thickness.

Posterior to the septum lies the preaponeurotic orbital fat. Pressure applied to the lower eyelid can force the fat to prolapse, which helps to differentiate this from descended retro-orbicularis fat and from fatty degeneration of the levator muscle and/or Müller's muscle. The preaponeurotic fat is a key landmark in upper eyelid surgery. The levator aponeurosis lies immediately beneath it (Figs. 15.5 and 15.12).

There are two main fat pads in the upper eyelid, a central pad and a nasal pad. The nasal fat pad is generally paler (Fig. 15.13).

It is extremely important to be able to distinguish the lacrimal gland from the orbital fat (Fig. 15.14).

The levator muscle gives rise to the levator aponeurosis at the level of Whitnall's ligament. The aponeurosis inserts onto the anterior surface of the superior two-thirds of the tarsus. The medial and lateral horns of the aponeurosis insert in the region of the medial and lateral canthal tendons. The lateral horn divides the lacrimal gland into orbital and palpebral lobes. Intraoperative damage to the medial horn can give rise to a lateral shift of the tarsus with an eyelid peak lying temporal to the pupil.

Whitnall's ligament supports the levator muscle complex, acting as a fulcrum for the action of the levator muscle, and should not be disturbed during surgery. It is a variably developed structure that runs from the lacrimal gland to the region of the trochlea (Fig. 15.15).

KEY POINT

Whitnall's ligament supports the levator muscle complex and should not be disturbed during surgery.

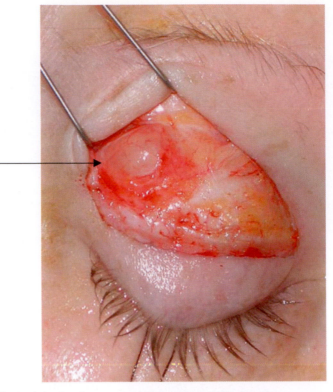

A prolapsed lacrimal
gland

Figure 15.9 A right lacrimal gland prolapse as seen during an upper lid blepharoplasty.

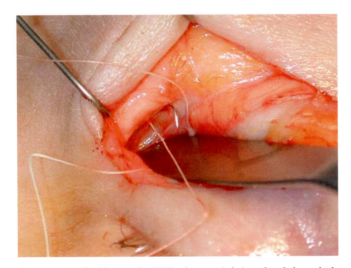

Figure 15.10 A double-armed 5/0 Vicryl suture is being placed through the periorbita of the lacrimal gland fossa.

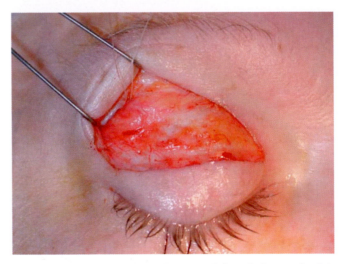

Figure 15.11 The Vicryl suture has been passed through the capsule of the lacrimal gland and tied, repositioning the gland into the lacrimal gland fossa.

The Lower Eyelids

The lower eyelid can be considered to consist of three lamellae:

- Anterior—skin and the orbicularis oculi muscle
- Middle—the orbital septum and the inferior eyelid retractors
- Posterior—the tarsus and conjunctiva

The lower eyelid skin crease is variable but is usually situated approximately 4 to 5 mm below the eyelid margin. The lateral canthal angle normally sits approximately 1 mm higher than the medial canthal angle.

The orbicularis oculi muscle is immediately deep to the skin of the lower lid. This muscle extends from just below the ciliary margin, past the inferior orbital rim, and onto the cheek.

Ptosis of the orbicularis oculi muscle commonly occurs over time and is responsible for the typical appearance of the malar crescent or malar mound in the aged face (Fig. 15.23).

Deep to the orbicularis oculi muscle lies the orbital septum which serves to retain orbital fat within the orbit. The septum is composed of inelastic fibrous tissue. Atrophy of the septum with age permits orbital fat to herniate anteriorly creating typical lower lid "bags" (Fig. 15.1B). The sub-orbicularis fascia, a plane of loose, fibrous connective tissue, lies between the orbicularis and orbital septum and provides a very good, relatively bloodless dissection plane. The orbital septum extends from the inferior border of the tarsus to fuse inferiorly with the periosteum of the infraorbital margin. This inferior attachment of the orbital septum to

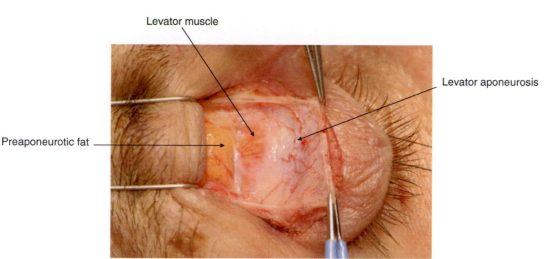

Levator muscle

Levator aponeurosis

Preaponeurotic fat

Figure 15.12 An intraoperative photograph demonstrating the levator muscle and its aponeurosis lying immediately beneath the pre-aponeurotic fat.

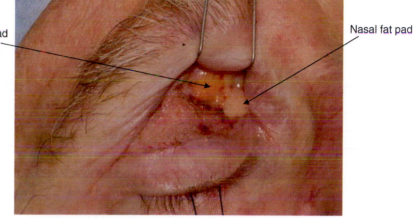

Central fat pad

Nasal fat pad

Figure 15.13 The nasal fat pad is paler than the central fat pad.

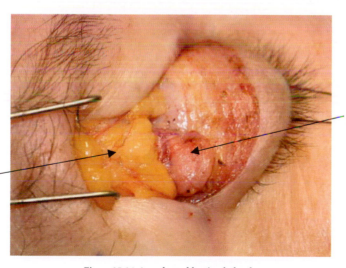

A prolapsed lacrimal gland

Preaponeurotic fat

Figure 15.14 A prolapsed lacrimal gland.

the periosteum, where there is a condensation of tissue, is referred to as the arcus marginalis (Fig. 15.16).

The arcus marginalis is strongest and best defined medially, where it attaches to the anterior lacrimal crest. As it extends laterally, the arcus marginalis becomes thinner and weakens. It also assumes a more inferior and anterior insertion; thus, medially, it runs along the inner aspect of the rim, but laterally,

it attaches approximately 2 mm inferior to the rim on the facial aspect of the zygomatic bone.

The tarsus in the lower eyelid is approximately 4 to 5 mm in height. The lower eyelid retractors are analogous to the levator aponeurosis in the upper eyelid. The smooth inferior tarsal muscle is analogous to Müller's muscle in the upper eyelid. The lower eyelid retractors, collectively referred to as

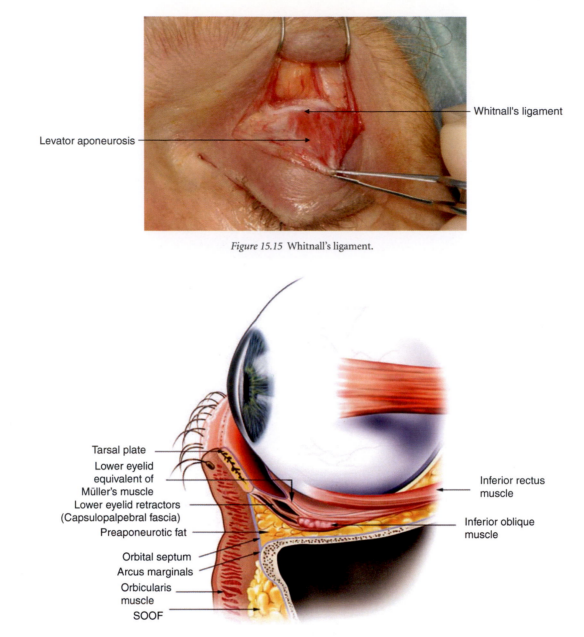

Figure 15.15 Whitnall's ligament.

Figure 15.16 A diagram illustrating the anatomy of the lower eyelid region.

the capsulo-palpebral fascia, run from the inferior rectus muscle and split to envelop the inferior oblique muscle. This fascia then inserts into the inferior border of the tarsus (Figs. 15.16 and 15.17). A deep layer of the fascia attaches to the conjunctival fornix as the suspensory ligament of the fornix.

Isolated shortening of the anterior lamella of the lower eyelid results in ectropion, of the middle lamella results in eyelid retraction with scleral show (Fig. 15.18), and of the posterior lamella results in entropion.

There are three fat compartments in the lower eyelid: medial, central, and lateral. Many delicate fibrous septa invest these compartments. The fat compartments lie between the capsulo-palpebral fascia and the orbital septum. As the capsulo-palpebral fascia (the lower eyelid retractor) is analogous to the levator aponeurosis in the upper eyelid, the fat lying in front of the capsulo-palpebral fascia can be considered to be analogous to the preaponeurotic fat in the upper eyelid. As in the upper eyelid, locating this fat is key to locating the eyelid retractor.

The inferior oblique muscle, originating from the antero-medial orbital wall, separates the medial and central fat compartments as it extends postero-laterally under the globe (Fig. 15.19).

KEY POINT

The inferior oblique muscle lies between the medial and central fat pads.

The arcuate expansion, an extension of the fascial sheath of the inferior oblique, continues laterally to attach to the lateral orbital rim and separates the central and lateral compartments (Fig. 15.20). Subtle differences exist among the 3 orbital fat pads. The fat of the medial compartment is typically white and membranous, while that of the central and lateral compartments appears yellow and soft. The lateral fat compartment contains more septa than the medial and central compartments and is therefore less prone to herniate anteriorly. It is

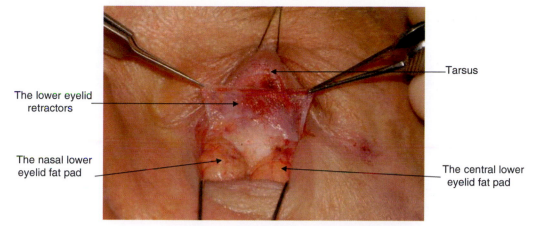

Figure 15.17 The lower eyelid retractors detached from the inferior border of the tarsus.

The lower eyelid retractors

Tarsus

The nasal lower eyelid fat pad

The central lower eyelid fat pad

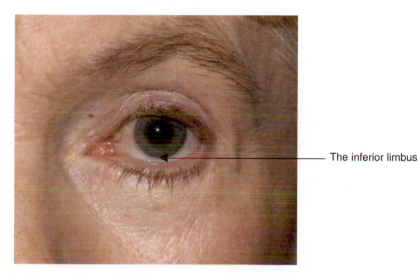

Figure 15.18 Middle lamellar scarring following a lower eyelid blepharoplasty resulting in lower eyelid retraction and scleral "show" below the inferior limbus.

The inferior limbus

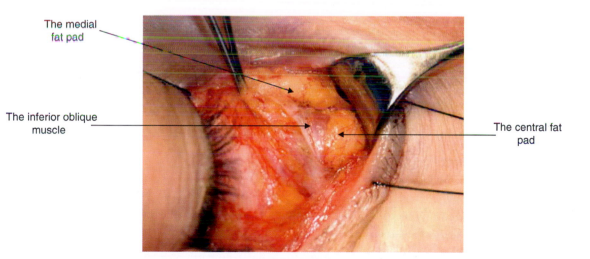

The medial fat pad

The inferior oblique muscle

The central fat pad

Figure 15.19 The inferior oblique muscle lying between the medial and central fat pads.

important to note that inferior palpebral vessels travel directly through the medial fat compartment.

Fat seen below the inferior orbital margin posterior to the orbicularis oculi muscle and just anterior to the periosteum is the SOOF (Fig. 15.21).

With increasing age, the orbicularis oculi muscle and the SOOF move inferiorly, leading to a double convexity of the lower eyelid. The superior convexity is caused by a herniation of orbital fat through a weakened orbital septum above the inferior orbital margin (Fig. 15.22A and B). The orbital margin itself is

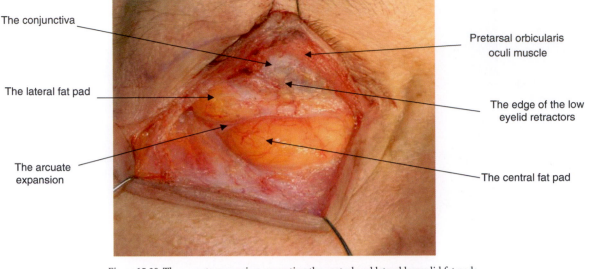

The conjunctiva

Pretarsal orbicularis
oculi muscle

The lateral fat pad

The edge of the low
eyelid retractors

The arcuate
expansion

The central fat pad

Figure 15.20 The arcuate expansion separating the central and lateral lower lid fat pads.

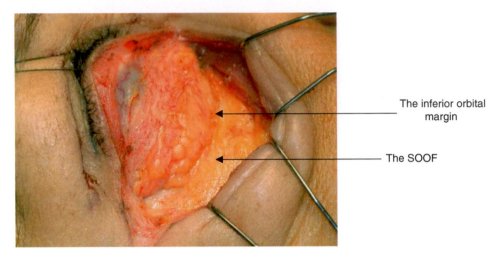

The inferior orbital
margin

The SOOF

Figure 15.21 The sub-orbicularis oculi fat (SOOF).

responsible for the horizontal concavity and the SOOF, which has moved inferiorly, is responsible for the second convexity.

The Mid-Face
Knowledge of the anatomy of the mid-face is essential for the understanding of the morphological changes which occur at the lower eyelid-cheek junction with advancing age.

The prezygomatic space is a triangular space overlying the zygomatic and maxillary bones with its apex toward the nose and is limited superiorly by the orbitomalar ligament. It contains:

- Fat overlying the orbital part of the orbicularis muscle
- The orbital part of the orbicularis muscle
- The SOOF
- Pre-periosteal fat deep to the origin of the lip elevator muscles
- Retaining ligaments

There are a number of retaining ligaments in the face, which are condensations of fibrous connective tissue and which act to anchor the superficial tissue layers to firmer underlying structures. These ligaments are divided into true and false retaining ligaments.

- True retaining ligaments

True retaining ligaments link the dermis to the underlying periosteum (zygomatic, orbital, orbito-malar, and mandibular ligaments).

- False retaining ligaments

False retaining ligaments link the deep facial fascia to the superficial facial fascia and the subcutaneous tissue (masseteric and platysma-auricular ligaments).

The zygomatic retaining ligament ("McGregor's patch") arises from the zygomatic arch and from the body of the zygoma, passes through the superior aspect of the malar fat pad, and inserts into the dermis of the overlying skin. The ligament is well-defined. The orbital retaining ligament lies over the fronto-zygomatic suture.

The orbito-malar ligament arises from a thickened area of periosteum a few millimeters below the inferior orbital margin, and passes through the superficial musculo-aponeurotic system and overlying fat to insert into the dermis.

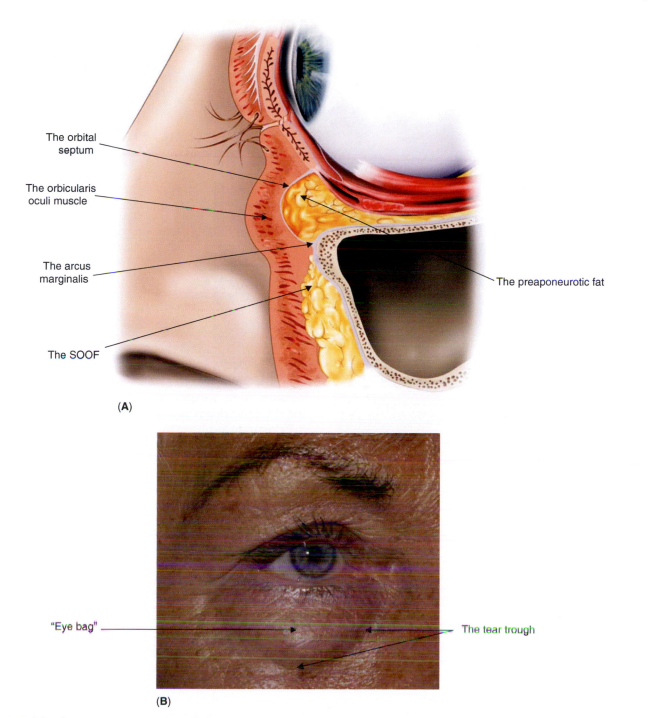

Figure 15.22 (**A**) A diagrammatic representation of bulging preaponeurotic fat through a weakened orbital septum with a secondary concavity over the inferior orbital margin responsible for the complaint of "eyebags" and for a tear trough deformity or "dark circle." (**B**) A patient demonstrating the typical "eyebag" and tear trough extending along the whole length of the inferior orbital margin.

The orbito-malar ligament, the levator labii superioris, and the levator alaeque nasi muscles are responsible for defining the tear trough. The tear trough extends into the upper central cheek as a triangular groove between these muscles as the malar fat descends with age.

"Malar mounds" are the result of edema within the fat of the prezygomatic space (Fig. 15.23). The malar fat pad is subcutaneous, triangular, and distinct from the "malar mounds." This fat pad contributes to the fullness of the mid-face. Elevation of the malar fat pad and the "malar mounds" contributes greatly to the aesthetic appearance of the mid-face and can improve the appearance of the tear troughs.

DERMATOCHALASIS

Dermatochalasis describes a common, physiologic condition seen clinically as sagging of the upper eyelid skin. It is typically bilateral and most often seen in patients over 50 years of age, but may occur in some younger adults. Examination of these patients' eyelids reveals redundant, lax skin with poor adhesion to the underlying orbicularis oculi muscle. An excess fold of skin in the upper eyelid is characteristic, which obscures the normal upper eyelid skin crease which may be lost (Fig. 15.24).

Dermatochalasis is often confused with blepharochalasis although the disorders are quite different both in their presentation and etiology. Blepharochalasis is a rare inflammatory

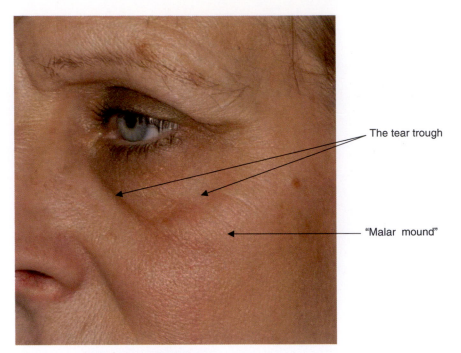

Figure 15.23 Typical age-related changes at the eyelid-cheek junction.

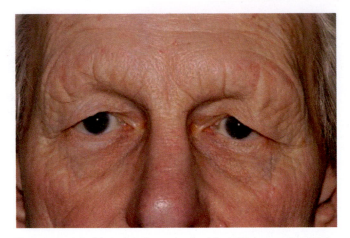

Figure 15.24 A female patient demonstrating bilateral brow ptosis and bilateral upper eyelid dermatochalasis. This patient complained of visual field limitation and headaches towards the evening (due to frontalis muscle fatigue).

condition that typically affects only the upper eyelids, and may be unilateral as well as bilateral. It occurs more often in younger patients. The condition is characterized by exacerbations and remissions of eyelid edema, which results in a "stretching" and subsequent atrophy of the eyelid tissue. The secondary effects of blepharochalasis include conjunctival hyperaemia and chemosis, entropion, ectropion, blepharoptosis, medial fat pad atrophy, and thinning of eyelid skin.

Pathophysiology
The tissue changes seen in dermatochalasis are similar to the normal aging changes of the skin seen elsewhere in the body. There is thinning of the epidermal tissue with a loss of elastin, resulting in laxity, redundancy, and hypertrophy of the skin. The tissue changes of dermatochalasis appear to be due to repeated facial expressions combined with the effects of gravity over many years. A number of systemic disorders such as thyroid eye disease, Ehlers-Danlos syndrome, cutis laxa, renal failure, and amyloidosis may hasten the development of dermatochalasis. In addition, some patients may have a genetic predisposition toward the development of dermatochalasis at a younger age.

By contrast, blepharochalasis stems from recurrent bouts of painless eyelid swelling, each instance of which may persist for several days. The swelling most likely represents a form of localized angiedema, although this remains speculative. Ultimately, after numerous episodes, the skin of the lids becomes thin and atrophic, and damage to the levator aponeurosis ensues. Blepharoptosis then develops (Fig. 15.25). Blepharochalasis is idiopathic in most cases, though it has been linked to kidney agenesis, vertebral abnormalities, and congenital heart defects in rare instances.

UPPER EYELID BLEPHAROPLASTY
The goals of an upper eyelid blepharoplasty are:

1. To remove an appropriate amount of excess upper eyelid skin alone, or skin and orbicularis muscle, in order to achieve the best cosmetic and functional result for the patient.
2. To remove or sculpt herniated orbital fat only where appropriate.
3. To create a symmetrical upper lid skin crease at an appropriate height for the individual patient.
4. To avoid visible scarring.
5. To avoid a secondary lagophthalmos or an incomplete blink.
6. To avoid exacerbating an associated brow ptosis.

An additional goal in the oriental patient is to create a visible upper eyelid crease.

Preoperative Patient Evaluation
History
A careful history should be obtained. The patient's complaints, goals, and expectations should be determined. The patient may be concerned about:

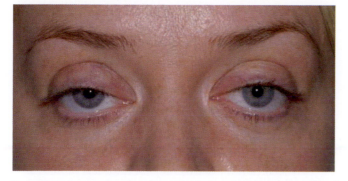

Figure 15.25 A young female patient with blepharochalasis showing bilateral blepharoptosis with raised skin creases, thinning of the upper eyelid skin, and atrophy of the preaponeurotic fat pads. She also demonstrates a bilateral pseudoproptosis from high axial myopia.

- An overhang of excess upper eyelid skin causing a loss of the superior visual field
- Excess upper lid skin causing cosmetic problems
- Upper lid fat herniation
- Upper lid "fullness"
- "Hooding" of the upper eyelids
- "Drooping eyelids"
- Headaches from frontalis muscle fatigue
- A tired appearance commented on by friends or relatives

The complaint of droopy upper eyelids may simply be due to severe dermatochalasis causing a pseudoptosis with the underlying eyelid height being normal. The lid position should be carefully evaluated, however, as a true blepharoptosis may also be present. If a true blepharoptosis is present, the patient must be carefully evaluated to diagnose the underlying cause of the blepharoptosis, e.g., an aponeurotic dehiscence from contact lens wear, a Horner's syndrome, myasthenia gravis, or chronic progressive external ophthalmoplegia (chap. 7—"Blepharoptosis"). Similarly, a severe dermatochalasis, often combined with a brow ptosis, may obstruct the patient's superior visual field.

Patients who have a moderate-to-severe brow ptosis and dermatochalasis are obliged to use their frontalis muscle to overcome the superior visual field defect. Such patients commonly develop deep forehead furrows (Fig. 15.26). This leads to fatigue of the frontalis muscle, which in turn can cause a headache.

Occasionally, upper eyelid dermatochalasis and a lateral brow ptosis can lead to a secondary mechanical misdirection of eyelashes causing chronic ocular discomfort.

The cosmetic effects of upper eyelid dermatochalasis and brow ptosis can lead to complaints of a tired appearance. Lower eyelid fat herniation can also lead to similar complaints (Fig. 15.1B).

Patients should be specifically questioned about previous eyelid surgery. Patients who have previously undergone a cosmetic blepharoplasty or a facelift may omit such information, particularly if accompanied by a new partner. A history of contact lens wear, dry eye, facial palsy, or thyroid dysfunction identifies a patient at risk of exposure keratopathy symptoms following an upper lid blepharoplasty.

KEY POINT

A history of contact lens wear, dry eye, facial palsy, or thyroid dysfunction identifies a patient at risk of exposure keratopathy symptoms following an upper lid blepharoplasty.

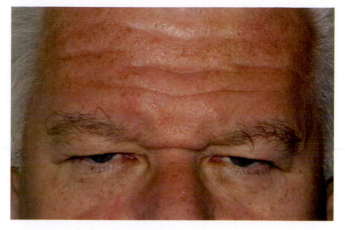

Figure 15.26 A patient with a severe bilateral brow ptosis and dermatochalasis causing visual field problems and headaches from frontalis overaction.

It is important to exclude a bleeding disorder, as a postoperative hemorrhage following a blepharoplasty can be potentially sight-threatening. The use of aspirin or non-steroidal anti-inflammatory agents should be discontinued if the patient's medical status permits this. Any other non-prescription medications or dietary supplements that may predispose to excessive bleeding should also be discontinued, e.g., vitamin E supplements.

KEY POINT

It is important to exclude a bleeding disorder, as a postoperative hemorrhage following a blepharoplasty is potentially sight-threatening. The use of aspirin or non-steroidal anti-inflammatory agents should be discontinued 2 weeks preoperatively.

Any allergies should be carefully noted.

Examination
The patient should undergo a complete ophthalmic examination:

- The patient's best corrected visual acuity should be recorded.
- The palpebral fissures should be measured and the position of the skin creases documented after lifting the upper lid excess skin.
- The height and curvature of the upper eyelids relative to the pupils should be noted, and the marginal reflex distance-1(MRD-1) and marginal reflex distance-2 (MRD-2) should be measured and recorded, looking for any evidence of true blepharoptosis.

KEY POINT

The patient seeking or referred to for a blepharoplasty should undergo a complete ophthalmic examination.

MRD-1 is the distance between the center of the pupillary light reflex and the upper eyelid margin with the eye in primary gaze. A measurement of 4 to 5 mm is considered normal. MRD-2 is the distance between the center of the pupillary light reflex and the lower eyelid margin with the eye in primary gaze.

- The amount of pretarsal skin "show" should be measured and recorded along with the amount of skin present from the lash line to the lowermost portion of the eyebrow, medially, centrally, and laterally. This can be difficult in patients who pluck or tattoo their eyebrows (Fig. 15.27).
- Any asymmetries should be noted. (It is important to make the patient aware of any preoperative asymmetries, which the patient may not have noticed. The patient will certainly notice asymmetries postoperatively!) Any frontalis overaction should be noted, and the position and shape of the brows observed after asking the patient to relax the frontalis muscle as much as possible. *The secondary effects of brow ptosis on the upper eyelids must be recognized* (Fig. 15.24) (see chap. 16).

- An assessment of the tear meniscus should be made using a slit lamp, and the tear film break-up time after the instillation of a drop of fluorescein should be documented.
- The upper lids should be everted to exclude the presence of any subtarsal lesions, e.g., papillae seen in atopy or with contact lens wear.
- The presence or absence of a Bell's phenomenon should be recorded.
- The degree of upper eyelid laxity is assessed to ensure that a "floppy eyelid syndrome" is not overlooked. This is done by pulling downwards on the eyelid after grasping the eyelid margin and the eyelashes in the lateral aspect of the eyelid. Excessive eyelid laxity is also evident if eversion of the upper eyelid is very easy to perform.
- Any herniation of the medial and central preaponeurotic fat pads is noted in the upper eyelids, and of the

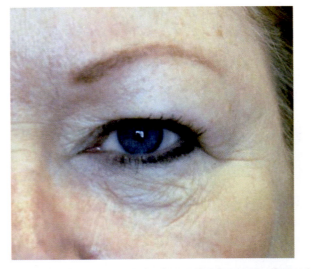

Figure 15.27 A patient with a plucked and tattooed eyebrow camouflaging the effects of a brow ptosis and a descent of the "ROOF."

medial, central, and lateral preaponeurotic fat pads in the lower eyelids.
- The degree of excess upper eyelid skin is assessed and measured.
- The degree of any associated brow ptosis is noted along with any asymmetry. Any overaction of the eyebrow depressor muscles is also determined by noting the extent of glabellar frown lines and lateral canthal rhytids.
- The skin quality and degree of actinic damage is assessed. Specific dermatological disorders should be excluded, e.g., atopic dermatitis.
- The ocular motility should be assessed and recorded along with cover and alternate cover tests to exclude any horizontal or vertical ocular muscle imbalance.
- Any proptosis or pseudo-proptosis due to axial myopia is noted. It may be much more difficult to achieve the desired surgical goals in such patients.

Preoperative photographs must be taken. Preoperative photographs are essential for patients who are to undergo any facial plastic and reconstructive surgery. They serve a number of useful purposes:

- A learning and teaching aid for the surgeon.
- A verification of the patient's disorder for health care insurance companies.
- An aid to defence in a medico-legal claim.
- To jolt the memory of the forgetful patient about their preoperative appearance.

Written patient consent should be obtained before the photographs are taken. It should be made clear to the patient how the photographs are to be used.

The limitations of an upper eyelid blepharoplasty performed alone in the presence of significant brow ptosis should be explained. Under these circumstances, an upper eyelid blepharoplasty should be very conservative in order to prevent further lowering of the brow and an unsatisfactory appearance. The patient should be carefully questioned to ascertain the patient's expectations of surgery. Some patients with a mild degree of brow ptosis and upper lid dermatochalasis are better managed with the use of botulinum toxin injections, which, if used correctly, can create a satisfactory and pleasing brow lift. The injection can be given into the lateral rhytids and tail of the eyebrow (30 to 60 units of Dysport per side given as four to five separate intramuscular injections), and can be combined with injections into the glabella

(80–120 units of Dysport given as four to six separate intramuscular injections) paralyzing the brow depressors and allowing the frontalis muscle to act unopposed. If an unwanted temporal peaking of the brows occurs, 5 to 10 units of botulinum toxin can be injected 1 to 2 cm above the lateral brow into the over-acting frontalis.

If botulinum toxin injections are to be used as a trial prior to surgery, this should be undertaken 2 weeks beforehand. The injections should not be given at the time of surgery as postoperative edema will cause the toxin to spread to other muscles, e.g., to the levator muscles causing a blepharoptosis.

KEY POINT

Botulinum toxin injections should not be given at the time of surgery.

Where a brow ptosis is significant, it is much preferable to address this by one of a number of surgical approaches, depending on the degree of brow ptosis and the age and preferences of the patient.

The management of eyebrow ptosis is discussed in detail in chapter 16.

Figure 15.28A illustrates the problem posed by a female patient requesting an upper eyelid blepharoplasty who demonstrates a marked bilateral brow ptosis. A blepharoplasty alone would be inappropriate. Figure 15.28B demonstrates her postoperative appearance 2 months following a bilateral upper eyelid skin/muscle blepharoplasty combined with a bilateral direct brow lift.

Informed Consent

The advantages, disadvantages, risks, and potential complications should be discussed with the patient in great detail. The siting of incisions and anticipated scars should be explained. The risks and the incidence of complications need to be outlined in an open and honest manner. The consequences of complications and their management should also be outlined. The patient should also be provided with a formal document which outlines the potential complications of blepharoplasty surgery, their management, and the financial responsibilities that would be incurred.

The description of any blepharoplasty procedure as "basic," "straightforward," "simple," "minor," or "routine" should be avoided.

Many patients seeking cosmetic blepharoplasty request that their general practitioner is not informed. A detailed letter outlining the patient's complaints, the clinical findings, the management options which have been discussed, the risks and potential complications of surgery, advice about the discontinuation of aspirin or anti-inflammatory drugs, the anticipated recovery period, and aftercare instructions should, however, be sent to the patient and retained in their

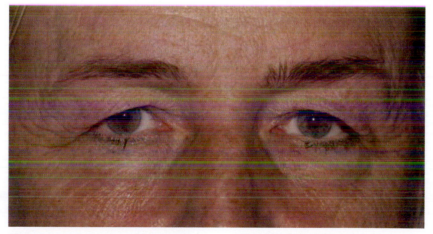

(A)

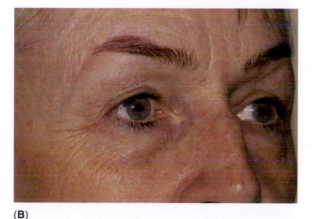

(B)

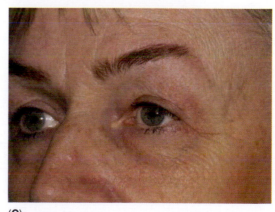

(C)

Figure 15.28 (**A**) A female patient with bilateral brow ptosis and upper eyelid dermatochalasis. (**B,C**) The same patient 2 months following a bilateral temporal direct brow lift and upper lid blepharoplasty. The height of the brows was overcorrected at the patient's request.

clinical records. This allows the patient to further consider the options discussed before making a decision to proceed with surgery. It also avoids any misunderstandings on the part of the patient.

Surgical Technique

Marking the upper eyelid skin crease with the patient sitting upright, before the injection of any local anesthetic solution, is the first very important step in a successful upper eyelid blepharoplasty. A drop of Proxymethacaine is instilled into each eye. The upper eyelid skin is cleaned with an alcohol wipe, and the skin crease marked with a cocktail stick, which has been dipped into a gentian violet marker block. A calliper should be used to measure the height of the crease. The fellow eyelid should be marked simultaneously, ensuring precise symmetry. The skin crease should be marked at a lower level in a male patient.

The skin above the crease centrally is gently pinched with a pair of fine toothed forceps. Great care should be taken to ensure that the eyelids can close passively. Any temptation to remove more than 8 to 10 mm of skin should be resisted particularly in the presence of an uncorrected brow ptosis. The superior aspect of the pinched skin is marked and an ellipse is drawn (Fig. 15.29).

The relative dimensions of this area divided into thirds should be remembered to maintain a good aesthetic appearance. (The distance between the inferior aspect of the eyebrow and the upper lid skin crease on down gaze should be approximately two-thirds of the distance from the inferior aspect of

the eyebrow to the eyelid margin. Likewise, the distance from the skin crease to the eyelid margin in down gaze should be one-third of the distance from the inferior aspect of the eyebrow to the eyelid margin.) In general at least 10 to 12 mm of skin should be left between the inferior aspect of the eyebrow and the superior skin excision marking (Fig. 15.30). It is important not to carry the incision markings into the medial canthal area to avoid webbed scars.

If there is no temporal hooding of skin, the lateral aspect of the incision should be kept within the orbital margin (Fig. 15.30). If there is temporal hooding, a lateral wing can be added to the crescent leaving the resulting scar running in a horizontal direction (Fig. 15.31). The patient should be warned that this lateral scar will be visible and will not be hidden with the upper lid skin crease.

If a patient is to undergo a simultaneous brow lift procedure the desired postoperative position of the brow is mimicked by an assistant raising the brow with a finger. The skin measurements, the skin pinch, and the markings are made with the brow maintained in the desired position.

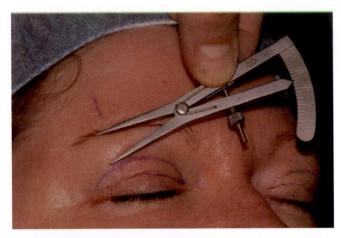

Figure 15.30 Twelve millimeters of skin has been left between the inferior aspect of the eyebrow and the superior skin excision marking.

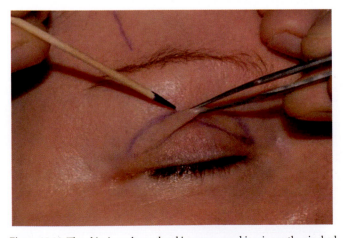

Figure 15.29 The skin just above the skin crease marking is gently pinched with toothed forceps ensuring that passive closure of the eye is not compromised. This is repeated medially and laterally and the proposed skin excision is marked.

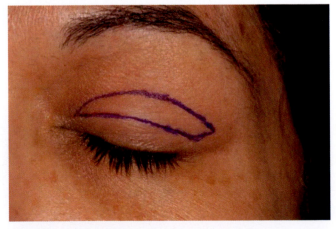

Figure 15.31 The desired position of the upper eyelid skin crease has been marked with a cocktail stick dipped into a gentian marker block. The skin above the crease has been gently pinched while asking the patient to passively close the eye. The markings are not taken medially beyond the limit of the skin crease. Laterally, a small "wing" has been added to prevent a "dog ear." A distance of at least 12 mm has been left between the inferior aspect of the brow and the superior aspect of the blepharoplasty.

Anesthesia

The procedure may be undertaken under either general anesthesia, local anesthesia, or local anesthesia with intravenous sedation. Local anesthesia, preferably with carefully titrated intravenous sedation provided by an anesthetist, is advantageous as it allows voluntary levator muscle function to be used to assist in the identification of eyelid structures. This is particularly important when an upper eyelid blepharoplasty is being performed in conjunction with a levator aponeurosis advancement procedure to correct blepharoptosis.

The patient should be kept in a semi-recumbent position with the head elevated at least 30° to reduce venous engorgement and bleeding. Normal saline sachets should be kept available in the refrigerator and used to moisten 4 × 4 gauze swabs, which are applied to the operated side while the fellow side is undergoing the same procedure.

Surgical Procedure

1. Approximately 2 to 3 ml of 0.5% Bupivacaine with 1:200,000 units of adrenaline mixed 50:50 with 2% Lidocaine with 1:80,000 units of adrenaline are injected just beneath the skin with a single pass of the needle if possible, avoiding the underlying orbicularis oculi muscle in order to prevent the occurrence of a hematoma. The needle is inserted temporally and advanced nasally while slowly injecting the solution. Immediate pressure should be applied for a few minutes. Ten minutes are allowed for the adrenaline to take effect.

2. The patient is prepped and draped, ensuring that the drapes do not place any downward pressure on the eyebrows.

3. A 4/0 silk traction suture is inserted along the gray line of the upper eyelid and fixated to the face drapes with a curved artery clip, providing downward traction on the eyelid. This makes the skin incision easier to undertake, and provides protection for the eye.

4. The skin incision is made along the gentian violet markings with a Colorado needle.

5. The incision is deepened through the orbicularis muscle to the plane of the orbital septum.

6. A myocutaneous flap is developed and dissected off the orbital septum (Fig. 15.32). If the patient merely requires the removal of excess skin and orbicularis muscle for functional reasons, the skin can be closed with simple interrupted 7/0 Vicryl sutures. This surgical procedure is quick and relatively simple to perform and does not expose the patient to the small risks of a postoperative intraorbital hemorrhage.

In patients who are at an increased risk of exposure keratopathy, a simple skin excision alone can be performed, preserving the underlying orbicularis muscle. In some patients, however, this can result in some bunching of the orbicularis muscle with a less satisfactory aesthetic result. Alternatively, a central 3 to 5 mm strip of orbicularis muscle can be removed.

7. If the patient requires the removal, sculpting, or redraping of orbital fat, the orbital septum is opened along its entire length.

8. The central preaponeurotic fat is allowed to prolapse. This can be sculpted with the Colorado needle using the coagulation mode and any larger vessels cauterized with bipolar cautery. The fascial septa around and within the medial fat pad can be gently opened and separated using the Colorado needle.

9. If fat needs to be removed, the fat should be carefully clamped using a small curved artery clip. The artery clip should be held carefully by the assistant. Great care should be taken to avoid anterior traction on the fat that can lead to rupture of posterior orbital vessels and a sight-threatening retrobulbar hematoma. The fat is removed using the Colorado needle on cautery mode. The artery clip should be released very slowly and carefully, and immediately reapplied if any vessels bleed. This is particularly important when removing fat medially. Great care should also be taken not to damage the medial horn of the levator muscle, or the trochlea. It

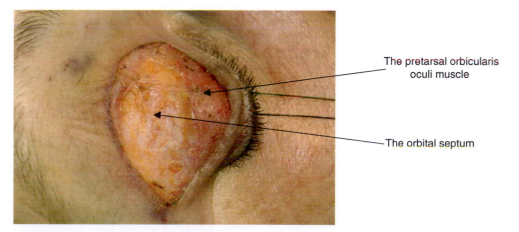

The pretarsal orbicularis oculi muscle

The orbital septum

Figure 15.32 The skin and orbicularis muscle have been removed in this patient whose pretarsal orbicularis muscle has also been partially exposed. (This patient has undergone a skin–muscle blepharoplasty prior to the completion of an orbicularis myectomy procedure for the management of essential blepharospasm.)

should be noted, however, that fat removal should be undertaken very conservatively, if at all, in the upper lid so as to avoid a secondary hollowing of the upper eyelid which can result in a very aged appearance. The fat should be retained within a swab moistened with sterile saline as it may be divided into small fat pearls and used as a free graft in the opposite upper eyelid to address an asymmetry or in the lower eyelid to assist in the camouflage of a tear trough defect.

10. The skin is closed with interrupted 7/0 Vicryl sutures, taking bites of the very edges of the skin. The type of skin closure is determined by the type of skin crease that is required. If this is to be a soft, less well-defined crease, the skin can be closed as above. If a higher well-defined crease is required, usually in a female patient, the skin is closed with interrupted 7/0 Vicryl sutures that incorporate a bite of the underlying levator aponeurosis. It is sometimes advantageous to remove a strip of orbicularis muscle from the inferior skin wound edge but this can lead to bleeding particularly if the effects of the adrenaline have begun to wear off.

KEY POINT

It should be noted that fat removal should be undertaken very conservatively, if at all, in the upper lid so as to avoid a secondary hollowing of the upper eyelid which can result in a very aged appearance.

Postoperative Care

Postoperatively the patient is prescribed a topical antibiotic ointment to the upper lid wounds three times a day for 2 weeks and Lacrilube ointment 1 to 2 hourly to the eyes for 48 hours and at bedtime. The Lacrilube ointment is then changed to preservative-free topical lubricant drops to be used hourly during the day and Lacrilube is continued at bedtime until the degree of lagophthalmos has improved. The frequency of the lubricants is then gradually reduced over the course of the next few weeks. The patient is instructed to sleep with the head of the bed elevated for 4 weeks and to avoid lifting any heavy weights for 2 weeks. Clean cool packs are gently applied to the eyelids intermittently for 48 hours. The patient should be reviewed in clinic within 2 weeks and again within 4 to 6 weeks. The upper lid skin sutures are removed after 2 weeks.

LOWER EYELID BLEPHAROPLASTY

The goals of a lower eyelid blepharoplasty are:

1. To remove an appropriate amount of excess lower eyelid skin and muscle if required
2. To remove or reposition herniated fat where appropriate
3. To avoid middle lamellar scarring and eyelid retraction
4. To address any associated lower eyelid or lateral canthal tendon laxity
5. To avoid any postoperative ectropion and secondary epiphora

An emerging concept in cosmetic surgery holds that the face develops the characteristics of aging as a result of not only elastosis and sagging but also soft tissue atrophy. The evolution of this concept is well illustrated in the field of lower lid blepharoplasty, in which the traditional approach to the surgical improvement of lower eyelid "bags" has been to resect the herniating preaponeurotic fat. While this method can indeed remove "bags," in many patients it may also eliminate the soft tissue that conceals the inferior orbital margins, creating a hollow, skeletonized appearance. This is in contrast to the appearance of the youthful face, in which soft tissue fullness creates a smooth transition from the cheek to the lower eyelid. The inferior bony orbital margin is concealed. The traditional approach of resecting orbital fat is therefore unlikely to produce a full, youthful lower lid contour and conflicts with the concept that facial aging is partly a consequence of soft tissue atrophy.

A number of alternative surgical approaches have been devised to address this problem. One such technique that has gained prominence is the arcus marginalis release, in which preaponeurotic fat is advanced and repositioned rather than resected, in order to reconstruct the soft tissue of the lower eyelids. This technique is designed to conceal the underlying bony structure of the inferior orbit in an attempt to impart a more youthful contour to the periorbital area. Alternatively, a "SOOF" lift or a mid-face lift may be undertaken in conjunction with a lower eyelid blepharoplasty in order to achieve the same goals, but the patient then has to accept a more extensive surgical dissection and a longer period of recuperation with more postoperative bruising and swelling.

Preoperative Patient Evaluation

History

The patient's complaints, goals, and expectations should be determined. The patient may be concerned about:

- Loose folds of skin
- Lower eyelid "bags"
- Dark circles beneath the eyes
- Skin wrinkles and/or signs of photo damage
- Malar mounds
- Lower eyelid "festoons"

Examination

As for an upper eyelid blepharoplasty, the patient should undergo a complete ophthalmic examination.

- The patient's best-corrected visual acuity should be recorded.
- The palpebral fissures should be measured and the position of the lower eyelid with respect to the inferior limbus noted. The MRD-1 and MRD-2 should be measured and recorded.
- Any asymmetries or scleral show should be noted.
- The patient's lower lid appearance at rest and on smiling should be compared.

KEY POINT

The patient should undergo a complete ophthalmic examination preoperatively.

- The relationship of the globe to the inferior orbital margin should be noted, particularly the degree to which the globe protrudes beyond the inferior orbital margin in profile view. A globe, which protrudes beyond the inferior orbital margin, is referred to as a "negative vector" configuration. Such patients are more at risk of postoperative problems with eyelid retraction and scleral show following a lower eyelid transcutaneous blepharoplasty.

- An assessment of tear production and the tear film should be undertaken using a slit lamp and the findings documented.

- Any "herniation" of the lower eyelid fat pads is noted and their positions documented. The skin quality and degree of actinic damage is assessed.

- The degree of lower eyelid laxity is assessed. This can be quite subjective but, as a general rule, if the lower eyelid can be distracted from the globe by more that 6 to 8 mm or if the eyelid does not return to its position after release without a blink (a positive "snap test"), the eyelid can be considered to have sufficient laxity to warrant a lower eyelid tightening procedure.

- Any proptosis or pseudo-proptosis due to a large globe is noted. It may be more difficult to achieve the surgical goals in such patients. *The patient should be examined specifically to exclude the possibility of thyroid eye disease.*

KEY POINT

The patient should be examined specifically to exclude the possibility of thyroid eye disease.

- The appearance of the infraorbital margin is carefully assessed. Almost any patient seeking a lower eyelid blepharoplasty with lower eyelid "bags" and/or a skeletonization of the inferior orbital margin is a candidate for an arcus marginalis release. In contrast, however, younger patients with a congenital excess of orbital fat are less likely to benefit from this technique. These patients are better managed using a traditional resection of the excess fat via a transconjunctival approach, with the use of CO_2 skin resurfacing or a chemical peel to manage any associated lower eyelid skin wrinkling and photo damage.

Just as the upper lid cannot be properly assessed without also taking into consideration the position of the eyebrow, the lower lid should not be examined in isolation but account should be taken of any associated mid-face ptosis and mid-face fat atrophy. Such a patient may require a SOOF lift, or a mid-face lift and/or volume augmentation of the cheek and tear trough using dermal fillers or structural fat grafting.

Surgical Approaches

A lower eyelid blepharoplasty procedure should ideally be tailored to the individual requirements of a patient. The surgical approach selected depends on a preoperative assessment of fat "herniation," the degree of skeletonization of the inferior orbital margin, the presence of a lower lid double convexity, the amount of excess lower eyelid skin, the degree of static wrinkling and actinic damage, the degree of orbicularis oculi muscle ptosis, the presence and degree of mid-face ptosis and mid-face fat atrophy, the presence of "malar mounds" or festoons, and the degree of lower eyelid or lateral canthal tendon laxity. The procedure may be performed in conjunction with another surgical procedure, e.g., an orbital decompression procedure in thyroid eye disease.

The patient should also be carefully evaluated to determine whether or not alternative non-surgical treatments might be better suited to their needs. This will depend on the patient's individual circumstances and age. Some patients with the complaint of lateral canthal rhytids ("laughter lines") and lateral eyelid skin wrinkling alone may be better managed with botulinum toxin injections. These can be given into the lateral rhytids (30 to 60 units of Dysport per side given as four to five injections) with the addition of tiny amounts to the lateral lower lid orbicularis muscle (two to three injections of two to three units of Dysport). Injections should not be given in the medial aspect of the lower eyelid, as this is associated with the risk of spread to involve the inferior oblique muscle. In addition, higher doses should be avoided in the lower eyelid to avoid undue weakness to the orbital portion of the orbicularis muscle with the risk of the patient developing a malar "bag."

Hyaluronic acid filler injections (e.g., Restylane or Juvéderm) can be used to camouflage the tear troughs in suitable candidates (Fig. 15.33). Alternatively, a Jessner's/trichloro-acetic acid peel (TCA) or CO_2 laser resurfacing can be considered to treat age and solar related skin wrinkling in the lower eyelids (Figs. 15.34 and 15.35).

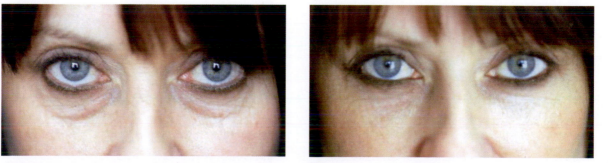

(A) (B)

Figure 15.33 (**A**) Bilateral lower eyelid "tear tough" defects. (**B**) The appearance of the same patient 2 weeks following the injection of a hyaluronic acid filler (Restylane) along the inferior orbital margins.

For patients who are better suited to surgical management there are two main surgical approaches:

- Transcutaneous lower lid blepharoplasty
- Transconjunctival lower lid blepharoplasty

These procedures can be supplemented by other techniques to enhance the result:

1. Horizontal eyelid tightening procedure
2. "Pinch" technique skin resection (in the case of a transconjunctival lower lid blepharoplasty)
3. CO_2 laser resurfacing
4. A Jessner's/TCA peel
5. Botulinum toxin injections
6. The injection of dermal fillers or autogenous fat to provide soft tissue enhancement
7. A "SOOF" lift
8. A mid-face lift
9. The placement of a cheek implant

A transconjunctival approach is preferred for patients with "fat herniation" but no significant skin excess. This approach avoids an external scar and is also ideal for patients who have previously undergone a transcutaneous blepharoplasty but who require revision surgery for residual fat "herniation." It can be combined with CO_2 laser resurfacing or with a Jessner's/TCA peel to deal with skin wrinkling in those patients who are prepared to cooperate with the more onerous postoperative care and the avoidance of sun exposure (Fig. 15.36).

Surgical Technique
A lower eyelid blepharoplasty can be performed under general anesthesia, local anesthesia, or local anesthesia with intravenous sedation. Local anesthesia affords the surgeon the opportunity of asking the patient to look up and to open the mouth to avoid excessive skin resection during a transcutaneous blepharoplasty. The patient should be draped using non-adhesive drapes to allow free movement of the lower eyelid and cheek. The upper lid skin crease may need to be marked or, if the procedure is to be combined with an upper lid blepharoplasty, the upper lid skin excision should be marked as described above.

TRANSCUTANEOUS BLEPHAROPLASTY WITH ARCUS MARGINALIS RELEASE, FAT REPOSITIONING AND ORBICULARIS OCULI MUSCLE SUSPENSION
The patient is advised preoperatively that the lateral aspect of the lower eyelids will be unnaturally high for the first 2 to 3 weeks following this procedure. As the absorbable 5/0 Vicryl suture holding the orbicularis muscle flap in place begins to give way, the lateral aspect of each lower eyelid gradually assumes its normal position.

Surgical Procedure
1. Approximately 2 to 3 ml of 0.5% Bupivacaine with 1:200,000 units of adrenaline mixed 50:50 with 2% Lidocaine with 1:80,000 units of adrenaline are injected with aouipl single injection just beneath the skin along the lower eyelid just below the tarsus and a further 2 ml is injected along the upper lid skin crease. The needle is inserted temporally and advanced nasally while slowly injecting the solution. Immediate pressure is applied. Ten minutes are allowed for the adrenaline to take effect.
2. The patient is prepped and draped.
3. A 4/0 silk traction suture is placed through the gray line of the lower eyelid and fixated to the head drape with a curved artery clip. A subciliary incision is made with a Colorado needle 1.5 mm below the eyelid margin to avoid damaging the eyelash follicles. This is commenced just beneath the

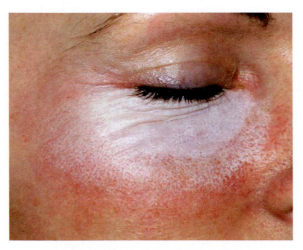

Figure 15.34 A lower eyelid 35% Jessner's/TCA peel.

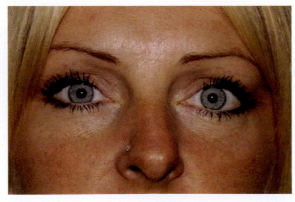

(A)

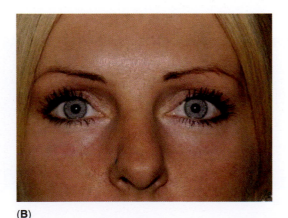

(B)

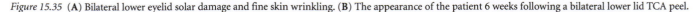

Figure 15.35 (**A**) Bilateral lower eyelid solar damage and fine skin wrinkling. (**B**) The appearance of the patient 6 weeks following a bilateral lower lid TCA peel.

inferior punctum and extends to the lateral canthus where it is continued within a lateral rhytid for a few millimeters (Figs. 15.37 and Fig. 15.38). The dissection plane first passes subcutaneously for a few millimeters until the inferior margin of the tarsus is reached, at which point the dissection plane passes deep to the orbicularis oculi muscle (Fig. 15.38). In this way, the pretarsal orbicularis oculi muscle is preserved, thereby minimizing the risk of denervation and, consequently, a paralytic lower eyelid ectropion.

4. A skin–muscle flap is dissected from the underlying orbital septum down to the inferior orbital margin.

5. Now exposed, the arcus marginalis is incised using the Colorado needle from a medial to lateral direction along the infraorbital rim, taking care to avoid the inferior oblique muscle and the lateral canthal tendon (Fig. 15.38).

6. The septum and released preaponeurotic fat are then advanced over the inferior orbital margin. If necessary, the lateral fat pad may be trimmed as it may not be possible to reposition this adequately. It is very important to avoid undue traction on the fat pads in order to avoid tearing deep orbital veins which can in turn lead to a sight-threatening retrobulbar hemorrhage. The fat should not be discarded, however, as it can be placed over the inferior orbital margin and used to further recontour the nasojugal groove and the lateral tear trough. Likewise, fat removed during the course of a simultaneous upper lid blepharoplasty should not be discarded. Any fat removed should be kept in a swab moistened with saline and re-implanted without undue delay.

7. The fat pads may need to be sculpted to achieve a smooth contour. Meticulous technique is critical at this stage, since irregularities in the contour of the advanced fat pads are noticeable through the skin. The advanced septum and orbital fat are reset (as a unit) onto the periosteum of the maxilla and zygoma inferior to the orbital rim with interrupted 5/0 Vicryl sutures (Figs. 15.39 and 15.40).

8. The septum should be reset under minimal tension to avoid scleral show or an ectropion. If resetting the septum results in any eyelid retraction, the fat alone can be repositioned and sutured.

9. A lateral upper lid skin incision is made using the Colorado needle. The dissection is carried down through the orbicularis muscle to the orbital septum. This is then traced to the lateral orbital margin where the periosteum is exposed.

10. Stevens scissors are then used to bluntly dissect beneath the lateral orbicularis oculi muscle creating a tunnel (Fig. 15.41).

11. A lateral tightening procedure may be required depending on the degree of lower lid laxity and should be performed before the septum is repositioned in order to establish and stabilize the position of the eyelid (Fig. 15.42). (This is in fact very rarely required in patients under the age of 60 years.) Using a no. 15 blade a tiny incision is made at the lateral commissure. A double-armed 5/0 Prolene suture on a round bodied needle is passed through the incision emerging through the lateral upper lid incision. Each needle is then passed through the periosteum of the internal aspect of lateral orbital wall in a medial to lateral direction and tied on the external surface of the lateral orbital wall, burying the knot (Fig. 15.42). Greater degrees of laxity of the lower eyelid and lateral canthal tendon should be addressed using a lateral tarsal strip procedure.

12. The orbicularis oculi muscle is now repositioned. With the use of this maneuver, lateral eyelid tightening is rarely if ever required in patients under the age of 60 years. From the dissection plane already created superficial to the septum and arcus marginalis, the lower lateral orbicularis is elevated off the underlying malar eminence with Westcott scissors, extending inferiorly in the submuscular plane as far as necessary to free the muscle's inferior border.

13. After separating the orbicularis oculi muscle from the skin of the lower lateral eyelid using Westcott scissors, a triangular muscle pedicle is created, with the base anchored inferolateral to the lateral canthus (Fig. 15.43). Any redundant orbicularis muscle medial to the pedicle is removed with Westcott scissors.

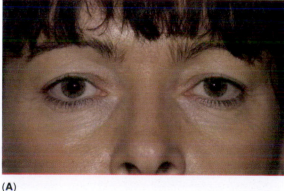
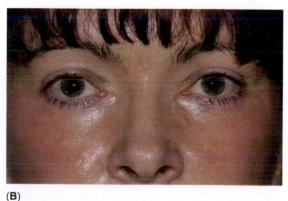

 (A) (B)

Figure 15.36 (A) The preoperative appearance of a patient with moderate lower eyelid rhytids. (B) The postoperative appearance of the same patient 2 weeks following a bilateral upper eyelid blepharoplasty and lower eyelid CO_2 resurfacing (prior to the application of camouflage mineral make-up) demonstrating improvement in skin wrinkling but with typical post laser erythema.

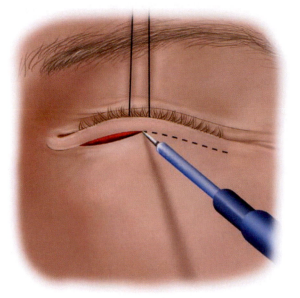

Figure 15.37 A subciliary incision is made with a Colorado needle with the lower eyelid placed on traction.

14. A double-armed 5/0 Vicryl suture on a half circle needle is passed through the orbicularis flap and the suture is passed under the bridge of skin and orbicularis muscle at the lateral canthus.

15. The needles are passed through the periosteum of the superolateral orbital margin from medial to lateral and tied (Fig. 15.44).

16. Moderate tension is maintained on the lower eyelid traction suture to prevent an over-resection of skin. If the surgery has been performed under local anesthesia, the patient is asked to look up and to open the mouth to further assist in ensuring that an over-resection of skin is avoided. The skin is incised vertically at the lateral canthus using straight iris scissors. The redundant skin is then excised medial and lateral to the vertical incision using the same straight scissors (Fig. 15.45). Care is taken to manage any residual dog-ear at the temporal aspect of the wound.

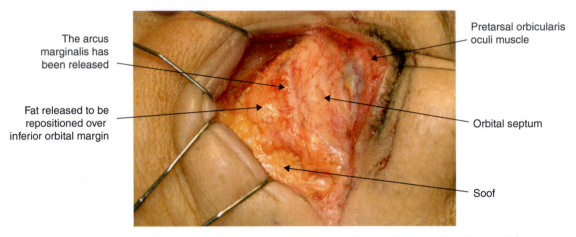

The arcus marginalis has been released

Fat released to be repositioned over inferior orbital margin

Pretarsal orbicularis oculi muscle

Orbital septum

Soof

Figure 15.38 The arcus marginalis has been released allowing pre-aponeurotic fat to prolapse over the inferior orbital margin.

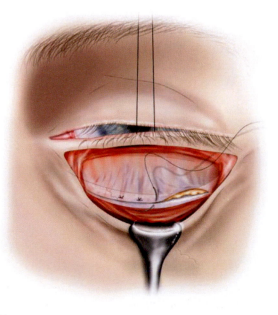

(A)   **(B)**

Figure 15.39 (**A**) A diagram showing the septum and fat being advanced over the inferior orbital margin and sutured to the periosteum just below the inferior orbital margin. (**B**) An intraoperative photograph of the septal reset procedure.

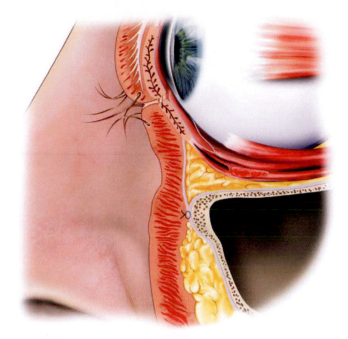

Figure 15.40 A more convex eyelid-cheek junction is created as the septal reset is performed and the orbicularis muscle is moved superolaterally.

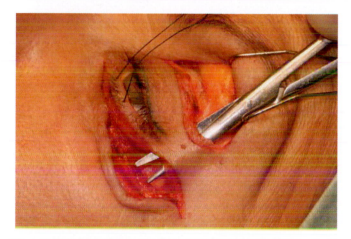

Figure 15.41 Stevens scissors are used to create a tunnel under the lateral orbicularis oculi muscle. In this patient, the lower eyelid blepharoplasty is being combined with an upper eyelid blepharoplasty.

KEY POINT

No skin should be removed from the medial 2/3 of the eyelid in the vast majority of cases. The skin resection should always be conservative.

17. The skin edges are then re-apposed using interrupted 7/0 Vicryl sutures.
18. The traction suture is removed.
19. The upper lid blepharoplasty wound is closed with interrupted 7/0 Vicryl sutures.

Postoperative Care

Postoperatively the patient is prescribed a topical antibiotic ointment to the upper and lower lid wounds three times a day for 2 weeks and Lacrilube ointment 1 to 2 hourly to the eyes for 48 hours and at bedtime. The Lacrilube ointment is then changed to a preservative-free topical lubricant gel to be used hourly during the day and Lacrilube is continued at bedtime until the degree of lagophthalmos has improved. The frequency of the lubricants is then gradually reduced over the course of the next few weeks. The patient is instructed to sleep with the head of the bed elevated for 4 weeks and to avoid lifting any heavy weights for 2 weeks. Clean cool packs are gently applied to the eyelid intermittently for 48 hours. The patient should be reviewed in clinic within 2 weeks and again within 4 to 6 weeks. The upper and lower lid skin sutures are removed at 10 to 14 days postoperatively. The patient is instructed to commence massage to the lower eyelids 2 weeks postoperatively. The patient should apply Lacrilube ointment to the skin and massage in an upward direction for 2 to 3 minutes three times a day for 4 to 6 weeks. This is important to help to avoid lower eyelid retraction.

An example of a patient who has undergone this procedure is shown in Figure 15.46.

For patients who also have mild malar mounds, the lower eyelid transcutaneous blepharoplasty can be combined with a SOOF lift using the same incisions. Likewise, for patients with malar bags and a mid-face ptosis with descent of the malar fat pads, the transcutaneous blepharoplasty can be combined with a mid-face lift, again using the same incisions (Fig. 15.47).

STRUCTURAL FAT GRAFTING

If structural fat grafting to the cheeks, temples, or other facial areas is to be undertaken in conjunction with a lower eyelid blepharoplasty, this should be undertaken initially. It is important that the fat is injected as soon as possible after it has been harvested. This increases its chances of survival. The fat should be placed at different depths in the tissues by injecting only 0.1 ml of fat with each pass of the cannula. Multiple passes are required. The injection technique should be meticulous. Structural fat grafting is described in detail in chapter 13.

SOOF LIFT
Surgical Procedure

1. This is undertaken after repositioning or removing lower eyelid fat.
2. The SOOF is mobilized by dissecting in the preperiosteal plane using blunt-tipped Westcott scissors, taking care to avoid damage to the infraorbital neurovascular bundle.
3. The SOOF is then sutured to the arcus marginalis and the periosteum of the lateral orbital margin with 4/0 Vicryl sutures (Fig. 15.48).
4. The blepharoplasty is then completed as described above.

MID-FACE LIFT
Surgical Procedure

1. This is undertaken after repositioning or removing lower eyelid fat medially.
2. The periosteum is incised 2 mm below the inferior orbital margin and a sub-periosteal dissection is performed using a Freer periosteal elevator, over the

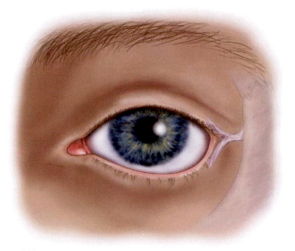

(A)

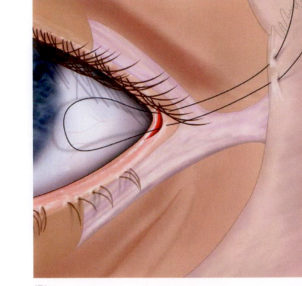

(B)

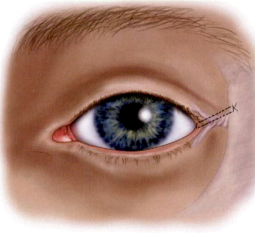

(C)

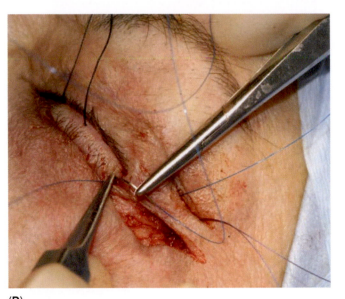

(D)

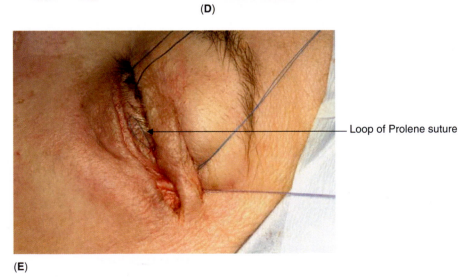

Loop of Prolene suture

(E)

Figure 15.42 (**A**) Laxity of the lower eyelid with inferior scleral "show". (**B, C**) A lateral canthal tightening suture. The lateral canthal tendon and the lateral orbital margin are exposed via a lateral upper lid skin crease incision. (**D**) An intraoperative photograph showing the placement of the Prolene suture through a small incision at the lateral commissure. (**E**) The loop of the Prolene suture is seen between the upper and lower eyelids laterally before the suture is tightened. (*Continued*)

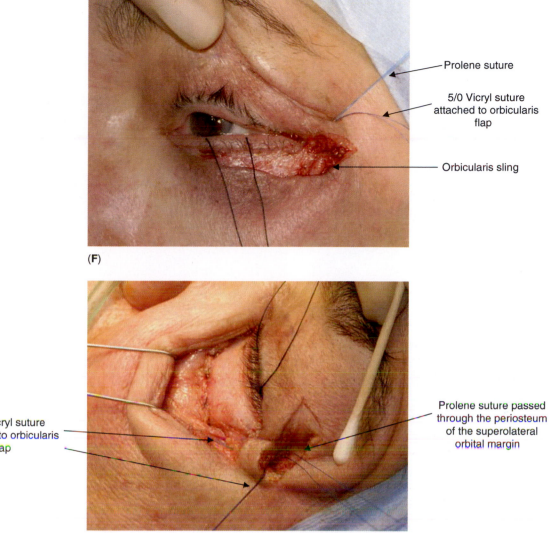

(F)

(G)

Figure 15.42 (Continued) (**F**) The Prolene suture has been tightened. The lower eyelid contour and height is checked to ensure that these are satisfactory. (**G**) The placement of the Prolene suture through the periosteum of the superolateral orbital margin is demonstrated.

surface of the maxilla and zygoma, taking care to avoid damage to the infraorbital neurovascular bundle.

3. The periosteum is divided close to the buccal sulcus using Stevens scissors or the sharp end of a Freer periosteal elevator. In some patients, a buccal sulcus incision can be used to aid the subperiosteal dissection and mobilization of the mid-face.

4. Next, the periorbita is raised over the inferior and inferolateral orbital margin and into the orbit for a few millimeters using the Freer periosteal elevator.

5. Two to three drill holes are made through the inferior and inferolateral orbital margin, protecting the orbital contents with a malleable retractor.

6. A 3/0 Prolene suture is passed through the superior edge of the mobilized periosteum and through the ptotic malar fat pad. This suture is then passed through the drill holes in the bony margin and tied (Fig. 15.49A). The suture knot is rotated into the drill hole. Additional sutures are placed as required.

7. The blepharoplasty is then completed as described above.

As an alternative option, the ptotic mid-face can be lifted with the use of a mid-face Endotine implant although this adds considerable expense to the procedure. The implant is positioned so that the tines at the inferior end of the implant engage the ptotic cheek fat pad and the other end is fixated to the lateral orbital margin using one or two titanium screws or biodegradable screws (Fig. 15.50). The stem of the implant is then severed just above the securing screw using a no. 15 Bard Parker blade.

The Endotine implant gradually biodegrades over a period of approximately 6 to 9 months. The implant can provide a very powerful and effective mid-face lift. The patient should be warned that a mid-face lift can result in considerable postoperative swelling which can take 2 to 3 months to subside.

Postoperative Care
This is as described above.

CHEEK IMPLANT
Although a variety of cheek implants are available, e.g., Medpor implants, and these can certainly provide augmentation of the mid-face, the author does not advocate the use of any cheek

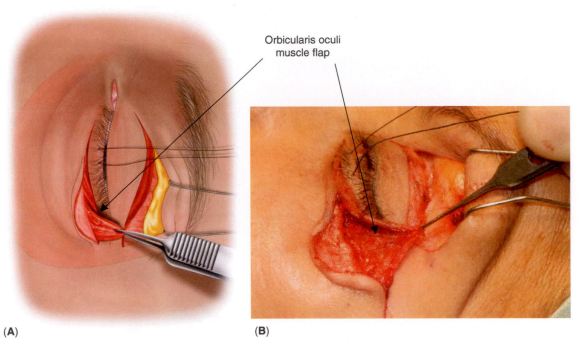

Orbicularis oculi
muscle flap

(A)   (B)

Figure 15.43 (**A**) A diagram demonstrating the creation of an orbicularis oculi muscle flap. (**B**) An intraoperative photograph showing a triangular flap of orbicularis oculi muscle being held with forceps. The redundant skin has been folded back on itself.

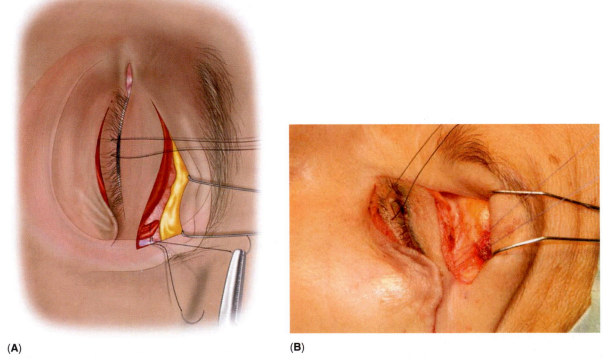

(A)   (B)

Figure 15.44 (**A**) The Vicryl sutures with the attached orbicularis flap are passed beneath the intact bridge of skin and muscle laterally. The sutures are passed through the periosteum of the superolateral orbital margin. (**B**) An intraoperative photograph demonstrating the effect achieved when tension is applied to the sutures which are attached to the orbicularis flap.

implants as these can lead to an unsatisfactory appearance after the patient has developed age-related soft tissue deflation in the area overlying and adjacent to the implant after some years.

TRANSCUTANEOUS BLEPHAROPLASTY WITH FAT DEBULKING

For the majority of patients seeking a lower lid blepharoplasty, usually in the age group 45 to 60 years of age, the transcutaneous blepharoplasty with arcus marginalis release, fat repositioning,

and an orbicularis oculi muscle suspension provides a very good cosmetic result with minimal risks. It is, however, time consuming. For older patients with greater degrees of fat herniation, the fat will need to be formally debulked, paying very careful attention to hemostasis and avoiding traction on the fat. In such patients, a transcutaneous approach gives excellent access to the lower lid fat pads, which can be debulked with a very conservative removal of skin. An orbicularis muscle sling can be avoided but a lateral tarsal strip procedure will usually

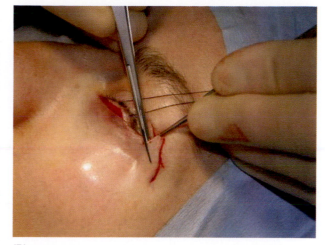

(A)   **(B)**

Figure 15.45 (**A**) A vertical incision is made in the central aspect of the lateral skin flap with straight iris scissors. (**B**) The excess skin is trimmed keeping some tension on the lower lid traction suture to prevent an inadvertent over-resection of skin.

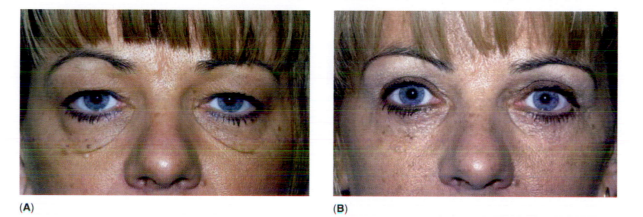

(A)   **(B)**

Figure 15.46 (**A**) Preoperative appearance. (**B**) Postoperative appearance 4 months after undergoing a bilateral upper lid blepharoplasty with sculpting of the medial and central fat pads, and a bilateral lower lid transcutaneous blepharoplasty with an arcus marginalis release, fat repositioning, and an orbicularis oculi muscle suspension.

be required. This procedure is quicker to perform and the patients who are suitable for this procedure tend to be less demanding and critical of slight asymmetries.

Such older patients should also be carefully screened for systemic co-morbidities, e.g., undiagnosed essential hypertension. Such patients are at an increased risk of a retrobulbar hematoma with its potential visual morbidity.

Steatoblepharon refers to a situation, usually in an older patient, where the orbital septum has become very lax with marked herniation of the lower eyelid fat pads (Fig. 15.51). This can occasionally occur in younger patients as a familial trait. In older patients it tends to accompany dermatochalasis, eyelid laxity, and ptosis. Prolapse of fat through a weakened Tenon's capsule may also accompany steatoblepharon. This fat can be resected via a lateral vertical conjunctival incision made directly over the prolapsed fat using Westcott scissors. The supero-lateral fornix should be avoided to prevent intra-operative damage being caused to the lacrimal gland ductules.

TRANSCONJUNCTIVAL BLEPHAROPLASTY

A transconjunctival blepharoplasty is ideally suited to the younger patient who has mild to moderate lower eyelid fat

herniation but with no or minimal skin or eyelid laxity. It is also suited to the patient with thyroid eye disease and can be combined with an orbital decompression procedure. For patients who have marked fat pad enlargement, the fat can be debulked, but for patients with lesser degrees of fat herniation and who are concerned about the appearance of lower eyelid dark circles due to tear trough defects, fat can be repositioned over the inferior orbital margins.

The patient should be warned preoperatively that postoperative chemosis is to be expected following this surgical approach, particularly in the patient with preoperative conjunctivochalasis, and that this usually takes 1 to 2 weeks to resolve. In some patients, however, this can take several weeks to resolve.

Surgical Procedure

The patient is examined in a sitting position and the prolapsed preaponeurotic fat pads are outlined using gentian violet. It is particularly important to outline a lateral fat pad as the position of the fat pad and the extent of the prolapse can be difficult to judge following the injection of local anesthetic solution and with the patient in a semi-recumbent position.

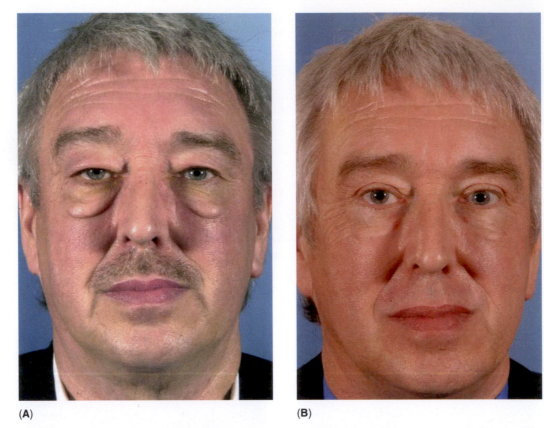

(A)   **(B)**

Figure 15.47 (**A**) The preoperative appearance of patient with marked bilateral lower eyelid festoons and bilateral upper eyelid dermatochalasis with no evidence of thyroid eye disease or other predisposing systemic disorder. (**B**) The postoperative appearance of the same patient 1 year following a bilateral upper lid blepharoplasty and transblepharoplasty internal browpexy and bilateral lower eyelid transcutaneous blepharoplasties combined with an orbicularis oculi muscle suspension. Note that this patient still has some lower lid festoons which are extremely difficult to eradicate completely

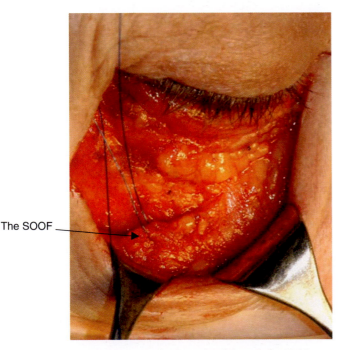

The SOOF ——————————→

Figure 15.48 A 4/0 Vicryl suture has been placed through the SOOF

Fat Repositioning

1. Approximately 2 to 3 ml of 0.5% Bupivacaine with 1:200,000 units of adrenaline mixed 50:50 with 2% lidocaine with 1:80,000 units of adrenaline are injected with a single injection just beneath the skin along the lower eyelid just below the tarsus. The needle is inserted temporally and advanced nasally while slowly injecting the solution. Immediate pressure is applied. Ten minutes are allowed for the adrenaline to take effect. Local anesthetic containing adrenaline is not injected subconjunctivally to avoid its effect on the pupil.

2. The patient is prepped and draped.

3. A 4/0 silk traction suture is placed through the gray line of the lower eyelid and everted over a medium Desmarres retractor.

4. A conjunctival incision is made with a Colorado needle 3 to 4 mm below the inferior border of the tarsus from the level of the punctum to the lateral canthus entering the plane between the orbital septum and the orbicularis oculi muscle. The orbital fat will remain contained behind the orbital septum as long as the incision is made above the line of fusion of the septum and the capsulopalpebral fascia.

5. 4/0 silk traction sutures are placed through the medial and lateral edges of the conjunctiva and the lower eyelid retractors and fixated to the head drapes using small curved artery clips in order to protect the cornea (Fig. 15.52A).

6. Dissection proceeds down the plane between the septum and the orbicularis and onto the anterior surface of the infraorbital rim. This bloodless dissection is greatly aided by the use of the Colorado needle.

7. A pocket is created beneath the orbicularis muscle over the inferior orbital margin.

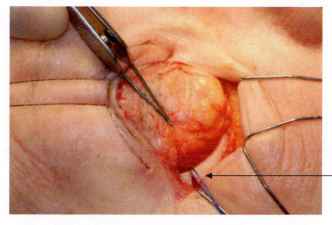

A 3/0 Prolene suture passed through a drill hole in the inferolateral orbital margin

Figure 15.49 A 3/0 Prolene suture has been passed through a drill hole in the inferolateral orbital margin.

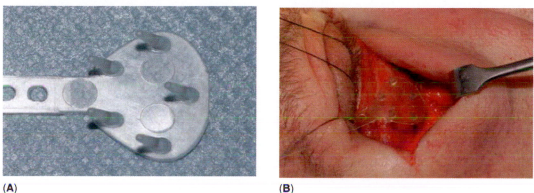

(A)

(B)

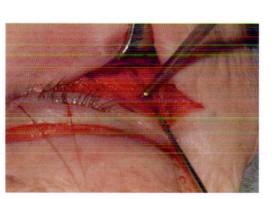

(C)

(D)

Figure 15.50 (**A**) The head of the mid-face Endotine implant with the protruding tines. (**B**) The implant is about to be placed in the mid-face. (**C**) The implant has been placed. The stem of the implant has been passed under the lateral canthal raphé and brought out through the upper eyelid wound in this example. The stem is then pulled in a superolateral direction until the desired height and contour of the mid-face have been achieved. The stem is being secured to the lateral orbital margin with a 1.5 × 4 mm titanium screw. (**D**) A drawing showing the location of the Endotine implant.

8. The arcus marginalis is incised with the Colorado needle from medial to lateral along the infraorbital rim, taking care to avoid the inferior oblique muscle medially (located directly behind the medial third of the septum) and the lateral canthal tendon laterally (Fig. 15.52A and B).

9. Next, a double-armed 5/0 Prolene suture is passed through the prolapsed fat medially. The needles are passed beneath the orbicularis muscle over the anterior lacrimal crest medially, through the full thickness of the eyelids to exit through the skin and are then tied over a silicone bolster, pulling the fat forward and the orbicularis upward over the inferior orbital margin. Further sutures are placed and passed just anterior to the periosteum over the anterior surface of the inferior orbital margin centrally and laterally (Fig. 15.53).

10. The conjunctival retraction sutures are removed and the conjunctiva and eyelid retractors are re-apposed with two to three interrupted 7/0 Vicryl sutures.

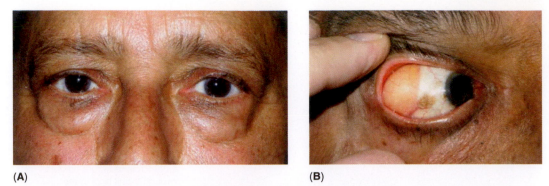

(A)   (B)

Figure 15.51 (**A**) Steatoblepharon and upper lid dermatochalasis. (**B**) A prolapse of orbital fat through a weakened Tenon's capsule in the same patient.

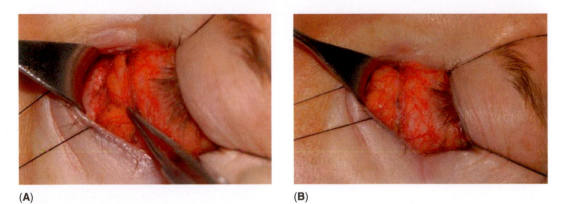

(A)   (B)

Figure 15.52 (**A**) The arcus marginalis has been opened allowing the preaponeurotic fat to prolapse. The inferior orbital margin has been exposed. (**B**) The fat is now prolapsing over the inferior orbital margin prior to placement of the double-armed Prolene sutures.

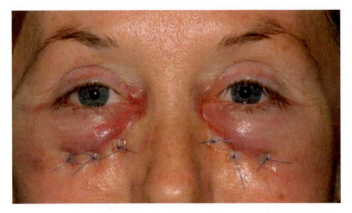

Figure 15.53 Three 5/0 double-armed Prolene sutures have been passed from the fat through the full thickness of the lower eyelids and tied over silicone bolsters.

An example of a patient who has undergone this procedure is shown in Figure 15.54.

Postoperative Care

Postoperatively the patient is prescribed a topical antibiotic ointment to the eyes three times a day for 2 weeks and Lacrilube ointment 2 hourly to the eyes for 48 hours and at bedtime. The Lacrilube ointment is then changed to a preservative-free topical lubricant gel to be used 2 hourly during the day and Lacrilube is continued at bedtime until any postoperative chemosis has resolved. Postoperative steroid drops are unnecessary. The patient is instructed to sleep with the head of the bed elevated for 2 weeks and to avoid lifting any heavy weights for 2 weeks. Clean cool packs are gently applied to the eyelid intermittently

for 48 hours. The patient should be reviewed in clinic within three to four days when the Prolene sutures are removed, and again within 4 to 6 weeks. The conjunctival sutures should drop out spontaneously within 2 weeks. Massage to the lower eyelid/cheek junction for 3 min three times per day can be commenced using Lacrilube ointment as soon as the Prolene sutures have been removed. This is continued for 2 to 3 weeks.

Fat Removal

In patients with a true fat excess a more traditional fat resection is required. In these patients gentle pressure is applied to the globe to allow the orbital fat pads to herniate into the wound.

The operation is as per stages 1 to 5.

6. The orbital septum is opened using the Colorado needle over the points of maximum convexity caused by the bulging of the fat with pressure applied to the globe. The fat will prolapse through the openings in the septum.
7. The fat is then very carefully excised after clamping the fat with a curved artery clip. Strict attention is paid to meticulous hemostasis (Fig. 15.55).
8. No undue traction should be exerted on the fat. The fat is removed commencing with the nasal fat pad, moving to the central, and then to the lateral fat pads.
9. The residual fat should be left flush with the orbital margin to prevent over resection with a subsequent "skeletonized" look.
10. The Desmarres retractor is removed and the eyelids inspected to ensure adequacy of fat removal

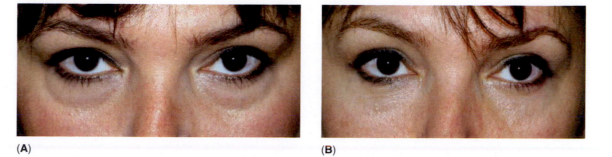

(A)   **(B)**

Figure 15.54 (**A**) Preoperative appearance. (**B**) Postoperative appearance following a bilateral lower lid transconjunctival blepharoplasty with arcus marginalis release and fat repositioning.

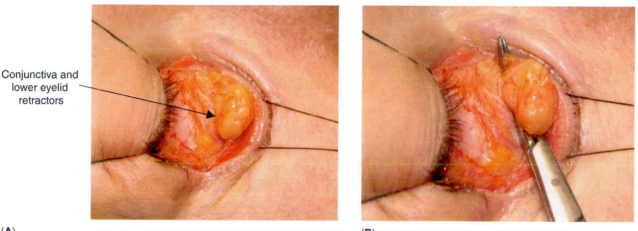

Conjunctiva and lower eyelid retractors

(A)   **(B)**

Figure 15.55 (**A**) The central eyelid fat pad has prolapsed into the wound after opening the orbital septum. (**B**) The central fat pad has been clamped with a curved artery clip.

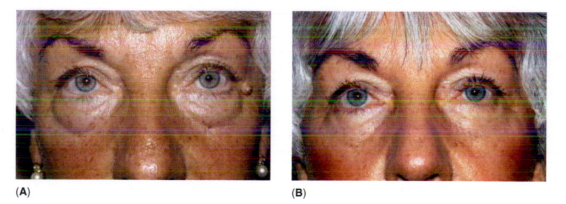

(A)   **(B)**

Figure 15.56 (**A**) The preoperative appearance. (**B**) The postoperative appearance of the same patient 12 months following a bilateral transconjunctival blepharoplasty with fat debulking and removal of a left lateral canthal skin lesion.

and symmetry. If there is concern that too much fat has been removed this can be replaced as a free graft over the inferior orbital margin.

11. The conjunctival retractor sutures are removed and the conjunctiva and eyelid retractors are re-apposed with two to three interrupted 7/0 Vicryl sutures.

An example of a patient who has undergone this procedure is shown in Figure 15.56.

In some patients a minimal skin excess can be addressed at this stage by adding a simple "pinch" skin resection. The lower lid skin is gently pinched into a fold in the lateral aspect of the eyelid using Castroviejo 0.3 mm toothed forceps and this is marked out using a cocktail stick impregnated with gentian violet solution ensuring that the eyelid position is not affected even with upgaze and with mouth opening. The skin alone is resected with a Colorado needle and the skin edges reapproximated with interrupted 7/0 Vicryl sutures.

Postoperative Care

Postoperatively the patient is prescribed a topical antibiotic ointment to the eyes three times a day for 2 weeks and Lacrilube ointment 2 hourly to the eyes for 48 hours and at bedtime. The Lacrilube ointment is then changed to a preservative-free topical lubricant gel to be used 2 hourly during the day and Lacrilube is continued at bedtime until any postoperative chemosis has resolved. Postoperative steroid drops are unnecessary. The patient is instructed to sleep with the head of the bed elevated for 2 weeks and to avoid lifting any heavy weights for 2 weeks. Clean cool packs are gently applied to the eyelid intermittently for 48 hours. The patient should be reviewed in clinic within 2 weeks, and again within 4 to 6 weeks. The conjunctival sutures should drop out spontaneously within 2 weeks. If a pinch skin excision has been performed the skin sutures are removed in clinic after 2 weeks.

If the surgery has been performed under general anesthesia it is wise to apply a compressive dressing for 30 minutes until the patient has recovered. This prevents oozing into the eyelids if the patient performs a Valsalva maneuver following extubation. The dressings are then removed and ice packs applied intermittently for 24 to 48 hours postoperatively. Significant postoperative pain is rare, and most patients are comfortable with a mild non-aspirin analgesic. *Significant postoperative pain should, however, raise concerns about the possibility of a retrobulbar hemorrhage and the patient should be examined to ensure that this has not occurred.*

Increased pigmentation from hemosiderin deposition is sometimes observed in patients with excessive bruising. To minimize this postoperative problem, patients should be instructed to avoid postoperative sun exposure until the ecchymosis has completely resolved.

Eyelids are extremely sensitive to allergenic insult, and any pre-existing atopy can be aggravated by surgery. Patients should therefore not use cosmetics for at least 10 days after surgery in order to avoid an allergic reaction. Mineral make-ups can be used 10 to 14 days postoperatively. Patients should also be made aware of the symptoms and signs of allergy to topical antibiotic ointments prescribed for application to the wounds at home after discharge.

For patients who have undergone a more extended lower eyelid blepharoplasty with resuspension of the orbicularis oculi muscle and a SOOF or midface lift, the patient and surgeon must be prepared to wait several weeks for postoperative swelling to resolve and healing to take place before judging the final outcome, since a complete recovery takes significantly longer after this procedure than after a more traditional blepharoplasty. Preoperative counseling of the patient is vital to ensure that such a prolonged period of convalescence is acceptable to the individual patient.

KEY POINT

Significant postoperative pain following a blepharoplasty should raise concerns about the possibility of a retrobulbar hemorrhage, and the patient should be examined immediately to ensure that this has not occurred.

Complications of Blepharoplasty Surgery

A number of complications can occur following blepharoplasty surgery (Table 15.1). Fortunately, serious complications are rare. The vast majority of complications are ophthalmic in nature and for this reason an increasing number of well-informed patients requesting blepharoplasty surgery seek the skills of appropriately trained and experienced oculoplastic surgeons for their preoperative evaluation and for their surgery.

Table 15.1 Complications of blepharoplasty

1. Blindness
2. Bradycardia or other dysrhythmias from the oculocardiac reflex
3. Dry eye
4. Lower eyelid retraction
5. Lower eyelid ectropion
6. Rounding of the lateral canthus
7. Hollowing of the eyelids
8. Epiphora
9. Lagophthalmos
10. Asymmetrical upper lid creases
11. Diplopia
12. Blepharoptosis
13. Chemosis
14. Corneal abrasion
15. Injury to branches of the facial nerve
16. Sensory loss in the distribution of the infraorbital or zygomaticofacial nerves
17. Irregular
18. Fat necrosis

Many of these complications can be avoided by careful preoperative patient evaluation and selection of the most appropriate surgical procedure for the patient as outlined above.

- *By far the most serious complication of blepharoplasty surgery is blindness.* This is usually due to the sudden occurrence of a postoperative orbital hemorrhage. Although rare (the precise incidence is unknown due to under-reporting of this complication but is estimated to be approximately 0.05%), this is a devastating complication of an operation performed most commonly to improve a patient's cosmetic appearance. The patient should be counseled about such a risk preoperatively. The surgery must be meticulously performed with strict attention to intra-operative hemostasis. Undue traction on orbital fat must be avoided. It is important to ensure that all risk factors for bleeding are addressed preoperatively. No patient should undergo blepharoplasty surgery involving the removal of orbital fat if hypertension is uncontrolled, if there is a history of a bleeding disorder, or if the patient is taking antiplatelet drugs. The patient must be given postoperative instructions about restrictions on activity following surgery. The patient must be able to return to hospital immediately in the event of any sudden orbital pain, proptosis, or decrease in vision. The patient with a retrobulbar hematoma usually complains of a steady, lancinating pain, similar to that of acute angle closure glaucoma. The patient may also report scintillating scotomas or complete visual loss and may exhibit mydriasis with a relative afferent pupil defect, proptosis with resistance to retropulsion, and hemorrhagic chemosis.

KEY POINT

By far the most serious complication of blepharoplasty surgery is blindness.

If a patient develops a sudden orbital hemorrhage with proptosis, subconjunctival hemorrhage and decreased visual acuity, the wound must be opened immediately to drain the hematoma and a lateral canthotomy and inferior cantholysis should be performed to achieve an emergency orbital decompression. Because the consequences of a retrobulbar hemorrhage are so severe, aggressive intervention is required. If possible the surgeon should not wait for signs of optic nerve compression (i.e., reduced visual acuity, visual field loss, an afferent pupillary defect) to arise, because permanent damage may have occurred by that time. Rather, excessive pain and proptosis necessitate immediate surgical decompression. The incision should be opened and carefully explored. Medical decompression of the orbit with corticosteroids (methylprednisolone 100 mg i.v. (intravenous)), carbonic anhydrase inhibition (acetazolamide 500 mg i.v.) should be organized straight away and if necessary osmotic diuresis (mannitol 50–100 g i.v. over 30 min) may also be used. The patient's intraocular pressure should be monitored using a Perkin's tonometer or a Tonopen and the patient's fundus should be examined to ensure patency of the central retinal artery.

- The oculocardiac reflex, characterized by intraoperative bradycardia or dysrhythmia, can be triggered by traction on the extraocular muscles or orbital fat pads. A profound bradycardia or even asystole can occur. Younger patients are more susceptible to the severe effects of this reflex. The anesthetist monitoring the patient should be aware of the possibility of a dysrhythmia occurring and should alert the surgeon who should in turn release any tissue to which traction is being applied. Atropine or glycopyrolate should be kept drawn up in a syringe and available immediately in the event of a severe dysrhythmia.
- Keratoconjunctivitis sicca (dry eye syndrome) is most often seen in patients who have a pre-existing tear film insufficiency. This should be specifically examined preoperatively and the patient should be counseled accordingly. This can be particularly important in patients who have undergone corneal refractive procedures, e.g., LASIK or who wear contact lenses. The consistent, continued use of frequent artificial tears is imperative in these patients who may also require additional procedures at a later date, e.g., punctal plug placement or punctal cautery. Patients who require artificial tears more frequently than three to four times per day should use a preservative free preparation.
- Mild lower eyelid retraction may be managed conservatively with postoperative eyelid massage. The eyelid should be massaged in an upward direction after applying Lacrilube ointment to the skin. A "SOOF" lift or mid-face lift combined with a lateral canthal resuspension may prevent the need for a full-thickness skin graft following an over resection of skin leading to lower eyelid retraction. Middle lamellar contracture resulting in lower eyelid retraction (Fig. 15.18) may, however, require division of the scar tissue and placement of a hard palate graft or a dermal graft.

- A temporary lower eyelid ectropion can occur, particularly laterally, as a result of postoperative wound edema, wound contraction, and/or hypotonicity of the orbicularis oculi muscle. A frank ectropion occurs when significant lower eyelid laxity has not been addressed or where caution has not been exercised in resetting of the orbital septum or in the degree of skin resection. This will usually require a lateral canthal tightening procedure and in some patients this will have to be combined with a skin graft.
- Rounding of the lateral canthus occurs following the excessive resection of skin and orbicularis oculi muscle as a triangle laterally, particularly in a patient whose eyelid laxity has not been appropriately addressed. This can prove to be very challenging to correct, and may require a mid-face lift combined with a lid tightening procedure.
- Hollowing of the eyelids occurs if too much orbital fat is removed, particularly in older patients with very thin eyelid skin. In the lower eyelids care should be taken to resect the fat flush with the inferior orbital margin and to avoid pulling the fat anteriorly during the resection. In general, fat removal from the upper eyelids should be avoided wherever possible. Hollowing of the eyelid can be addressed by the placement of fat pearls harvested from the periumbilical area, or by means of structural fat grafting.
- Epiphora is common in the first few postoperative days. Corneal irritation, which triggers hypersecretion of tears, and lower eyelid ectropion, which removes the inferior punctum from the surface of the globe, usually causes epiphora. Continued epiphora following blepharoplasty surgery may occur as a consequence of lagophthalmos with a secondary punctate keratopathy and hypersecretion of tears and/or a malposition of the inferior punctum. A subtle vertical positioning of the inferior punctum may result in epiphora. This is seen on careful slit lamp examination and may occur some years after surgery as the lower eyelid tarsoligamentous support becomes more lax. Conjunctivochalasis, a redundant fold of bulbar conjunctiva, may lie over the inferior punctum obstructing tear flow. This is again a subtle abnormality requiring careful slit lamp examination. It can respond to a conservative resection of the redundant conjunctiva. Persistent epiphora due to malposition of the inferior punctum requires further surgery to reposition the punctum.
- Lagophthalmos following an upper eyelid blepharoplasty is avoided by ensuring a conservative skin resection in the upper eyelids. Over zealous resection may require a skin graft if exposure symptoms do not respond to conservative treatment.
- The appearance of the upper eyelid skin creases has a profound effect on the cosmetic outcome of an upper eyelid blepharoplasty. The skin crease should be higher in a female and well defined in contrast to a male in which this should be lower and more subtle. Complications are avoided by meticulous preoperative planning and marking. Postoperatively it is

easier to raise a skin crease which is unsatisfactory than it is to lower it.

- Diplopia is a rare complication following lower eyelid blepharoplasty. This is usually due to surgical trauma to the inferior oblique muscle. A good knowledge of anatomy, a meticulous surgical dissection, and an avoidance of the excessive use of cautery should prevent such a complication. A permanent ocular motility disturbance caused by blepharoplasty is much rarer than a preexisting phoria, which may decompensate following surgery. For this reason it is imperative to perform a detailed preoperative ophthalmic examination in order to diagnose the problem and to protect the surgeon from unfair blame.

- A blepharoptosis may occur if the levator muscle, the horns of the levator muscle complex, or Whitnall's ligament are damaged during surgery. These should be carefully identified and avoided. Any preexisting ptosis should be addressed at the time of an upper eyelid blepharoplasty by means of a levator aponeurosis advancement. This should be performed under local anesthesia to facilitate an intraoperative adjustment of the height and contour of the upper eyelid(s) with the benefit of the patient's cooperation.

- Chemosis (Fig. 15.57), which is more commonly seen following a transconjunctival blepharoplasty, usually resolves after 10 to 14 days following the liberal use of topical lubricants. On very rare occasions it may last for some weeks postoperatively. The use of topical steroids to treat this should be avoided because of the risk of cataract, glaucoma, and predisposition to infection. If the chemosis does not resolve, a redundant fold of forniceal conjunctiva may need to be removed and the cut edges sutured to the episclera using 8/0 Vicryl sutures. The occurrence of postoperative chemosis can be predicted in the patient who has preoperative conjunctivochalasis (Fig. 15.58). Such a patient should undergo the simultaneous resection of the redundant conjunctiva at the time of the blepharoplasty.

- All precautions must be taken to prevent a corneal abrasion, which can be extremely painful. Care should be taken when placing eyelid and conjunctival traction sutures to avoid causing a corneal abrasion. Most corneal abrasions heal rapidly without any long-term sequelae but in some patients a recurrent corneal abrasion syndrome can occur. Diabetic patients and patients with corneal dystrophies (which may have been previously undiagnosed) are at particular risk of a recurrent corneal abrasion syndrome. If an abrasion does occur the patient must be treated with frequent topical antibiotics and should undergo a daily review with slit lamp examinations until the abrasion has completely healed. A topical lubricant ointment should be prescribed at night for a minimum period of 6 weeks to help to prevent a recurrent corneal abrasion syndrome.

- Injury to branches the facial nerve, particularly the zygomatic branch to the inferior orbicularis, is a potential hazard of dissecting below the orbicularis oculi muscle. This can lead to a loss of tone in the muscle with loss of lower eyelid symmetry, lower eyelid ectropion, or lagophthalmos. A subperiosteal dissection minimizes the risk of this complication.

- Sensory loss in the distribution of the infraorbital or zygomaticofacial nerves is usually temporary. Care should be taken when cauterizing branches of the infraorbital artery over the inferior orbital margin.

- Irregular lower eyelid lumps can occur following fat repositioning. This is usually temporary and the lumps often respond to a period of postoperative massage. The use of steroid injections should be avoided.

- Fat necrosis is rare and manifests as small, painful, indurated nodules. Massage can hasten their resolution. Injection of steroids into the lesions is effective but carries the risk of subcutaneous atrophy and hypopigmentation.

MEDICOLEGAL PITFALLS

Most complications of blepharoplasty surgery stem from an inadequate preoperative patient evaluation. From a medicolegal perspective, a thorough history and meticulous ophthalmic examination, good documentation, informed consent with the

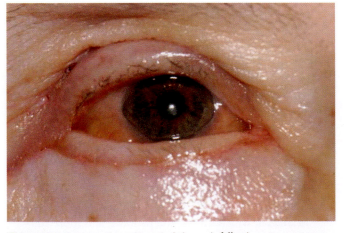

Figure 15.57 Postoperative conjunctival chemosis following a transcutaneous lower eyelid blepharoplasty.

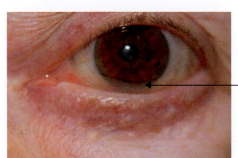

Figure 15.58 Conjunctivochalasis.

provision of detailed information about the pros, cons, risks and potential complications and their management, and excellent patient communication are crucial.

KEY POINTS

- A thorough understanding of the surgical anatomy of the eyebrows, eyelids, and mid-face is essential prior to performing a blepharoplasty.
- The distance between the inferior aspect of the eyebrow and the upper lid skin crease on down gaze should be approximately two-thirds of the distance from the inferior aspect of the eyebrow to the eyelid margin. It is important to maintain these dimensions. In general, a minimum distance of 10 to 12 mm should be left between the inferior aspect of the eyebrow and the upper eyelid skin crease when performing an upper lid blepharoplasty.
- It is very important to be able to distinguish the lacrimal gland from orbital fat.
- Whitnall's ligament supports the levator muscle complex and should not be disturbed during surgery.
- The inferior oblique muscle lies between the medial and central fat pads.
- A history of contact lens wear, previous corneal laser refractive surgery, a dry eye, facial palsy, or thyroid dysfunction identifies a patient at risk of exposure keratopathy symptoms following an upper lid blepharoplasty.
- It is important to exclude a bleeding disorder, as a postoperative hemorrhage following a blepharoplasty is potentially sight-threatening. The use of aspirin or non-steroidal anti-inflammatory agents should be discontinued 2 weeks preoperatively.
- The patient should undergo a complete preoperative ophthalmic examination.
- The secondary effects of brow ptosis on the upper eyelids must be recognized.
- The patient should be examined specifically to exclude the possibility of thyroid eye disease.
- For purely elective, cosmetic procedures, the patient should be encouraged to consider the information carefully before making a decision to proceed. This may necessitate a further consultation or an attendance at a pre-assessment clinic to obtain fully informed consent and to answer any residual queries.
- The patient should not be asked to sign a consent form for an elective cosmetic procedure on the day of surgery. The risks and potential complications that have been discussed should be documented in the patient's records, on the patient's consent form and in a letter addressed to the patient. The patient should also be provided with a formal document which outlines the potential complications of blepharoplasty surgery, their management, and the financial responsibilities that would be incurred.
- It should be noted, however, that fat removal should be undertaken very conservatively, if at all, in the upper lid so as to avoid a secondary hollowing of the upper eyelid which can result in a very aged appearance.
- No skin should be removed from the medial 2/3 of the eyelid in the vast majority of cases. The skin resection should always be conservative.
- By far the most serious complication of blepharoplasty surgery is blindness.

FURTHER READING

1. Adamson PA, Strecker HD. Transcutaneous lower blepharoplasty. Facial Plast Surg 1996; 12: 171–83.
2. Adamson PA, Tropper GJ, McGraw BL. Extended blepharoplasty. Arch Otolaryngol Head Neck Surg 1991; 117: 606–9.
3. Aiache AE, Ramirez OH. The suborbicularis oculi fat pads: an anatomic and clinical study. Plast Reconstr Surg 1955; 95: 37–42.
4. Aiache AE, Ramirez OH. The suborbicularis oculi fat pads: an anatomic and clinical study. Plast Reconstr Surg 1995; 95: 37–42.
5. Albert DM, Lucarelli MJ. Aesthetic and functional surgery of the eyebrow and forehead ptosis. In: Clinical Atlas of Procedures in Ophthalmic Surgery. Chicago, MI: AMA Press, 2004: 263–83.
6. Alt TH. Blepharoplasty. Dermatol Clin 1995; 13: 389–430.
7. Anderson RL. The tarsal strip procedure. Arch Ophthalmol 1979; 97: 2192.
8. Atiyeh BS, Hayek SN. Combined arcus marginalis release, preseptal orbicularis muscle sling, and SOOF plication for midfacial rejuvenation. Aesthetic Plast Surg 2004; 28(4): 197–202.
9. Barker DE. Dye injection studies of orbital fat compartments. Plast Reconstr Surg 1977; 59: 82–5.
10. Barton FE, Ha R, Awada M. Fat extrusion and septal reset in patients with the tear trough triad: a critical appraisal. Plast Reconstr Surg 2004; 113(7): 2115–21; discussion 2122–3.
11. Baylis HI, Goldberg RA, Kerivan KM, Jacobs JL. Blepharoplasty and periorbital surgery. Dermatol Clin 1997; 15: 635–47.
12. Baylis HI, Long JA, Groth MJ. Transconjunctival lower eyelid blepharoplasty: technique and complications. Ophthalmology 1989; 96: 1027–32.
13. Baylis HI, Long JA, Groth MJ. Transconjunctival lower eyelid blepharoplasty. Technique and complications. Ophthalmology 1989; 96: 1027–32.
14. Ben Simon GJ, McCann JD. Cosmetic eyelid and facial surgery. [Review] [139 refs] Source Survey Ophthalmol 2008; 53(5): 426–42.
15. Berman WE. To do or not to do the conjunctival approach lower eyelid blepharoplasty. Ear Nose Throat J 1994; 73: 932–3.
16. Bernardi C, Dura S, Amata PL. Treatment of orbicularis oculi muscle hypertrophy in lower lid blepharoplasty. Aesthetic Plast Surg 1998; 22: 349–51.
17. Bosniak SL. Cosmetic Blepharoplasty. New York, NY: Raven Press, 1990.
18. Carraway J. The prevention and treatment of lower lid ectropion following blepharoplasty. Plast Reconstr Surg 1990; 971–81.
19. Carraway JH, Mellow CG. The prevention and treatment of lower lid ectropion following blepharoplasty. Plast Reconstr Surg 1990; 85: 971–81.
20. Castanares S. Blepharoplasty for herniated orbital fat. Anatomical basis for a new approach. Plast Reconstr Surg 1951; 8: 46–58.
21. Chen WPD, Khan JA, McCord CD. Colour Atlas of Cosmetic Oculofacial Surgery. Philadelphia, PA: Butterworth-Heinemann, 2004.
22. Chen WPD, Khan JA, McCord CD, eds. The Colour Atlas of Cosmetic Oculofacial Surgery. Philadelphia, PA: Elsevier, 2004.
23. Chisholm BB, Lew D. Modified brow lift: an adjunct to blepharoplasty. J Oral Maxillofac Surg 1996; 54: 281–4.
24. Coleman, Sydney R. Structural fat grafting: more than a permanent filler. Plast & Reconstr Surg 2006; 118(3 Suppl): 108S–120S.
25. Constantinides MS, Adamson PA. Aesthetics of blepharoplasty. Facial Plast Surg 1994; 10: 6–17.
26. Dodenhoff TG. Transconjunctival blepharoplasty: further applications and adjuncts. Aesthetic Plast Surg 1995; 19: 511–7.
27. Doxanas MT. The lateral canthus in lower eyelid blepharoplasty. Facial Plast Surg 1994; 10: 84–9.
28. Dutton JJ. Atlas of Clinical and Surgical Orbital Anatomy. Philadelphia, PA: W.B. Saunders, 1994.

29. Dutton JL. Atlas of Clinical and Surgical Orbital Anatomy. Philadelphia, PA: W.B. Saunders, 1994.

30. Dutton JL. Atlas of Opthalmic Surgery. Volume II: Oculoplastic, Lacrimal, and Orbital Surgery. St Louis, MO: Mosby Year Book, 1992.

31. Weiss DD, Carraway, JH. Eyelid rejuvenation: a marriage of old and new. Curr Opin Otolaryngol Head Neck Surg 2005; 13: 248–54.

32. Fagien S, Brandt FS. Primary and adjunctive use of botulinum toxin type A (Botox) in facial aesthetic surgery: beyond the glabella. Clin Plast Surg 2001; 28(1): 127–48.

33. Fagien S, ed. Puttermann's Cosmetic Oculoplastic Surgery, 4th edn. Philadelphia, PA: Elsevier, 2008.

34. Fedok FG, Perkins SW. Transconjunctival blepharoplasty. Facial Plast Surg 1996; 12: 185–95.

35. Flowers RS, Flowers SS. Precision planning in blepharoplasty. The importance of preoperative mapping. Clin Plast Surg 1993; 20: 303–10.

36. Flowers RS. Canthopexy as a routine blepharoplasty component. Clin Plast Surg 1993; 20: 351–65.

37. Frankel AS, Kamer FM. The effect of blepharoplasty on eyebrow position. Arch Otolaryngol Head Neck Surg 1997; 123: 393–6.

38. Friedland JA, Jacobsen WM, TerKonda S. Safety and efficacy of combined upper blepharoplasties and open coronal browlift: a consecutive series of 600 patients. Aesthetic Plast Surg 1996; 20: 453–62.

39. American Academy of Ophthalmology. Functional indications for upper and lower eyelid blepharoplasty. Ophthalmology 1995; 102: 693–5.

40. Gasperoni C, Salgarello M, Gargani G. Subperiosteal lateral browlift and its relationship to upper blepharoplasty. Aesthetic Plast Surg 1993; 17: 243–6.

41. Gausas RE. Complications of blepharoplasty. Facial Plast Surg 1999; 15(3): 243–53.

42. Ghabrial R, Lisman RD, Kane MA, Milite J, Richards R. Diplopia following transconjunctival blepharoplasty. Plast Reconstr Surg 1998; 102: 1219–25.

43. Goldberg RA, Edelstein C, Shorr N. Fat repositioning in lower blepharoplasty to maintain infraorbital rim contour. Facial Plast Surg 1999; 15(3): 225–9.

44. Goldberg RA, McCann JD, Fiaschetti D, Simon GJ. What causes eyelid bags? Analysis of 114 consecutive patients. Plast Reconstr Surg 2005; 115(5): 1395–402; discussion 1403–4.

45. Goldberg RA. Transconjunctival orbital fat repositioning:transposition of orbital fat pedicles into a sub-periosteal pocket. Plast Reconstr Surg 2000; 105: 743–8, discussion 745–51.

46. Goldberg RA, McCannjd, Fiaschetti D, et al. What causes eyelid bags? Analysis of 114 consecutive patients. Plast Reconstr Surg 2005; 115: 1395–402, discussion 1403–4.

47. Hamra ST. Arcus marginalis release and orbital fat preservation in midface rejuvenation. Plast Reconstr Surg 1995; 96(2): 354–62.

48. Hamra ST. The role of orbital fat preservation in facial aesthetic surgery. A new concept. Clin Plast Surg 1996-; 23(1): 17–28.

49. Hamra ST. The role of the septal reset in creating a youthful eyelid-cheek complex in facial rejuvenation. Plast Reconstr Surg 2004; 113(7): 2124–41; discussion 2142–4.

50. Hamra ST. The zygorbicular dissection in composite rhytidectomy: an ideal midface plane. Plast Reconstr Surg 1998; 102(5): 1646–57.

51. Hanira ST. Arcus marginalis release and orbital fat preservation in midface rejuvenation. Plast Reconstr Surg 1995; 96: 354–62.

52. Hoenig JA, Shorr N, Shorr J. The suborbicularis oculi fat in aesthetic and reconstructive surgery. Int Ophthal Clin 1997; 37: 179–91.

53. Hugo NE, Stone E. Anatomy for a blepharoplasty. Plast Reconstr Surg 1974; 53: 381–3.

54. Jelks GW, Jelks EB. Preoperative evaluation of the blepharoplasty patient. Bypassing the pitfalls. Clin Plast Surg 1993; 20: 213–23.

55. Jordan D. The tarsal tuck procedure: avoiding eyelid retraction after lower blepharoplasty. Plast Reconstr Surg 1990; 85: 22.

56. Kikkawa DO, Kim JW. Lower-eyelid blepharoplasty. Int Ophthalmol Clin 1997; 37: 163–78.

57. Kikkawa DO, Lemke BN, Dortzbach RK. Relations of the superficial musculoaponeurotic system to the orbit and characterization of the orbitomalar ligament. Ophthal Plast Reconstr Surg 1996; 12: 77–88.

58. Knize DM. Limited-incision forehead lift for eyebrow elevation to enhance upper blepharoplasty. Plast Reconstr Surg 1996; 97: 1334–42.

59. Koch RJ. Laser resurfacing of the periorbital region. Facial Plast Surg 1999; 15(3): 263–70.

60. Kopelman JE, Keen MS. Lower eyelid blepharoplasty and other aesthetic considerations. Facial Plast Surg 1994; 10: 129–40.

61. Larrabee WF, Makielski KH. Surgical Anatomy of the Face. New York, NY: Raven Press, 1993.

62. Loeb R. Fat pad sliding and fat grafting for levelling lid depressions. Clin Plast Surg 1981; 8(4): 757–76.

63. Lowry JC, Bartley GB. Complications of blepharoplasty. Surv Ophthalmol 1994; 38: 327–50.

64. Lyon DB, Raphtis CS. Management of complications of blepharoplasty. Int Ophthalmol Clin 1997; 37: 205–16.

65. Mahe E. Lower lid blepharoplasty—the transconjunctival approach: extended indications. Aesthetic Plast Surg 1998; 22: 1–8.

66. Matarasso A. The oculocardiac reflex in blepharoplasty surgery. Plast Reconstr Surg 1989; 83(2): 243–50.

67. Mauriello JA. Techniques of Cosmetic Eyelid Surgery: A Case Study Approach. Philadelphia, PA: Lippincott Williams & Wilkins, 2004.

68. May JW, Fearon J, Zingarelli P. Retro-orbicularis oculi fat (ROOF) resection in aesthetic blepharoplasty: 6 year study in 63 patients. Plast Reconstr Surg 1990; 86: 682–9.

69. McCord CD, Doxanas MT. Browplasty and browpexy: an adjunct to blepharoplasty. Plast Reconstr Surg 1990; 86: 248–54.

70. McGraw BL, Adamson PA. Postblepharoplasty ectropion. Prevention and management. Arch Otolaryngol Head Neck Surg 1991; 117: 852–6.

71. McKinney P, Zukowski ML. The value of tear film breakup and Schirmer's tests in preoperative blepharoplasty evaluation. Plast Reconstr Surg 1989; 84: 572–6.

72. Mendelson BC, Hartley W, Scott M, McNab A, Granzow JW. Age-related changes of the orbit and midcheek and the implications for facial rejuvenation. Aesthetic Plast Surg 2007; 31(5): 419–23.

73. Mendelson BC, Muzaffar AR, Adams WP Jr. Surgical anatomy of the midcheek and malar mounds. Plast & Reconstr Surg 2002; 110(3): 885–96; discussion 897–911.

74. Mendleson B, Muzaffar AR, Adams WP, et al. Surgical anatomy of the mid cheek and malar mounds. Plast Reconstr Surg 2002; 110: 805.

75. Millay DJ, Larrabee WF Jr. Ptosis and blepharoplasty surgery. Arch Otolaryngol Head Neck Surg 1989; 115: 198-201.

76. Millay DJ. Upper lid blepharoplasty. Facial Plast Surg 1994; 10: 18–26.

77. Morax S, Touitou V. Complications of blepharoplasty. Orbit 2006; 25(4): 303–18.

78. Murakami CS, Plant RL. Complications of blepharoplasty surgery. Facial Plast Surg 1994; 10: 214–24.

79. Netscher DT, Patrinely JR, Peltier M, Polsen C, Thornby J. Trans-conjunctival versus transcutaneous lower eyelid blepharoplasty: a prospective study. Plast Reconstr Surg 1995; 96: 1053–60.

80. Neuhaus RW. Lower eyelid blepharoplasty. J Dermatol Surg Oncol 1992; 18: 1100–09.

81. Older JJ. Ptosis repair and blepharoplasty in the adult. Ophthal Surg 1995; 26: 304–8.

82. Palmer FR 3rd, Rice DH, Churukian MM. Transconjunctival blepharoplasty. Complications and their avoidance: a retrospective analysis and review of the literature. Arch Otolaryngol Head Neck Surg 1993; 119: 993–9.

83. Papel ID. Muscle suspension blepharoplasty. Facial Plast Surg 1994; 10: 147–9.

84. Pastorek N. Upper-lid blepharoplasty. Facial Plast Surg 1996; 12: 157–69.

85. Patel BC. Midface rejuvenation. Facial Plast Surg 1999; 15(3): 231–42.

86. Perkins SW, Dyer WK 2nd, Simo F. Transconjunctival approach to lower eyelid blepharoplasty. Experience, indications, and technique in 300 patients. Arch Otolaryngol Head Neck Surg 1994; 120: 172–7.

87. Perman KI. Upper eyelid blepharoplasty. J Dermatol Surg Oncol 1992; 18: 1096–9.

88. Pessa JE, Garza JR. The malar septum: the anatomic basis of malar mounds and malar edema. Aesthetics Surg J 1997; 17: 1.

89. Pontius AT, Williams EF 3rd. The evolution of midface rejuvenation: combining the midface-lift and fat transfer. Arch Facial Plast Surg 2006; 8(5): 300–5.

90. Saylan Z, et al. VS-lift: less is more. Aesthetic Surg J 1999; 19: 406.

91. Scaccia FJ, Hoffman JA, Stepnick DW. Upper eyelid blepharoplasty. A technical comparative analysis. Arch Otolaryngol Head Neck Surg 1994; 120: 827–30.

92. Schaefer AJ. Lateral canthal tendon tuck. Ophthalmology 1979; 86: 1879.

93. Seiff SR. Complications of upper and lower blepharoplasty. Int Ophthalmol Clin 1992; 32: 67–77.

94. Siegel RJ. Essential anatomy for contemporary upper lid blepharoplasty. Clin Plast Surg 1993; 20: 209–12.

95. Stambaugh KI. Upper lid blepharoplasty: skin flap vs pinch. Laryngoscope 1991; 101: 1233–7.

96. Starck WJ, Griffin JE Jr, Epker BN. Objective evaluation of the eyelids and eyebrows after blepharoplasty. J Oral Maxillofac Surg 1996; 54: 297–302.

97. Stephenson CB. Upper-eyelid blepharoplasty. Int Ophthalmol Clin 1997; 37: 123–32.

98. Structural Fat Grafting S.R. Coleman Quality Medical Publishing, Inc. 2004 (ISBN: 1-57626-133-6).

99. Thornton WR. Combined approach of ptosis and blepharoplasty surgery. Facial Plast Surg 1994; 10: 177–84.

100. Tonnard P, Verpaele A, Monstreys, et al. Minimal access cranial suspension lift: a modified S-lift. Plast Reconstr Surg 2002; 109: 2074–86.

101. Trussler AP, Rohrich RJ. MOC-PSSM CME Article: Blepharoplasty, Plast Reconstr Surg 2008; 121: 1.

102. Waldman SR. Transconjunctival blepharoplasty: minimizing the risks of lower lid blepharoplasty. Facial Plast Surg 1994; 10: 27–41.

103. Webster RC. Suspending sutures in blepharoplasty. Arch Otolaryngol 1979; 105: 601.

104. Weinberg DA, Baylis HI. Transconjunctival lower eyelid blepharoplasty. Dermatol Surg 1995; 21: 407–10.

105. Yousif NJ, Sonderman P, Dzwierzynski WW, Larson DL. Anatomic considerations in transconjunctival blepharoplasty. Plast Reconstr Surg 1995; 96: 1271–6.

106. Zarem HA, Resnick JI, Carr RM, Wootton DG. Browpexy: lateral orbicularis muscle fixation as an adjunct to upper blepharoplasty. Plast Reconstr Surg 1997; 100: 1258–61.

107. Zarem HA, Resnick JI. Expanded applications for transconjunctival lower lid blepharoplasty. Plast Reconstr Surg 1991; 88: 215–20.

108. Zarem HA, Resnick JI. Minimizing deformity in lower blepharoplasty. The transconjunctival approach. Clin Plast Surg 1993; 20: 317–21.

109. Zarem HA, Resnick JI. Operative technique for transconjunctival lower blepharoplasty. Clin Plast Surg 1992; 19: 351–6.

16 The management of brow ptosis

INTRODUCTION

The position of the eyebrows affects facial expression and influences the way in which a patient's mood and personality are judged by others. There are a variety of eyebrow shapes. In general, the female eyebrow has a higher arch than a male's, which tends to be flatter (Fig. 16.1). The eyebrow position tends to become lower with age from the effects of gravity, tissue deflation, and the action of the depressors of the eyebrow (the corrugator supercilii, the depressor supercilii, the procerus, and the orbicularis oculi muscles). The brow may become ptotic to a very variable degree (Fig. 16.2).

Patients often attempt to raise the ptotic eyebrows by using the frontalis muscle. This action eventually becomes involuntary and leads to a paradoxical rise in the central eyebrow of some older patients. Brow ptosis creates a skin redundancy in the upper eyelids and medial and lateral canthi. This can lead to the appearance of more severe upper eyelid dermatochalasis centrally, hooding of the eyelids temporally and skin redundancy medially. It is important to recognize brow ptosis and to determine its most appropriate management for the individual patient. This may also include accepting the brow ptosis, particularly in a male patient, but modifying an upper eyelid blepharoplasty to prevent the brow from being drawn down more to meet the upper eyelid incision. This can otherwise lead to a very unsatisfactory postoperative appearance.

APPLIED ANATOMY
Eyebrow

The applied anatomy of the eyebrows, the eyebrow elevators and depressors, the scalp, the temple, and the facial nerve is presented in detail in Chapter 2—"Applied Anatomy." This anatomy should be carefully reviewed.

PREOPERATIVE PATIENT EVALUATION
History

The patient's complaints should be carefully noted. The patient may complain of:

- Drooping or hooding of the upper eyelids
- A loss of the superior visual field
- A tired appearance commented on by colleagues, friends or relatives
- Headaches
- Ocular discomfort

The complaint of drooping of the upper eyelids may simply be due to severe dermatochalasis causing a pseudoptosis with the underlying eyelid height being normal. The lid position should be carefully evaluated, however, as a true blepharoptosis may also be present. Similarly, a severe dermatochalasis, often combined with a brow ptosis, may obstruct the patient's superior visual field. Often, patients will have a more significant lateral brow ptosis than true dermatochalasis of the upper

eyelids and a brow lift combined with an upper eyelid blepharoplasty may be required for such a patient.

Patients who have a moderate-to-severe brow ptosis and dermatochalasis are obliged to use their frontalis muscle to overcome the superior visual field defect. Such patients commonly develop deep forehead furrows (Fig. 16.3).

This leads to fatigue of the frontalis muscle, which in turn can cause a headache. The cosmetic effects of upper eyelid dermatochalasis and a brow ptosis can lead to complaints of a tired appearance. Occasionally, upper eyelid dermatochalasis and a severe lateral brow ptosis can lead to a secondary mechanical misdirection of eyelashes, causing chronic discomfort.

Patients should be specifically questioned about previous periocular botulinum toxin injections and facial rejuvenation surgery. Patients who have previously undergone such injections, a cosmetic blepharoplasty or a facelift may omit such information, particularly if accompanied by a new partner. A history of contact lens wear, dry eye, facial palsy or thyroid dysfunction identifies a patient at risk of exposure keratopathy symptoms following an upper lid blepharoplasty. It is important to exclude a bleeding disorder, as a postoperative hemorrhage following a blepharoplasty is potentially sight threatening. Hypertension should be excluded. Allergies should be excluded. The use of aspirin or nonsteroidal anti-inflammatory agents (NSAIAs) should be discontinued 2 weeks prior to surgery.

Examination

The patient should undergo a complete ophthalmic examination. The patient's best-corrected visual acuity should be recorded. The patient should be assessed in a sitting position with the eyes looking straight ahead. The palpebral apertures should be measured and the position of the skin creases recorded as described in Chapter 15—"Blepharoplasty." Any asymmetries should be noted. Any frontalis overaction should be noted and the position and shape of the brows assessed after preventing frontalis overaction. The degree of mobility of the brows associated with gentle downward traction of the upper eyelids is assessed. Any subcutaneous soft tissue atrophy is sought immediately above the brow and in the adjacent temple. The secondary effects of brow ptosis on the upper eyelids must be recognized. In addition, it may be difficult to ascertain the true position of the brow in patients who pluck their eyebrows or who have their eyebrows threaded or tattooed.

The position of the hairline should be noted and any thinning of the hair documented. The vertical height of the forehead from the apex of the brow to the hairline is noted as well as any undue prominence of the frontal bone. (A patient with a high forehead, thinning of the hair and a prominent frontal bone may be an unsuitable candidate for an endoscopic brow lift procedure. Such a procedure is more difficult to perform in such a patient and the procedure risks causing permanent damage to hair follicles).

An assessment of tear production and the tear film should be documented. The degree of upper eyelid laxity is assessed.

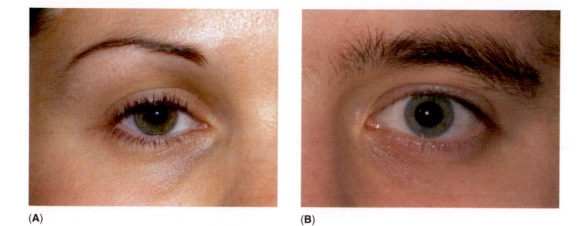

Figure 16.1 (**A**) Female brow in a young patient. (**B**) Male brow in a young patient.

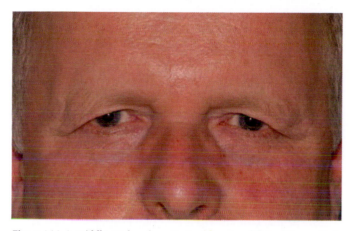

Figure 16.2 A middle-aged male patient with severe bilateral brow ptosis causing a visualfield restriction.

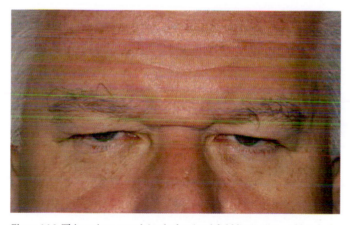

Figure 16.3 This patient complained of a visual field limitation and headache toward the evening due to frontalis muscle fatigue. He demonstrates deep forehead furrows from the effects of frontalis overaction.

Any herniation of medial and central preaponeurotic fat is noted. The degree of excess upper eyelid skin is assessed. Any prolapse of the lacrimal gland is noted. The skin quality and degree of actinic damage is assessed.

Surgical Planning

The options for surgical and nonsurgical management should be discussed in detail with the patient. Some patients, in particular dysthyroid patients with medial brow ptosis and deep glabellar frown lines, may prefer the use of botulinum toxin instead of surgery. This is highly effective for such patients, whose glabellar furrows can create an aggressive appearance. It has the disadvantage, however, of being expensive and temporary in its effects. It has to be repeated every 3 to 4 months. The use of botulinum toxin in the cosmetic patient does offer the following advantages:

- Botulinum toxin injections to the brow depressors can effect a "chemical brow lift" in some patients without the need for surgery.
- Botulinum toxin injections to the brow depressors given 2 weeks prior to an endoscopic brow lift procedure, or a transblepharoplasty browpexy/brow lift procedure can enhance the long-term results of the procedure (the injections should not be given at the time of the procedure as postoperative edema can carry the toxin to other muscle groups, e.g., the levator palpebrae superioris resulting in a blepharoptosis).

The author uses Dysport for these injections. This treatment is described in detail in Chapter 14—"The Evaluation and Management of the Cosmetic Patient."

Botulinum toxin injections can be combined with the use of a dermal filler or structural fat grafting to re-inflate the tail of the brow and to address any associated hollowing of the adjacent temple. This is discussed in Chapter 14—"The Evaluation and Management of the Cosmetic Patient."

The goals, limitations, risks, and potential complications of surgery should be fully discussed with the patient. The patient should be fully informed about the sitting of incisions. Risks specific to the surgical approach should be explained: infection, hematoma, neurosensory loss or annoying paraesthesiae and itching in the distribution of the supraorbital and supratrochlear nerves, loss of hair around scalp incisions, palpability of implants, frontalis palsy from damage to the temporal branch of the facial nerve, and persistent headache. The limitations of upper eyelid blepharoplasty performed alone in the presence of significant brow ptosis should be explained. Under these circumstances, an upper eyelid blepharoplasty should be very conservative to prevent further lowering of the brow and an unsatisfactory appearance. Patients should be carefully questioned to ascertain their expectations of surgery.

KEY POINT

Consider the potential benefits of botulinum toxin injections in patients with a brow ptosis, either as an alternative to surgery or to supplement the effects of surgery.

Anesthesia
Brow lift procedures may be undertaken under either general or local anesthesia, or under local anesthesia with intravenous sedation. The patient should be kept in a semi-recumbent position with the head elevated at least 30° to reduce venous engorgement and bleeding.

SURGICAL PROCEDURES FOR THE MANAGEMENT OF BROW PTOSIS
The surgical approaches to the management of eyebrow ptosis are:

1. The direct brow lift
2. The "gull-wing" direct brow lift
3. The mid-forehead brow lift
4. The temporal eyebrow lift
5. The transblepharoplasty browpexy
6. The transblepharoplasty brow lift
7. The endoscopic brow lift
8. The coronal forehead and brow lift
9. The pretrichial forehead and brow lift

The Direct Brow Lift
The direct brow lift is a simple surgical technique that is suitable for older patients in whom the surgical scar can be hidden within natural creases, and for the patient with a severe brow ptosis due to a facial palsy. It can be performed quickly under local anesthesia with or without sedation and can be combined with an upper lid blepharoplasty. A temporal direct brow lift to manage a temporal brow ptosis is particularly effective and can also yield a good cosmetic result (Fig. 16.4).

The resultant scar, confined to the lateral half of the eyebrow only, is far preferable to a scar which extends to the medial aspect of the brow. In addition, a temporal direct brow lift poses no risk to the supraorbital and supratrochlear nerves. If a significant amount of tissue has to be resected, however, temporal peaking of the brows can occur, particularly if the patient continues to exhibit involuntary frontalis overaction. The procedure offers the advantage of a long-lasting result.

Surgical Procedure
1. With the patient in a sitting position, an incision is marked just above the eyebrow with a gentian violet marker pen. The brow is mechanically elevated to the desired level and then released. A mark is then made on the forehead at a point that represented the leading edge of the raised brow (Fig. 16.5A).
2. A slight overcorrection is desirable. An elliptical incision is then drawn out (Fig. 16.5B).
3. If the brow lift is to be combined with an upper lid blepharoplasty, the proposed blepharoplasty incisions should be marked out with an assistant raising the brow to the desired position to avoid an over-resection of upper eyelid skin.
4. The shape of the proposed area for excision can be adjusted according to the desired shape of the brow. For a marked temporal brow ptosis, the incision can be modified and kept over the lateral brow only (Fig. 16.4). A lateral "dog ear" can be addressed with a "winged" extension to the incision.
5. The marked out area is infiltrated with 8 to 10 ml of 0.5% Bupivacaine with 1:200,000 units of adrenaline mixed 50:50 with 2% Lidocaine with 1:80,000 units of adrenaline.
6. A perpendicular incision is made through the skin and subcutaneous tissue with a no. 15 Bard Parker blade down to the level of the frontalis and orbicularis muscles (Fig. 16.5C). Great care should be taken medially to avoid any damage to the supraorbital and supratrochlear neurovascular bundles.
7. The ellipse of tissue is excised and the wound is closed with deep buried interrupted subcutaneous 5/0 Vicryl sutures. The skin is closed with interrupted 7/0 Vicryl sutures (Fig. 16.5D). These do not leave visible suture marks in the skin. (Alternatively the skin can be closed with a subcuticular 5/0 Nylon suture.) The skin closure is reinforced with sterile adhesive tape (Fig. 16.6).

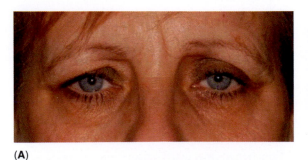

(A)

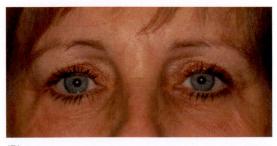

(B)

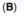

Figure 16.4 (**A**) A female patient with a bilateral brow ptosis. (**B**) The appearance of the same patient 3 months postoperatively following a bilateral temporal direct brow lift and conservative bilateral upper and lower eyelid blepharoplasties. She had also undergone botulinum toxin injections to the glabella.

Postoperative Care

Postoperatively the patient is prescribed a topical antibiotic ointment to the brow wounds three times a day for 2 weeks. The patient is instructed to sleep with the head of the bed elevated for 4 weeks and to avoid lifting any heavy weights for 2 weeks. Clean cool packs are gently applied to the brow intermittently for 48 hours. The patient is instructed to remove the adhesive tape from the wounds after 3 days. The patient should be reviewed in clinic within 2 weeks and again within 4 to 6 weeks. The skin sutures are removed at 10 to 14 days postoperatively.

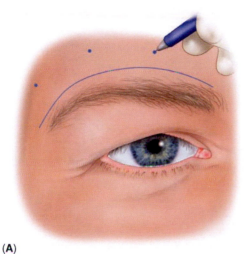

(A)

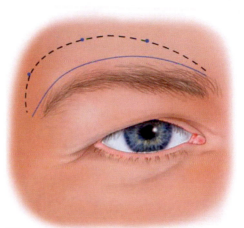

(B)

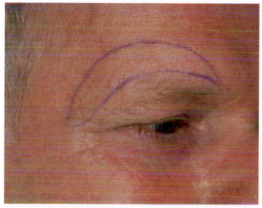

(C)

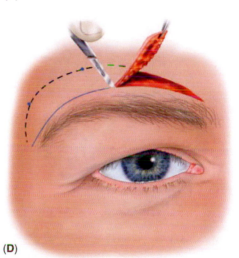

(D)

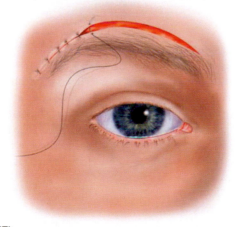

(E)

Figure 16.5 (**A**) A fine incision line is marked just above the eyebrow. It is preferable to keep the incision as temporal as possible to leave a relatively unobtrusive scar (Fig. 16.4). The brow is raised and then released. Marks are made at the desired position of the brow. (**B**) The tissue to be removed is marked out and the ends tapered. (**C**) The maximum height of the ellipse should correspond to the desired peak of the brow. (**D**) The incisions are made down to the underlying muscle. The tissue resection is then completed with Stevens scissors. (**E**) The skin is closed with interrupted 7/0 Vicryl sutures. Alternatively the skin can be closed with a continuous subcuticular 5/0 Nylon suture.

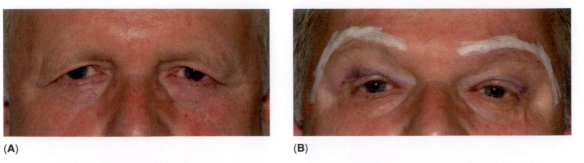

Figure 16.6 (**A**) A male patient with a severe bilateral brow ptosis. (**B**) The same patient immediately following a bilateral direct brow lift and very conservative bilateral upper lid blepharoplasties. His wound closure has been reinforced with the application of Steristrips.

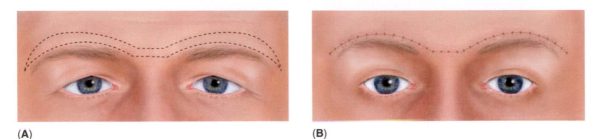

Figure 16.7 (**A**) A "gull-wing" direct brow lift marked out. (**B**) A "gull-wing" direct brow lift sutured.

KEY POINT

If a brow lift is to be combined with an upper lid blepharoplasty, the proposed blepharoplasty incisions should be marked out with an assistant raising the brow to the desired position to avoid an over-resection of upper eyelid skin.

The "Gull-Wing" Direct Brow Lift

This surgical procedure extends the direct brow lift into the glabellar region in a "gull-wing" fashion (Fig. 16.7). It is suitable for older patients who have a marked brow ptosis that affects the medial aspect of the brows in addition to the lateral aspect. It does, however, leave a much more obtrusive scar which patients must be warned about (Fig. 16.8).

The Mid-Forehead Lift

This procedure is used very infrequently and reserved for older patients with a marked medial as well as a temporal brow ptosis and prominent glabellar frown lines, who have thin, non-sebaceous type of skin with deep forehead furrows. In this procedure, an incision is made through one of the deep forehead furrows in the mid-forehead area extending to a point just medial to each temporal crest. This approach allows direct access to the central depressors of the brows, which can be dissected and weakened, taking great care to avoid cutting the adjacent sensory nerves. A section of the mid-forehead skin and subcutaneous tissue is removed.

Surgical Procedure
1. With the patient in a sitting position, the proposed incision is marked along a mid-forehead furrow with a gentian violet marker pen (Fig. 16.9A).

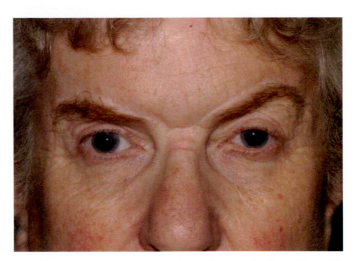

Figure 16.8 A 70-year-old patient who has undergone a "gull-wing" brow lift.

2. The mid-forehead is mechanically elevated to the desired level and then released. A mark is then made on the forehead at a point that represented the leading edge of the raised skin. A slight overcorrection is desirable. A rectangular incision is then drawn out with tapered lateral ends (Fig. 16.9B).
3. If the brow lift is to be combined with an upper lid blepharoplasty, the proposed blepharoplasty incisions should be marked out with an assistant raising the brow to the desired position to avoid an over-resection of upper eyelid skin.
4. The marked out area is infiltrated with 8 to 10 ml of 0.5% Bupivacaine with 1:200,000 units of adrenaline mixed 50:50 with 2% Lidocaine with 1:80,000 units of adrenaline. In addition,

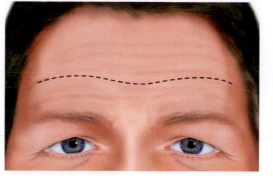
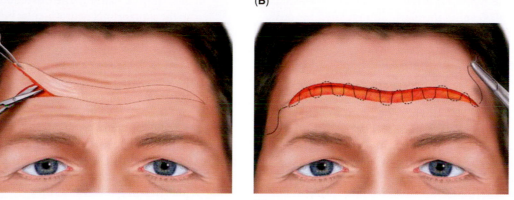

(A)   **(B)**

(C)   **(D)**

Figure 16.9 (**A**) A drawing showing the position of the initial skin marking along a central forehead crease for a mid-forehead brow lift. (**B**) A drawing showing the approximate position of the incisions for a mid-forehead brow lift. (**C**) The block of forehead tissue is excised with Stevens scissors down to the level of the frontalis muscle. (**D**) A drawing showing the forehead wound being closed with a subcuticular suture.

supraorbital and supratrochlear nerve blocks are performed.

5. A perpendicular incision is made through the skin and subcutaneous tissue with a no. 15 Bard Parker blade down to the level of the frontalis muscle.
6. The block of tissue is excised with Stevens scissors (Fig. 16.9C).
7. The subcutaneous layer is closed with interrupted 4/0 polydioxanone (PDS) sutures.
8. The skin is closed with interrupted 7/0 Vicryl sutures. (Alternatively the skin can be closed with a subcuticular 5/0 Nylon suture (Fig. 16.9D). The skin closure is reinforced with sterile adhesive tape.

Postoperative Care
The postoperative care is as described for a direct brow lift above.

The Temporal Eyebrow Lift
The temporal lift may be used to supplement the effect of a transblepharoplasty brow lift procedure (see transblepharoplasty brow lift below).

Surgical Procedure
1. The hair is parted with a comb and tied to expose the proposed temporal incisions which are marked with a gentian violet marker pen. The incisions, measuring approximately 2.5 to 3 cm in length, are centered on a line joining the alar base and the lateral canthus

as it runs into the temporal hair, and are placed approximately 2 to 3 cm posterior to the hairline.

2. The blepharoplasty incisions should be marked out with an assistant raising the brow to the desired position to avoid an over-resection of upper eyelid skin.
3. The marked out area is infiltrated with 3 to 4 ml of 0.5% Bupivacaine with 1:200,000 units of adrenaline mixed 50:50 with 2% Lidocaine with 1:80,000 units of adrenaline.
4. The temporal regions are then infiltrated with a tumescent solution made up of 500 ml of Ringer's lactate, 25 ml of 0.25% Bupivacaine with 1:200,000 units of adrenaline, 25 ml of 2% Lidocaine with 1:80,000 units of adrenaline, 0.5 ml of 1:10,000 adrenaline, 5 ml of triamcinolone 10 mg/ml, and 1500 units of hyaluronidase. The solution is injected using a 20-ml Luer lock syringe and a 21-gauge needle. Approximately, 10 to 15 ml of the solution are injected into the temples, with every effort made to inject into the plane between the temporo-parietal fascia and the temporal fascia. The solution is allowed at least 10 min to work.
5. A perpendicular incision is made through the skin and temporo-parietal fascia with a no. 15 Bard Parker blade down to the glistening fibers of the temporal fascia.
6. If the superficial temporal vessels are encountered toward the posterior aspect of the wound they should be ligated.

7. A blunt-tipped periosteal dissector then is used to develop the plane between the temporo-parietal fascia and the temporal fascia while the skin edge is elevated with a large double-pronged skin hook.

8. The plane is dissected toward the temporal crest ensuring that the dissector is inclined toward the temporal fascia and deep to the temporo-parietal fascia to avoid damage to the frontal branch of the facial nerve.

9. A sharper-tipped periosteal dissector is then used to break through the periosteal confluence along the temporal crest, in a lateral to medial direction, keeping the elevator angulated toward the bone.

10. The dissection now meets the subperiosteal dissection pocket over the frontal bone performed via the upper lid blepharoplasty incision, and the lateral orbital margin dissection also performed via the upper lid blepharoplasty incision (see below).

11. After the completion of the transblepharoplasty brow lift using an Endotine implant (see below), the temporo-parietal fascia is elevated by suturing the cut edge of the fascia to the temporal fascia at the posterior aspect of the wound using a 3/0 Monocryl horizontal mattress suture.

12. The temporal skin wound is closed with interrupted 4/0 Nylon sutures. Alternatively, skin staples can be used. In some patients, a small ellipse of hair-bearing skin is excised if this is redundant.

13. A compressive dressing supported by a bandage is applied around the head for 18 to 24 hours.

Postoperative Care
Postoperatively the patient is prescribed a topical antibiotic ointment to the temporal wounds three times a day for 2 weeks. The patient is instructed to sleep with the head of the bed elevated for 4 weeks and to avoid lifting any heavy weights for 2 weeks. Clean cool packs are gently applied to the brow intermittently for 48 hours. The patient should be reviewed in clinic within 2 weeks and again within 4 to 6 weeks. The skin sutures (or staples) are removed at 10 to 14 days postoperatively.

The Transblepharoplasty Browpexy
This procedure does not raise the brows but stabilizes the brows centrally and laterally to prevent descent of the brow following an upper lid blepharoplasty.

Surgical Procedure
1. With the patient in a sitting position, the skin is marked just above the peak of the eyebrow with a gentian violet marker pen.

2. With the brow stabilized, the upper lid blepharoplasty is marked out.

3. The upper eyelid is infiltrated with 2 to 3 ml of 0.5% Bupivacaine with 1:200,000 units of adrenaline mixed 50:50 with 2% Lidocaine with 1:80,000 units of adrenaline.

4. A further 3 to 5 ml of the same solution is injected subcutaneously above the brow.

5. The blepharoplasty skin (and where appropriate orbicularis muscle) excision is performed using a Colorado needle.

6. Using the Colorado needle and Paufique forceps, a plane of dissection is created underneath the orbicularis muscle and continued superiorly to a position just above the supraorbital margin.

7. Next, a Desmarres retractor is used to retract the skin–muscle flap. Using the Colorado needle the retro-orbicularis oculi muscle fat is entered and a pre-periosteal plane dissected for 3 to 4 cm above the supraorbital margin. The dissection is kept medial to the supraorbital neurovascular bundle, bearing in mind that a deep lateral branch may be present. The lateral orbital retaining ligament is released.

8. Next, a 3/0 Prolene suture is passed through the periosteum with a double bite 2 to 3 cm above the supraorbital margin in line with the marked peak of the brow (Fig. 16.10). The suture is then passed through the retro-orbicularis oculi fat and subcutaneous tissue of the brow and tied with multiple knots. If needed, an additional suture can be placed.

9. The blepharoplasty skin wound is then closed with interrupted 7/0 Vicryl sutures.

10. Normal saline sachets should be kept available in the refrigerator and used to moisten 4 × 4 gauze swabs which are applied to the first operated side while the fellow side is undergoing the same procedure.

Postoperative Care
Postoperatively the patient is prescribed a topical antibiotic ointment to the upper lid wounds three times a day for 2 weeks and Lacrilube ointment 1 to 2 hourly to the eyes for 48 hours and at bedtime. The Lacrilube ointment is then changed to a preservative-free topical lubricant gel to be used hourly during the day and Lacrilube is continued at bedtime until the degree of lagophthalmos has improved. The frequency of the lubricants is then gradually reduced over the course of the next few weeks. The patient is instructed to sleep with the head of the bed elevated for 4 weeks and to avoid lifting any heavy weights

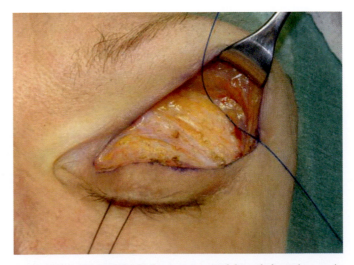

Figure 16.10 A browpexy 3/0 Prolene suture passed through the periosteum in line with the peak of the brow.

for 2 weeks. Clean cool packs are gently applied to the eyelid intermittently for 48 hours. The patient should be reviewed in clinic within 2 weeks and again within 4 to 6 weeks. The upper lid skin sutures are removed at 2 weeks.

The Transblepharoplasty Endotine Brow Lift

This procedure raises the lateral aspect of the brow and relies on a temporary biodegradable implant (an Endotine implant) to maintain the elevated brow position during the healing phase. The implant is placed into a small partially thick hole made in the frontal bone just above the brow with a dedicated non-powered drill (Fig. 16.11).

The implant can, however, take several months to disappear during which time it is palpable and can be tender to touch. Its use is not suitable for patients with thin skin and poor subcutaneous tissue above the brow. The brow is dissected and released via an upper lid blepharoplasty approach although the effects can be supplemented by the additional use of a temporal brow lift as described above. The best results are seen in those patients who have a moderate temporal brow ptosis and who are willing to undergo preoperative periocular botulinum toxin injections to weaken the brow depressors, and who are also willing to undergo long term maintenance injections every 3 to 4 months.

Surgical Procedure

1. With the patient in a sitting position, the skin is marked just above the peak of the eyebrow with a gentian violet marker pen.
2. With the brow raised to the desired position, the upper lid blepharoplasty is marked out.
3. The upper eyelid is infiltrated with 2 to 3 ml of 0.5% Bupivacaine with 1:200,000 units of adrenaline mixed 50:50 with 2% Lidocaine with 1:80,000 units of adrenaline.
4. The frontal and temporal regions are then infiltrated with a tumescent solution made up of 500 ml of Ringer's lactate, 25 ml of 0.25% Bupivacaine with 1:200,000 units of adrenaline, 25 ml of 2% Lidocaine with 1:80,000 units of adrenaline, 0.5 ml of 1:10,000 adrenaline, 5 ml

of triamcinolone, 10 mg/ml, and 1500 units of hyaluronidase. The solution is injected using a 20-ml Luer lock syringe and a 21-gauge needle. Approximately 15 to 20 ml of the solution are first injected subperiosteally over the frontal bone and pressure is then applied to diffuse the solution. Next a further 15 to 20 ml of the solutions are injected into the temples, with every effort made to inject into the plane between the temporoparietal fascia and the temporal fascia. The solution is allowed at least 10 min to work.

5. The blepharoplasty skin (and where appropriate orbicularis muscle) excision is performed using a Colorado needle.
6. Using the Colorado needle and Paufique forceps, a plane of dissection is created underneath the orbicularis muscle and continued superiorly to a position just above the supraorbital margin.
7. Next, a Desmarres retractor is used to retract the skin–muscle flap. Using the Colorado needle the retro-orbicularis oculi muscle fat is entered and the periosteum exposed.
8. The periosteum is then opened along the supraorbital margin, taking care to avoid the supraorbital neurovascular bundle medially and bearing in mind that a deep lateral branch may be present, and to the superior aspect of the lateral orbital margin laterally. The lateral orbital retaining ligament is released.
9. The subperiosteal dissection is continued over the whole of the frontal bone on the same side using a blunt-tipped periosteal dissector (Fig. 16.12).
10. The plane between the temporo-parietal fascia and the temporal fascia is then dissected under direct visualization for distance of 5 to 6 cm. The periosteal dissector is inclined towards the temporal fascia

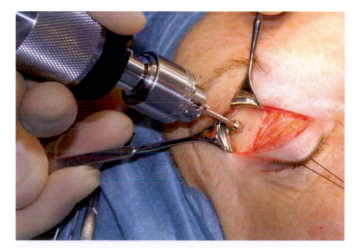

Figure 16.11 A drill hole being made in the frontal bone using a dedicated non-powered drill.

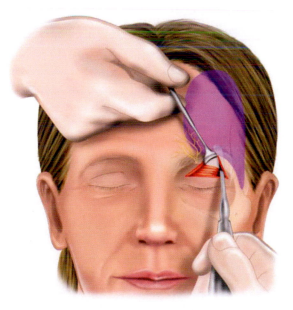

Figure 16.12 A drawing showing a shaded area depicting the area of subperiosteal dissection over the frontal bone, the release of the conjoint fascia over the temporal crest, and the release of the orbital retaining ligament laterally.

and deep to the temporo-parietal fascia to avoid damage to the frontal branch of the facial nerve.

11. A sharper-tipped periosteal dissector is then used to break through the periosteal confluence along the temporal crest, in a lateral to medial direction, keeping the elevator angulated towards the bone.

12. The brow is now quite mobile.

13. Next the frontal bone is exposed 2 to 3 cm above supraorbital margin using a Desmarres retractor. A gentian violet mark is placed on the frontal bone in the desired location of the Endotine implant.

14. The non-powered drill is used to create a hole in the frontal bone (Fig. 16.13). The drill bit is specially guarded to ensure that the drill hole cannot exceed the preset depth (Fig. 16.14). It is essential that the drill is held perpendicular to the bone. The bone debris is sucked from the hole with a Yankauer sucker.

15. Next, a 4/0 Nylon suture is passed through the medial and lateral holes of the implant (Fig. 16.15).

16. The implant, which comes preloaded on its inserter (Fig. 16.16), is pushed into the hole in the correct orientation with the apex of the implant facing inferiorly (Fig. 16.17). The implant should "click" into position. The inserter is then twisted anti-clockwise releasing the implant. The implant should lie flush with the frontal bone.

17. The periosteum should be draped above the protruding tines of the implant (Fig. 16.15).

18. The Nylon suture is then passed through the adjacent retro-orbicularis oculi fat and subcutaneous tissue and tied. (The use of the Nylon suture is optional but this does offer additional security of fixation during the healing phase.) The tissues are engaged with the tines of the implant.

19. Additional fixation can be secured with the use of Tisseell® sprayed over the exposed frontal bone but this incurs yet further expense.

20. The blepharoplasty skin wound is then closed with interrupted 7/0 Vicryl sutures.

21. Normal saline sachets should be kept available in the refrigerator and used to moisten 4 × 4 gauze swabs which are applied to the first operated side while the fellow side is undergoing the same procedure.

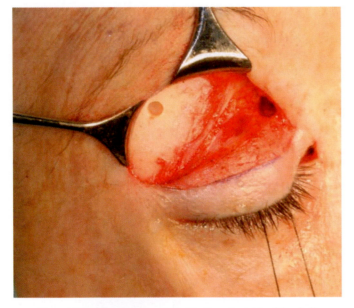

Figure 16.13 A hole has been drilled in the outer table of the skull.

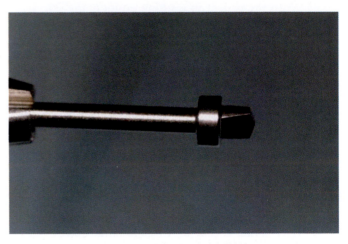

Figure 16.14 The guarded drill bit.

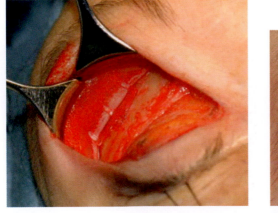

(A)

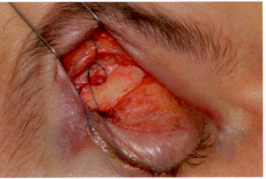

(B)

Figure 16.15 (**A**) The periosteum has been hooked behind the tines. In this case a Nylon suture fixation has not been undertaken. (**B**) In this case a Nylon suture has been passed through the holes of the implant and through the "ROOF."

Postoperative Care

The postoperative care is as described under transblepharoplasty browpexy above.

An example of a patient who has undergone this procedure is seen in Figure 16.18.

The Endoscopic Brow Lift

This procedure has to a large extent eliminated the need for a large coronal or pretrichial scar with its associated morbidity for patients seeking brow lift surgery. It is suitable for most patients who require a brow lift but who are unsuitable for a less invasive transblepharoplasty brow lift or a direct brow lift. It is not, however, suitable for patients whose brows are very heavy and severely ptotic.

The most suitable patients for an endoscopic brow lift are those with a relatively short flat forehead and a thick non-receding hairline, mild-to-moderate forehead skin rhytids, and minimal skin excess. Although the procedure can be undertaken under local anesthesia with sedation, most patients elect to undergo an endoscopic brow lift under general anesthesia.

Many surgeons have now abandoned the dissection of the brow depressors in the glabella as part of this procedure, given the associated morbidity, particularly as the use of botulinum toxin injections in this area achieves very good results. Botulinum toxin injections should be given to the glabella and lateral canthal rhytids 2 weeks prior to surgery. Some surgeons have also abandoned the use of the endoscope for this procedure. A lot of the periosteal dissection at the supraorbital margin can be undertaken via the upper lid blepharoplasty incisions if the brow lift is performed in conjunction with an upper lid blepharoplasty. This has simplified the instrumentation required for this procedure. The procedure can be performed satisfactorily and safely without endoscopic equipment and without endoscopic scissors, punches, and graspers.

Surgical Procedure

1. With the patient in a sitting position, the skin is marked just above the desired peak of the eyebrow with a gentian violet marker pen.
2. If an upper lid blepharoplasty is to be performed, the upper lid blepharoplasty is marked out with an assistant raising the brows to ensure that too much skin is not resected.
3. Five incisions are planned (Fig. 16.19). Three incisions are marked in the anterior frontal scalp commencing at the hairline and running vertically for a distance of 1.5 to 2 cm. The first incision is placed

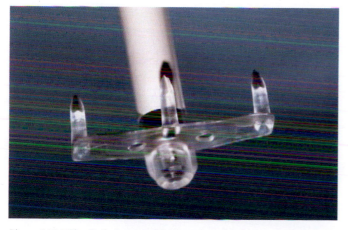

Figure 16.16 The Endotine transblepharoplasty implant preloaded on its inserter.

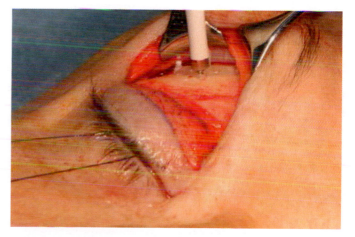

Figure 16.17 The Endotine implant is inserted.

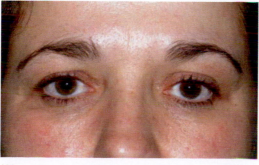

(A)

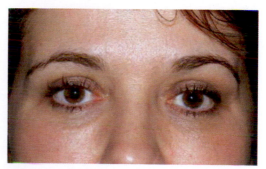

(B)

Figure 16.18 (A) The preoperative appearance of a patient complaining of hooded upper eyelid. (B) The postoperative appearance following a bilateral upper lid blepharoplasty and transblepharoplasty Endotine implant brow lift.

in the midline and the other two are placed in line with the skin markings above the desired peak of the eyebrow. The remaining incisions are placed in the temple The incisions, measuring approximately 2.5 to 3 cm in length, are centered on a line joining the alar base and the lateral canthus as it runs into the temporal hair, and are placed approximately 2 to 3 cm posterior to the hairline.

4. The hair is prepared with Hibiscrub solution and then carefully parted with a comb exposing the areas for the proposed scalp incisions (Fig. 16.20). The hair is not tied to avoid undue stress to the hair follicles. It is instead stapled to the scalp with a few staples.

5. The frontal and temporal regions are then infiltrated with a tumescent solution made up of 500 ml of Ringer's lactate, 25 ml of 0.25% Bupivacaine with 1: 200,000 units of adrenaline, 25 ml of 2%

Lidocaine with 1:80,000 units of adrenaline, 0.5 ml of 1:10,000 adrenaline, 5 ml of triamcinolone 10 mg/ml, and 1500 units of hyaluronidase. The solution is injected using a 20-ml Luer lock syringe and a 21-gauge needle. Approximately 40 to 50 ml of the solution are first injected subperiosteally over the frontal bone and pressure is then applied to diffuse the solution. Next a further 15 to 20 ml of the solution are injected into the temples, with every effort made to inject into the plane between the temporo-parietal fascia and the temporal fascia. The solution is allowed at least 10 min to work.

6. The head drapes are secured to the scalp behind the incisions using a few skin staples.

7. The surgeon sits or stands at the head of the patient with the endoscopic stack system positioned to the side of the patient (Fig. 16.21).

8. The frontal scalp incisions are made with a no. 15 Bard Parker blade. The incisions are carried straight through all layers of the scalp to the frontal bone.

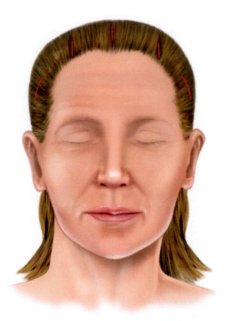

Figure 16.19 The location of the incisions for an endoscopic brow lift.

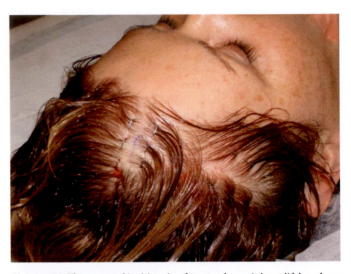

Figure 16.20 The proposed incision sites for an endoscopic brow lift have been prepared.

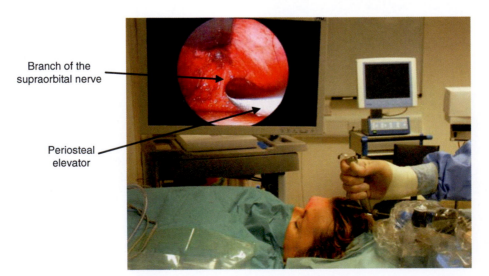

Branch of the supraorbital nerve

Periosteal elevator

Figure 16.21 The endoscopic stack system is positioned at the side of the patient with the surgeon operating at the head of the patient. In this patient's case, an endoscopic brow lift alone is being undertaken. The endoscope has been inserted into a special retractor which helps to maintain a "visualization pocket."

9. Through these incisions a no. 2 periosteal elevator is inserted and used to elevate the periosteum in a blind fashion over the whole frontal area to a position approximately 1 cm above the supraorbital margin inferiorly and to the conjoint fascia at the temporal crest (Fig. 16.22).

10. The head is then gently turned to the side and the temporal incision is made.

11. A perpendicular incision is made through the skin and temporo-parietal fascia with a no. 15 Bard Parker blade down to the glistening fibers of the temporal fascia.

12. If the superficial temporal vessels are encountered toward the posterior aspect of the wound they should be ligated.

13. A blunt-tipped periosteal dissector then is used to develop the plane between the temporo-parietal fascia and the temporal fascia while the skin edge is elevated with a large double-pronged skin hook.

14. The plane is dissected toward the temporal crest ensuring that the dissector is inclined toward the temporal fascia and deep to the temporo-parietal fascia to avoid damage to the frontal branch of the facial nerve.

15. A sharper-tipped periosteal dissector is then used to break through the periosteal confluence along the temporal crest, in a lateral-to-medial direction, keeping the elevator angulated towards the bone (Fig. 16.23). This can be done under direct vision using a headlight and a Sewall retractor or with the endoscope.

16. The dissection now meets the subperiosteal dissection pocket over the frontal bone. An optical cavity continues with the subperiosteal dissection in the forehead is now present. The 0° endoscope with an irrigation/retraction sleeve is now inserted through one of the central scalp incisions and the subperiosteal dissection continued to the arcus marginalis and root of the nose, and along the superolateral orbital margin beyond the zygomatico-frontal suture. (If an endoscope is not to be used the periosteum just above the supraorbital margins is broken and released using an angulated periosteal elevator which is levered upward. This manoeuver breaks the periosteum in a blind fashion but does not cut the supraorbital neurovascular bundle which is instead stretched. Alternatively, most of the periosteum along the superior and lateral orbital margins can be opened and released under direct visualization via the upper lid blepharoplasty incisions if an upper lid blepharoplasty has also been performed, leaving just the periosteum over the root of the nose to be opened using the angulated periosteal elevator.)

17. If the endoscope is used a no. 7 periosteal dissector with an upward angulated cutting edge is used to split open the periosteum (Fig. 16.24A). The periosteum is also lifted, exposing the brow depressors. If any bleeding is encountered the grasping forceps can be used to grasp the bleeding vessel, and hemostasis is achieved by touching the insulated forceps with a monopolar cautery.

18. Although the corrugator supercilii and procerus muscles can be gently dissected with endoscopic scissors and graspers, it is essential that the sensory nerve branches within the corrugator supercilii are preserved (Fig. 16.24B). Overly aggressive removal of these muscles will leave a depression in the brow. Given the potential morbidity associated with this aspect of the procedure, it is preferable to avoid surgery to the brow depressors and to instead rely on chemodenervation using botulinum toxin injections.

19. The next step is to provide scalp fixation. A variety of fixation methods have been described. The preferred options are:
   - The placement of drills holes creating a bone tunnel in the outer table of the skull
   - The use of Endotine implants
   - The use of microplates
   - (The use of implants, microplates or Tisseell® adds significant expense to the procedure)

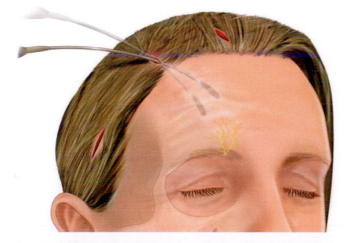

Figure 16.22 The periosteum is elevated over the frontal bone without the use of an endoscope.

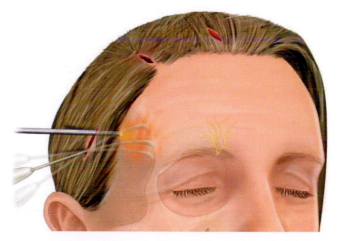

Figure 16.23 The conjoint fascia is divided from the temporal approach.

20. If drill holes are used, a 2.4-mm rose head burr on a powered irrigating drill is required. The holes are drilled in the outer table of the skull via each lateral frontal scalp incision. The drill is angulated at approximately 45° in the sagittal plane and the skull is drilled to the diploë. The drill is then brought from the opposite direction and the skull drilled again to create a bone tunnel. Bone dust is irrigated away with saline.

21. A 2/0 clear PDS suture is passed through the periosteum at the anterolateral aspect of the frontal wound and then passed through the anterior drill hole through to the posterior drill hole.

22. The assistant then draws the scalp upwards taking the tension off the suture as this is tied. This is achieved by applying tension to the posterior aspect of the scalp wound with a large skin hook.

23. Great care should be taken to ensure that the wound is closed meticulously over the buried PDS suture. A number of 5/0 Vicryl sutures are used for the subcutaneous closure and interrupted 4/0 Nylon sutures are used for the skin closure.

24. Alternatively, a triangular Endotine implant, which is specially designed for this procedure, can be placed in the skull at the inferior aspect of the two paramedian scalp wounds (Fig. 16.25). A gentian violet mark is placed on the frontal bone in the desired location of the Endotine implant.

25. The non-powered drill is used to create a hole in the frontal bone. The drill bit is specially guarded to ensure that the drill hole cannot exceed the preset depth. It is essential that the drill is held perpendicular to the bone. The bone debris is sucked from the hole.

26. The implant, which comes preloaded on its inserter, is pushed into the hole in the correct orientation with the apex of the implant facing superiorly. The implant should "click" into position. The inserter is then twisted anti-clockwise releasing the implant. The implant should lie flush with the frontal bone (Fig. 16.26).

27. The scalp is then drawn upwards using a large skin hook and the periosteum manipulated over

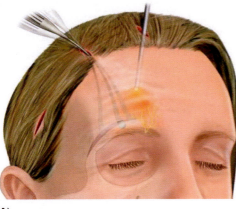 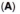 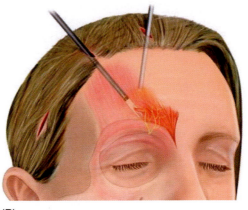

(A) (B)

Figure 16.24 (**A**) The periosteum just above the superior orbital margin is split open with an angulated periosteal elevator. (**B**) A drawing showing the disinsertion and removal of fibers of the corrugator supercilii muscle.

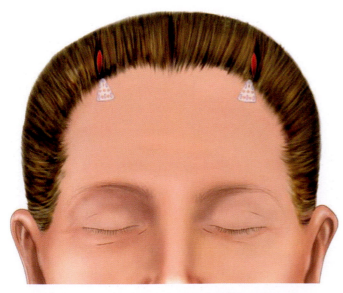

Figure 16.25 The Endotine implants have been positioned.

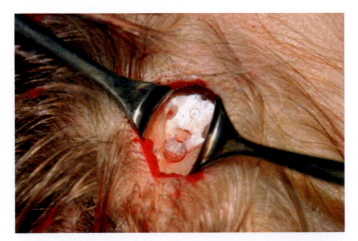

Figure 16.26 An Endotine implant lying flush with the frontal bone.

the tines of the implant. The height of the brow elevation can be adjusted as required by releasing the scalp from the implant and repositioning the periosteal attachment onto the implant. Great care should be taken to ensure that the wound is closed meticulously over the implants.

28. Another alternative is to place a small linear titanium microplate on the skull using small screws. The scalp can be elevated and fixated to the microplate using the same suture fixation described above for the bone tunnel fixation method.

29. After the frontal scalp wounds have been sutured, the temple wounds are closed. The temporoparietal fascia is elevated by suturing the cut edge of the fascia to the temporal fascia at the posterior aspect of the wound using a 3/0 Monocryl horizontal mattress suture.

30. The temporal skin wound is closed with interrupted 4/0 Nylon sutures. Alternatively, skin staples can be used. In some patients, a small ellipse of hair-bearing skin is excised if this is redundant.

31. If necessary, a single microsuction drain can be placed via the central frontal scalp incision and removed the following morning.

32. The hair is thoroughly washed.

33. A compressive dressing supported by a bandage is applied around the head for 18 to 24 hours.

Postoperative Care

Postoperatively the patient is prescribed a topical antibiotic ointment to the wounds three times a day for 2 weeks and Lacrilube ointment 1 to 2 hourly to the eyes for 48 hours and at bedtime. The Lacrilube ointment is then changed to a preservative-free topical lubricant gel to be used hourly during the day and Lacrilube is continued at bedtime until the degree of lagophthalmos has improved (if the patient has also undergone an upper lid blepharoplasty). The frequency of the lubricants is then gradually reduced over the course of the next few weeks. The patient is instructed to sleep with the head of the bed elevated for 4 weeks and to avoid lifting any heavy weights for 2 weeks. Clean cool packs are gently applied to the eyelids intermittently for 48 hours. The patient should be reviewed in clinic within 2 weeks and again within 4 to 6 weeks. The skin sutures are removed at 10 to 14 days postoperatively.

KEY POINTS

- Select the best candidate for this procedure
- Consider the use of botulinum toxin injections to the glabella rather than brow depressor stripping/extirpation
- Tumescent anesthesia greatly facilitates this surgery with minimal intraoperative bleeding and a reduced risk of postoperative hematoma
- Minimize the risk of damage to the frontal branch of the facial nerve by dissecting along the plane of the temporal fascia, staying below the level of the temporo-parietal fascia
- Take immense care if utilizing a bone tunnel for scalp fixation

---

The Coronal Forehead and Brow Lift

The coronal lift involves the use of an incision behind the hairline extending from ear to ear. It can be extended into a face lift incision if required. It involves the development of a scalp-forehead flap in a subgaleal plane over the glabella and the supraorbital margins. The frontalis muscle can be scored to reduce horizontal forehead furrows and the glabellar brow depressors can be weakened under direct vision reducing the frown lines. The coronal lift can be effective in raising the brow medially. It does, however, involve a very extensive incision, and leaves an area of sensory loss posterior to the incision, which may be permanent. Its use is reserved for patients with very heavy brows in whom the extensive scar can be hidden behind the hairline. It is not suitable for the patient who has a high hairline as this will be moved further posteriorly. In addition, the scar can adversely affect the growth pattern of the hair and the way this falls when wet. It can also cause some alopecia. With an excessive degree of elevation, the scalp and forehead skin can stretch again. Few patients now accept such an approach and the coronal lift is used far less frequently with the advent of the less invasive endoscopic brow lift.

The Pretrichial Forehead and Brow Lift

The pretrichial lift uses an incision just in front of the hairline, or just within the hairline, with the advantage that the hairline is not raised but lowered. This procedure can therefore be considered for the patient with a high forehead who is unsuitable for any other brow lift procedure. It can be combined with an upper lid blepharoplasty. The surgery can be undertaken under local anesthesia with sedation or under general anesthesia. The incision is still lengthy and is associated with an area of sensory loss posterior to the incision extending to the vertex of the scalp. Patients with a history of hypertrophic scarring should be excluded.

Surgical Procedure

With the patient in a sitting position, a geometric skin incision is marked out with a gentian violet skin marker just below the hairline extending to each temporal crest. The amount of forehead and brow lift is estimated by manually elevated both brows before marking the inferior incision (Fig. 16.27).

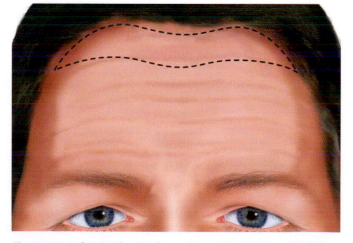

Figure 16.27 A drawing showing the position of the incision markings for a pretrichial brow lift.

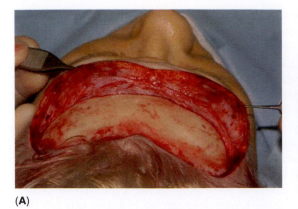
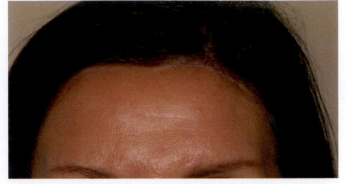

(A)   **(B)**

Figure 16.28 (**A**) The forehead flap is elevated in the sub-periosteal plane to the glabella and to the supraorbital margins. (**B**) A pre-trichial brow and forehead lift scar.

1. The incision line is infiltrated with 8 to 10 ml of 0.5% Bupivacaine with 1:200,000 units of adrenaline mixed 50:50 with 2% Lidocaine with 1:80,000 units of adrenaline.
2. The frontal region is then infiltrated with a tumescent solution made up of 500 ml of Ringer's lactate, 25 ml of 0.25% Bupivacaine with 1:200,000 units of adrenaline, 25 ml of 2% Lidocaine with 1:80,000 units of adrenaline, 0.5 ml of 1:10,000 adrenaline, 5 ml of triamcinolone 10 mg/ml, and 1500 units of hyaluronidase. The solution is injected using a 20-ml Luer lock syringe and a 21-gauge needle. Approximately 15 to 20 ml of the solution are first injected subperiosteally over the frontal bone and pressure is then applied to diffuse the solution. The solution is allowed at least 10 min to work.
3. The patient is prepped and draped.
4. The patient is placed into 30° to 40° of a reversed Trendelenburg position to help to reduce bleeding.
5. The skin incisions are made along the markings with a no. 15 Bard Parker blade.
6. The use of bipolar cautery is kept to a minimum.
7. The scalp-forehead flap is elevated in the subperiosteal plane to the glabella and to the supraorbital margins (Fig. 16.28A).
8. It is not usually necessary to extend the dissection beyond the temporal crest into the temples. If this proves to be necessary, the same plane of dissection is followed as described above for a temporal brow lift.
9. The periosteum just above the supraorbital margins is divided horizontally using a periosteal elevator. The periosteum is opened with the elevator exposing the brow depressors as described for an endoscopic brow lift. (An endoscope can be used to assist this process. Alternatively, if an upper eyelid blepharoplasty is also being performed simultaneously, the periosteum can be released under direct vision from below.)
10. The orbital ligament is released. (If an upper lid blepharoplasty is also being performed the lateral brow can be released quite easily from below.)
11. The glabellar brow depressors are then weakened if necessary as described for an endoscopic brow lift.
12. The wound is then closed in layers.
13. The subcutaneous layer is closed with interrupted 4/0 PDS sutures.
14. The skin is closed with a continuous subcuticular 5/0 Nylon suture.

Figure 16.28(B) shows the appearance of a typical scar 12 months postoperatively.

Postoperative Care
This is as described for an endoscopic brow lift. The sutures are removed after 10 to 14 days.

COMPLICATIONS OF BROW LIFT SURGERY
A number of complications can occur from brow lift surgery. The potential complications must be discussed with the patient prior to surgery.

Facial Nerve Trauma
A meticulous surgical technique and a very good knowledge of anatomy of the temporal region will help to avoid iatrogenic damage to the temporal branch of the facial nerve. The plane of dissection in the temple must be kept on the temporal fascia and deep to the temporo-parietal fascia.

Sensory Nerve Trauma
Care must be taken to recognize and avoid damage to the supraorbital and supratrochlear nerves during all types of brow lift procedures. During an endoscopic brow lift procedure, it is preferable to avoid muscle dissection in the glabellar region which can result in sensory loss in the forehead.

Hematoma
Great care should be taken to avoid intraoperative damage to the "sentinel" vein just above the zygomatic arch and to the supraorbital and supratrochlear vessels to prevent bleeding and the occurrence of a postoperative hematoma. If bleeding is encountered the vessel should be identified and cauterized. A drain should be used in patients who show intraoperative oozing or bleeding during an endoscopic brow lift. In practice, this is rarely required. Precautions should be taken to prevent intraoperative and postoperative bleeding by the preoperative discontinuation of aspirin and anti-inflammatory drugs, the adequate control of

hypertension, the appropriate use of local and tumescent anesthesia, raising the patient's head during surgery, meticulous wound closure, and the use of appropriate dressings.

Scarring

Visible incisions should be camouflaged appropriately and closed very carefully to avoid unsightly scars. The type of brow lift selected will influence the position and degree of resultant scarring. It is important to select the type of procedure that is most appropriate for the individual patient.

Alopecia

Care must be taken to avoid the inappropriate use of cautery in the region of scalp hair follicles to prevent undue hair loss. In addition, no dissection should be undertaken in a posterior direction during an endoscopic brow lift.

FURTHER READING

1. Albert DM, Lucarelli MJ. Aesthetic and functional surgery of the eyebrow and forehead ptosis. In: Clinical Atlas of Procedures in Ophthalmic Surgery. Chicago, IL: AMA Press, 2004: 263–83.
2. Brown BZ. Blepharoplasty. In: Levine MR, ed., Manual of Oculoplastic Surgery, 3rd edn. Boston, MA: Butterworth-Heinemann, 2003: 77–87.
3. Chen WPD, Khan JA, McCord CD, eds. The Color Atlas of Cosmetic Oculofacial Surgery. Philadelphia, PA: Elsevier, 2004.
4. De Cordier BC, DelaTorre JI, AL-Hakeem MS, et al. Endoscopic forehead lift: review of technique cases, and complications. Plast Reconstr Surg 2002; 110: 1558–68, discussion 1569–70.
5. Dutton JJ. Atlas of Clinical and Surgical Orbital Anatomy. Philadelphia, PA: W.B. Saunders, 1994.
6. Fagien S, ed. Chapters 2–6 through 2–12. In: Putterman's Cosmetic Oculoplastic Surgery, 4th edn. Philadelphia, PA: Elsevier, 2008: 67–145.
7. Jones BM, Grover R. Facial Rejuvenation Surgery. Philadelphia, PA: Mosby Elsevier, 2008 (ISBN: 978-0-3230-48309).
8. Jones BM, Grover R. Endoscopic brow lift: a personal review of 538 patients and comparison of fixation techniques. Plast Reconstr Surg 2004; 113: 1242–50, discussion 1251–2.
9. Jordan DR, Anderson RL. The facial nerve in eyelid surgery. Arch Ophthalmol 1989; 107: 1114–15.
10. Lemke BN, Stasior OG. The anatomy of eyebrow ptosis. Arch Ophthalmol 1982; 100: 981–6.
11. Nerad JD, Carter KD, Alford MA: Brow ptosis. In: Rapid Diagnosis in Ophthalmology-Oculoplastic and Reconstructive Surgery. Philadelphia, PA: Mosby Elsevier, 2008: 68–9.
12. Patel BCK. Endoscopic brow lifts Über Alles. Orbit 2006; 25: 4267–301.
13. Seery GE. Surgical anatomy of the scalp. Dermatol Surg 2002; 28(7): 581–7.
14. Shorr N, Hoenig JA, Cook T. Brow lift. In: Levine MR, ed. Manual of Oculoplastic Surgery, 3rd edn. Boston, MA: Butterworth-Heinemann, 2003: 61–75.
15. Shorr N, Hoenig JA. Brow lift. In: Levine M, ed., Manual of Oculoplastic Surgery. Newton MA: Butterworth-Heinmann, 1996: 47–62.
16. Tardy ME, Willianis EF, Boyee PG. Rejuvenation of the aging eyebrow and forehead. In: Putterman AE, ed., Cosmetic Oculoplastic Surgery. Philadelphia, PA: WB Saunders, 1994.
17. Tyers AG. Brow lift via the direct and trans-blepharoplasty approaches. Orbit 25: 4261–5.
18. Wobig JL, Dailey RA. Surgery of the upper eyelid and brow. In: Wobig JL, Dailey RA, eds., Oculofacial Plastic Surgery, Face, Lacrimal System and Orbit. New York, NY: Thieme, 2004: 34–53.

17 Orbital disorders

INTRODUCTION

This chapter deals with the evaluation of patients presenting with an orbital disorder. Such patients pose a potential diagnostic challenge and are encountered by most ophthalmic surgeons relatively infrequently. While it is tempting to save time in the evaluation of such a patient by routinely ordering orbital imaging, this should only be done where specifically indicated after a careful clinical evaluation of the patient. Likewise, the surgeon who is referred a patient who has already undergone orbital imaging may be tempted to examine the scans before seeing the patient. This is a bad habit which should be avoided, as it can cloud the surgeon's mind and lead to shortcuts that adversely affect patient management. The scans taken may not have imaged the appropriate area satisfactorily and may not have been the imaging modality most suited to the patient's orbital disorder.

The presentation and management of a number of specific orbital disorders are discussed. The disorders which have been selected are those more commonly encountered and which can be considered as very important in clinical practice.

EVALUATION OF ORBITAL DISEASE

The surgeon should approach the patient presenting with an orbital disorder with the basic clinical patterns of orbital disease in mind:

1. Thyroid-related orbitopathy
2. Neoplastic disorder
3. Inflammatory disorder
4. Vascular disorder
5. Structural disorder
6. Degeneration/deposition

Although the patient's disorder may occasionally fall into more than one category, this framework allows the surgeon to proceed with the evaluation of the patient in a stepwise and logical manner.

Thyroid-related orbitopathy is the most frequently encountered orbital disorder. It is the most common cause of unilateral or bilateral proptosis in an adult. It should always be considered in the differential diagnosis of a patient presenting with proptosis or orbital inflammatory signs (Fig. 17.1). Although its classic presentation is easily recognized, it can have a variable and asymmetric presentation, making it difficult to diagnose in some patients.

KEY POINT

Thyroid-related orbitopathy is the most common cause of unilateral or bilateral proptosis in an adult.

Tumors may be primary or secondary, benign, or malignant. They may spread to the orbit from the globe, from the eyelids, or from the paranasal sinuses. They may originate elsewhere in the body and metastasize to the orbit, e.g., from the breast. Cavernous hemangioma is the most commonly encountered benign orbital tumor. Lacrimal gland tumors represent a small but significant proportion of orbital disease. Lymphomas and metastatic tumors are the most commonly encountered malignant tumors in adults. In a child a history of rapidly progressive proptosis demands the urgent exclusion of rhabdomyosarcoma as the cause.

Many orbital disorders have inflammation as their pattern of presentation. Pain is frequently an accompanying symptom. The inflammatory process may be acute, subacute, or chronic. Acute inflammation is typified by orbital cellulitis. Subacute inflammation may be seen with nonspecific orbital inflammatory syndrome, whereas a chronic inflammatory process is seen with idiopathic sclerosing inflammatory syndrome, or Wegener's granulomatosis. It is important to bear in mind that some tumors may present with signs of orbital inflammation which may respond to treatment with steroids. Such masquerade syndromes are important to exclude by means of a biopsy.

Vascular lesions which may be encountered include high- and low-flow arteriovenous fistulas, orbital varices, and lymphangiomas. These lesions may mimic other orbital disorders, e.g., a low-flow arteriovenous shunt can mimic the appearance of thyroid eye disease.

Structural disorders may be congenital—e.g., dermoid cysts, sphenoid wing hypoplasia in neurofibromatosis, encephalocoele, microphthalmia with orbital cyst – or acquired, e.g., orbital wall blowout fracture, silent sinus syndrome.

Degenerations and depositions are rarer disorders. Examples include amyloidosis, scleroderma, and hemifacial atrophy.

The functional effect of the pathophysiological orbital process on the patient should also be considered. The patient may have a number of functional deficits:

- Visual disturbance
- Ocular motility restriction with diplopia
- Pain
- Neuro-sensory loss

It is important to be aware that orbital disease occurring in childhood has little overlap with that occurring in adulthood, although the approach to patient evaluation is very similar. Orbital cellulitis is the most commonly encountered orbital disorder of childhood. Malignant tumors, e.g., rhabdomyosarcoma and neuroblastoma, are very rare but rhabdomyosarcoma must be considered in any child presenting with a rapidly progressive orbital or eyelid mass and proptosis. Choristomas, e.g., dermoid cysts, and hamartomas, e.g., capillary hemangiomas, are the commonest orbital lesions encountered in childhood. In contrast to adulthood, thyroid eye disease is very rarely encountered in childhood.

KEY POINT

Rhabdomyosarcoma must be considered in any child presenting with a rapidly progressive proptosis or orbital/eyelid mass.

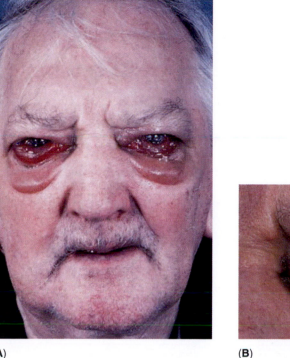
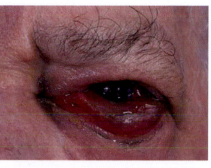

(A)   (B)

Figure 17.1 (**A**) A patient presenting with a rapidly progressive bilateral orbital inflammation and visual loss. He had "malignant" thyroid eye disease with severe compressive optic neuropathy. (**B**) A close-up photograph of the patient's left eye showing severe chemosis with conjunctival prolapse.

HISTORY

The history should be recorded in detail. It is important to listen carefully to the patient. Specific questions should be asked:

- What is the time course of the disorder? Acute, subacute, or chronic?
- Have there been any visual symptoms? Visual disturbance, gaze-evoked amaurosis?
- Has there been any pain?
- Has the patient experienced diplopia?
- Has the patient experienced any periorbital neurosensory loss?
- Has there been a history of trauma?
- Is the patient aware of any bruits?
- Are the symptoms aggravated by any specific maneuver, e.g., coughing, straining, nose blowing?

The history may suggest a specific diagnosis. A sudden dramatic proptosis with conjunctival prolapse in a child with a recent upper respiratory tract infection suggests a hemorrhage into a lymphangioma. Gaze-evoked amaurosis may be associated with an orbital apex tumor. Pain associated with a short history of a mass in the region of the lacrimal gland suggests a diagnosis of a malignant lesion, e.g., an adenoid cystic carcinoma, in contrast to a long history of a gradually progressive painless mass in the region of the lacrimal gland suggestive of a benign pleomorphic adenoma. Periorbital neurosensory loss in the absence of trauma suggests a malignant lesion. A history of "tinnitus" described by the patient may indicate an arteriovenous shunt. Proptosis provoked by straining may suggest orbital varices. A history of spontaneous unilateral periorbital bruising in an adult may suggest amyloidosis. Spontaneous bilateral bruising in a child may suggest a diagnosis of

neuroblastoma. A history of acquired enophthalmos in a female patient with a past history of breast carcinoma suggests a scirrhous orbital metastasis.

A full past ophthalmic, medical, and surgical history should be taken. A multitude of systemic disorders can affect the orbit. Unless prompted, the patient may omit details of a previous thyroid disorder, ear, nose, and throat (ENT) disorder, or treatment for a previous malignancy, e.g., breast carcinoma.

Old photographs may be helpful in evaluating the patient. It is always helpful to suggest that these are brought to any consultation.

EXAMINATION

The patient should undergo a full ocular examination, a specific orbital examination, and, where indicated, a full general physical examination. A careful examination of the globe and ocular adnexa may provide important clues to the underlying diagnosis, e.g., dilated episcleral vessels may suggest an arteriovenous shunt (Fig. 17.2); opticociliary shunt vessels may suggest an optic nerve sheath meningioma (Fig. 17.3); a "salmon patch" lesion beneath the upper eyelid may indicate the presence of an orbital lymphoma (Fig. 17.4), although such a lesion can also be seen in amyloidosis, sarcoidosis, leukemia, lymphoid hyperplasia, and rhabdomyosarcoma; eversion of the upper eyelid may reveal a waxy yellow infiltrate with tortuous vessels suggesting an amyloid lesion; an S-shaped deformity of upper eyelid may suggest a plexiform neurofibroma (Figs. 17.5 and 7.24).

Specific Orbital Examination

Proptosis/Enophthalmos Should be Assessed and Measured Using an Exophthalmometer

As a general rule, any asymmetry greater than 2 mm is considered pathological. Pseudo proptosis (unilateral and bilateral)

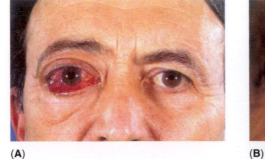
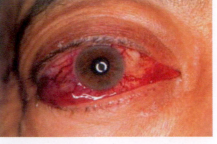

(A)   **(B)**

Figure 17.2 A patient with an acquired right arteriovenous malformation.

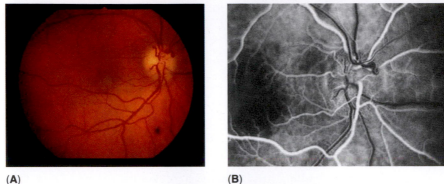

(A)   **(B)**

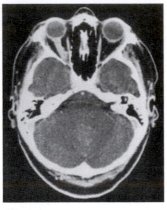

(C)

Figure 17.3 (**A**) Opticociliary shunt vessels on optic disc in a patient with an optic nerve sheath meningioma. (**B**) A fluorescein angiogram of the same patient. (**C**) An axial CT scan of the same patient demonstrating an optic nerve sheath meningioma.

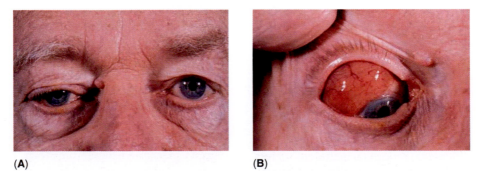

(A)   **(B)**

Figure 17.4 (**A**) A patient referred with acquired right ptosis. (**B**) Raising the upper eyelid revealed a large "salmon patch" lesion biopsy confirmed the diagnosis of orbital lymphoma.

from high myopia, contralateral enophthalmos, or facial asymmetry should be excluded (Fig. 17.6).

It should be noted if the proptosis is axial or non-axial. Axial proptosis usually suggests the presence of an intraconal mass.

Non-axial proptosis indicates an extraconal lesion. The globe is pushed in the opposite direction to the orbital mass lesion, e.g., a frontoethmoidal mucocele causes an inferolateral displacement of the globe (Fig. 17.7).

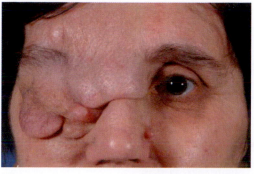
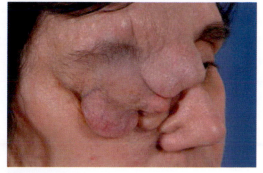

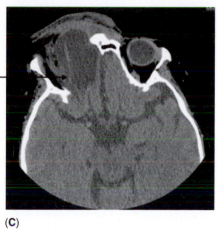

Large sphenoid wing defect

(C)

Figure 17.5 (**A,B**) A patient with type 1 neurofibromatosis. She has a large plexiform neurofibroma. (**C**) An axial CT of the same patient demonstrating a sphenoid wing defect and a large orbital encephalocoele.

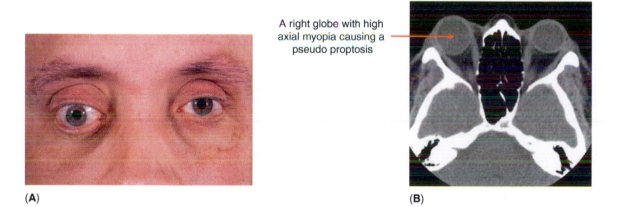

A right globe with high
axial myopia causing a
pseudo proptosis

(A) (B)

Figure 17.6 (**A**) Pseudoproptosis from axial myopia. This patient has a "heavy eyeball syndrome." (**B**) An axial CT scan demonstrating an enlarged right globe to be the cause of a pseudo proptosis.

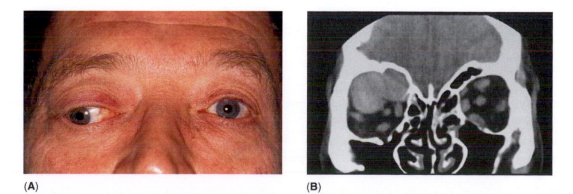

(A) (B)

Figure 17.7 (**A**) A patient presenting with a right nonaxial proptosis. (**B**) A coronal CT scan demonstrating a right frontal sinus mucocele.

Unilateral proptosis can have a multitude of specific causes but bilateral proptosis, in general, has a more well-defined differential diagnosis. In general, the most common causes of bilateral proptosis include:

- Thyroid orbitopathy (Fig. 17.8),
- Nonspecific orbital inflammatory syndrome
- Lymphomas
- Leukaemias
- Myeloma (Fig. 17.9)
- Metastatic lesions
- Congenital craniofacial disorders (Fig. 17.10)
- Arteriovenous shunts

Enophthalmos may be subtle, presenting as a pseudoptosis or as a cosmetic asymmetry from the development of an upper lid sulcus. The causes are numerous and include:

- Orbital wall blowout fracture
- Silent sinus syndrome (Fig. 17.11)
- Metastatic carcinoma (Fig. 17.12)
- Parry–Romberg syndrome (Fig. 17.13)
- Linear scleroderma (Fig. 17.65)
- Lipodystrophy
- Orbital irradiation

The Resistance to Retropulsion Should be Assessed
A solid orbital tumor will cause marked resistance to retropulsion. This assessment of orbital compliance can help to determine the approach to orbital decompression in a patient with thyroid eye disease.

The Orbital Margins and Eyelids Should be Palpated
An orbital mass may be palpable. Its characteristics should be noted: e.g., smooth or irregular, soft or hard, mobile or fixed, tender or non-tender. A cystic mass may transilluminate. A clinical diagnosis may be suggested from these findings, e.g., a small firm, smooth, fixed, non-tender lesion in the supero-temporal quadrant of the orbit which has gradually increased in size in an infant suggests a dermoid cyst. A smooth inferior orbital mass in an infant with microphthalmia and a coloboma suggests microphthalmia with orbital cyst, a developmental anomaly. A fullness in the adjacent temple may suggest the presence of a sphenoid wing meningioma.

The Patient Should be Observed for Spontaneous Ocular Pulsations
The orbit should be palpated for thrills and auscultated for bruits.

The Patient Should be Asked to Perform a Valsalva Maneuver
The effect on the globe position or a surface vascular lesion is observed at the same time (Fig. 17.14).

The Intraocular Pressure Should be Recorded in Upgaze as well as in the Primary Position
A rise in intraocular pressure may be seen in patients with restrictive myopathy, e.g., thyroid eye disease.

General Physical Examination
The Patient's Skin and Oropharynx Should be Assessed
The presence of cutaneous or intraoral vascular lesions may suggest an orbital lymphangioma (see Fig. 17.60B). The presence of café au lait spots suggests neurofibromatosis (Fig. 17.15).

The Regional and Distant Lymph Nodes Should Be Palpated
The presence of a generalized lymphadenopathy suggests a systemic lymphoproliferative disorder.

Cranial Nerve Examination
A cranial nerve examination should be performed, including an assessment of periorbital and corneal sensation.

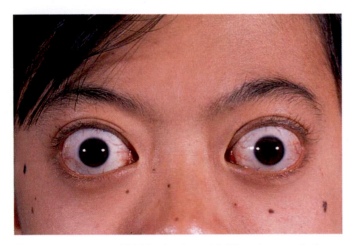

Figure 17.8 A 12-year-old Malaysian boy with bilateral proptosis due to thyroid eye disease. His proptosis is exaggerated by the presence of axial myopia and shallow orbits.

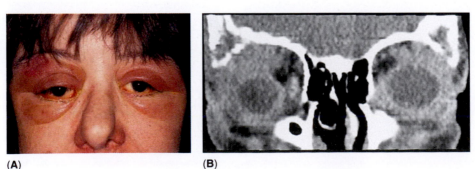

(A)   (B)

Figure 17.9 (**A**) A patient with multiple myeloma with nonaxial proptosis and orbital inflammatory signs. (**B**) A coronal CT scan demonstrating bilateral orbit masses.

Examination of Chest and Abdomen
An examination of the patient's chest and abdomen is important wherever there is the possibility of a systemic malignancy, e.g., undiagnosed breast carcinoma.

LABORATORY INVESTIGATIONS
A number of laboratory investigations may assist in establishing the diagnosis of an orbital disorder, particularly where the disorder is a manifestation of a systemic disease. These include:

- Chest X-ray: sarcoidosis, bronchial carcinoma, Wegener's granulomatosis

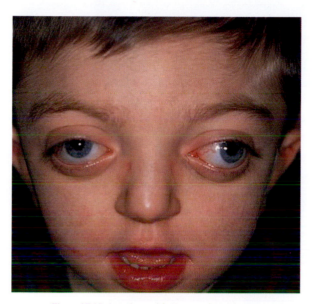

Figure 17.10 A patient with Crouzon's syndrome.

- Thyroid function tests/thyroid antibodies: Graves' disease
- Angiotensin-converting enzyme: sarcoidosis
- Antinuclear cytoplasmic antibody (c-ANCA): Wegener's granulomatosis
- Renal function tests: Wegener's granulomatosis
- Immunology screen: systemic lupus erythematosus (SLE)

ORBITAL IMAGING
Orbital imaging has become a cornerstone of orbital diagnosis and surgical planning. As orbital imaging technology continues to improve, the orbital surgeon has been able to refine preoperative differential diagnoses based on the imaging findings. Good communication between the surgeon and the radiologist is essential in obtaining appropriate studies. The better defined the differential diagnosis following a good history and clinical examination, the more appropriate the imaging will be. The selection of the appropriate type of scan, the area to be scanned and whether to use contrast media are crucial in obtaining the required information. Misinterpretation of images can result when the necessary information required could not be provided by the actual type of scan performed; consequently, it is essential that the surgeon reviews the scans and discusses them with the radiologist to ensure that the appropriate studies have been performed.

The imaging modalities available for the assessment of the patient with an orbital disorder are:

1. Ultrasonography (USG)
2. Computed tomography (CT)
3. Magnetic resonance imaging (MRI)

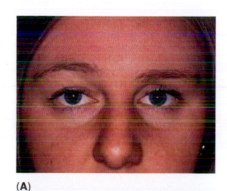

(A)

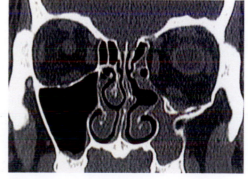

(B)

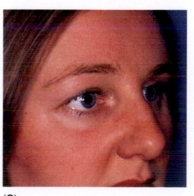

(C)

(D)

Figure 17.11 (**A–C**) A patient presenting with a history of a gradual left enophthalmos. (**D**) A coronal CT scan demonstrating the features of a "silent sinus syndrome" with a small opacified left maxillary antrum, an inferiorly bowed orbital floor, and a secondary increase in the volume of the left orbit.

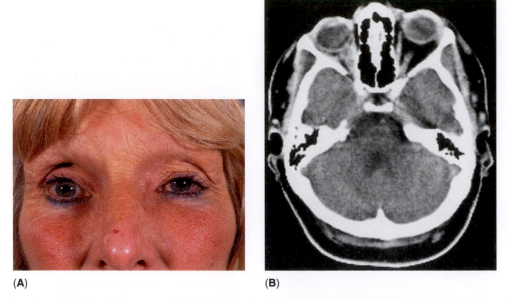

(A)   (B)

Figure 17.12 (**A**) A patient presenting with a right upper eyelid sulcus deformity. She had 3 mm of enophthalmos. (**B**) An axial CT scan demonstrated a right cicatrizing orbital mass and enophthalmos. She was found to have carcinoma of the breast. The orbital mass was a metastatic deposit.

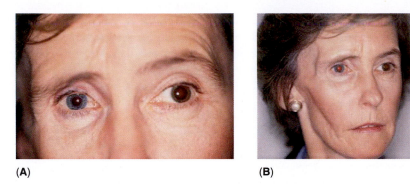

(A)   (B)

Figure 17.13 A patient with Parry-Romberg syndrome.

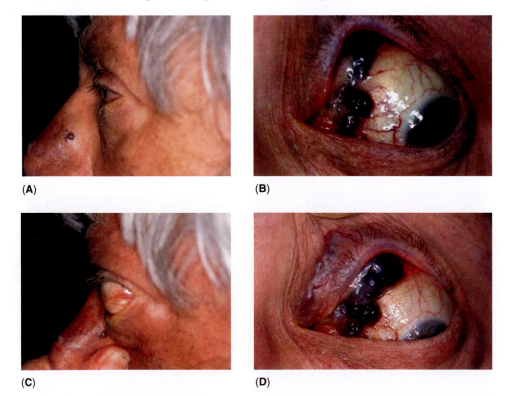

(A)   (B)

(C)   (D)

Figure 17.14 (**A**) A patient with a left orbital venous anomaly. (**B**) A lesion visible on elevating the left upper eyelid. (**C**) The patient performing a Valsalva maneuver with immediate proptosis. (**D**) The lesion increasing in size on performing a Valsalva maneuver.

4. Magnetic resonance angiography (MRA)
5. Arteriography

Ultrasonography (USG)

USG has a number of potential advantages. It is relatively cheap and can be repeated at regular intervals. It provides dynamic information. It has good resolution in the area of the optic nerve and sclera. Color-flow Doppler USG demonstrates vascular flow very well. These advantages can be exploited in the assessment of selected orbital disorders, e.g., it can be used to assist in the differentiation of posterior scleritis from other orbital inflammatory syndromes.

It has a number of disadvantages. It requires a skilled and experienced operator and it may be difficult for the surgeon to interpret the findings. The modality has poor resolution in the posterior orbit. For these reasons orbital USG has been largely replaced by CT and MRI, except in highly selected situations, e.g., to assist in the assessment of the response of a capillary hemangioma of the orbit to treatment with steroids or Propranolol.

Computed Tomography

CT is a medical imaging modality which employs tomography created by computer processing. CT produces a volume of data which can be manipulated, through a process referred to as "windowing," in order to demonstrate various bodily structures based on their ability to block an X-ray beam. Modern scanners allow this volume of data to be reformatted in a variety of planes or even as three-dimensional representations of structures.

It is the single most useful orbital imaging modality. It is relatively inexpensive, faster, and easier to obtain than MRI in most centers. The scans can provide good resolution and soft tissue contrast in addition to superior assessment of bone. It is ideal as an imaging modality to assess orbital trauma and lesions affecting bone. It does, however, expose the patient to ionizing radiation and this should be borne in mind when ordering repeated CT imaging. Its major limitation is the loss of resolution at the orbital apex where soft tissue is enveloped by bone. MRI is preferred for the evaluation of lesions involving the apex of the orbit.

Pixels in an image obtained by CT scanning are displayed in terms of relative radiodensity. The pixel itself is displayed according to the mean attenuation of the tissue(s) that it corresponds to on a scale from +3071 (most attenuating) to −1024 (least attenuating) on the Hounsfield scale. Pixel is a two-dimensional unit based on the matrix size and the field of view. When the CT slice thickness is also factored in, the unit is known as a Voxel (a volumetric pixel), which is a three-dimensional unit. Water has an attenuation of 0 Hounsfield units (HU) while air is −1000 HU, cancellous bone is typically +400 HU, while cranial bone can reach 2000 HU or more and can cause artifacts. The attenuation of metallic implants depends on the atomic number of the element used. Titanium usually has an amount of +1000 HU. Iron and steel can completely extinguish the X-ray and are therefore responsible for well-known line-artifacts in computed tomograms.

A single film does not have enough range of gray scale to display all the data from a scan. The data can be split and displayed on different films as soft tissue and bone windows. This is now done by computer manipulation of images stored on discs and viewed on computer screens. Bone windows should be reviewed wherever a bone lesion is suspected (Fig. 17.16). Some lesions have very typical imaging characteristics seen with CT, e.g., the "ground glass" appearance typical of fibrous dysplasia (Fig. 17.17).

Spiral CT can produce volume data sets in the axial plane. These data sets can then be retrospectively reconstructed into thin sections in any other required plane, which minimizes the radiation dose in the acquisition of multiplanar images. It also overcomes problems of patient positioning in the scanner, as axial images are obtained in the supine position. Reconstruction is of most value in the coronal plane, which allows more detailed assessment of the inferior and superior recti and also the orbital floor. Spiral technology provides rapid image acquisition and therefore reduces problems with movement artifact. This is particularly useful when scanning younger patients.

CT can detect very small intraorbital metallic foreign bodies. Larger nonmetallic foreign bodies such as glass, some plastic materials, and dry wood may also be visible on CT. With multiplanar imaging, CT can also accurately localize foreign bodies.

CT is generally sufficient for the assessment of tumors of the lacrimal gland. In this situation, the important factors to be assessed are the effects of the lesion on the adjacent orbital bone as well as the size, shape, and consistency of the lesion. A benign pleomorphic adenoma tends to be smooth and regular in outline, homogenous, and causes indentation with remodeling of the lacrimal fossa. In contrast, a lacrimal gland carcinoma

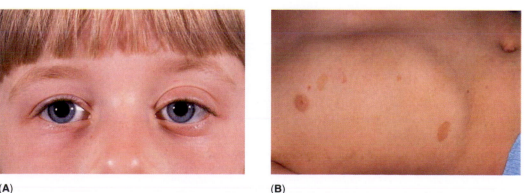

(A) (B)

Figure 17.15 (**A**) A patient presenting with a left axial proptosis. (**B**) A general physical examination revealed multiple cafe au lait spots. The patient had neurofibromatosis and an optic nerve glioma.

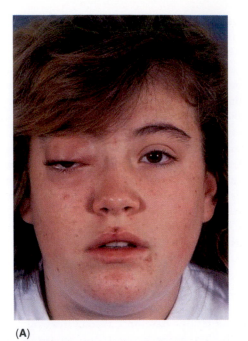

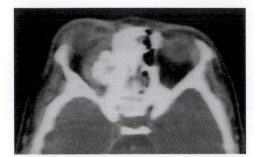

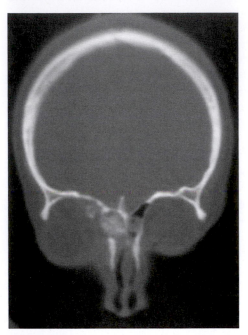

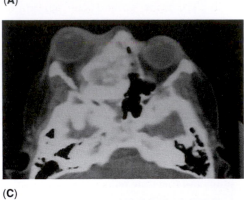

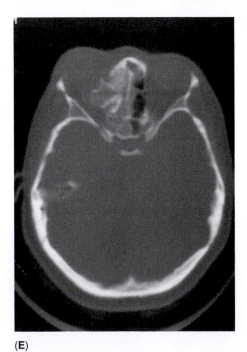

Figure 17.16 (**A**) A patient presenting with an acute right orbital cellulitis. She had experienced no previous symptoms. (**B, C**) Axial CT scans demonstrating an orbito-ethmoidal mass. (**D, E**) Coronal and axial CT scans – bone windows. The true extent of the bony mass is clarified. The lesion proved to be a benign fibro-osseous tumor which had obstructed the sinus ostea, leading to a sinusitis and a secondary orbital cellulitis.

is irregular, with areas of enhancement and non-enhancement with contrast, and may cause irregular bone destruction (Fig. 17.18).

The injection of intravenous contrast media can provide more information about orbital inflammatory lesions and tumors, e.g., the intraorbital and intracranial soft tissue extension of a sphenoid wing meningioma is better seen after the use of contrast. In many cases, however, it is unnecessary, given the wide range of intrinsic tissue contrast provided by various intraorbital structures against the hypodense background of orbital fat. The use of iodinated contrast media may, however, be contraindicated: e.g., with renal dysfunction, or a history of allergy to iodine-containing contrast media. An acute anaphylactic reaction can be potentially life threatening. The newer low-osmolar contrast media have an extremely low complication rate.

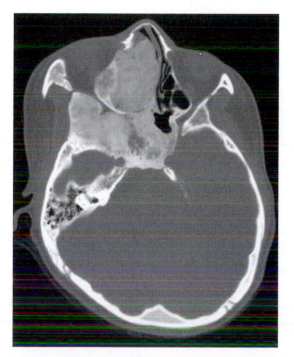

Figure 17.17 An axial CT scan showing extensive fibrous dysplasia in a 20-year-old female.

Magnetic Resonance Imaging

Although MRI technology is continuing to improve, it is still more expensive than CT. It is more uncomfortable and claustrophobic for the patient. Magnetic resonance imaging is adversely affected by patient movement: it does not, however, expose the patient to ionizing radiation, and has the advantage of allowing scans to be performed in any plane without the need to reposition the patient. MRI provides excellent soft tissue detail but, because bone is not differentiated from air, it is not a useful imaging modality for the evaluation of orbital fractures or lesions of bone. MRI is the preferred modality for imaging the intracanalicular and intracranial portions of the optic nerve. It is less sensitive for the detection of calcification.

For optic nerve tumors and orbital apex lesions, both CT and MRI may provide complementary information (Fig. 17.19).

An MRI image is generated based on the movement of protons in tissues when a patient is placed into the magnetic field of a scanner and then subjected to a series of radio wave pulses. The radio wave pulses are varied by the radiologist to generate T1- and T2-weighted scans. A T1-weighted scan is recognized by the dark appearance of the vitreous in contrast to the very bright appearance of the vitreous on a T2-weighted scan (see Fig. 17.20). T1-weighted scans provide the best anatomical detail. Fluid creates a bright signal on T2-weighted scans. A "fluid void" is seen in areas of high vascular flow where the protons are moving too rapidly to be imaged. Cortical bone appears as a dark area on MRI scans, as the protons are too tightly bound to generate a signal.

The use of surface coil techniques can improve resolution in the orbit, but these are more sensitive to patient movement. A number of fat suppression techniques can be used to suppress the bright signal from orbital fat on T1-weighted images that can interfere with the signal from adjacent extraocular muscles and the optic nerve. The use of these techniques is essential in post-contrast imaging to prevent enhancing lesions from getting "lost" against the background of orbital fat. The use of intravenous gadolinium as a contrast medium in combination

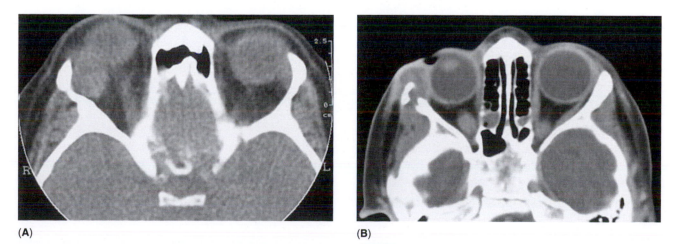

(A) **(B)**

Figure 17.18 (**A**) An axial CT scan demonstrating a pleomorphic adenoma of the lacrimal gland with local remodelling of the bone of the lacrimal fossa. (**B**) An axial CT scan demonstrating bony destruction from an adenoid cystic carcinoma of the lacrimal gland.

with fat suppression is particularly useful in the evaluation of optic nerve sheath meningiomas.

There are a number of contraindications to the use of MRI:

- Iron-containing intraocular foreign bodies
- Cochlear implants
- Intracranial vascular clips

- Cardiac pacemakers
- Older styles of prosthetic cardiac valves
- Claustrophobia

If an intraorbital foreign body is suspected, a plain X-ray of the orbit should be performed initially to ensure that an MRI scan is safe to perform.

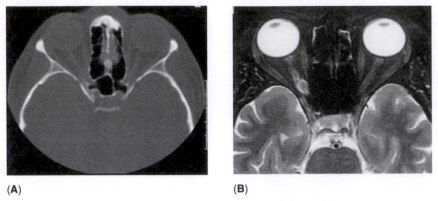

(A)   (B)

Figure 17.19 (**A**) An axial CT scan demonstrating an ill-defined orbital apical lesion in a patient presenting with a visual field defect. (**B**) An axial MRI scan clearly demonstrating the presence of an orbital apical lesion which was compressing the optic nerve. This proved to be a small cavernous hemangioma.

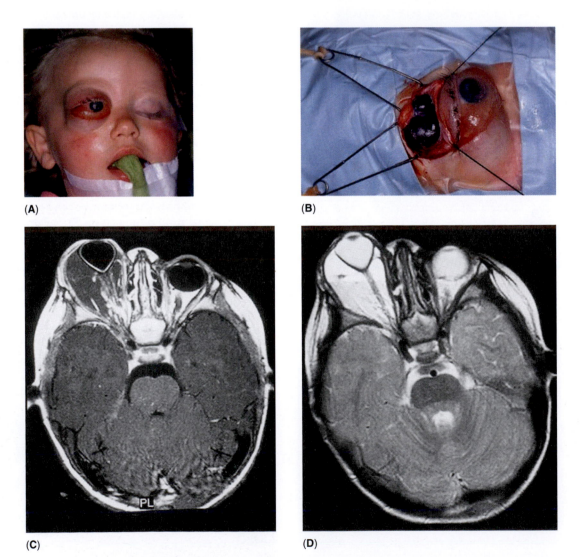

(A)   (B)

(C)   (D)

Figure 17.20 (**A**) An infant presenting with an acute proptosis following an upper respiratory tract infection. (**B**) The appearance at surgical exploration confirms the presence of a lymphangioma. (**C**) An axial T1-weighted MRI scan demonstrating extreme proptosis with tenting of the posterior pole of the globe with an extensive orbital mass. (**D**) The cystic nature of the lesion is demonstrated on the axial T2-weighted MRI scan with a fluid level visible.

Magnetic Resonance Angiography

There are a number of imaging modalities available for the investigation of orbital vascular lesions. For many years, conventional (i.e., digital subtraction) arteriography has been considered the gold standard because of its ability to provide both spatial and temporal information about orbital vascular lesions. Arteriography can provide detailed information about the arterial blood supply and venous drainage of orbital vascular lesions, the caliber of blood vessels, the collateral circulation, flow velocity, arteriovenous shunting, and the presence of flow-related aneurysms. This imaging modality is, however, invasive and carries a small risk of a cerebro-vascular accident and an ophthalmic artery thrombosis or embolization resulting in blindness.

Magnetic resonance imaging can provide greater soft tissue detail about the structure of orbital vascular lesions than can be provided by CT scanning but it is more susceptible to motion artifact from ocular movement due to the longer scanning times involved. MRA and venography can provide non-invasive static views of the orbital vasculature and some limited indirect information about blood flow. While traditional MRA provides excellent spatial resolution, it cannot visualize smaller blood vessels very well and can only provide indirect flow information about larger arterial vessels.

Imaging modalities are constantly improving and new ones are being developed. A new imaging modality, known as "Time-Resolved Imaging of Contrast KineticS" (TRICKS), uses extremely rapid acquisition of MRIs to provide dynamic images of intravascular contrast flow. TRICKS delivers relatively high spatial resolution and also provides dynamic flow information that has not been previously available without more invasive studies, such as interventional angiography. This imaging modality may improve the evaluation of certain orbital vascular lesion.

Arteriography

Arteriography can be regarded as the gold standard to diagnose and characterize certain orbital vascular lesions, e.g., arteriovenous fistulae. It is not, however, without its risks and potential complications. Interventional radiologists can also treat many of these lesions by the placement of intralesional coils via transarterial or transvenous routes. Occasionally, the orbital surgeon can assist such procedures by the placement of a cannula into the superior ophthalmic vein (Fig. 17.59).

Review of Images

The surgeon should review the images in a systematic fashion. The basic preliminary data provided on the scan should be examined:

- The patient's name
- The date of the scan
- The technique performed
- Contrast or non contrast
- Right–left orientation

The scout film should be examined. This shows the slices as sectioned by the computer (Fig. 17.21), which assists in orientation of the plane of scanning performed. The images should be examined systematically, comparing both sides for any asymmetry. It is important to look for any rotation of the head that can lead to misleading asymmetries of no diagnostic significance. The bone structures are examined first, followed by the soft tissues. Interpretation of the images requires practice and experience. It is extremely helpful to review the images with an experienced radiologist.

A number of lesions can be categorized according to their imaging characteristics, e.g., cystic lesions (dermoid cysts, mucoceles, lymphangiomas, parasitic cysts), isolated lesions (cavernous hemangioma, schwannoma), hyperostotic lesions (sphenoid wing meningioma, metastatic prostatic carcinoma), and lesions with calcification (varices, optic nerve sheath meningioma). This can aid in the differential diagnosis (Figs. 17.20, 17.22, and 17.23).

Extraocular muscle enlargement, for example, suggests a number of potential differential diagnoses:

- Thyroid orbitopathy (Fig. 17.24)
- Myositis (Fig. 17.25)
- Metastases (Fig. 17.26)
- Lymphoma
- Arteriovenous shunts
- Amyloidosis
- Chronic lymphatic leukemia

ORBITAL BIOPSY

Direct communication with the pathologist prior to surgery is extremely useful. Advice should be sought about any special handling of the tissue and the use of special fixatives. A fresh specimen may be required for certain immunohistochemical studies. Previous biopsy material obtained elsewhere may need to be reviewed by the pathologist and may aid in making a diagnosis.

An orbital biopsy may be incisional or excisional or may be obtained by fine-needle aspiration. An open incisional biopsy is performed with the intention of obtaining a diagnostic tissue sample with as little damage to adjacent structures as possible. It is very important to be aware of situations where this would be inappropriate, e.g., a pleomorphic adenoma of the lacrimal gland. In this situation, a complete extirpative excisional biopsy should be performed. An incisional biopsy

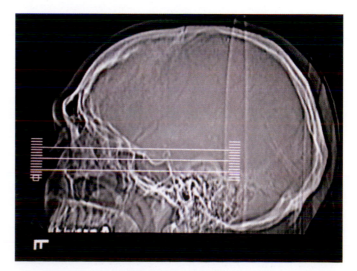

Figure 17.21 A scout film.

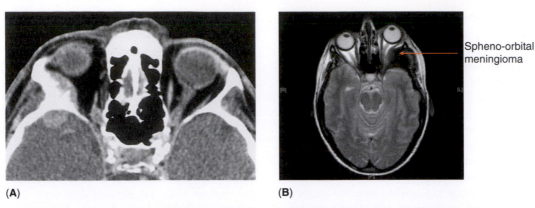

(A)   **(B)**

Spheno-orbital
meningioma

Figure 17.22 (**A**) An axial CT scan with contrast demonstrating a right sphenoid wing meningioma. Marked hyperostosis of the zygoma and greater wing of sphenoid is clearly seen. (**B**) An axial MRI scan showing a left spheno-orbital meningioma.

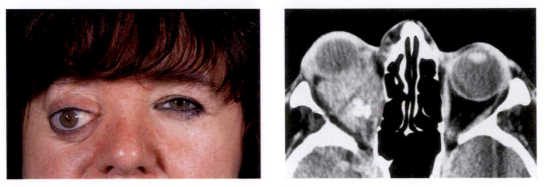

(A)   **(B)**

Figure 17.23 (**A**) This patient presented with an unrelated visual problem affecting the left eye. Her right nonaxial proptosis was long-standing. (**B**) An axial CT scan demonstrated orbital calcification within her orbital mass. This was a congenital venous anomaly.

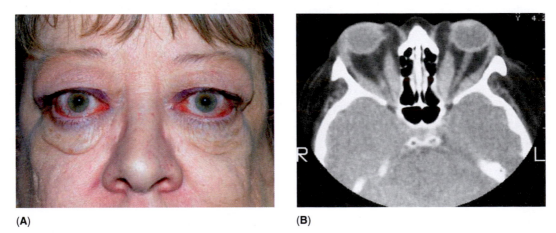

(A)   **(B)**

Figure 17.24 (**A**) This patient with bilateral proptosis and known thyrotoxicosis presented with a rapidly progressive visual loss. (**B**) An axial CT scan demonstrates marked enlargement of the horizontal recti muscle bellies with sparing of the tendons of insertion on the globe. The medial recti are particularly enlarged, with secondary remodeling of the posterior lamina papyracea. The optic nerves are stretched and the orbital apices are crowded. Swelling of the orbital fat compartment also contributes to the marked proptosis. The findings are typical of dysthyroid orbitopathy with compressive optic neuropathy.

requires careful preoperative planning and experience. It is essential to ensure that a representative sample is obtained which is sufficient for the pathologist to be able to examine. This can be difficult in situations where normal orbital anatomy is obscured by edema and hemorrhage.

Fine-needle aspiration biopsy is appropriate for some situations but requires the services of a skilled and experienced cytopathologist. The tissue obtained may, however, be misleading: e.g., a mistaken diagnosis of nonspecific orbital inflammatory disease may be made from small samples of a lesion which is due to the presence of a parasite. Such misdiagnosis can have grave repercussions for the patient.

The biopsy material obtained must be handled carefully to avoid crush artifact. All histopathology forms accompanying the specimen must provide the pathologist with all relevant information.

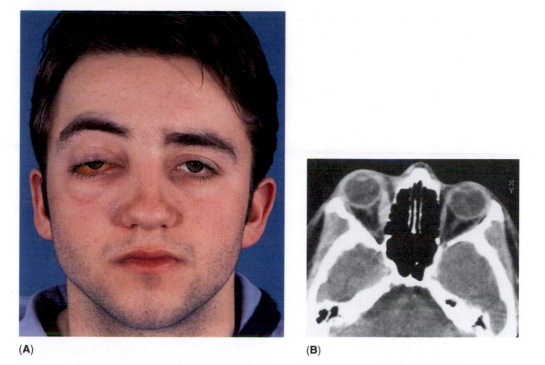

(A)　　　　　　　　　　　　　　(B)

Figure 17.25 (**A**) This patient presented with an acute painful ophthalmoplegia. He has unilateral orbital inflammatory signs. (**B**) An axial CT scan demonstrates enlargement of the right medial rectus muscle. In contrast to the patient with thyroid eye disease, the tendon of insertion is not spared. This patient had acute orbital myositis, which rapidly responded to a short course of systemic steroid treatment.

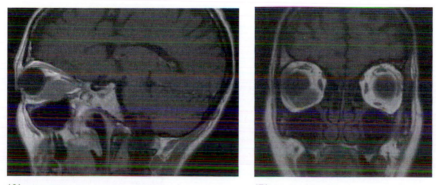

(A)　　　　　　　　　　　　　　(B)

Figure 17.26 (**A**) A sagittal coronal MRI scan demonstrating a mass within the inferior rectus muscle. (**B**) A coronal MRI scan of the same patient. The patient had a small intestine carcinoid tumour with metastases.

SELECTED ORBITAL DISORDERS

A comprehensive discussion of all orbital disorders is beyond the scope of this text. A number of disorders have been selected which represent either common or very important orbital problems.

Orbital Inflammation

A significant proportion of orbital disorders present with a picture of acute/subacute inflammation. The disorders most commonly encountered are:

- Acute thyroid orbitopathy
- Orbital cellulitis
- Non-specific orbital inflammatory disease
- Specific orbital inflammatory disease

Acute Thyroid Orbitopathy

Thyroid-related orbitopathy is the most common orbital inflammatory disease, accounting for approximately 50% of cases seen. This disorder, in view of its unique character, has been addressed separately in chapter 19.

Orbital Cellulitis

Orbital cellulitis is an inflammation of the orbital or periorbital tissues. Microbial orbital cellulitis is a true ophthalmic emergency, requiring hospital admission and the immediate administration of antibiotics. Although the morbidity and mortality associated with orbital cellulitis have dramatically improved since the advent of antibiotics, serious complications may still occur including blindness, meningitis, cavernous sinus thrombosis, brain abscess, and death. The ophthalmic surgeon must play an active role in helping to establish the diagnosis and must be responsible for monitoring visual function. Where this has to be delegated to non-ophthalmic nursing staff, e.g., on an ENT ward, it is the ophthalmologist's responsibility to ensure that the nurses know how to monitor visual function and whom to communicate with in the event of deterioration of visual function.

KEY POINT

Orbital cellulitis should be treated as an ophthalmic emergency.

Etiology

The most common cause is the spread of bacterial infection from a paranasal sinusitis. Children frequently present with a history of a recent upper respiratory tract infection. The locus of disease is usually ethmoidal and maxillary in children, in contrast to adults, who typically have disease in the fronto-ethmoidal complex. Many such adults have a previous history of polyps, allergy, or trauma. Additional causes include contiguous spread from infections of the eyelid or face, e.g., dacryocystitis and dacryoadenitis, panophthalmitis, metastatic infection, foreign bodies, trauma, infected orbital implants, and dental abscesses. Occasionally, orbital cellulitis can complicate surgery, e.g., retinal reattachment surgery. General medical conditions may predispose some patients to infection, e.g., diabetes mellitus.

The organisms responsible for microbial orbital cellulitis secondary to sinusitis are:

- Staphylococcal species
- Streptococci
- Hemophilus influenzae
- Diphtheroids
- Escherichia coli
- Pseudomonas species
- Polymicrobial aerobes and anaerobes

Hemophilus influenza is more common in children, whereas anaerobes are more frequently seen in adults. In debilitated or immuno-compromised patients, the possibility of fungal infection, in particular mucormycosis, should be considered.

Clinical Features

The presentation and progress vary, depending on the virulence of the organism(s) responsible for the infection. Preseptal cellulitis is typified by eyelid edema and erythema with a white eye and no orbital signs (Fig. 17.27). It should not, however, be regarded as benign but should be regarded as stage 1 orbital cellulitis.

Orbital cellulitis is typified by:

- Malaise
- Pyrexia
- Eyelid oedema and erythema
- Chemosis (Fig. 17.28)
- Axial proptosis
- Restriction of ocular motility
- Increased intraocular pressure

As the condition worsens, the retinal veins may become engorged and the patient may develop optic disc edema. The development of non-axial proptosis should raise the suspicion that the patient has developed a subperiosteal abscess (Fig. 17.29). The patient may then develop a reduction in visual acuity and a relative afferent pupil defect. The progression to a frank intraorbital abscess is heralded by increased proptosis, increased chemosis, ophthalmoplegia, increased malaise, and spiking of the patient's temperature. The development of cavernous sinus thrombosis is heralded by severe headache, delirium, bilateral orbital signs, cranial nerve palsies, neurosensory loss, optic disc edema, and dusky discoloration of the eyelids.

A well-known classification of the stages of orbital cellulitis is that of Chandler.

1. Group I—Preseptal cellulitis
2. Group II—Orbital cellulitis
3. Group III—Subperiosteal abscess
4. Group IV—Orbital abscess
5. Group V—Cavernous sinus thrombosis

KEY POINT

Preseptal cellulitis should not be regarded as benign but should be regarded as stage 1 orbital cellulitis.

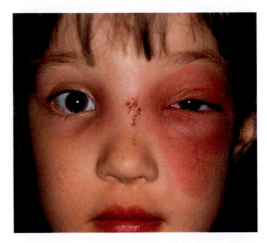

Figure 17.27 A child with an acute "preseptal cellulitis" secondary to local skin trauma. This should be regarded as Stage 1 orbital cellulitis.

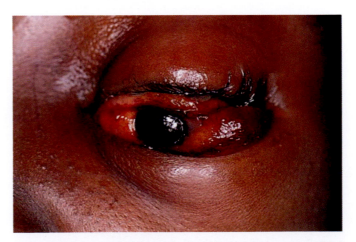

Figure 17.28 A 12-year-old boy with a rapidly progressive severe orbital cellulitis secondary to acute ethmoiditis.

Diagnosis

The diagnosis of orbital cellulitis is made on the history and clinical examination findings. The patient should undergo an urgent CT scan of the orbit and paranasal sinuses to determine the underlying cause and to exclude the development of complications such as an orbital abscess. In children it is important to exclude the possibility of a foreign body within the orbit or within the nasal passages. A CT scan demonstrates the location and extent of the inflammatory process and can be repeated if the clinical situation deteriorates. If the intraconal space is predominantly involved in the absence of associated sinus disease, an intraorbital foreign body should be suspected.

A subperiosteal abscess usually occurs adjacent to sinus disease. It is most commonly seen medially, secondary to ethmoiditis, and occasionally superomedially, secondary to a frontal sinusitis. As the abscess increases in size, the periorbita, which is loosely attached to the orbital bones except at suture lines, bows away from the orbital walls, assuming a convex configuration (Fig. 17.30).

Small subperiosteal abscesses in children may respond to antibiotic treatment alone. By contrast, subperiosteal abscesses in adults require prompt drainage. Undue delay in such management can result in severe morbidity. A frank intraorbital abscess may be identified as a poorly defined mass with variable enhancement with intravenous contrast.

It is important to be aware that immuno-compromised patients may have minimal signs of orbital inflammation, as they are unable to mount an adequate white cell response. Such patients may also show less aggressive CT scan signs.

Management

The patient should be admitted to hospital and antibiotic treatment commenced *without delay*. The patient should be kept nil by mouth in case a need for surgical intervention develops. There has been a tendency in the past to regard preseptal cellulitis as relatively benign and a separate entity to orbital cellulitis. Preseptal cellulitis should, however, be regarded as a potentially serious infection, particularly where this complicates an adjacent sinusitis. It should instead be considered as stage 1 orbital cellulitis. Spread into the orbit with serious consequences can occur.

KEY POINT

Preseptal cellulitis should be regarded as a potentially serious infection, particularly where this complicates an adjacent sinusitis. It should be considered as stage 1 orbital cellulitis. Spread into the orbit can occur rapidly, with serious consequences.

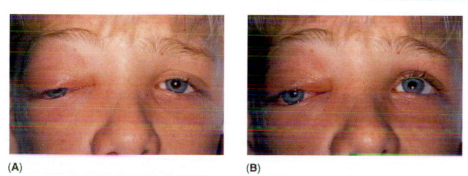

(A)   (B)

Figure 17.29 (**A**) A 13-year-old boy with orbital cellulitis and a nonaxial proptosis. (**B**) He has marked limitation of up gaze. A subperiosteal abscess should be suspected.

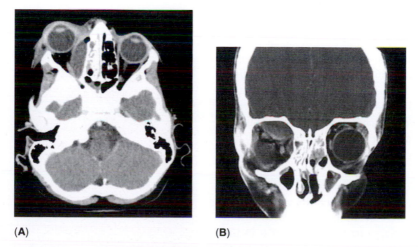

(A)   (B)

Figure 17.30 (**A**) An axial CT scan demonstrates a small medial subperiosteal abscess and extensive ethmoiditis. (**B**) The coronal CT scan demonstrates a large subperiosteal abscess along the roof of the orbit responsible for the globe displacement seen in Figure 16.28. The attachment of the periorbita at the fronto-ethmoidal suture line is visible.

It is essential that the patient is monitored at least on an hourly basis during the first 24 to 48 hours following admission. The following should be assessed:

- Visual acuity
- Pupil reactions
- Changes in proptosis
- Non-axial displacement of the globe
- Intraocular pressure
- Conjunctival chemosis
- Eyelid closure
- Ocular motility
- Fundal appearance
- Central nervous system (CNS) function

The assessment of visual acuity and pupil reactions in a fractious child with severe eyelid edema can be extremely difficult. Under these circumstances, the assessment of the other parameters assumes an even greater importance.

With increasing orbital edema, the conjunctiva may prolapse. This must be lubricated frequently to prevent drying and ulceration. Occasionally, a lower eyelid Frost suture is required, but care should be taken to ensure that this does not abrade the cornea.

The patient's condition can deteriorate very rapidly. Repeated imaging studies are required if the clinical signs worsen. Facilities for surgical management should be available and prepared to accept the patient at short notice.

In patients with eyelid disease, wounds or foreign bodies, swabs should be taken of any discharging wound. Where sinusitis is the underlying cause, swabs should be taken from the nasopharynx and blood cultures taken. Specimens should be placed in both aerobic and anaerobic culture media and submitted without delay. Blood should also be drawn for a full blood count, glucose, and biochemistry screen. An intravenous line should be inserted and intravenous antibiotics commenced. It has generally been accepted that broad spectrum intravenous (i.v.) antibiotics are required to manage the most likely causative organisms, namely streptococci species, staphylococcus aureus, hemophilus influenza, and the anaerobic bacteria of the upper respiratory tract.

There is, however, growing interest in the role of oral antibiotics where the oral bioavailability is similar to the i.v. preparation. The oral form of ciprofloxacin is nearly bioequivalent to the i.v. form (70–80%). In adults an oral dose of 500 mg and an i.v. dose of 400 mg have been found to provide an equivalent serum level. The oral bioavailability of clindamycin is 90%. Both ciprofloxacin and clindamycin have a broad spectrum of activity against Gram-positive and Gram-negative organisms, with clindamycin having additional activity against Gram-negative anaerobic organisms. The oral preparations can certainly offer more rapid delivery of the first dose, can result in fewer interruptions in the treatment delivery, and can simplify treatment delivery, especially in children.

Antibiotics are commenced on an empirical basis initially (Table 17.1) and altered according to bacteriology results. It is helpful to discuss the choice of antibiotics to be used with a local infectious diseases' specialist or with a specialist in the microbiology department whenever possible. Antibiotic treatment should be continued until all signs of infection have completely subsided.

Nasal decongestants and adequate analgesia should be provided. If sinusitis is present, an ENT surgeon should be consulted. If the clinical signs deteriorate in spite of appropriate medical treatment, surgical intervention may be required urgently to drain a subperiosteal/orbital abscess.

Subperiosteal abscesses along the medial orbital wall and orbital floor have traditionally been drained via an external skin incision at the medial canthus (Fig. 17.31). This is referred to as a Lynch incision. This has largely been replaced

Table 17.1 Initial Antibiotic Regimen for Orbital Cellulitis

Clinical variety	Likely organisms	Recommended antibiotics
Preseptal	Gram positives Staphylococcus	Clindamycin and ciprofloxacin
	Streptococcus	Clindamycin and rifampicin
Sinusitis related	Gram positives Staphylococcus	Clindamycin and ciprofloxacin
	Streptococcus	Clindamycin and rifampicin
	Hemophilus Anaerobes rarely	
Trauma or foreign body related	Gram positives	Clindamycin and ciprofloxacin
	Anaerobes more likely	

Doses recommended: For orbital cellulitis in adults maximal doses are recommended; in children, liaison with a pediatrician is advised.
[a]Clindamycin: the incidence of pseudomembranous colitis is no greater than with other broad-spectrum antibiotics. Clindamycin has the advantage of greater soft tissue penetration as well as excellent Gram-positive and anaerobic cover.
Ciprofloxacin: this provides good Gram-positive cover (although less for streptococcal species), excellent Gram-negative cover and some anaerobic cover. It is well tolerated and considered safe in children.
Empirically, this combination is very broad spectrum, offering excellent tissue penetration and can be used in all situations. Alternatives such as Augmentin (co-amoxiclav) and metronidazole offer a similar spectrum of cover but do not achieve as high soft tissue concentrations.
[b]Rifampicin is useful if Gram-positives are suspected, but it should never be used as a single therapy.

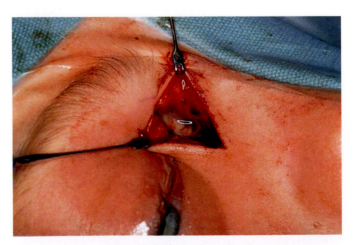

Figure 17.31 A subperiosteal abscess being drained via a Lynch incision.

by the transcaruncular approach which offers the following advantages:

1. It avoids a permanent cutaneous scar in a very visible location
2. It avoids the risk of a "bow string" scar
3. It avoids the risk of postoperative medial canthal dystopia from disturbance of the medial canthal tendon
4. It reduces the risk of inadvertent iatrogenic injury to the lacrimal sac or trochlea
5. It is quicker to perform

Such abscesses can also be drained via an endoscopic transnasal approach but this is not advocated in the majority of cases as the nasal congestion associated with such infections makes this surgical approach particularly challenging and potentially dangerous.

The role of a sinus washout in such patients remains controversial and lacks good evidence to support its use. Advocates of this treatment claim that it reduces the bacterial load on the patient while opponents draw attention to the potential morbidity associated with such intervention.

A corrugated drain should be placed and left in place until drainage of any pus, blood, or exudate has ceased. Attention should also be paid to adequate postoperative treatment of the sinuses to re-establish appropriate drainage. Occasionally, orbital abscesses may occur that require repeated drainage before a satisfactory response to antibiotic treatment is seen (Fig. 17.32).

In rare circumstances where the intraorbital tension is very high in the absence of an abscess, a formal orbital decompression may have to be undertaken to prevent optic nerve/ocular ischemia and exposure keratopathy.

Complications

The risk of serious complications following orbital cellulitis is greater in adults than children. Complications are more likely to follow inadequate or inappropriate treatment. The potential complications are:

- Exposure keratopathy
- Neurotrophic keratopathy
- Conjunctival ulceration
- Optic neuropathy
- Septic uveitis
- Panophthalmitis
- Blindness
- Cavernous sinus thrombosis
- Meningitis
- Intracranial abscess
- Death

KEY POINTS

There should be no delay in the administration of antibiotics to a patient with microbial orbital cellulitis. The patient should undergo hourly monitoring of visual function and frequent repeated clinical examinations as the situation can rapidly deteriorate (see Table 17.2).

Non-specific Orbital Inflammatory Disease

A number of orbital inflammations currently elude specific diagnosis and are grouped under the term idiopathic or non-specific orbital inflammatory syndrome. This syndrome was formerly known by the outdated term "pseudotumor." Patients tend to present with acute or sub-acute inflammation. Histologically, the syndrome is characterized by polymorphous infiltrations of inflammatory cells. The inflammation can vary in location, being either diffuse or localized to a specific orbital structure, e.g., an extraocular muscle (Fig. 17.25) or centered on the lacrimal gland (Fig. 17.33). Orbital apex disease can lead to an orbital apex syndrome with visual deterioration and cranial nerve palsies (Tolosa–Hunt syndrome). Patients usually respond to systemic corticosteroids or radiotherapy but a high index of suspicion for the possibility of an alternative pathological process—e.g., lacrimal gland carcinoma or lymphoproliferative disease—must be maintained. A biopsy is usually required, with the exception of most cases of orbital

Table 17.2 Protocol for the Management of Orbital Cellulitis

Initial management

1. Empirical antibiotic cover with oral ciprofloxacin and clindamycin
2. Hospital admission
3. Keep nil by mouth
4. Urgent CT scan of the paranasal sinuses, orbit, and brain
5. Full blood count, urea, and electrolytes
6. Blood cultures
7. Hourly monitoring of visual function and pupil reactions
8. Frequent clinical examinations to detect proptosis and reduced ocular motility
9. Liaison with ENT colleagues where sinusitis is present
10. Liaison with infectious disease/microbiology specialist

Indications for surgical intervention include

1. Signs of optic nerve dysfunction
2. Orbital or subperiosteal abscess on CT (particularly if an orbital roof abscess is present)
3. Failure to improve on medical treatment
4. Gas within the abscess space (anaerobic infection)
5. Concurrent chronic sinusitis
6. Concurrent dental infection

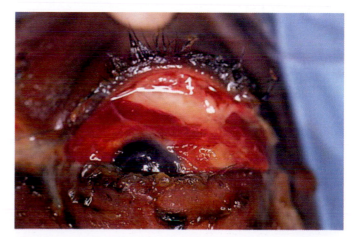

Figure 17.32 A patient with severe orbital cellulitis and orbital abscess formation.

myositis where a biopsy can result in loss of function. Failure to perform a biopsy may delay appropriate treatment and lead to avoidable morbidity.

Specific Orbital Inflammatory Disease

The specific orbital inflammatory diseases can be broadly divided into:

1. Vasculitides, e.g., Wegener's granulomatosis, poly-arteritis nodosa, hypersensitivity angiitis, Churg–Strauss syndrome
2. Granulomatous disorders, e.g., sarcoidosis, xantho-granulomatous disorders, ruptured dermoid cyst
3. Idiopathic sclerosing inflammation

Vasculitides

Vasculitis includes a wide range of angiodestructive inflammatory processes. The major orbital diseases in this category are Wegener's granulomatosis, polyarteritis nodosa, and hypersensitivity angiitis. Although these disorders may have distinct systemic symptoms and clinical signs, it can prove to be difficult to diagnose them and to differentiate them from non-specific orbital inflammatory diseases if they are restricted to the orbit during the early stages of the disease. It is extremely important, however, to make the correct diagnosis as early as possible as these disorders can have life-threatening consequences.

Wegener's granulomatosis deserves particular attention. It can occur as a systemic or as a localized disease. It can affect patients of varying age, including children. The main systemic features are:

- Sinonasal disease
- Lower respiratory tract disease
- Renal failure from necrotizing glomerulonephritis

The major clinical signs in orbital Wegner's disease are:

- Proptosis associated with a destructive orbital inflam-matory mass
- Uveitis, keratitis, and necrotizing scleritis
- Optic neuropathy

Extensive orbital infiltration may be associated with a yellowish discoloration of the eyelids. Involvement of the lac-rimal gland may be associated with eyelid edema and a brawny discoloration of the eyelid skin.

The CT scan findings may include:

- Diffuse orbital disease, which may be bilateral, with infiltration and obliteration of the fat planes
- Bone erosion with midline disease

The diagnosis of orbital Wegener's disease should be based on a combination of clinical signs, radiological features, hema-tological investigations (c-ANCA testing) and histopathologi-cal findings. In the presence of an orbital mass the diagnosis should be established with the help of a biopsy, although the histopathological findings alone may not establish the diagno-sis. C-ANCA may be negative, particularly in the localized orbital form.

The histopathological features which are suggestive of Wegener's granulomatosis include:

- A mixed inflammatory infiltrate
- A mixed granulomatous inflammation
- Areas of fat necrosis
- A vasculitis
- Fibroplasia

The patient should be managed by a multidisciplinary team. The management usually involves the use of systemic steroids and cyclophosphamide, and in some cases anti- tumor necro-sis factors (TNFs), e.g., Infliximab, may play a role.

Granulomatous Disorders

The major orbital diseases in this category are: foreign body granulomas, sarcoidosis, xanthogranulomatous disorders, and ruptured dermoid cysts.

Patients with sarcoidosis usually present with little clinical evidence of orbital inflammation but exhibit more of a mass effect. The lacrimal glands are often involved (Fig. 17.34).

Idiopathic Sclerosing Inflammation

A specific variety of nonspecific orbital inflammatory syn-drome is idiopathic sclerosing inflammation of the orbit. This entity has a characteristic pathological appearance with desmo-plasia and considerable fibrosis, which results in an orbital mass lesion that slowly enlarges. Anatomically it can present in the lacrimal gland area (Fig. 17.44), in the apical aspect of the orbit or it can affect the orbit diffusely. It shows histopatho-logical similarities to retroperitoneal fibrosis. The clinical fea-tures are dominated by cicatricial changes, mass effect, and only mild inflammatory signs. Patients present with pain. The typical clinical signs include: proptosis, mild lid swelling, ocu-lar motility restriction, ocular injection, and ptosis. As the dis-ease progresses there may be severe loss of visual function with potentially significant cosmetic deformity, and therefore early and aggressive treatment with a combination of corticoste-roids, radiotherapy, and cytotoxic drug therapy is required. Surgical debulking may be required. Advanced disease with a blind eye, chronic pain, and disfiguring proptosis may even require an orbital exenteration.

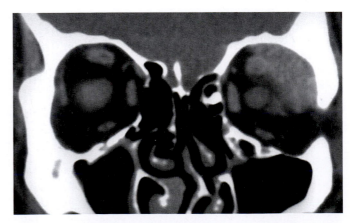

Figure 17.33 A coronal CT scan of a patient with non-specific orbital inflam-matory disease localized to the lacrimal gland.

Orbital Tumors

A multitude of benign and malignant tumors can occur in the orbit. This section describes those which are commonly encountered.

Cavernous Hemangioma

Cavernous hemangiomas are the most common benign orbital tumors in adults. They typically affect patients between the ages of 30 and 70 years. They are usually intraconal and cause slowly progressive proptosis. They may cause choroidal folds. Those tumors located at the orbital apex can cause compressive optic neuropathy. Gaze-evoked amaurosis may occur. Many asymptomatic cavernous hemangiomas are picked up as an incidental finding on head scans performed for unrelated indications.

Histologically, the lesions consist of large endothelial-lined channels with abundant loosely arranged smooth muscle fibers in the vascular wall. The lesions are surrounded by a fine capsule.

The lesions have very low-flow characteristics in contrast to infantile capillary hemangiomas.

A scan USG shows medium reflectivity and medium acoustic attenuation. The capsule demonstrates a high reflective spike (Fig. 17.35A). B scan USG demonstrates a well-circumscribed usually regular mass, which is homogenous (Fig. 17.35B). A CT scan typically demonstrates a

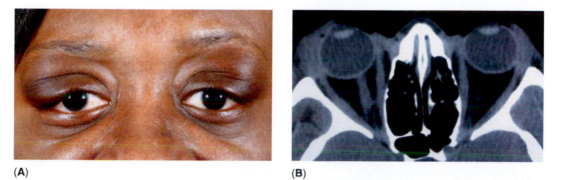

(A)   (B)

Figure 17.34 (A) A patient with bilateral lacrimal gland enlargement. This patient had sarcoidosis. (B) The appearance of the enlarged lacrimal glands seen on an axial CT scan.

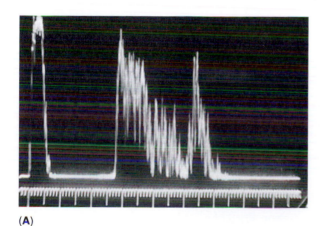
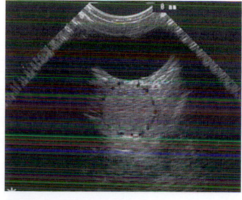

(A)   (B)

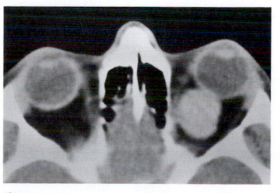

(C)

Figure 17.35 (A) A scan echography of a cavernous hemangioma showing a high reflective initial spike from the capsule, medium internal reflectivity, medium acoustic attenuation, and a second high spike from the capsule. (B) B scan echography of a cavernous hemangioma showing a relatively homogenous mass. (C) An axial CT scan demonstrating a well-defined, oval intraconal mass enhancing with contrast.

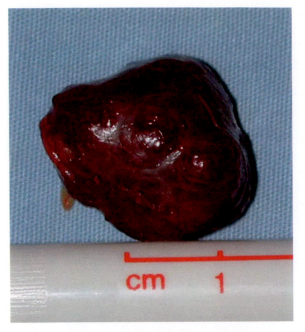

Figure 17.36 A typical cavernous hemangioma.

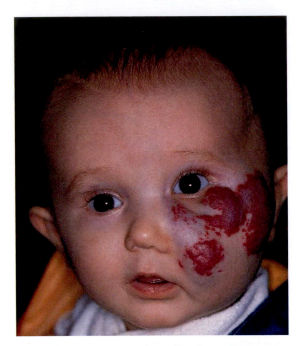

Figure 17.37 An extensive capillary hemangioma.

well-defined, round, or oval mass with a smooth outline that enhances with contrast (Fig. 17.35C). More than one tumor is occasionally present.

The management is surgical removal for the majority of these tumors. This carries the risk of significant visual morbidity, however, where the tumor is located at the orbital apex. In this location the alternative management is an endoscopic orbital apical decompression. At surgery the lesion has a typical slightly nodular appearance with a plum color and vascular channels on its surface (Fig. 17.36). It is usually easily separated from adjacent structures by careful blunt dissection. Delivery of the tumor may be aided by the use of a cryoprobe.

Other benign orbital tumors which may mimic a cavernous hemangioma include the schwannoma, fibrous histiocytoma, and solitary fibrous tumor.

> **KEY POINT**
>
> Cavernous hemangiomas are the most common benign orbital tumors in adults.

Capillary Hemangioma

Capillary hemangiomas represent the most common ocular adnexal tumors of childhood (Fig. 17.37). These vascular hamartomas typically appear during the perinatal period, enlarge rapidly over the next few months, remain stable for a period of several months, and then begin to involute spontaneously. Resolution of the lesion usually begins in the second year of life and is complete in 60% of cases by 4 years of age and in 76% of cases by 7 years of age. No treatment is therefore advocated unless the lesion threatens to cause amblyopia. The lesion can cause amblyopia by ocular occlusion or by inducing marked astigmatism. In this case, treatment is necessary and usually involves the administration of local or systemic corticosteroids (Fig. 17.38).

Intralesional corticosteroid injections are preferred to avoid the numerous side effects associated with oral corticosteroids. A 50:50 mixture of triamcinolone (40 mg/ml) and betamethasone (6 mg/ml) is used; 1 to 2 ml is injected within the substance of the hemangioma. A 27-gauge needle should be used and aspiration should be carried out prior to injection in the attempt to avoid intravascular injection. Use of a 10-cm³ syringe reduces the hydraulic pressure and thus the likelihood of flow reversal if inadvertent intravascular injection should occur.

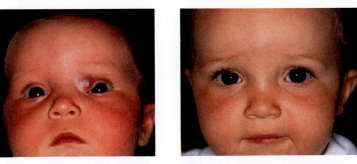

(A)   (B)

Figure 17.38 (**A**) A small upper eyelid capillary hemangioma in an infant causing five diopters of astigmatism. (**B**) The same patient 6 months after a local steroid injection with complete resolution of the hemangioma and the astigmatism.

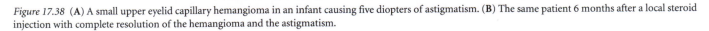

The response to the corticosteroid injections is usually evident within 1 to 3 days, and the most marked involution occurs in the first 1 to 2 weeks. Gradual but slow involution may continue for 6 to 8 weeks. If the response to the first injection is inadequate, a second injection can be given approximately 8 weeks later. The mechanism of action of intralesional steroid injection is not fully understood, but corticosteroids are thought to produce intralesional vascular constriction, facilitating capillary closure with resultant local tissue hypoxia.

Although safer than systemic steroid administration, intralesional corticosteroid injection has also been associated with complications. These include visible subcutaneous deposits, fat atrophy, eyelid skin necrosis, and inadvertent intravascular injection with central retinal artery occlusion, adrenal suppression, and growth retardation. CT should be performed prior to injection into deep orbital tumors for guidance. In such cases, however, oral steroids should be considered (prednisone, 1 to 2 mg/kg/day). Such treatment should be undertaken in conjunction with a pediatrician and the parents must be fully counseled about all the potential side effects of systemic steroid use.

The lesion may enlarge noticeably after the injection because of the bulk of medication and, rarely, hemorrhage, but mild pressure over the area assures hemostasis. The retinal vessels should be examined during and after the injection for possible compromise of the central retinal artery.

If the hemangioma is very large and requires an unacceptably high dose of corticosteroid, the injection should be limited to the most critical area, such as the upper lid when ptosis is obstructing the visual axis.

Surgical excision is occasionally effective for small, relatively localized adnexal hemangiomas that are unresponsive to pharmacological therapy and are causing amblyopia, and for the removal of remnants after regression. Occasionally, larger eyelid lesions can be safely removed surgically, but such surgery requires skill and experience (Fig. 17.39). The Colorado needle is particularly useful in ensuring that such surgery is relatively bloodless.

Treatment with interferon alpha-2a has been generally reserved for life- or sight-threatening corticosteroid-resistant hemangiomas. The response to interferon therapy may be slow and often not rapid enough to alleviate impending amblyopia. Since daily injections for weeks or months may be required and the effect of interferon therapy is often mild, this treatment has enjoyed limited popularity for orbital lesions. Side effects are common and patients must be closely monitored during treatment.

The use of oral Propranolol is also being investigated and has shown some very promising results. This treatment may obviate the need for steroid treatment. Possible methods of action of this non-selective beta-blocker on capillary hemangiomas are:

1. Vasoconstriction
2. Down-regulation of the RAF-mitomycin-activated protein kinase pathway with decreased expression of VEGF and bFGF genes

KEY POINT

The use of oral Propranolol may obviate the need for steroid treatment in patients with capillary hemangiomas.

Optic Nerve Sheath Meningioma

This tumor typically affects middle-aged adults. The tumor arises from the optic nerve meningeal sheath, leading to optic nerve compression usually before noticeable proptosis occurs. Patients usually present with slowly progressive painless visual loss. Unilateral optic disc edema, optic disc atrophy, and optico-ciliary shunt vessels may be seen (Fig. 17.3A and B). These shunt vessels represent a dilatation of pre-existing venous channels occurring in response to obstruction of venous blood flow by a mass compressing the intraorbital portion of the optic nerve.

A CT scan may demonstrate subtle enlargement of the optic nerve. Occasionally an exophytic tumor may be present and may present a diagnostic challenge that requires a biopsy. Calcification may be seen very occasionally. A "tram-track" sign is sometimes seen on an axial CT scan, where parallel radiodense lines are seen along the optic nerve sheath (see Fig. 17.3C). A radiodense ring is seen on a coronal scan. This sign is diagnostic of an optic nerve sheath meningioma.

An MRI scan is performed to delineate the posterior extent of the lesion. A lesion confined to the optic canal can present a diagnostic challenge. Although benign, this lesion in patients under the age of 40 may behave more aggressively and may require surgical excision. Cystic forms of the tumor may spread into the orbit, making surgical excision extremely difficult. Stereotactic radiotherapy may be considered for patients

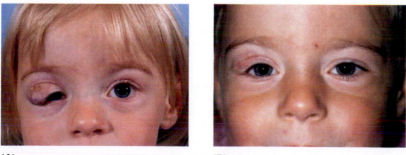

(A)   (B)

Figure 17.39 (**A**) A right upper eyelid capillary hemangioma unresponsive to steroid injections. (**B**) The appearance 2 months following a debulking of the lesion, wedge excision, and levator advancement.

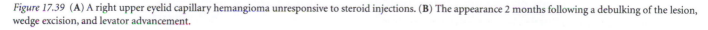

who demonstrate growth of the lesion in order to preserve useful visual function for a longer period of time. Surgical excision is usually performed in younger patients who demonstrate active growth that threatens to extend intracranially. It may also be performed for patients with disfiguring proptosis and a blind eye. Such surgery requires a transcranial approach, with removal of the nerve from the chiasm to the globe.

Sphenoid Wing Meningioma

A sphenoid wing meningioma is more commonly encountered than an optic nerve sheath meningioma. The growth of hyperostotic bone into the orbit usually causes a slowly progressive painless proptosis with inferior displacement of the globe. The degree of proptosis can become marked before visual loss from optic nerve compression occurs. Temporal "fullness" is seen as the hyperostotic bone extends into the temporal fossa. The hyperostotic bone is readily seen on a CT scan but the full extent of the associated soft tissue lesion requires the use of an intravenous contrast agent (see Fig. 17.22A).

The tumor can be debulked but cannot be removed completely. Radiotherapy is occasionally used and can be very effective in controlling the progress of the tumor and protecting visual function, but some tumors are not very radiosensitive. Recurrences are common and repeated surgery is required over the course of the patient's life.

Spheno-orbital meningiomas are considered by some to be a separate entity to the sphenoid wing meningioma. These are defined by a distinct periorbital component (Fig. 17.22B). They can more rapidly extend to the orbital apex and cavernous sinus and cause optic nerve compression. Recurrences following surgery are very common and radiotherapy may have to be used to protect visual function.

Optic Nerve Glioma

An optic nerve glioma, in contrast to an optic nerve sheath meningioma, is an intrinsic optic nerve tumor originating from the optic nerve tissue. It is usually seen initially in children under the age of 10 years. In contrast to an optic nerve sheath meningioma, which causes compression of the optic nerve and gradual loss of visual function, vision is usually reasonably well preserved in children with an optic nerve glioma. The lesion is considered to be a hamartoma rather than a true tumor. Patients tend to develop a very slowly progressive painless axial proptosis. Mucinous degeneration of the lesion can rarely lead to a more rapid progression.

Most optic nerve gliomas are unilateral. Approximately 25% of patients have neurofibromatosis. Bilateral optic nerve glioma is diagnostic of neurofibromatosis.

A CT scan usually shows fusiform enlargement of the optic nerve, although eccentric enlargement of the nerve may also be seen (Fig. 17.40). In contrast to an optic nerve meningioma, there is an absence of calcification. An MRI scan should be performed to assess the posterior extent of the lesion. The optic chiasm may be affected in up to 50% of patients. Other intracranial areas can be affected and may be associated with a poor prognosis.

An incisional biopsy may be performed in those cases where the clinical diagnosis is uncertain or if the proptosis suddenly progresses. For most patients observation with serial MRI scans is appropriate. Surgical excision of the lesion is usually

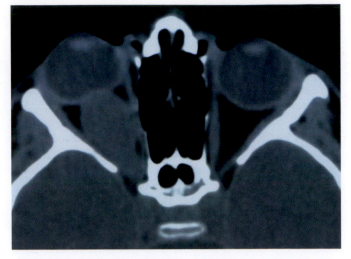

Figure 17.40 An axial CT scan showing a fusiform lesion in the right intraconal space. The patient had an optic nerve glioma.

Table 17.3 Examples of space-occupying Lesions of the Lacrimal Fossa

Category	Intrinsic	Extrinsic
Neoplastic	Epithelial tumor/lymphoma	Myeloma
Inflammatory	Sarcoidosis	Granuloma
Structural	Dacryocoele	Dermoid cyst

only required in patients with unsightly proptosis and a blind eye. For most patients this requires a transcranial approach.

Lacrimal Gland Tumors

The major steps in the management of lesions of the lacrimal gland consist of accurate clinical and investigative categorization into neoplastic, inflammatory, and structural processes. These processes may be intrinsic or extrinsic (Table 17.3).

The structural lesions—e.g., inclusion cysts, dermoid cysts, and dermolipomas—are not usually difficult to differentiate from the other processes (Figs. 17.41 and 17.42).

The inflammatory lesions (Fig. 17.43), particularly those with a subacute or chronic course and imaging characteristics which suggest a non-destructive localized infiltration, should be subjected to an incisional biopsy (Fig. 17.44). The management is based on the histological findings.

It has been generally held that approximately 50% of all intrinsic neoplastic lesions of the lacrimal gland are epithelial tumors and 50% lymphomas. Of the epithelial tumors, 50% are pleomorphic adenomas and 50% are carcinomas. Of the carcinomas, 50% are adenoid cystic carcinomas, with the remainder divided between mixed tumors and other carcinomas. Although useful as an aide-memoire, these figures have been challenged.

The main goal in the management of epithelial tumors of the lacrimal gland is the differentiation between pleomorphic adenoma (benign mixed cell tumor) and carcinomas. This can, however, be far from straightforward. In general, pleomorphic adenoma is characterized by a long history and an absence of pain. It tends to occur between the ages of 20 and 50 years. An orbital CT scan usually demonstrates a well-defined, regular, homogenous mass that causes pressure erosion of the bone of the lacrimal fossa (Fig. 17.45B).

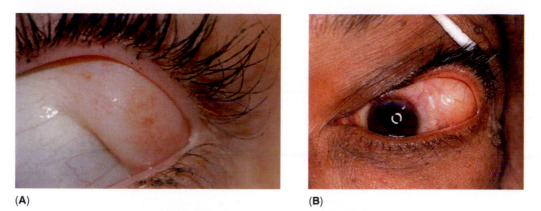

(A)   **(B)**

Figure 17.41 (**A**) A typical dermolipoma. The visible portion represents the "tip of the iceberg." The lesion typically extends deep into the orbit. Attempted surgical excision risks damage to the lacrimal ductules, resulting in a dry eye; the lateral rectus muscle, resulting in diplopia; the levator aponeurosis, resulting in ptosis; and the conjunctiva, with scarring and a restriction of ocular motility. (**B**) The typical appearance of a prolapse of orbital fat through a dehiscence in Tenon's capsule. This appearance should be differentiated from a prolapsed lacrimal gland, whose appearance is much paler.

In contrast, the carcinomas have a short history and are associated with pain in approximately 30% of cases. Adenoid cystic carcinoma has a peak incidence in the fourth decade. An orbital CT scan may show an irregular lesion with infiltration of adjacent structures, destruction of bone, and calcification (Fig. 17.46), although these features tend to be absent in younger patients (Fig. 17.47).

The major goal is to identify the characteristic clinical and investigative features of the pleomorphic adenoma in order to ensure that complete en bloc surgical removal is the initial management and that incisional biopsy is avoided. This can be difficult in some patients who do not present with textbook symptoms and signs (Fig. 17.48). Surgical intervention for diagnostic purposes in all other lesions involving the lacrimal fossa (with the exception of well-defined, non-infiltrative lesions, e.g., dermoid cysts) should be incisional biopsy.

The prognosis following appropriate management of a pleomorphic adenoma is excellent. There is, however, a high recurrence rate following incomplete excision or incisional biopsy. Recurrence following incomplete excision may be delayed for many years and may be associated with malignant transformation.

The prognosis for adenoid cystic carcinoma is very poor. The tendency to perineural invasion, which may extend centimeters beyond the apparent margins of the solid mass, is a dominant factor in the prognosis. The clinical course is one of painful local and regional recurrence followed by systemic spread. The median disease-free survival is 3 years and overall median survival is approximately 10 years.

When preoperative evaluation indicates a malignant tumor of the lacrimal gland, the recommended therapy is surgical with an initial transeptal diagnostic biopsy followed by exenteration, or en bloc resection, and radiotherapy. The role of radiotherapy is controversial.

KEY POINT

The major goal in the management of lacrimal gland tumors is to identify the characteristic clinical and investigative features of the pleomorphic adenoma in order to ensure that complete en bloc surgical removal is the initial management and that an incisional biopsy is avoided.

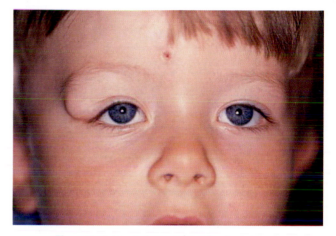

Figure 17.42 A typical external angular dermoid cyst.

Lymphoma

Orbital lymphoma is a rare presentation of extranodal non-Hodgkin's lymphoma (NHL), accounting for less than 1% of the total. Lymphomas form the largest group of lymphoproliferative disorders seen in the orbit. Approximately 55% of malignant tumors arising in the orbit are lymphomas. Approximately 75% of orbital lymphomas are unilateral and 25% bilateral; approximately 50 to 60% of orbital lymphomas present as isolated orbital lesions; 30 to 35% have evidence of systemic disease on presentation. Hence, all patients with ocular lymphoma should be fully investigated to rule out systemic lymphoma. Of those patients who present with isolated orbital disease, approximately 15% subsequently develop systemic disease.

Advances in imaging techniques, improved biopsy techniques, and newer classification systems are likely to have contributed to an apparent increase in the incidence of lymphoma. The aging population, the increasing usage of immunosuppressive drugs, and the AIDS epidemic have also contributed to the apparent increased incidence of NHL.

Over the years, different classification systems have been used to differentiate lymphomas, including the Rappaport Classification (used until the 1970s), the Working Formulation, the National Cancer Institute Working Formulation, and the Revised European-American Lymphoma Classification (REAL).

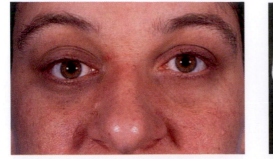
(A)

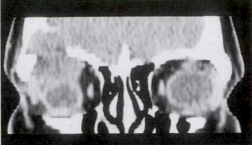
(B)

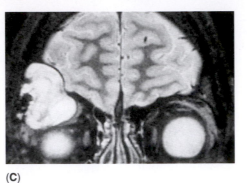
(C)

Figure 17.43 (**A**) A patient who presented with a palpable mass in the region of the right lacrimal gland and a right hypoglobus. (**B**) A coronal CT scan demonstrating a lesion within the right frontal bone extending into the orbit responsible for the patient's hypoglobus. (**C**) A coronal MRI scan of the same lesion. The patient's prior history of blunt trauma to the area suggested the diagnosis of a cholesterol granuloma. This was confirmed histologically after surgical removal.

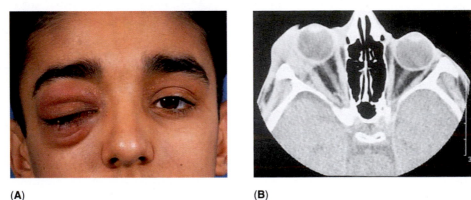
(A)   (B)

Figure 17.44 (**A**) A 15-year-old patient with a chronic orbital inflammatory mass. (**B**) An axial CT scan demonstrating a mass in the region of the right lacrimal gland. A biopsy confirmed the diagnosis of an idiopathic sclerosing inflammation of the orbit.

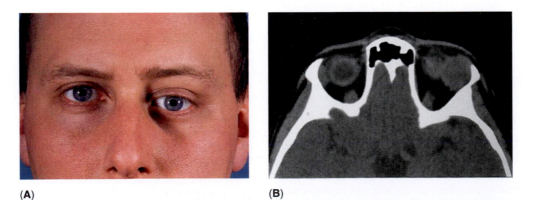
(A)   (B)

Figure 17.45 (**A**) A patient presenting with a 2-year history of a gradual painless nonaxial proptosis. (**B**) An axial CT scan demonstrating a well-defined mass in the left lacrimal fossa with pressure erosion of the adjacent bone. The preoperative diagnosis of a pleomorphic adenoma was confirmed histologically.

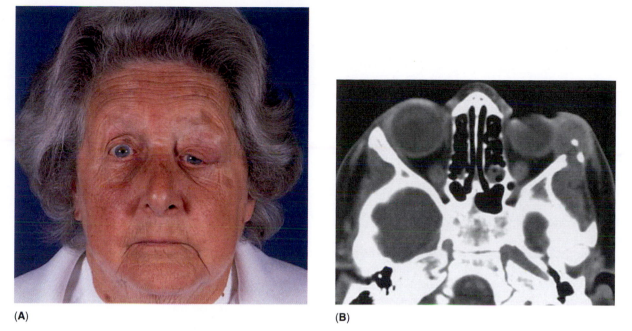

(A) (B)

Figure 17.46 (A) An elderly patient presenting with a rapidly progressive nonaxial proptosis with pain. (B) An axial CT scan demonstrating a mass in the region of the lacrimal fossa with destruction of adjacent bone. A transeptal biopsy confirmed the diagnosis of adenoid cystic carcinoma of the lacrimal gland.

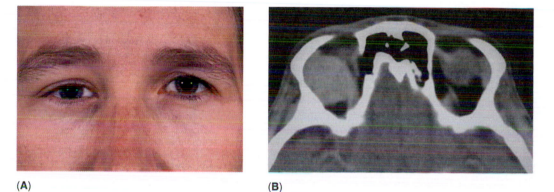

(A) (B)

Figure 17.47 (A) A 40-year-old patient presenting with a 4-month history of a palpable mass in the region of the right lacrimal gland. (B) An axial CT scan showed a large but well-defined mass without any adjacent bony erosion or destruction. The lesion proved to be an adenoid cystic carcinoma.

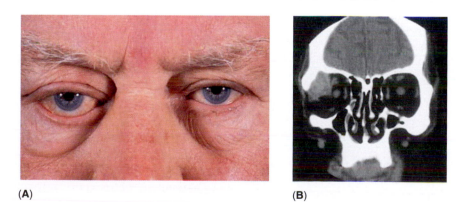

(A) (B)

Figure 17.48 (A) A 66-year-old patient presenting with a 4-month history of a painless nonaxial proptosis. (B) A coronal CT scan demonstrated remodelling of the bone of the lacrimal fossa and a large irregular mass. The lesion was removed en bloc via a lateral orbitotomy. It proved to be a pleomorphic adenoma with malignant transformation affecting only the central core of the tumor.

In 2001, a modern comprehensive classification system was published under the World Health Organization (WHO), which represented the first worldwide consensus document on the classification of lymphoma. This was updated in 2008. The prognosis depends on the histological type and stage of lymphoma and treatment. In general, with modern treatment of patients with NHL, the overall survival rate at 5 years is approximately 60%.

Extranodal marginal zone B-cell lymphoma of mucosa associated lymphoid tissue (MALT lymphoma) is the most common, accounting for 38%, followed by follicular center lymphoma at 29%, diffuse large B-cell lymphoma at 19%, and mantle cell lymphoma at 7%. Peripheral T-cell lymphoma, and natural killer cell lymphoma have also been reported to affect the orbit.

These lesions usually affect patients over the age of 50 years. Orbital lymphomas present with painless proptosis. A gradual onset with slow painless progression is typical. Typically, they occur in the anterior, superior, or lateral aspects of the orbit extraconally. The mass is usually rubbery to firm on palpation with no palpable bony destruction. The lacrimal gland, lacrimal sac, and extraocular muscles can also be similarly involved.

Conjunctival lymphoma has a characteristic salmon pink appearance (Fig. 17.49). Conjunctival lymphoma may be an extension of orbital or intraocular lymphoma. Lymphomatous lesions can also involve the preseptal portion of the eyelid.

On CT scan examination they tend to mould themselves to the shape of the globe and to the adjacent orbital bone. They may involve the lacrimal gland. They tend to have a similar density on CT to that of the extraocular muscles (Fig. 17.50).

Obtaining an adequate safe biopsy is the key to management of orbital lymphoma. Two tissue samples should be submitted for histopathological assessment. One sample should be sent fixed in formalin for hematoxylin and eosin staining and the other sample should be sent fresh for immunohistochemical evaluation.

The patient is referred to an oncology team with expertise in lymphoma management for systemic investigations to stage the disease. The patients undergo:

- A complete physical examination
- Dilated fundoscopy
- Full blood count
- Biochemistry profile
- Liver function tests
- Orbital CT/MRI scanning
- CT scanning of abdomen, thorax, and pelvis
- Bone marrow aspiration
- GI tract endoscopy
- Total body PET scanning (if available)

Radiotherapy is a well-established treatment modality for orbital lymphoma. Lymphomas are markedly radiosensitive. Primary chemotherapy has minimal efficacy in localized low-grade orbital lymphoma and is not therefore advocated as a first-line treatment. Different radiation techniques can be used depending on the extent of involvement. Long-term local control of orbital lymphoma can usually be achieved with radiation therapy, but recurrences are common as well as a risk of distant relapse. Chemotherapy is used for more aggressive histology sub-types and for patients with systemic disease.

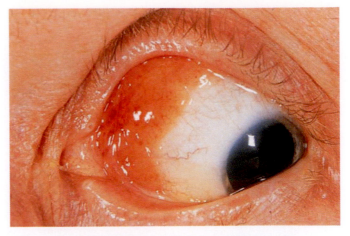

Figure 17.49 A typical "salmon patch" lesion.

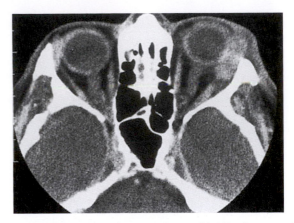

Figure 17.50 An axial CT scan demonstrating an orbital lymphoma moulding itself to adjacent structures.

Conjunctival lymphoma is known to have the lowest rate of extraorbital spread and lymphoma-related death. The rate of extraorbital spread and lymphoma-related death is sequentially greater for patients with predominantly deep orbital lymphoma, lacrimal gland lymphoma, or eyelid lymphoma.

Metastases

The pathophysiology of orbital metastases reflects the character of the primary tumor. A metastasis may present as a rapidly progressive mass with proptosis, infiltrative signs, and bone destruction or may present with an insidious cicatrization of soft tissues. The patient may already have a known primary tumor or may have had treatment for a tumor many years previously. Occasionally, the primary tumor is occult.

Some tumors show a tendency to metastasize to particular orbital structures, e.g., breast carcinoma to extraocular muscle, prostatic carcinoma to bone. Some tumors present with unusual systemic features, e.g., carcinoid tumor presenting as an orbital mass and features of carcinoid syndrome from the release of 5-hydroxytryptamine (5-HT) (Fig. 17.51).

The tumors which most frequently metastasize to the orbit are:

- Breast carcinoma
- Bronchial carcinoma

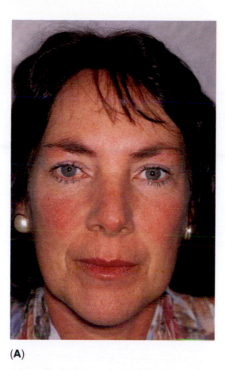
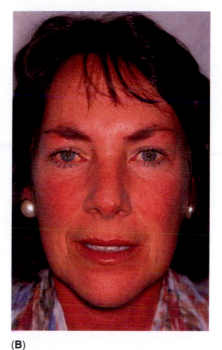

(A)   (B)

Figure 17.51 (A) Patient presenting with diplopia and a right proptosis. (B) The same patient 5 min later, experiencing symptoms of carcinoid syndrome from release of 5-HT. She had a small intestine carcinoid tumor with hepatic metastases and a metastasis to the right inferior rectus muscle (see Figure 16.25).

- Neuroblastoma
- Prostatic carcinoma
- Gastrointestinal tract carcinomas
- Renal carcinoma
- Melanoma
- Thyroid carcinoma
- Carcinoid tumor
- Ewing's sarcoma

CT scans show typically infiltrative masses which envelop the globe or encase the retrobulbar soft tissues. There may be an extension into the paranasal sinuses or into the cranial cavity.

The role of the orbital surgeon is to perform a safe orbital biopsy. The patient should be referred to an oncology team for further investigations and appropriate management. The goal of management is usually palliative therapy, although long-term survival for some patients can be achieved.

Rhabdomyosarcoma

Rhabdomyosarcoma is the most common primary malignant orbital tumor in children. Although it has been reported from birth to the seventh decade, the majority of cases occur before the age of 10 years. The most common presentation is a rapidly progressive proptosis with an inferolateral displacement of the globe. Associated inflammatory signs may lead to an initial misdiagnosis. The tumor may also masquerade as other lesions making the diagnosis difficult (Figs. 17.52 and 17.53).

On CT scans, the tumor is often relatively well circumscribed but with associated destruction of bone (Fig. 17.54). There may be extraorbital or intracranial extension.

The differential diagnosis of rhabdomyosarcoma is:

- Orbital cellulitis
- Neuroblastoma
- Chloroma

- Lymphangioma
- Capillary hemangioma
- Ruptured dermoid cyst
- Eosinophilic granuloma

Recognition of this tumor is extremely important. The tumor is lethal without urgent treatment. A biopsy of the lesion should be performed as soon as possible. The patient should be referred without delay to a pediatric oncology team for staging of the disease and treatment involving chemotherapy and radiotherapy. The prognosis for survival is approximately 95% over 5 years.

Secondary Orbital Tumors

The orbit may be invaded by benign or malignant tumors arising from adjacent structures, e.g., the paranasal sinuses, the globe, and the eyelids. Neglected eyelid tumors, e.g., squamous cell carcinomas, basal cell carcinomas, particularly morphea-form tumors occurring at the medial canthus, can invade the orbit and present with proptosis and diplopia. The ocular motility disturbance may be due to a mechanical restriction from the tumor mass itself or it may be paretic from cranial nerve involvement. Orbital exenteration may be required to effect a cure. Such surgery may need to be supplemented by radiotherapy in appropriate cases.

Extrascleral orbital extension of a choroidal melanoma may present with proptosis (Fig. 17.55). Small to moderate extensions can usually be managed by plaque radiotherapy, enucleation with conjunctivectomy/Tenonectomy, or enucleation with a lateral orbitotomy and complete careful extirpation of the orbital mass. For larger orbital extensions, a skin-sparing exenteration is required.

Tumors of the paranasal sinuses may extend into the orbit and present with non-axial proptosis. The direction of

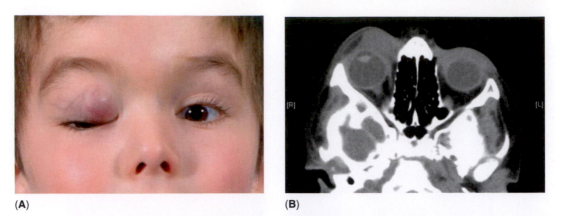

Figure 17.52 (**A**) A child who presented with a rapidly enlarging right upper eyelid lesion which was initially misdiagnosed as a capillary hemangioma. An excisional biopsy of the lesion was performed and it proved to be a rhabdomyosarcoma. (**B**) An axial CT scan of the same patient demonstrating the preseptal location of the tumor.

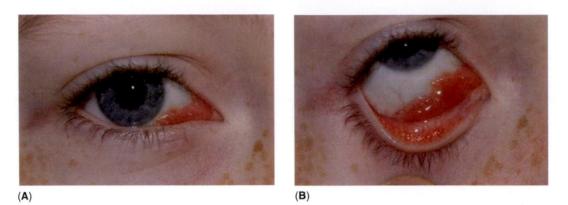

Figure 17.53 (A, B) A child referred with a conjunctival "papilloma." An incisional biopsy of the lesion proved this to be a rhabdomyosarcoma.

displacement of the globe reflects the location of the tumor and its extension into the orbit. Such lesions should be referred to an ENT colleague for biopsy. The management of such tumors may require the skills of a multidisciplinary team and may involve the use of surgical resection, radiotherapy, and chemotherapy.

Vascular Disorders

Orbital vascular lesions are common and include cavernous hemangioma, capillary hemangioma, lymphangioma, varices, and arteriovenous malformation. These vascular abnormalities are classified according to their hemodynamic properties based on clinical and imaging criteria. A correct diagnosis is important because the natural history and proper management are often dramatically different among no-flow, slow-flow, and higher-flow lesions.

Orbital vascular lesions can be classified into three types:

- Type 1 (no flow) lesions have essentially little connection to the vascular system and include lymphangiomas or combined venous lymphatic malformations, and cavernous hemangiomas.
- Type 2 (venous flow) lesions appear as either distensible lesions with a direct and rich communication with the venous system or non-distensible anomalies that have a minimal communication with the venous system. Types 1 and 2 can be combined with

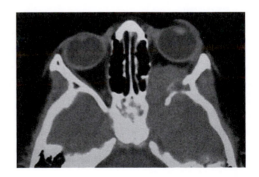

Figure 17.54 An axial CT scan of a child with a rhabdomyosarcoma involving the posterior orbit with local bone destruction and extension to the middle cranial fossa.

both features of distensible and non-distensible hemodynamics.

- Type 3 (arterial flow) include arteriovenous malformations characterized by direct high flow through the lesion to the venous side.

Arteriovenous (a–v) Shunts

Arteriovenous shunts may be congenital or acquired. They can follow trauma or occur spontaneously. They are classified hemodynamically as high flow or low flow. The high-flow shunts are usually post-traumatic caroticocavernous fistulas or a–v malformations, whereas the low-flow shunts are spontaneous dural a–v fistulas of the cavernous sinus region.

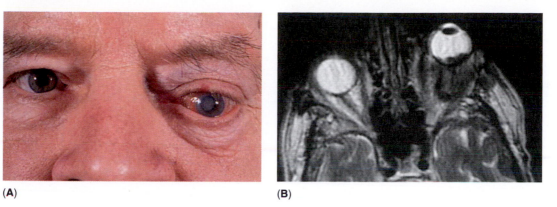

(A) (B)

Figure 17.55 (**A**) A patient referred with a painful left nonaxial proptosis. He had a mature cataract and rubeotic glaucoma. The patient had a dark discoloration of his left upper eyelid. (**B**) An MRI scan demonstrated an intraocular lesion at the posterior pole and a large irregular intraorbital mass. The patient had a choroidal melanoma with massive extrascleral extension.

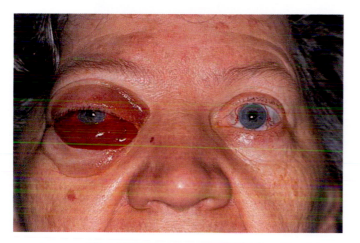

Figure 17.56 A carotico-cavernous fistula.

The clinical features of high-flow shunts are dramatic (Fig. 17.56):

- Pulsatile proptosis
- Bruit
- Eyelid edema
- Reduced visual acuity
- Chemosis/conjunctival prolapse
- Raised intraocular pressure secondary to raised episcleral venous pressure
- Retinal vascular dilatation
- Cranial nerve palsy

By contrast, the clinical features of low-flow shunts are far less dramatic and can lead to misdiagnosis (Fig. 17.57).

- A red eye with episcleral venous dilation
- Mild proptosis
- Mildly raised intraocular pressure

This clinical presentation often leads to misdiagnoses of conjunctivitis, episcleritis, and thyroid eye disease.

CT scan images demonstrate proptosis, enlargement of the superior ophthalmic vein (Fig. 17.58), and enlargement of the extraocular muscles. Recognition of enlargement of the superior ophthalmic vein is important, as enlargement of the extraocular muscles in a patient with a red eye can reinforce the misdiagnosis of thyroid eye disease. Enlargement of the cavernous sinuses is an important radiological feature of a caroticocavernous fistula.

The diagnosis is confirmed by arteriography. This also aids in planning treatment.

High-flow shunts usually require treatment, whereas low-flow shunts can be managed conservatively and the patient's visual status monitored as many low-flow shunts spontaneously resolve. The patient can be advised to perform carotid massage on the affected side, which may help the shunt to close spontaneously. Treatment of shunts requires the expertise of the interventional neuro-radiologist. Closure of shunts is usually achieved via the endovascular route, either arterial or venous, depending on the type of fistula and the hemodynamics. Embolic agents include balloons and coils for direct high-flow lesions and particles for low-flow fistulae. These techniques have significantly advanced the treatment of these lesions with relatively low complication rates. The associated risks of a cerebrovascular accident or blindness must, however, be taken into account.

For the management of some fistulae, the neuro-radiologist requires access via the superior ophthalmic vein. The oculoplastic surgeon plays an important role in gaining access to the vein. This is carefully exposed via an upper lid skin crease incision and control of the vein is gained with the use of 2/0 silk sutures (Fig. 17.59A). A small nick is made in the wall of the vein and a catheter is passed along the vein and into the cavernous sinus (Fig. 17.59B). The catheter is secured into position and used by the neuro-radiologist to pass a guide wire and coils under radiological guidance.

For some patients, an arterio-venous malformation can be initially embolised by the neuro-radiologist, allowing the safe removal of the residual mass by the surgeon.

Varices

Orbital varices may be hemodynamically active or inactive. Active lesions have large connections with the systemic venous system and demonstrate enlargement in response to changes in venous pressure. Patients may present with intermittent proptosis and orbital pain aggravated by straining. Inactive lesions are more hemodynamically isolated and are characterized by stasis of blood, which can lead to thrombosis or occasionally hemorrhage, usually in an older patient. Such a patient may present with an acute proptosis, which slowly resolves spontaneously.

Varices can be extremely difficult to manage. The indications for intervention are severe hemorrhage that causes pain and visual deterioration that is not amenable to conservative management, and severe cosmetic disfigurement. Lesions that are hemodynamically active must be approached with respect and caution (see Fig. 17.14).

Lymphangioma
Lymphangiomas are hemodynamically isolated thin-walled, endothelially lined vascular hamartomas. They are not affected

by a Valsalva maneuver. They may be superficial and/or deep and tend to be diffuse. Superficial lesions may be confined to the conjunctiva and/or eyelid and may be amenable to resection if necessary. Deep lesions tend to present in infancy or early childhood as a gradually enlarging mass with decreased vision or as a sudden dramatic acute proptosis following a spontaneous hemorrhage into a previously unrecognized lesion. This typically occurs in the context of an upper respiratory tract infection. Deep orbital lesions, which have a superficial component, are readily diagnosed clinically. A deep lesion

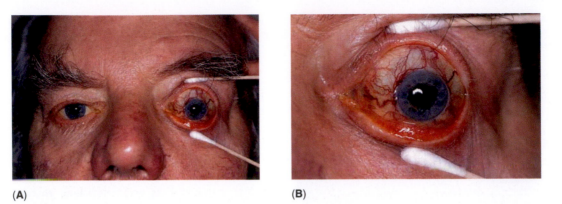

(A)   (B)

Figure 17.57 (**A**) A patient with a low-flow arteriovenous shunt. (**B**) A close-up photograph of the patient's left eye demonstrating diffuse episcleral vascular engorgement.

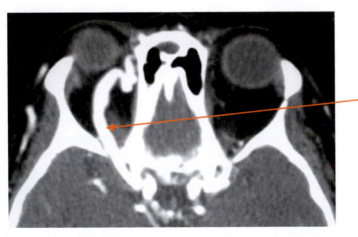

A grossly enlarged superior ophthalmic vein

Figure 17.58 An axial CT scan showing a grossly enlarged superior ophthalmic vein.

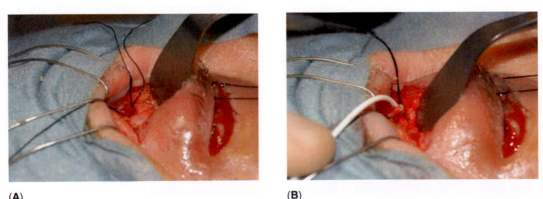

(A)   (B)

Figure 17.59 (**A**) The superior ophthalmic vein has been isolated and sutures placed to exert control over bleeding. (**B**) A catheter has been introduced into the vein and secured into position with a suture.

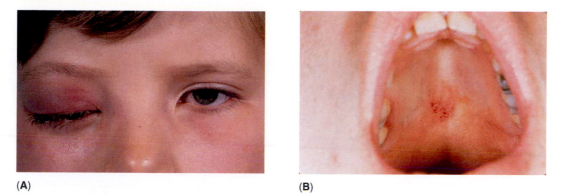

(A)   **(B)**

Figure 17.60 (**A**) A 10-year-old patient presenting with an acute right proptosis. (**B**) Examination of the patient's hard palate revealed a vascular anomaly. The orbital lesion was a lymphangioma with an acute intralesional hemorrhage.

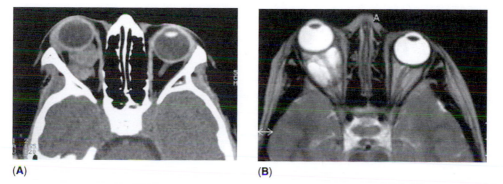

(A)   **(B)**

Figure 17.61 (**A**) An axial CT scan demonstrating the appearance of an orbital lymphangioma. (**B**) An axial T2-weighted MRI scan of the same patient.

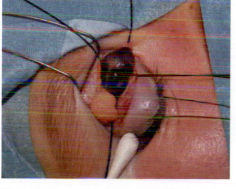 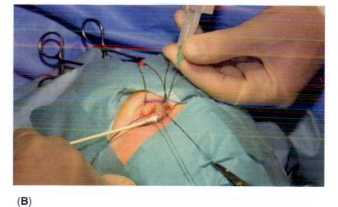

(A)   **(B)**

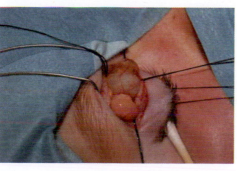 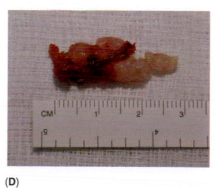

(C)   **(D)**

Figure 17.62 (**A**) A multilobulated medial orbital lymphangioma exposed via an anterior orbitotomy. (**B**) The lesion is being injected with Tisseel®. (**C**) The appearance of the lesion following the injection with Tisseel®. (**D**) The appearance of the lesion removed en bloc.

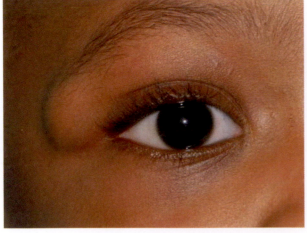

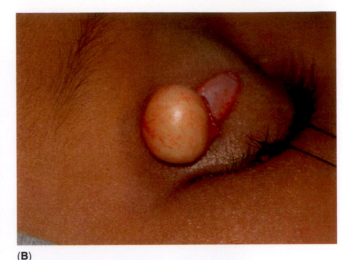

(A)   (B)

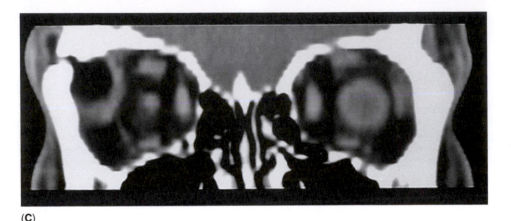

(C)

Figure 17.63 (**A**) A typical dermoid cyst based on the right fronto-zygomatic suture. (**B**) The dermoid cyst has been exposed via an upper lid skin crease incision. (**C**) An intraorbital dermoid cyst related to the frontozygomatic suture.

may present more of a diagnostic challenge. The patient may show other clues, which assist in the diagnosis, e.g., intraoral vascular lesions (Fig. 17.60).

The appearances on CT scans of deep lymphangiomas are typically low-density cystic masses in the intraconal and extraconal spaces. Contrast enhancement may occur around the lesions in approximately 50% of cases. The lesions delineate extremely well on MRI (Fig. 17.61).

The management of these lesions should be conservative wherever possible. Surgery may be required if an acute hemorrhage has caused compressive optic neuropathy or exposure keratopathy which is not amenable to conservative management alone. Surgery should be conservative and aimed at removal of the major macrocysts, which raise intraorbital pressure, cause extreme proptosis, or compress the optic nerve. Multiple surgical resections are associated with a poor final visual acuity.

Sclerosing agents, e.g., 5% sodium morrhuate, have been advocated for the management of some orbital lymphangiomas. It is essential to ensure that the lesion is hemodynamically isolated using dynamic contrast-enhanced MRA (CEMRA)before such agents are used. A sclerosing agent can also be injected at the time of an orbitotomy, e.g., Tisseel® (a fibrin sealant), followed by immediate resection of the lesion (Fig. 17.62). This use of Tisseel is off-licence. The use of sclerosing agents represents an area of current controversy.

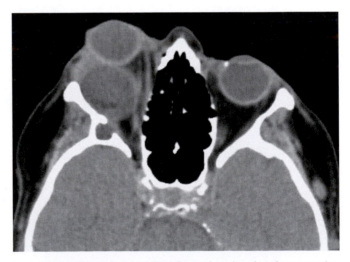

Figure 17.64 A large right intraorbital dermoid cyst based on the zygomaticosphenoidal suture.

Likewise, the use of systemic steroids for severe exacerbations is controversial.

Structural Disorders

Structural disorders may be congenital—e.g., dermoid cysts, sphenoid wing dysplasia in neurofibromatosis (Fig. 17.5),

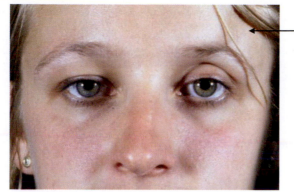

A depression in the soft tissue of the forehead

Figure 17.65 A patient with linear scleroderma en coup de sabre with a left upper lid sulcus and a typical depression running up from the left eyebrow.

encephalocoele, microphthalmia with orbital cyst—or acquired, e.g., orbital wall blowout fracture, silent sinus syndrome (Fig. 17.11). Of these disorders, the dermoid cyst is the one most frequently encountered in clinical practice.

Dermoid Cyst
A dermoid cyst is a choristoma, which contains skin and skin appendages, i.e., hairs, keratin, and sebaceous gland material. (An epidermoid cyst is very similar but does not contain skin appendages.) The lesion occurs in association with bony sutures, most commonly the fronto-zygomatic suture (Fig. 17.63). It usually presents in infancy as a smooth painless gradually enlarging cystic mass that lies outside the orbit (see Fig. 17.41). It may be freely mobile or it may be fixed to the underlying bony suture. It may, however, present with a gradually progressive painless axial or non-axial proptosis in a young adult if it arises from a deeper bony suture, e.g., the spheno-zygomatic suture. Rarely, the lesion may rupture following minor trauma and present with an acute orbital inflammation.

Superficial freely mobile lesions are simple to remove and require no preoperative imaging. Superficial lesions at the lateral aspect of the eyebrow or supero-medial orbit can be removed via an upper eyelid skin crease incision, avoiding a visible scar. Great care should be taken not to rupture the cyst during the surgical excision.

Lesions that are fixed to bone should be imaged with a CT scan. It is important to exclude the possibility of a "dumb-bell" dermoid cyst, which extends through the lateral orbital bone into the orbit. The surgical approach can then be selected to adequately remove the lesion in its entirety. This may require a formal lateral orbitotomy (Fig. 17.64). Failure to remove the entire lesion will lead to a recurrence, which will be more difficult to manage. A preoperative CT scan is certainly indicated for any lesion at the medial canthus. The differential diagnosis of a mass at the medial canthus includes an encephalocoele, which should be excluded.

DEGENERATIONS AND DEPOSITIONS
These are rarer orbital disorders. Examples include amyloidosis, scleroderma (Fig. 17.65), and hemifacial atrophy (Fig. 17.13).

FURTHER READING

1. Bernardini FP, Devoto MH, Croxatto JO. Epithelial tumors of the lacrimal gland: an update. Curr Opin Ophthalmol 2008; 19: 409–13.
2. Bonavolonta G. Anterior, medial, lateral and combined surgical approaches to orbital tumor resection. In: Bosniak S, ed. Principles and Practice of Ophthalmic Plastic and Reconstructive Surgery, vol. 11. Philadelphia, PA: WB Saunders, 1996: 1060–9.
3. Bonavolonta G. Surgical approaches to the orbit. In: Bosniak S, ed. Principles and Practice of Ophthalmic Plastic and Reconstructive Surgery, vol. 11. Philadelphia, PA: WB Saunders, 1996: 1050–5.
4. Bosniak S. Principles and Practice of Ophthalmic Plastic and Reconstructive Surgery. Philadelphia, PA: WB Saunders, 1996: 999–1006.
5. Brannan PA. A review of sclerosis idiopathic orbital inflammation. Cur Opin Ophthalmol 2007; 18: 402–4.
6. Brook I. Microbiology and antimicrobial treatment of orbital and intracranial complications of sinusitis in children and their management. Int J Ped Otorhinolaryngol 2009; 73(9): 1183–6.
7. Brown CL, Graham SM, Griffin MC, et al. Pediatric medial subperiosteal orbital abscess: medical management where possible. Am J Rhinol 2004; 18(5): 321–7.
8. Burkat CN, Lucarelli MJ. Rhabdomyosarcoma masquerading as acute dacryocystitis. Ophthal Plast & Reconstr Surg 2005; 21(6): 456–8.
9. Cannon PS, Mc Keag D, Ataullah, Leatherbarrow B. Our experience using primary oral antibiotics in the management of orbital cellulitis in a tertiary referral centre. Eye 2008; 23(3): 612–5.
10. Chandler JR, Langenbrunner DJ, Stevens ER. The pathogenesis of orbital complications in acute sinusitis. Laryngoscope 1970; 80: 1414–28.
11. Char DH, Miller T, Kroll S. Orbital metastases: diagnosis and course. Br J Ophthalmol 1997; 81: 386–90.
12. Coupland SE, Hummel M, Stein H. Ocular adnexal lymphomas: five case presentations and a review of the literature. Surv Ophthalmol 2002; 47(5): 470–90.
13. Rootman J. Diseases of the Orbit, A Multidisciplinary Approach, 2nd edn, Baltimore, MD: Lippincott Williams & Wilkins, 2003 (ISBN: 0-7817-1512-1).
14. Dutton J. Atlas of Clinical and Surgical Orbital Anatomy. Philadelphia, PA: WB Saunders, 1994.
15. Dutton JJ. Orbital imaging techniques. In: Yanoff and Duker, eds. Ophthalmology. London: Mosby, 2004: 649–54.
16. Eddleman CS, Liu JK. Optic nerve sheath meningioma: current diagnosis and treatment. Neurosurg Focus 2007; 23(5): E4.
17. Erb MH, Uzcategui N, See RF, Burnstine MA. Orbitotemporal neurofibromatosis: classification and treatment. Orbit 2007; 26(4): 223–8.
18. Garcia GH, Harris GJ. Criteria for nonsurgical management of subperiosteal abscess of the orbit: analysis of outcomes 1988–1998. Ophthalmol 2000; 107: 1454–8.
19. Garrity JA, Henderson JW, Cameron JD. Henderson's Orbital Tumours, 4th edn. Philadelphia, PA: Lippincott Williams & Wilkins, 2007.
20. Gordon LK. Orbital inflammatory disease: a diagnostic and therapeutic challenge. Eye 2006; 20: 1196–206.
21. Haik BG, Karcioglu ZA, Gordon RA, Pechous BP. Capillary hemangioma (infantile periocular hemangioma). Surv Ophthalmol 1994; 38: 399–426.
22. Harris GJ. Idiopathic orbital inflammation: a pathogenic construct and treatment strategy. Ophthal Plast Reconstr Surg 2006; 22(2): 79–86.

23. Harris GJ. Orbital vascular malformations: a consensus statement on terminology and its clinical implications. Orbital Society. Am J Ophthalmol 1999; 127: 453–5.

24. Harris NL, Jaffe ES, Diebold J, et al. The World Health Organization classification of neoplastic diseases of the haematopoietic and lymphoid tissues: report of the Clinical Advisory Committee Meeting. Airlie House, Virginia, November 1997. Histopathology, 2000; 36: 69–89.

25. Kahana A, Lucarelli MJ, Grayev AM, et al. Noninvasive dynamic magnetic resonance angiography with time-resolved imaging of contrast kinetics (TRICKS) in the evaluation of orbital vascular lesions. Arch Ophthalmol 2007; 125(12): 1635–42.

26. Krishnakumar S, Subramanian N, Mohan R, et al. Solitary fibrous tumor of the orbit: a clinicopathologic study of six cases with review of the literature. Surv Ophthalmol 2003; 48(5): 544–54.

27. Lacey B, Chang W, Rootman J. Nonthyroid causes of extraocular muscle disease. Surv Ophthalmol 1999; 44: 187–213.

28. Leibovitch I, Prabhakaran VC, Davis G, Selva D. Intraorbital injection of triamcinolone acetonide in patients with idiopathic orbital inflammation. Arch Ophthalmol 2007; 125(12): 1647–51.

29. Levin LA, Avery R, Shore JW, Woog JJ, Baker AS. The spectrum of orbital aspergillosis: a clinicopathological review. Surv Ophthalmol 1996; 41(2): 142–154.

30. Madge SN, Prabhakaran VC, Shome D, et al. Orbital tuberculosis: a review of the literature. Orbit 2008; 27: 4267–77.

31. McNab AA, Wright JE, Caswell AG. Clinical features and surgical management of dermolipomas. Austral NZ J Ophthalmol 1990; 18: 159–62.

32. McNab AA, Wright JE. Cavernous haemangiomas of the orbit. Austral NZ J Ophthalmol 1989; 17: 337–45.

33. McNab AA, Wright JE. Orbitofrontal cholesterol granuloma. Ophthalmology 1990; 97: 28–32.

34. McNab AA. Subconjunctival fat prolapse. Austral NZ J Ophthalmol 1999; 27: 33–6.

35. Nerad JA, Carter KD, Alford MA. Disorders of the orbit: infections, inflammations, neoplasms, vascular abnormalities. In: Rapid Diagnosis in Ophthalmology-Oculoplastic and Reconstructive Surgery. Philadelphia, PA: Mosby Elsevier, 2008: 160–239.

36. Pakrou N, Selva D, Leibovitch I. Wegener's granulomatosis: ophthalmic manifestations and management. Semin Arthritis Rheum 2006; 35: 284–92.

37. Leaute-Labreze C, et al. Propranolol for severe hemangiomas of infancy. N Engl J Med 2008; 358(24): 2649–51.

38. Rootman J, ed. Diseases of the Orbit. Philadelphia, PA: JB Lippincott, 1988.

39. Rootman J, Kao SC, Graeb DA. Multidisciplinary approaches to complicated vascular lesions of the orbit. Ophthalmology 1992; 99: 1440–6.

40. Rootman J, McCarthy M, White V, Harris G, Kennerdell J. Idiopathic sclerosing inflammation of the orbit. A distinct clinicopathologic entity. Ophthalmology 1994; 101: 570–84.

41. Rootman J. Why 'orbital pseudotumour' is no longer a useful concept. Br J Ophthalmol 1998; 82: 339–40.

42. Rootman J. Orbital Disease – Present Status and Future Challenges. Boca Raton, FL: Taylor and Francis, 2005.

43. Rootman J. Orbital Disease: Present Status and Future Challenges. Boca Raton, FL: Taylor & Francis, 2005.

44. Rose GE, Wright JE. Pleomorphic adenoma of the lacrimal gland. Br J Ophthalmol 1992; 76: 395–400.

45. Saeed P, Rootman J, Nugent RA, et al. Optic nerve sheath meningiomas. Ophthalmology 2003; 110(10): 2019–30.

46. Sato K, Yamaguchi T, Yokota H. A surgical technique with connective tissue repair for the management of subconjunctival orbital fat prolapse. Clin Exp Ophthalmol 2006; 34: 841–5.

47. Soparkar CN, Patrinely JR, Cuaycong MJ, et al. The silent sinus syndrome. A cause of spontaneous enophthalmos. Ophthalmology 1994; 101: 772–8.

48. Taban M, Goldberg RA. Propranolol for orbital hemangioma. Ophthalmology 2010; 117(1): 195–5.e4.

49. Tessier P. Anatomical Clssification of facial, crano-facial and latero-facial clefts. J Max Fac Surg 1976; 4: 69–92.

50. Thomas RD, Graham SM, Carter KD, Nerad JA. Management of the orbital floor in silent sinus syndrome. Am J Rhinol 2003; 17(2): 97–100.

51. Vaphiades MS, Horton JA. MRA or CTA, that's the question. Surv Ophthalmol 2005; 50: 406–10.

52. Walker RS, Custer PL, Nerad JA. Surgical excision of periorbital capillary hemangiomas. Ophthalmology 1994; 101: 1333–40.

53. Swerdlow SH, et al. WHO Classification of Tumours of Haematopoietic and Lymphoid Tissues, 4th edn. Lyon, France: IARC Press, 2008.

54. Wilhelm H. Primary optic nerve tumours. Curr Opin Neurol 2009; 22: 11–8.

55. Wobig JL, Dailey RA, eds. Oculofacial Plastic Surgery: Face, Lacrimal System, and Orbit. New York, NY: Thieme, 2004: 192–254.

56. Wright JE, Rose GE, Garner A. Primary malignant neoplasms of the lacrimal gland. Br J Ophthalmol 1992; 76: 400–7.

57. Wright JE, Stewart WB, Krohel GB. Factors affecting the survival of patients with lacrimal gland tumours. Can J Ophthalmol 1982; 17: 3–9.

18　Surgical approaches to the orbit

INTRODUCTION

This chapter describes the surgical approaches used in the management of orbital lesions. The surgical approaches used to achieve a decompression of the orbit in the management of thyroid eye disease are described in chapter 19. The surgical approaches used to manage orbital wall blowout fractures are described in chapter 25.

It is important to ensure that the patient has been properly prepared for surgery before proceeding with an orbitotomy, particularly with regard to the management of hypertension and the use of anti-platelet and anticoagulant agents. If significant blood loss is anticipated from the surgery, the patient should be grouped and saved and blood crossed matched and made available if necessary. A full blood count and platelet count should be undertaken prior to surgery along with a biochemical profile. Informed consent should be obtained ensuring that the patient understands the small risk of visual loss from intraoperative trauma to the optic nerve, or from postoperative intraorbital hemorrhage. Additional risks specific to the surgical approach should also be discussed, e.g., infection, bleeding, ptosis, diplopia, sensory loss, pupillary enlargement, cosmetic deformity, hypertrophic scarring, CSF leak, meningitis, and intracranial trauma. The correct side should be clearly marked by the surgeon after checking with the patient, after checking the consent form and after checking the orbital scans.

The anesthetist should understand the surgical approach and the requirements for head positioning, nasal packing, the use of vasoconstrictive agents, hypotension, the potential risk of the oculocardiac reflex, the potential risk of bleeding, the anticipated length of the surgical procedure and the requirements for postoperative analgesia. Simple anterior orbitotomies can be performed under local anesthesia, usually with intravenous sedation, but the more complex orbitotomies are performed under general anesthesia. A patient should be kept in hospital overnight for observation and regular visual function checks following any orbitotomy.

It is essential that the patient's computed tomography/magnetic resonance imaging (CT/MRI) scans are available. These should be clearly visible on a viewing/computer screen adjacent to the operating table. These should be reviewed before the orbitotomy is commenced and the correct side reconfirmed with the surgical team. The scans may need to be reviewed to confirm the location of the orbital lesion as the surgery proceeds.

The surgical plan should be coordinated with the nursing team in advance to ensure that the appropriate surgical instrumentation is available. A potential change in the surgical approach, depending on the intraoperative findings, should be anticipated and the necessary instrumentation made available. It is also important to liaise with the pathologist prior to surgery, particularly if urgent reporting of a biopsy is required. The pathologist must be provided with adequate clinical details.

If a multidisciplinary team is involved in the surgical management of the patient, it is important to define the responsibilities of each member in advance. This also relates to the postoperative care of the patient.

> **KEY POINTS**
> - Patient preparation—control of hypertension, discontinuation of anti-platelet drugs, informed consent, correct surgical site checking, and marking
> - Communicate with the anesthetist
> - Communicate with the operating department nursing staff
> - Communicate with the pathologist
> - Ensure all orbital scans are available in the operating room

SELECTION OF THE SURGICAL APPROACH

The choice of surgical approach to an orbital lesion will depend on:

- The anatomical location of the lesion
- The size and extent of the lesion
- The suspected pathology
- The goal of the surgery

The Anatomical Location of the Lesion

Orbital tumours that lie anterior to the equator of the globe are most commonly approached via an anterior orbitotomy. Tumours located posterior to the equator of the globe require a more complex deep surgical approach, which is also influenced by the relationship of the lesion(s) to the optic nerve.

> **KEY POINTS**
> A surgical approach should be selected which avoids crossing the optic nerve.

The Size and Extent of the Lesion

Most orbital lesions can be managed adequately via a single orbitotomy approach. Some orbital lesions require a combination of orbitotomy approaches, e.g., a medial transconjunctival orbitotomy can be combined with a lateral orbitotomy, which enables the globe to be retracted laterally. This can greatly improve safe surgical access to large or deep medial orbital lesions.

The Suspected Pathology

The surgical approach is influenced by the suspected pathology of the orbital lesion. For example, an incisional biopsy of a suspected lacrimal gland carcinoma should be performed via a trans-septal anterior orbitotomy. In contrast, a suspected pleomorphic adenoma of the lacrimal gland should not be subjected to an incisional biopsy if at all possible but should be removed as an extirpative excisional biopsy via a lateral orbitotomy.

The Goal of the Surgery

In the management of orbital tumors the goals of the surgery are usually to achieve, as safely as possible, an incisional biopsy, an excisional biopsy, a debulking or decompression of the tumor. In general, infiltrative processes suggest a malignant lesion and require an incisional biopsy to establish a histopathological diagnosis. Well-circumscribed lesions generally suggest a benign lesion that can be removed as an excisional biopsy, e.g., a cavernous hemangioma. Such surgery not only establishes a histopathological diagnosis but also serves as a curative treatment. Some benign orbital lesions may not be amenable to surgical excision but a debulking procedure may be beneficial, e.g., a plexiform neurofibroma. A small benign orbital apical tumor located medial to the optic nerve, causing compressive optic neuropathy, may be better managed by means of an endoscopic medial orbital wall decompression than by a more invasive procedure undertaken to remove the lesion with a risk of visual loss.

APPLIED ANATOMY

See chapter 2 for a detailed description of orbital anatomy. This should be carefully reviewed before undertaking any orbital surgery.

SURGICAL SPACES OF THE ORBIT

Anatomically, the orbital spaces are divided into:

- Sub-Tenon's space
- Intraconal space
- Extraconal space
- Subperiosteal space

A good understanding of the surgical spaces of the orbit is essential in order to select the most appropriate surgical approach and to assist in navigation within the orbit during surgery (Fig. 18.1).

Extraconal Space

The extraconal space contains the following:

- The lacrimal gland
- The oblique muscles
- The trochlea
- Orbital fat
- The superior and inferior ophthalmic veins
- Nerves and other vessels

The lacrimal gland is approached via an upper eyelid skin crease incision for an incisional biopsy for suspected lymphoma, non-specific orbital inflammatory syndrome or malignancy. A formal lateral orbitotomy with bone removal is required for the removal of a suspected lacrimal gland pleomorphic adenoma.

The extraconal fat includes the preaponeurotic fat that is important in the identification of the underlying eyelid retractors. Extraconal fat can be removed superiorly via an upper eyelid skin

crease incision. Medial, lateral and inferior extraconal fat can be removed via a transconjunctival incision.

The anterior portion of the superior ophthalmic vein lies in the extraconal space. This can be accessed via an upper eyelid skin crease incision. In patients with arteriovenous shunts the vein is dilated and can provide an alternative access for the insertion of platinum coils in conjunction with an interventional radiologist in selected cases.

Intraconal Space

The intraconal space lies within the recti and their intermuscular septa. The intraconal space contains the optic nerve, intraconal fat, nerves and vessels. Tumors of the optic nerve lie within this space.

The intraconal space may be accessed via a number of surgical approaches: e.g., in order to perform an optic nerve sheath fenestration, the optic nerve may be approached supero-medially via an upper eyelid skin crease incision (the preferred approach), medially via a conjunctival incision with disinsertion of the medial rectus muscle or laterally via a lateral orbitotomy, with or without bone removal. During a lateral orbitotomy approach with bone removal, the intraconal space is usually accessed by dissecting between the lacrimal gland and the lateral rectus muscle.

Subperiosteal Space

The subperiosteal space is a potential space that lies between the periorbita and the bony orbital walls. The periorbita covers all the bones of the internal orbit. Unlike the periosteum covering bones elsewhere, the periorbita is loosely adherent over the orbital walls, except at the orbital suture lines and along the orbital rims, where it is tightly adherent to the bone. The subperiosteal space is a potential space that can be filled with blood (a subperiosteal hematoma) or pus (a subperiosteal abscess). The periorbita is lifted from the walls of the orbit in a characteristic dome-shaped fashion that is limited by the orbital suture lines (Fig. 18.2).

The periorbita is dome-shaped below the roof and along the medial wall of the orbit, assuming a configuration limited by the attachment of the periorbita to the frontoethmoidal suture line.

The subperiosteal space is accessed surgically for the repair of orbital wall blowout fractures, for the drainage of subperiosteal abscesses or hematomas, for bony orbital decompression surgery or for the insertion of subperiosteal orbital implants in anophthalmic patients. This space can be accessed via a variety of transcutaneous or transconjunctival incisions.

Sub-Tenon's Space

Sub-Tenon's space is a potential space situated between the globe and Tenon's capsule. It is not commonly involved in pathological processes. The space may be enlarged with fluid visible on echography in posterior scleritis, by air (Fig. 18.1B), or by infiltration by extraocular extension of intraocular tumors, e.g., choroidal melanoma.

THE PRINCIPLES OF ORBITAL SURGERY

The prerequisites for successful atraumatic orbital surgery are:

- A thorough knowledge of eyelid and orbital anatomy
- A thorough knowledge of orbital disorders

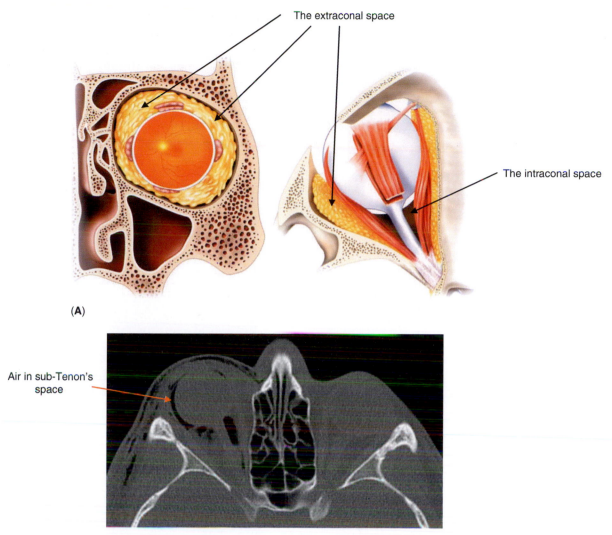

Figure 18.1 (A) The intraconal and extraconal spaces of the orbit. (B) An axial CT scan showing air within the sub-Tenon's space of the patient's right orbit following trauma.

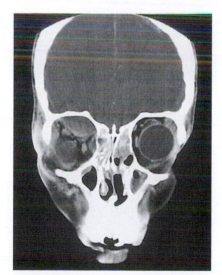

Figure 18.2 A coronal CT scan of a patient with ethmoiditis and right superior and medial subperiosteal orbital abscesses.

- A thorough understanding of orbital imaging techniques
- Familiarity with the surgical approaches to the orbit
- Familiarity with the required surgical instrumentation

- Proper illumination and magnification of the surgical field
- Adequate surgical exposure
- Meticulous surgical dissection
- Careful removal and presentation of biopsy specimens
- Good hemostasis

A Thorough Knowledge of Eyelid and Orbital Anatomy

It is essential to acquire a thorough knowledge of normal eyelid and orbital anatomy before undertaking surgical procedures in an orbit whose anatomy has been altered by a pathological process. It is imperative to observe and assist at a variety of orbitotomy approaches before embarking on such surgery. If possible, the opportunity to examine the orbital contents from above with the brain and orbital roof removed during a postmortem examination should not be missed. This is particularly helpful prior to performing any surgery on the orbital apex with a neurosurgical colleague.

A Thorough Knowledge of Orbital Disorders

The evaluation of the patient with an orbital disorder is discussed in chapter 17 which deals with both common and important orbital disorders. A differential diagnosis based on a thorough history, a meticulous physical examination, imaging and laboratory investigations should enable a decision about appropriate management to be made. For the appropriate management of many orbital inflammatory or neoplastic lesions, a biopsy will be required. As a general rule, an incisional biopsy will be required for an orbital lesion that is suggestive of malignancy or inflammation, whereas an excisional biopsy is indicated for the removal of a well-circumscribed orbital lesion suggestive of a benign process.

A Thorough Understanding of Imaging Techniques
Spending time with an experienced neuro-radiologist reviewing a variety of orbital CT and MRI images on a regular basis is an invaluable exercise.

Familiarity with the Surgical Approaches
This can only be gained by experience. It is essential to observe and assist at a variety of surgical approaches to the orbit before undertaking this surgery.

Familiarity with the Required Surgical Instrumentation and Equipment
This is also gained by experience. It is essential to understand the basic assembly of the drills and saws used in orbital surgery and the safety provisions for all members of the team. The drill hand-piece should have a safe mode that is activated and deactivated by the surgeon (Fig. 18.3). This avoids inadvertent activation of the drill/saw via a footswitch when attempting to use bipolar cautery. All members of the team should wear face guards to protect their eyes and faces from blood and bone fragments. Protection of the patient's globe from inadvertent injury by the instrumentation is the surgeon's responsibility. A variety of burr sizes (both rose head and diamond) should be available. A variety of bone rongeurs are also required (Fig. 18.4).

A microplating system and Medpor blocks and sheets are occasionally required to reconstruct complex bony orbitotomies, especially where additional bone has been removed to gain improved access to the orbit. A variety of orbital retractors should be available in different sizes (Sewall, Wright's and malleable ribbon retractors). The retractors have different purposes and must be used appropriately. Sewall retractors have a sturdy handle that enables the assistant to apply traction by hand (Fig. 18.5). These are used during subperiosteal dissection in orbital decompression procedures or orbital blowout fracture repairs. These retractors are particularly efficient if used with a sheet of Supramid that prevents the prolapse of fat around the edges of the retractor. This makes dissection of all margins of a large orbital floor blowout fracture much simpler.

It is essential to appreciate the pressure on the globe that can be generated with these retractors. This is particularly important if the globe's integrity has been compromised (previous penetrating keratoplasty, penetrating injury repair, peripheral corneal gutter, staphyloma, etc.). Traction on the retractors should be released at regular intervals during surgery and the pupil closely monitored.

Wright's retractors have more delicate handles, and blades that are more appropriate for the retraction of fat around orbital tumors (Fig. 18.6). These are held with the fingers, in contrast to the Sewall retractors. Malleable ribbon retractors are

particularly useful for protecting the globe and surrounding tissues when using the drill and saw.

Proper Illumination and Magnification of the Surgical Field
A comfortable fiberoptic headlight provides excellent illumination of the orbital structures during most orbitotomy procedures. This should be used in conjunction with surgical loupes that provide a comfortable working distance, good

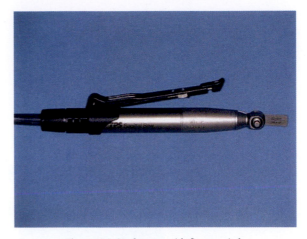

Figure 18.3 Stryker saw with finger switch.

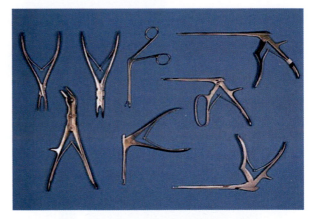

Figure 18.4 A variety of bone rongeurs used in orbital surgery.

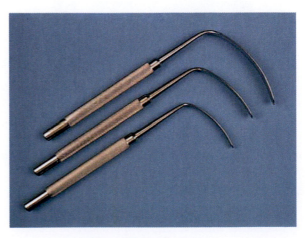

Figure 18.5 Sewall retractors.

magnification, a satisfactory depth of focus and an adequate field of view. It may be necessary for some orbital dissections to resort to the use of the operating microscope. This allows the surgical assistant and observers (via a VDU screen) to see precisely the same deeper orbital structures as the surgeon.

Adequate Surgical Exposure

The surgical incision should be of an adequate length. Although incisions are generally selected to achieve the best possible postoperative cosmetic result (Fig. 18.7), the main consideration is safe and adequate surgical access.

Traction sutures should be carefully placed at strategic positions. These can be supplemented with self-retaining Jaffe retractors.

Meticulous Surgical Dissection

Surgical dissection within the orbit requires a delicate and patient approach. Lesions can often be palpated with the tip of the little finger, which can greatly assist orientation. This can be done at regular intervals if the lesion cannot be easily identified. Gentle blunt dissection should be undertaken using Wright's retractors in a hand-over-hand dissection technique. Once the surface of the lesion has been exposed, the blunt tip of a Freer periosteal elevator can be used to gently separate the tissues and fat from the surface of the lesion. As the plane of dissection proceeds, the retractors can be repositioned (see Fig. 18.8A). The dissection can be further facilitated by the placement of neurosurgical cottonoids,

moistened with saline, into the wound (see Fig. 18.8B). The retractors are then placed over these to prevent the prolapse of orbital fat into the surgical field. This also enables the efficient use of suction with a Baron suction tip, which is applied against the cottonoid to prevent the suction tip from engaging orbital fat. The inadvertent application of suction directly to the orbital fat can cause undue trauma and orbital bleeding.

Careful dissection with blunt-tipped Westcott scissors or Stevens scissors can be used, where required. The assistant should apply counter traction with the orbital retractors,

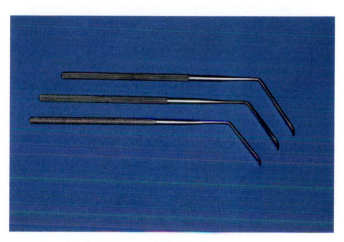

Figure 18.6 Wright's retractors.

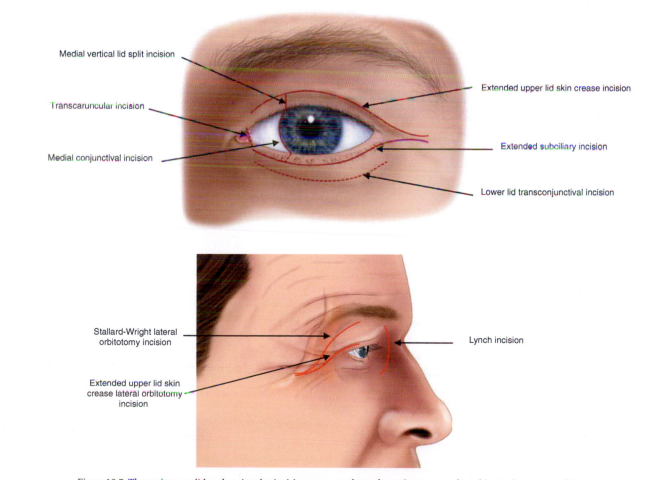

Figure 18.7 The various eyelid and periocular incisions commonly used to gain access to the orbit, singly or in combination.

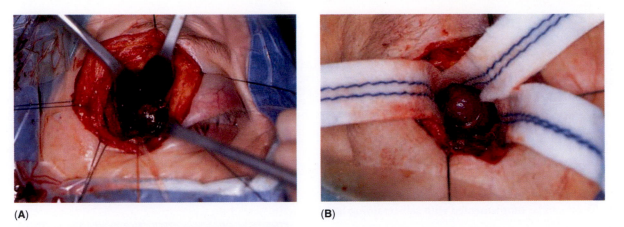

Figure 18.8 (**A**) An orbital cavernous hemangioma is carefully exposed using Wright's retractors to hold back the orbital fat. (**B**) Neurosurgical cottonoids are used to aid the maintenance of a surgical field free of blood and fat.

as the surgeon maneuvers the lesion away from the retractors with a cotton-tipped applicator, retractor or a combined Freer/suction elevator using the non-dominant hand. The tissues are gently dissected from the mass with the scissors in the dominant hand. For deep orbital dissection, blunt-tipped Yasargil neurosurgical scissors (curved or straight) may be used. Occasionally, a cryoprobe may assist the dissection by allowing the lesion to be gently pulled in different directions. A cystic lesion or a cavernous hemangioma may be decompressed with a needle and syringe to facilitate safe dissection from surrounding orbital structures.

Careful removal and Presentation of Biopsy Specimens

The management of many undiagnosed orbital lesions requires an orbitotomy procedure with an incisional biopsy to obtain an accurate diagnosis. It is essential to ensure that the pathologist is presented with tissue samples that are:

- Of adequate size
- Representative of the entire lesion
- Undamaged by cautery or surgical instruments
- Appropriately stored

It may be necessary to provide more than one tissue sample, depending on the appearance of the lesion. Great care should be taken to ensure that the tissue samples are not damaged. It is preferable to use a right-angled 66 Beaver blade to obtain biopsies from a solid lesion. Small cutting biopsy forceps are more appropriate for lesions that are friable. Very occasionally it is helpful to request a frozen section analysis of tissue samples taken from a small orbital lesion if there is any doubt about the adequacy of a specimen. The pathologist can then confirm that adequate material has been obtained. No management decisions, however, should ever be based on the frozen section analysis of orbital biopsies. If frozen section analysis may be required, it is important to communicate this to the pathologist in advance. The pathology requisition forms should be completed prior to the commencement of surgery and should provide appropriate clinical information about the patient. The tissue samples should be quickly

placed into the appropriate transport container to prevent desiccation. If fresh tissue samples are required by the pathologist, it is essential to communicate with the pathologist in advance and to ensure rapid transportation of the specimen(s) to the pathologist.

It is not appropriate to undertake fine-needle aspiration biopsies of orbital lesions on a routine basis. It can, however, be advantageous to perform an open approach fine-needle aspiration biopsy for deep orbital lesions from which it would be difficult and potentially dangerous to attempt to obtain a standard incisional biopsy. The surface of the lesion is carefully exposed. An 18-gauge needle (green) is attached to a 5-ml syringe. The needle is placed into the lesion and moved back and forth, while withdrawing on the plunger. The needle is carefully capped and the needle and syringe are sent to the cytopathologist.

KEY POINT

No management decisions should ever be based on the frozen section analysis of orbital biopsies.

Good Hemostasis

Good hemostasis is an extremely important prerequisite for successful orbital surgery. The fundamental principles underlying the successful achievement of good hemostasis are outlined in chapter 1. For orbital dissections, some points require emphasis:

- Only bipolar cautery should be used within the orbit
- Insulated bayonet bipolar forceps with delicate tips should be used
- The minimum power required for the cautery should be used
- The minimum amount of cautery required should be used

KEY POINT

It is essential that tissue to be submitted for histopathological examination is not damaged by cautery or by crush injury.

Gelfoam soaked with thrombin can be applied to the orbital wound during surgery and following removal of the orbital lesion to assist in hemostasis when there is generalized oozing without an identifiable source amenable to bipolar cautery. The gelfoam is carefully removed prior to closure of the wounds.

For some orbital procedures a safe degree of hypotension is advantageous. The anesthetist should be asked to restore a normal level of blood pressure following removal of an orbital lesion to ensure that intraoperative hemostasis is adequate before the orbit is closed. It is inevitable that the patient's venous pressure will rise on extubation. It is therefore reasonable to apply a compressive dressing supported by a bandage at the completion of surgery to tamponade the orbit and to remove this is in the recovery room as soon as the patient is awake and cooperative. The anesthetist should be warned about this, so that the anesthetic is not reversed too soon.

The patient's visual acuity and pupil reactions should be recorded in the recovery room as soon as the dressings have been removed. The team should be prepared to intervene straight away in the event of a retrobulbar hemorrhage.

THE ORBITOTOMY APPROACHES

The surgical approaches which are most commonly used to gain access to the orbital spaces are:

- Anterior orbitotomy
  - transcutaneous
  - transconjunctival
  - eyelid split
- Medial orbitotomy
  - transcutaneous (Lynch incision)
  - transconjunctival
  - transcaruncular
  - endoscopic
- Lateral orbitotomy
- Combined orbitotomies
- Transcranial orbitotomy
- Endoscopic orbitotomy

Anterior Orbitotomy

An anterior orbitotomy is used for the incisional or excisional biopsy of anterior orbital lesions, for the biopsy of more posteriorly placed orbital lesions and for the drainage of hematomas/abscesses (Fig. 18.9). It can also be used to gain access to the superior or inferior ophthalmic vein. An upper eyelid skin crease transseptal approach is used particularly for superior lesions, whereas a transconjunctival approach may be preferred for inferior lesions, as this avoids a visible cutaneous scar. A lower eyelid transconjunctival approach can be combined with a lateral canthotomy and inferior cantholysis to provide improved exposure of the inferior and lateral orbit. The conjunctival incision can be extended into a transcaruncular incision to gain further access to the medial orbit.

Both approaches can also be used to gain access to the subperiosteal space as well as to the extraconal space, e.g., for the management of an orbital wall blowout fracture or for a bony orbital decompression. It is important, however, not to disturb the periosteum when performing a biopsy on potentially malignant orbital lesions, as the periosteum is an important barrier to tumor spread and an important surgical excision margin. For the excision of more posteriorly placed lesions this approach may be combined with a lateral orbitotomy. Superomedial orbital lesions may be approached by an upper eyelid vertical split technique, where the upper eyelid is split vertically just lateral to the superior punctum (Fig. 18.10).

This approach can be used very effectively for lesions which are quite large (Fig. 18.11). A fair cosmetic result can also be achieved using this approach (Fig. 18.11).

Transcutaneous Anterior Orbitotomy
Surgical Procedure

1. A skin crease incision in the upper lid (or a subciliary or a skin crease incision in the lower lid) is marked with a cocktail stick dipped in a gentian violet marker. (A large superior lesion, which is readily palpable through the skin, may be more easily approached by means of a skin incision placed directly over the lesion, although this will leave a visible scar. This is not of concern with suspected orbital malignancies. A superior subperiosteal abscess should be approached via a sub-brow incision rather than via an upper lid skin crease incision, taking great care not to disturb the supraorbital and supratrochlear neurovascular bundles. Incisions over the inferior orbital margin should be avoided, as this leaves an unsightly scar and is associated with persistent postoperative lower eyelid lymphedema. An inferior subperiosteal abscess may be approached via a lower lid skin crease incision but the drain is brought through the skin overlying the inferior orbital margin.)
2. 1.5 to 2 ml of 0.5% Bupivacaine with 1:200,000 mixed 50:50 with 2% Lidocaine with 1:80,000 units of adrenaline is injected subcutaneously into the eyelid along the marked incision.
3. A gray line traction suture is placed and fixated to the drapes with a curved artery clip.
4. The skin and orbicularis are incised with a Colorado needle.
5. The orbital septum is opened and a Jaffe eyelid retractor is placed. (If the subperiosteal space is to be approached, the orbital septum is instead maintained intact and the periosteum is incised over the orbital margin and elevated using the sharp end of a Freer periosteal elevator.)
6. The lesion is dissected and removed or biopsied and hemostasis obtained.
7. The orbital septum is not repaired.
8. The skin is closed with interrupted 7/0 Vicryl sutures.
9. Topical antibiotic is applied to the wound.
10. A pressure dressing is applied.

Lower Eyelid Transconjunctival Anterior Orbitotomy
Surgical Procedure

1. Subconjunctival injections of local anesthetic solution containing adrenaline are avoided because of

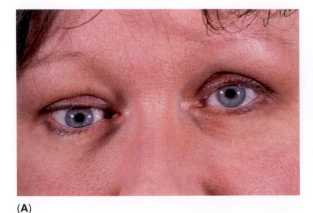

(A)

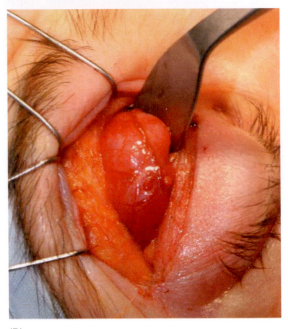

(B)

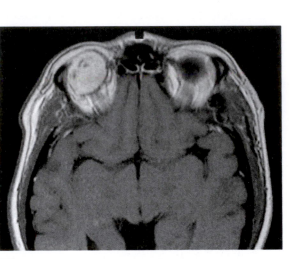

(C)

(D)

Figure 18.9 (A) A 40-year-old female patient who presented with a history of a gradual inferior displacement of the right globe. (B) A coronal MRI scan demonstrating a well-defined homogenous superior extraconal mass. (C) An axial MRI scan demonstrating that the lesion is anteriorly placed in the orbit. (D) The lesion was excised via an upper eyelid skin crease incision. A histopathological examination confirmed the lesion to be a solitary fibrous tumor.

the effects on the pupil. The local anesthetic injections are instead given just beneath the skin in the lower eyelid and at the lateral canthus.

2. A 4/0 silk traction suture is passed through the gray line of the lower eyelid.

3. A lateral canthal skin incision is made along the previously marked crease using a Colorado needle or no. 15 Bard Parker blade. The incision is deepened to expose the periosteum of the lateral orbital margin.

4. Next a lateral canthotomy is performed using the Colorado needle or using blunt-tipped Westcott scissors.

5. The lower eyelid is then everted over a small Desmarres retractor. The silk suture is fixated to the face drapes using a small curved artery clip.

6. A conjunctival incision is made immediately below the inferior border of the tarsus extending from just

below the inferior punctum to the lateral canthus using the Colorado needle.

7. Hemostasis is achieved using bipolar cautery when required.

8. A plane of dissection is created anterior to the orbital septum (Fig. 18.12). The orbicularis muscle is clearly seen using the bloodless approach with a Colorado needle and the dissection is continued keeping immediately posterior to this muscle.

9. This plane is dissected all the way to the inferior orbital margin. 4/0 silk traction sutures are placed through the medial and lateral aspects of the conjunctival/lower eyelid retractor complex. The sutures are then fixated to the forehead drapes using curved artery clips to protect the cornea during the rest of the surgery. Care is taken to ensure that the sutures themselves are placed medial and lateral to the globe so that they do not abrade the cornea.

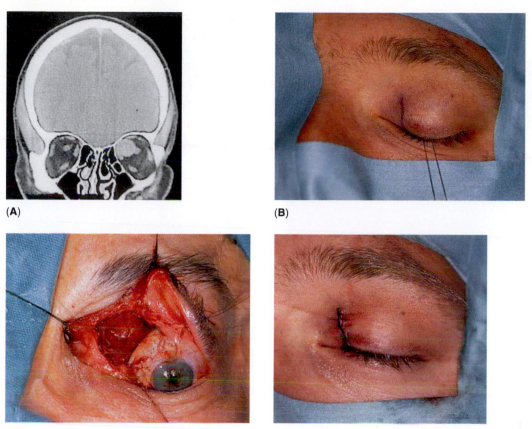

Figure 18.10 (**A**) A coronal CT scan demonstrating a superonasal orbital mass. (**B**) A vertical lid split incision has been marked nasal to the superior punctum extending into the superior fornix. (**C**) A cavernous hemangioma was exposed and an excision biopsy performed. (**D**) The eyelid split is carefully repaired.

10. One or two Jaffe lid retractors are inserted into the wound and fixated to the face drapes using a curved artery clip.
11. The orbital septum or the periorbita is opened, depending on the location of the lesion.
12. The lesion is exposed with the aid of Wright's retractors and removed or biopsied.
13. Hemostasis is obtained.
14. The conjunctiva is closed with interrupted 7/0 Vicryl sutures and the lateral canthotomy is repaired with a double-armed 5/0 Vicryl suture on a 1/2-circle needle passed from the tarsus to the lateral orbital periosteum. The skin is closed with interrupted 7/0 Vicryl sutures.
15. Topical antibiotic is applied to the wound.
16. A pressure dressing is applied.

Upper Eyelid Vertical Split Anterior Orbitotomy
Surgical Procedure
1. 1.5 to 2 ml of 0.5% Bupivacaine with 1:200,000 mixed 50:50 with 2% Lidocaine with 1:80,000 units of adrenaline are injected subcutaneously into the medial aspect of the upper eyelid.
2. The eyelid margin is incised 3 to 4 mm lateral to the superior punctum with a no. 15 Bard Parker blade.
3. The incision is extended to the superior fornix with straight iris scissors.

4. The lesion is exposed with the aid of Wright's retractors and removed or biopsied.
5. The eyelid is repaired in layers.
6. A single armed 6/0 black silk suture is passed through the eyelid margin along the line of the meibomian glands 2 mm from the wound edge emerging 1 mm from the surface. The needle is remounted and passed similarly through the opposing wound emerging 2 mm from the wound edge. The suture is cut leaving the ends long. The same suture is passed in a similar fashion along the lash line and cut leaving the ends long.
7. The silk sutures are then fixated to the head drapes using a small curved artery clip. This elongates the wound making it easier to place the subsequent sutures.
8. A single-armed 5/0 Vicryl suture on a 1/2-circle needle loaded on a Castroviejo needle holder is passed through the most superior aspect of the tarsus just below the black silk sutures, ensuring that the needle and suture are anterior to the conjunctiva to avoid contact with the cornea.
9. This suture is tied with a single throw and the eyelid margin approximation checked. If this is unsatisfactory, the suture is replaced and the process repeated. Proper placement of this suture will avoid the complications of eyelid notching and trichiasis, and wound dehiscence. Once the margin approximation is good, the suture is tied.

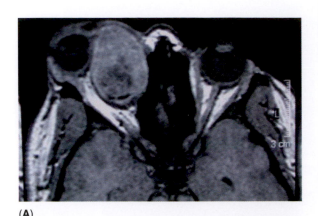

(A)

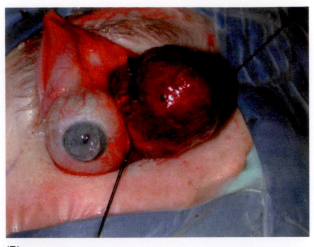

(B)

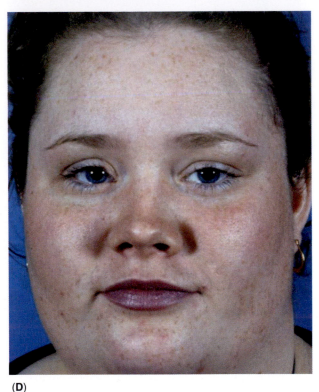

(C)

(D)

Figure 18.11 (**A**) An axial MRI scan showing a large right superomedial orbital mass. (**B**) The mass is being removed via an upper eyelid vertical split approach. (**C**) The preoperative appearance of the same patient. (**D**) The appearance of the same patient 3 months postoperatively.

10. Further 5/0 Vicryl sutures are passed through the tarsus and tied. Additional sutures are then passed through the orbicularis muscle and tied.

11. Next, the 6/0 silk sutures are tied with sufficient tension to cause eversion of the edges of the eyelid margin wound. A small amount of pucker is desirable initially, to avoid late lid notching as the lid heals and the wound contracts. The sutures are left long and incorporated into the skin closure sutures to prevent contact with the cornea.

12. The skin is closed with simple interrupted 6/0 black silk sutures.

13. Topical antibiotic is applied to the wound.

14. A pressure dressing is applied.

Medial Orbitotomy

Lynch Skin Incision Medial Orbitotomy

A Lynch incision can be used to approach the medial subperiosteal space, e.g., for the drainage of a subperiosteal abscess (Fig. 18.13), and to approach large lesions which may involve the nose and/or ethmoid sinus as well as the orbit (Fig.18.14). This approach for the management of a patient with a subperiosteal abscess has been largely superceded by the transcaruncular approach.

Surgical Procedure

1. The proposed skin incision is marked at the medial canthus midway between the medial commissure and the bridge of the nose with a cocktail stick

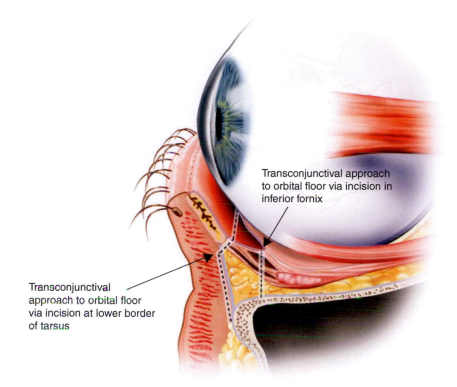

Figure 18.12 Surgical approaches to the orbit via lower eyelid conjunctival incisions.

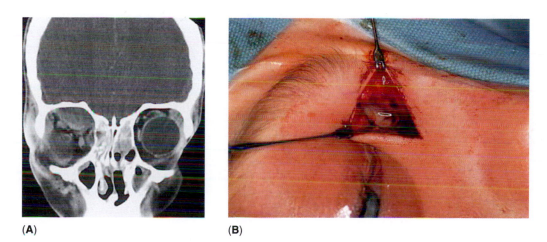

(A)   (B)

Figure 18.13 (**A**) A coronal CT scan demonstrating a large superior orbital subperiosteal abscess and a smaller medial wall subperiosteal abscess in a patient with an ethmoid sinusitis. The configuration of the subperiosteal abscess is determined by the attachment of the periorbita at the frontoethmoidal suture line. (**B**) A Lynch incision has bee made in the same patient to drain the abscess.

dipped in a gentian violet marker. The curvilinear incision commences at a position level with the medial aspect of the eyebrow and extends inferiorly to a position approximately 1 cm below the medial canthal tendon (Fig. 18.14).

2. 1.5 to 2 ml of 0.5% Bupivacaine with 1:200,000 mixed 50:50 with 2% Lidocaine with 1:80,000 units of adrenaline are injected subcutaneously along the marked incision line.

3. The skin incision is made using a no. 15 Bard Parker blade.

4. Blunt-tipped Stevens tenotomy scissors are then inserted into the centre of the wound and spread open along the line of the wound. These are used to dissect bluntly and bloodlessly through the orbicularis muscle down to the underlying periosteum. Alternatively, a Colorado needle can be used.

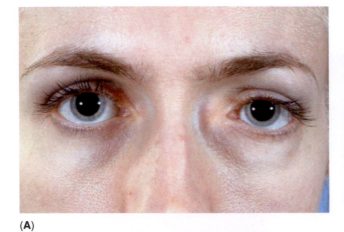

(A)

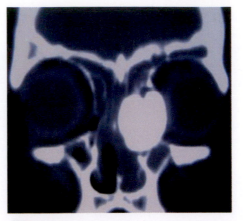

(B)

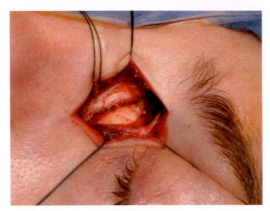

(C)

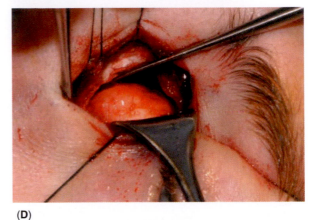

(D)

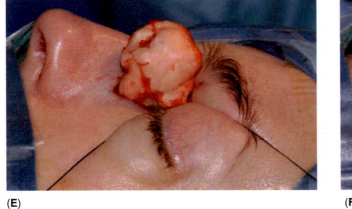

(E)

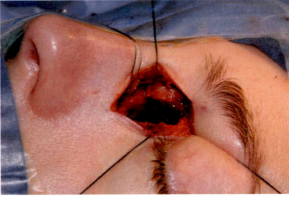

(F)

Figure 18.14 (**A**) A young female patient with a hard left medial canthal mass and a history of left constant epiphora. (**B**) A coronal CT scan demonstrating a left anterior ethmoidal ivory osteoma invading the medial aspect of the orbit. (**C**) A Lynch incision has been made to approach the lesion. The medial canthal tendon has been completely disinserted. (**D**) The lesion is being mobilized using a Freer periosteal elevator. (**E**) The large osteoma is being delivered via the Lynch incision. (**F**) An intraoperative photograph showing the resultant medial canthal bony defect and the lack of any fixation point for the medial canthal tendon. (*Continued*)

5. The angular vessels can be seen easily and cauterized with bipolar cautery wherever necessary to prevent bleeding.

6. The periosteum is then incised down to the bone with the no. 15 Bard Parker blade or with the Colorado needle.

7. The periosteum is then elevated off the frontal process of the maxilla and nasal bone using blunt dissection with a Freer periosteal elevator.

8. Next, 4/0 black silk traction sutures are used for retraction of the wound edges. The needle is passed deeply into the wound through the orbicularis and brought out just beneath the skin. Generally, four silk sutures are used.

9. The sutures are clamped to the drapes with curved artery clips. The use of the sutures greatly enhances visibility and hemostasis throughout the operation, particularly if a surgical assistant is not available to hold retractors.

10. Next, the periosteum is elevated toward the anterior lacrimal crest. The sutura notha is located 1 to 2 mm anterior to the anterior lacrimal crest.

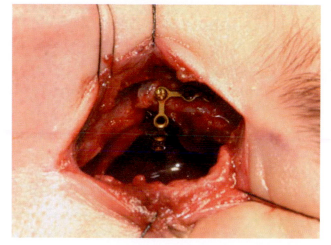

(G)

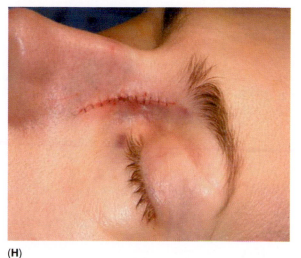

(H)

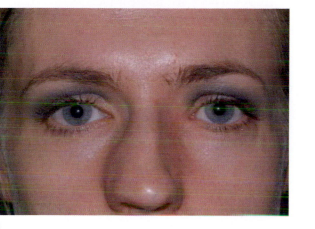

(I)

(J)

Figure 18.14 (*Continued*) (**G**) An L-shaped titanium microplate has been fixated to the nasal bone with titanium screws leaving the main limb of the microplate running posteriorly along the medial orbital wall. (**H**) The wound has been closed with interrupted 7/0 Vicryl sutures. (**I**) The appearance of the patient 3 months postoperatively following massage of the wound by the patient. (**J**) A lateral view of the patient showing a well healed cosmetically acceptable scar.

This is an important and consistent landmark, which should be recognized. Often, bleeding from a branch of the infraorbital artery, which travels in the groove, will occur.

11. Bone wax should be applied to the sutura notha for hemostasis.

12. The anterior limb of the medial canthal tendon may be removed from its bony attachment and sutured back into position following completion of the surgery. If the adjacent bone has had to be removed, including the posterior lacrimal crest, the medial canthal tendon can be attached to a titanium microplate. The microplate is anchored anteriorly on any available remaining bone (Fig. 18.14) with the main limb extending posteriorly. The medial canthal tendon is attached to the posterior limb of the microplate with a 5/0 Prolene suture. Alternatively, a bio-absorbable plate and screws can be used.

13. The remaining dissection depends on the nature and extent of the lesion to be removed.

14. Greater exposure requires the careful cauterization and division of the anterior ethmoidal vessels.

15. Great care must be taken in the region of the trochlea.

16. The wound is closed using interrupted subcutaneous 5/0 Vicryl sutures and interrupted 7/0 Vicryl sutures for the skin closure.

17. Topical antibiotic is applied to the wound.

18. A pressure dressing is applied.

Postoperative Care

The skin sutures are removed after 2 weeks. At this stage the patient is instructed to commence wound massage along the line of the wound for 3 minutes three to four times per day for a minimum period of 6 weeks using Lacrilube ointment. This is important to help to prevent the development of a "bow-string" scar (Fig. 18.14). A silicone gel preparation, e.g., Kelo-cote or Dermatix can also be used to help to prevent thickening of the wound.

Transconjunctival Medial Orbitotomy

A transconjunctival approach is used, often in conjunction with disinsertion of the medial rectus muscle, to remove intraconal lesions medial to the optic nerve or to perform an optic nerve fenestration procedure (Fig. 18.15). An alternative approach to an optic nerve sheath fenestration is via an upper eyelid skin crease incision. The optic nerve is approached from above, along the medial aspect of the levator muscle. This approach can be quick and does not adversely affect ocular motility in contrast to the medial orbitotomy approach.

A lateral orbitotomy can be combined with the medial orbitotomy to provide improved exposure if necessary.

Surgical Procedure

1. A Clark's speculum is placed and the cornea protected with Lacrilube ointment.
2. Subconjunctival injections of local anesthetic solution containing adrenaline are avoided because of the effect on the pupil.
3. A medial 180° peritomy is performed with blunt-tipped Westcott scissors and Moorfields forceps.
4. Radial relieving incisions are made in the conjunctiva.
5. 4/0 silk traction sutures are placed through the conjunctival edges superiorly and inferiorly.
6. Stevens tenotomy scissors are used to open Tenon's space, with a blunt spreading action, above and below the medial rectus muscle.
7. A muscle hook is inserted beneath the medial rectus muscle, which is drawn anteriorly.
8. A double-armed 5/0 Vicryl suture is passed through the medial rectus muscle 2 to 3 mm posterior to its insertion. Each needle is then reversed and passed beneath the muscle and brought through the muscle close to its centre. Each needle is then passed through the loop of suture at each end and pulled tight.
9. The medial rectus muscle is then disinserted from the globe with the Westcott scissors, leaving a short stump.
10. A 4/0 black silk suture is then passed carefully in a continuous fashion through the muscle stump and the needle is removed.

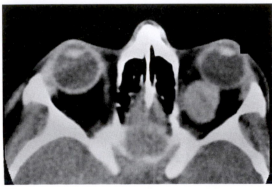

(A)

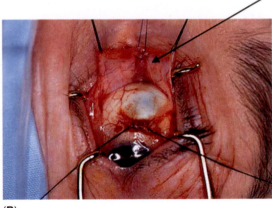

The medial rectus muscle

(B)

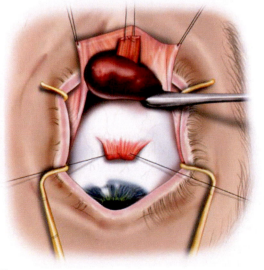

(C)

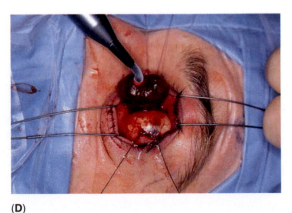

(D)

Figure 18.15 (**A**) An axial CT scan demonstrating a medial intraconal orbital mass. (**B**) The medial rectus muscle has been sutured, detached from its insertion and drawn medially. Traction sutures have been placed through the medial rectus stump and the globe rotated laterally. Traction sutures have also been placed through the conjunctiva and anterior Tenon's fascia after radial relieving incisions have been made. (**C**) Wright's retractors are used to gently expose the lesion, which is then gently dissected free. (**D**) A cryotherapy probe insulated to the tip is being used to assist delivery of the lesion, a cavernous hemangioma.

11. The ends of the silk sutures are fixated to the face drapes laterally, above and below the globe, with small curved artery clips, rotating the globe laterally.

12. The ends of the Vicryl sutures are fixated to the face drapes medially, above and below the globe, with small curved artery clips, drawing the medial rectus muscle medially.

13. Additional 4/0 silk traction sutures can be passed beneath the superior and inferior recti if required to provide better rotation of the globe.

14. The intraconal space is exposed using two pairs of Wright's retractors.

15. If an optic nerve sheath fenestration is to be performed, the assistant exposes the bulbar expansion of the optic nerve sheath just posterior to the globe using the Wright's retractors. The nerve sheath is very carefully opened using the tip of a myringotomy blade. A gush of CSF is usually seen. The optic nerve sheath is grasped with a pair of Castroviejo 0.12 toothed forceps and a 5 × 7 mm rectangular window of optic nerve sheath is removed with Westcott scissors.

16. The silk traction sutures are removed.

17. The medial rectus muscle is repositioned by passing the needles of the 5/0 Vicryl suture through the muscle stump at each end and again through the centre of the muscle stump. The muscle is drawn forward to its position and the suture is tied.

18. The conjunctiva is closed with interrupted 8/0 Vicryl sutures.

19. Topical antibiotic is instilled into the conjunctival sac.

20. A pressure dressing is applied.

Transcaruncular Medial Orbitotomy

A transcaruncular incision can be used to access lesions in the medial extraconal orbital space, to perform a medial orbital wall decompression for thyroid eye disease, to drain a medial subperiosteal hematoma or abscess, or to repair a medial orbital wall blowout fracture. (In carefully selected cases an endoscopic approach can be used as an alternative approach to gain access to the posterior aspect of the medial orbit for the decompression of benign apical tumors or for an incisional biopsy.)

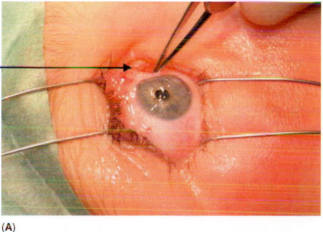

An incision has been made between the plica semilunaris and the caruncle

(A)

Tenon's fascia

The medial orbital wall

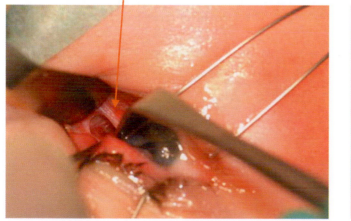

(B)

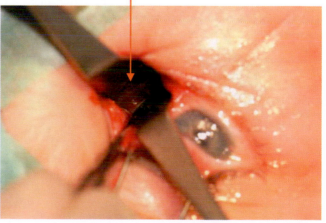

(C)

Figure 18.16 (**A**) An incision has been made between the plica semilunaris and the caruncle. (**B**) Wright's retractors are being used to assist in the exposure of the medial orbital wall. (**C**) The subperiosteal space has been entered and the medial orbital wall has been exposed.

Surgical Procedure

1. Subconjunctival injections of local anesthetic solution containing adrenaline are avoided because of the effect on the pupil.
2. An incision is made between the caruncle and the plica semilunaris using blunt-tipped Westcott scissors (Fig. 18.16A).
3. Blunt dissection with Stevens scissors is used to expose the medial orbital wall posterior to the posterior lacrimal crest. The posterior lacrimal crest can be palpated with the tips of the scissors.
4. 4/0 silk traction sutures are placed through the conjunctiva to improve exposure.
5. If access is required to the subperiosteal space, the periorbita is incised and elevated using the sharp end of a Freer periosteal elevator.
6. Wright's retractors or narrow Sewall retractors are used to gain exposure of the posterior aspects of the medial orbit (Fig. 18.16B).
7. The conjunctiva is closed with interrupted 8/0 Vicryl sutures at the completion of surgery.
8. Topical antibiotic is instilled into the conjunctival sac.
9. A pressure dressing is applied.

Lateral Orbitotomy

The lateral orbitotomy provides a very good approach to the intraconal space and to lesions lateral to the optic nerve. It can be combined with other approaches to the orbit, allowing the globe to be moved laterally to facilitate improved surgical exposure. It can also be used as part of an orbital decompression procedure. The lateral orbital wall can be approached by means of different surgical incisions:

1. The Berke–Reese approach
2. The Stallard–Wright approach
3. An upper eyelid skin crease approach
4. A bicoronal flap approach

The Stallard–Wright approach is the approach of choice (Fig. 18.17). The Berke–Reese approach leaves a less satisfactory scar and disturbs the lateral canthus. The upper eyelid skin crease approach can help to camouflage the scar but may leave the patient with a mechanical ptosis for

some weeks postoperatively due to prolonged pretarsal edema (Fig. 18.18).

The bicoronal flap requires much more operative time and exposes the patient to risks of hair loss, greater degrees of sensory loss and the risk of a frontalis palsy. The subsequent development of male pattern baldness will expose an extensive scar.

Stallard–Wright Lateral Orbitotomy
Surgical Procedure

1. The patient is placed into a reverse Trendelenburg position with the permission of the anesthetist.
2. The surgeon is seated at the side of the patient facing the lateral orbital margin.
3. The patient's head is turned slightly away from the surgeon.
4. The lateral orbitotomy incision is marked out with gentian violet. This should extend from just below the lateral aspect of the eyebrow to end in a rhytid over the anterior zygomatic arch (Fig. 18.17A).
5. Two to three milliliters of 0.5% bupivacaine with 1:200,000 units of adrenaline mixed 50:50 with 2% Lidocaine with 1:80,000 units of adrenaline are injected subcutaneously along the marked incision and further 3 to 4 ml are injected into the temporal fossa with the needle angulated horizontally to avoid any inadvertent injection directly into the orbit through a bony defect in the lateral orbital wall.
6. The cornea is protected with Lacrilube ointment.
7. A 4/0 silk suture is passed through the gray line of the upper eyelid and fixated to the face drapes inferiorly with a small curved artery clip.
8. A skin incision is made with a no. 15 Bard Parker blade.
9. The subcutaneous tissues are dissected down to the periosteum of the lateral orbital margin using a Colorado needle.
10. Multiple 4/0 silk traction sutures are placed through the subcutaneous tissues and fixated to the face drapes with small curved artery clips (Fig. 18.29).
11. The periosteum is then incised with a no. 15 Bard Parker blade 2 mm lateral to the orbital margin. The incision is carried superiorly above the

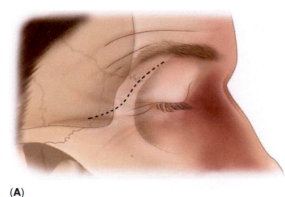

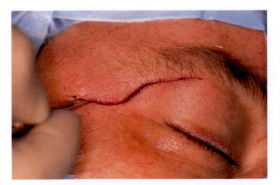

(A)   (B)

Figure 18.17 (A) A diagram demonstrating the position of a Stallard–Wright lateral orbitotomy incision in relation to the lateral orbital margin. (B) The lateral orbitotomy incision is being made in this patient.

fronto-zygomatic suture and inferiorly past the superior aspect of the zygomatic arch (Fig. 18.19). Posterior relieving incisions are made in the periosteum at the superior and inferior limits of the incision.

12. The periosteum and temporalis muscle are then reflected posteriorly using a Freer periosteal elevator, exposing the lateral wall of the orbit in the temporal fossa. Two or three 2 × 2 gauze swabs are inserted into the temporal fossa to aid in retraction and hemostasis (Fig. 18.20). These must be carefully

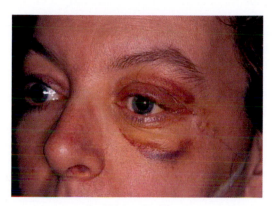

Figure 18.18 A patient 3 days after undergoing a lateral orbitotomy via an extended upper eyelid crease incision.

counted, recorded and removed at the end of the procedure. It is very easy to lose sight of a swab deep in the inferior aspect of the wound.

13. The periosteum is now very carefully reflected from the internal aspect of the lateral orbital wall using the sharp end of a Freer periosteal elevator (Fig. 18.21). Great care should be taken to maintain the periorbita intact at this stage.

14. The zygomatico-temporal and zygomatico-facial vessels are cauterized and divided as they are encountered. The periorbita does not need to be raised beyond the zygomatico-sphenoidal suture line.

15. Incision lines are drawn on the bone with gentian violet approximately 5mm above the fronto-zygomatic suture superiorly and just above the zygomatic arch inferiorly (Fig. 18.22).

16. A broad malleable retractor is inserted into the orbit to protect the orbital contents, while another is placed into the temporal fossa to protect the temporalis muscle and to prevent any swabs from being caught by the saw.

17. An oscillating saw with a straight blade is used to cut along the incision lines (Fig. 18.23A). It is important to use copious irrigation. Great care is taken to angulate the superior saw cut inferiorly to avoid any risk of entering the anterior cranial fossa.

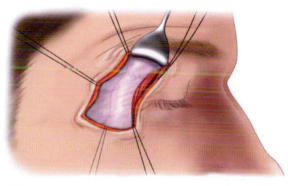

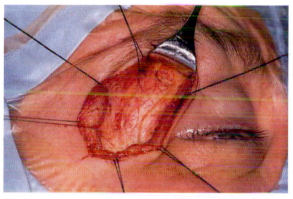

(A)   (B)

Figure 18.19 (**A**) The lateral orbital margin is exposed to a position approximately 2 cm above the frontozygomatic suture line superiorly and to a position level with the zygomatic arch inferiorly. (**B**) The periosteum is incised 2 mm lateral to the orbital rim with posterior relieving incisions at the superior and inferior aspects of the incision.

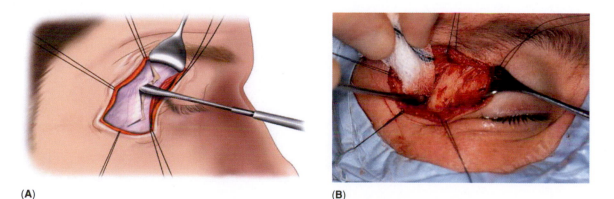

(A)   (B)

Figure 18.20 The periosteum is carefully reflected from the lateral orbital margin and internal aspect of the lateral orbital wall with a fine periosteal elevator.

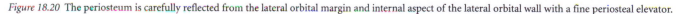

(It is preferable to place the superior incision at a slightly lower level, as the bony opening can always be enlarged if necessary with a burr and the superior drill hole repositioned).

18. Drill holes are now made through the bone with a wire pass burr above and below the saw cuts (Fig. 18.23B).

19. The lateral orbital wall is grasped with a large bone rongeur and gently rocked in an outward direction until it fractures posteriorly (Fig. 18.24). It is then removed (Fig. 18.25). It is safely stored in a large saline-soaked gauze swab (Fig. 18.26).

20. The irregular fracture line can be smoothed and further bone removed with a burr or a Belz lacrimal

rongeur (Fig. 18.27). The thick cancellous bone of the sphenoid is encountered, marking the posterior limit of any further bone removal.

21. Bone wax is applied to any bleeding points from the bone. The gauze swabs in the temporal fossa are removed and replaced. Hemostasis is secured before proceeding.

22. A T-shaped incision is made in the periorbita. A small initial incision is made with a no. 15 Bard Parker blade at the lower border of the lateral rectus muscle in an antero-posterior direction. This incision is enlarged posteriorly with blunt-tipped Westcott scissors. Vertical incisions are made anteriorly in a superior direction in front of the lacrimal gland and in an inferior direction towards the base of the orbitotomy.

23. The periorbita is grasped and gently dissected from the orbital contents with blunt-tipped Westcott scissors.

24. The lateral rectus muscle is identified after opening the perimuscular fascial sheaths by blunt dissection. A loop of O'Donoghue's lacrimal silicone tubing is carefully passed around the muscle, retracted inferiorly and fixated to the face drapes with a curved artery clip (Fig. 18.28).

25. The position of the orbital mass is confirmed by gentle digital palpation.

26. The orbital fat is gently retracted in a hand-over-hand fashion using Wright's retractors (Fig. 18.8A).

27. Blunt dissection over and around the lesion is aided by placing long rectangular neurosurgical cottonoid patties behind the retractors, which assists in keeping the orbital fat from the surgical field (Fig. 18.8B). These also absorb blood and allow gentle suction to be applied to them without frequent blockage of the suction tip by globules of fat. Suction of fat should be avoided to prevent the rupture of fine blood vessels.

28. Fine-tipped bayonet bipolar cautery forceps are used very carefully to achieve hemostasis where necessary.

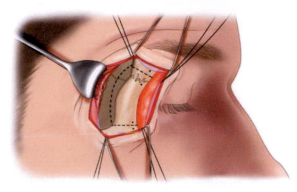

Figure 18.21 The position of the bone cuts is demonstrated in this diagram.

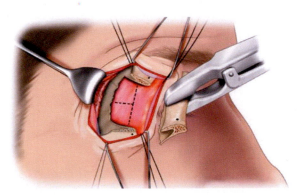

Figure 18.22 A diagram showing the removal of the bone from the lateral orbital wall and the position of the "T"-shaped incision in the periorbita.

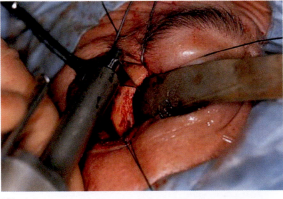

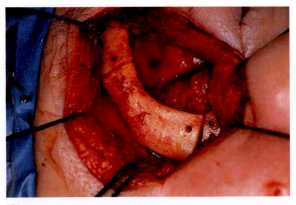

(A)   (B)

Figure 18.23 (A) Malleable retractors are used to protect the orbital contents and the temporal fossa when the saw cuts are made. The superior saw cut should be angled inferiorly. (B) Drill holes have been made above and below the saw cuts.

29. Operating loupes usually provide adequate magnification but the operating microscope may occasionally be required.
30. If the lesion is encapsulated it is bluntly dissected from the surrounding orbital tissues with a Freer periosteal elevator, keeping the dissection close to the capsule to avoid inadvertent injury to adjacent orbital structures. Pressure on the retractors should be released at regular and frequent intervals.
31. The patient's pupil should be checked at regular intervals.
32. Delivery of the lesion may be assisted by the use of a cryoprobe.
33. If the lesion is not encapsulated and cannot be removed safely, it should be biopsied or debulked as safely as possible.
34. Meticulous attention is paid to hemostasis with gentle cautery. Gelfoam and thrombin may be used but should be removed prior to closure of the orbitotomy.
35. Intravenous corticosteroid (8mg of dexamethasone) is given by the anesthetist to help to minimize postoperative orbital edema.
36. It may not be possible to close the periorbita at the end of the procedure. If the edges can be re-approximated, the periorbita is sutured with interrupted 5/0 Vicryl sutures.

37. The bone fragment is replaced and anchored into position with 3/0 Vicryl sutures (Fig. 18.29).
38. The periosteum is carefully reapproximated over the bone with interrupted 5/0 Vicryl sutures.
39. The swabs are removed from the temporal fossa and the bone and temporalis muscle checked for bleeding.
40. The subcutaneous tissue is closed with interrupted 5/0 Vicryl sutures.
41. The skin is closed with a continuous subcuticular 6/0 nylon suture or interrupted 7/0 Vicryl sutures passed in a vertical mattress fashion.
42. A suction drain should be placed into the temporal fossa and brought out through the skin posterior to the orbitotomy wound. The drain should be sutured to the skin with a 4/0 silk suture.
43. Topical antibiotic is applied to the wound.
44. A pressure dressing is applied.

ENDOSCOPIC ORBITOTOMY

A transethmoidal endoscopic approach to the medial orbital wall can be used to undertake a medial orbital wall decompression for the management of thyroid eye disease, but this can also be used to decompress small benign orbital apical lesions causing a compressive optic neuropathy. The posterior aspect of the lamina papyracea may be removed and the periorbita opened to allow the lesion to prolapse medially, relieving pressure on the optic nerve. This is a particularly useful approach for older patients

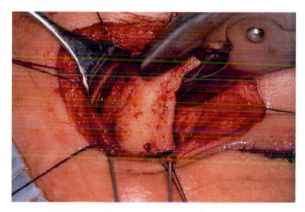

Figure 18.24 The lateral orbital bone is grasped with a large rongeur and gently rocked back and forth.

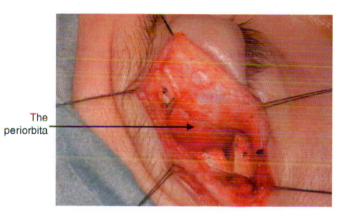

The periorbita →

Figure 18.26 The appearance of the intact periorbita.

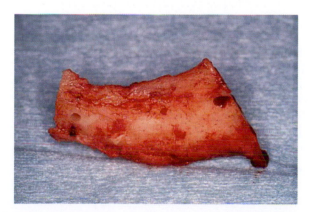

Figure 18.25 The appearance of the bone removed for a lateral orbitotomy.

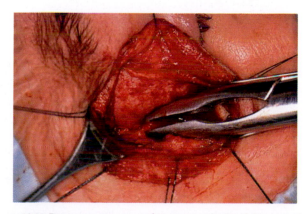

Figure 18.27 Bone rongeurs are used to remove further bone posteriorly, leaving a smooth edge.

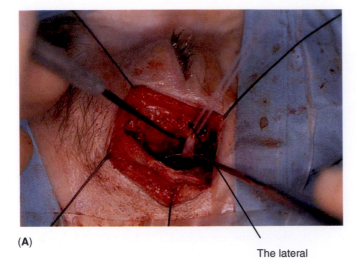

(A)

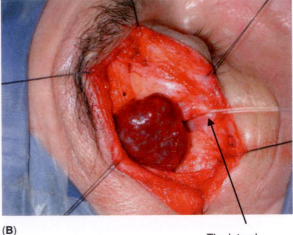

(B)

The lateral
rectus muscle

The lateral
rectus muscle

Figure 18.28 (**A**) The lateral rectus muscle has been isolated and looped with O'Donoghue's silicone tubing. (**B**) A cavernous hemangioma is being delivered via the lateral orbitotomy approach.

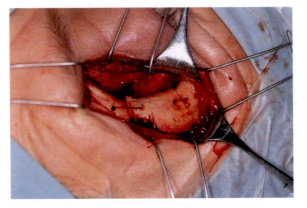

Figure 18.29 The bone is replaced and sutured into position with 3/0 vicryl sutures.

with cardiovascular problems in whom a more formal surgical exploration carries a significant risk of visual morbidity. This approach can also be used in selected cases in order to obtain a small biopsy of a medial orbital apical lesion. It is preferable to undertake such surgery in conjunction with an ENT surgeon skilled in functional endoscopic sinus surgery (FESS).

Combined Orbitotomies

The orbitotomies described above may be used in combination if necessary.

Transcranial Orbitotomy

A lesion at the orbital apex may require a transcranial approach to the orbit to gain adequate safe access. Such surgery is undertaken as a team approach involving a neurosurgeon. The patient must understand the risks and potential complications of such surgery: e.g., postoperative epilepsy, which may have major implications for the patient's occupation and driving. The patient should understand that a postoperative ptosis and an extraocular muscle palsy are frequently seen, but in most cases resolve spontaneously after a period of months.

There are two main transcranial approaches to the orbit:

- The transcranial frontal orbitotomy (Fig. 18.30A).
- The pterional craniotomy (Fig. 18.30B).

Frontal Craniotomy

A frontal craniotomy is undertaken by a neurosurgeon via a bicoronal or hemicoronal flap approach (Figs. 18.30–18.32). A frontal bone flap is removed and hinged laterally, still attached to the temporalis muscle and pericranium. The bone of the posterior orbital roof can be removed piecemeal with a rongeur to the optic canal. The bone flap can, however, include the superior orbital margin if a wider exposure is required. This approach provides very good exposure of the medial, superior and lateral orbital apex. Lesions that involve the inferior orbital apex may require a pterional craniotomy approach, sometimes combined with a lateral orbitotomy.

For lesions confined to the orbit, an extradural approach is undertaken. For orbitocranial tumors, e.g., an optic nerve sheath meningioma, an intradural approach is required. The frontal lobe is gently retracted with self-retaining retractors (Fig. 18.32).

The periorbita is then opened in a similar fashion to a lateral orbitotomy. The frontal nerve is identified, running in a postero-anterior direction over the levator muscle. The orbit should be entered medial to the optic nerve to avoid damaging the cranial nerves entering the orbit via the superior orbital fissure. The orbital lesion is identified and removed in a similar fashion to that described during the course of a lateral orbitotomy. The orbital roof is then reconstructed by using either an alloplastic material, e.g., porous polyethylene or by using a bone graft harvested from the inner table of the frontal bone flap.

This approach can be used for the management of the following:

- Tumors of the orbital apex, particularly those medial to the optic nerve that cannot be removed using an transnasal endoscopic approach or via a transcaruncular approach

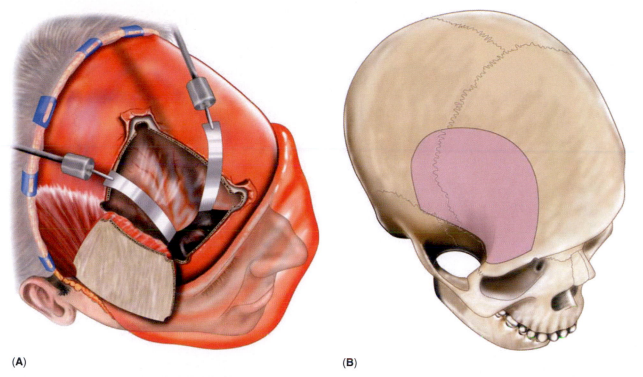

(A)   **(B)**

Figure 18.30 (**A**) A drawing depicting a transfrontal craniotomy with removal of the orbital roof permitting access to the superior orbital apex. In this example, the superior orbital margin has been left intact. (**B**) A drawing depicting the area of bone removed in a pterional craniotomy.

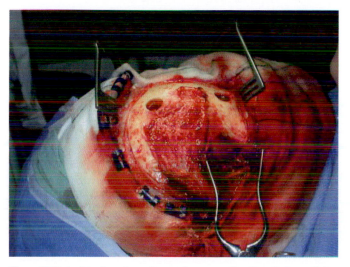

Figure 18.31 A right frontal craniotomy in preparation. Burr holes are being prepared. The bone flap with attached pericranium and temporalis muscle will be hinged laterally and kept moistened in a large swab during the orbital dissection.

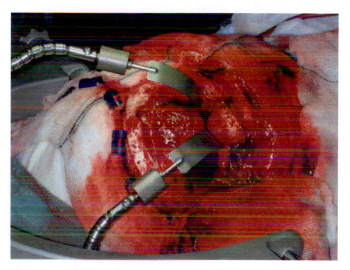

Figure 18.32 The frontal lobe is very gently retracted with self-retaining retractors. The orbital roof has been removed. The periorbita is intact. This will be opened and the orbital apical lesion exposed.

- Removal of an optic nerve meningioma or glioma from the globe to the optic chiasm
- An extensive orbitocranial tumor

A Pterional Craniotomy

A pterional craniotomy is a surgical approach with which neurosurgeons are most familiar as it is the most common neurosurgical approach for the microsurgical clipping of intracranial aneurysms. Typically, a 6 to 8 cm bone flap centered on the pterion is elevated. This approach provides excellent exposure of the lateral and apical aspects of the orbit. It is mostly utilized in orbitocranial surgery for the management of sphenoid wing or orbitosphenoid meningiomas. The

approach permits a decompression of the roof and lateral wall of the optic canal.

POSTOPERATIVE MANAGEMENT FOLLOWING ORBITAL SURGERY

1. Instructions are given for the patient's head to be elevated 30° to 45°.
2. The patient is instructed to avoid bending or lifting weights for at least 72 hours as this raises venous pressure with the risk of provoking an orbital hemorrhage.
3. The dressings are removed approximately 30 to 45 min following surgery and the patient's visual acuity and pupil reactions checked hourly for 12 hours.

4. An ice pack is applied to the periorbital area intermittently for 24 hours.

5. No opiates are prescribed for pain management. Any complaint of pain should be followed by the immediate examination of the patient to exclude signs of a retrobulbar hemorrhage.

6. The patient should be kept nil by mouth until the following day as a precaution. If a sudden retrobulbar hemorrhage were to occur causing an orbital compartment syndrome the patient would have to be returned to the operating room immediately for the orbit to be re-explored and the source of bleeding stopped. Should this occur, an immediate lateral canthotomy and inferior cantholysis should be performed and medical therapy given to lower the intraocular pressure without delay.

7. Systemic corticosteroids are prescribed for a period of 6 days following surgery (commencing at 60 mg of prednisolone and reducing by 10 mg per day) and topical antibiotic ointment for the wound.

8. Systemic antibiotics are only used for specific indications, e.g., previous infection, foreign bodies, exposure of the paranasal sinuses.

KEY POINT

No opiates are prescribed for pain management. Any complaint of pain should be followed by the immediate examination of the patient to exclude signs of a retrobulbar hemorrhage.

FURTHER READING

1. American Academy of Ophthalmology. Basic and Clinical Science Course: Orbit, Eyelids, and Lacrimal System, section 7. San Francisco, CA: The American Academy of Ophthalmology, 2006/7: 63–96.
2. De Potter P, Shields JA, Shields CL. MRI of the Eye and Orbit. Philadelphia, PA: JB Lippincott, 1995.
3. Dutton JJ. Atlas of Clinical and Surgical Orbital Anatomy. Philadelphia, PA: WB Saunders, 1994.
4. Goldberg RA. Mancini R. Demer JL. The transcaruncular approach: surgical anatomy and technique. Arch Facial Plast Surg 2007; 9(6): 443–7.
5. Housepian EM. Microsurgical anatomy of the orbital apex and principles of transcranial orbital exploration. Clin Neurosurg 1978; **25**: 556–73.
6. Nerad JA. (ISBN: 978-1-4377-0008-4). Philadelphia, PA: Elsevier Inc., 2010
7. Jordan DR, Anderson RL. Surgical Anatomy of the Ocular Adnexa: A Clinical Approach. Ophthalmology Monograph 9, San Francisco, CA: American Academy of Ophthalmology, 1996.
8. Kersten RC, Kulwin DR. Vertical lid split orbitotomy revisited. Ophthal Plast Reconstr Surg 1999; 15: 425–8.
9. Kersten RC, Nerad JA. Orbital surgery. In: Tasman W, Jaeger EA, eds., Duane's Clinical Ophthalmology, rev ed., vol. 5. Baltimore, MD: Lippincott, Williams & Wilkins, 1988: 1–36.
10. Kersten RC. The eyelid crease approach to superficial lateral dermoid cysts. J Pediatr Ophthalmol Strabismus 1988; 25: 48–51.
11. Rootman J, Stewart B, Goldberg RA. Orbital Surgery, A Conceptual Approach. Philadelphia, PA: Lippincott-Raven, 1995.
12. Rootman J. Orbital surgery. In: Rootman J, ed., Diseases of the Orbit, Philadelphia, PA: JB Lippincott, 1988: 579–612.
13. Shorr N, Baylis H. Transcaruncular–transconjunctival approach to the medial orbit and orbital apex. Oral presentation at the American Society of Ophthalmic Plastic and Reconstructive Surgeons, 24th Annual Scientific Symposium, Chicago, November 13, 1993.
14. Wobig JL, Dailey RA, eds. Oculofacial Plastic Surgery: Face, Lacrimal System and Orbit. New York, NY: Thieme, 2004: 192–254.
15. Zide BM, Jelks GW. Surgical anatomy around the orbit: the system of zones. In: Techniques in Ophthalmic Plastic Surgery—A Personal Tutorial. Philadelphia, PA: Williams & Wilkins, 2006: 429–60.

19 Thyroid eye disease

INTRODUCTION

Thyroid eye disease is the most common orbital inflammatory disorder and the commonest cause of unilateral or bilateral proptosis in an adult. Although it was described by Graves in 1835, the disorder remains an enigma with many major issues remaining unresolved. Over the years it has been known by a number of different terms: Graves' orbitopathy, Graves' eye disease, Graves' ophthalmopathy, thyroid-associated ophthalmology (TAO), thyroid exophthalmos, thyroid-related eye disease, and Von Basedow's ophthalmopathy.

It is a very variable disorder with a wide spectrum of clinical presentation which can result in initial misdiagnosis. Diagnostic accuracy has been improved by advances, both in laboratory investigations and orbital imaging techniques. Research continues to improve our understanding of the underlying pathogenesis of the disorder. The clinical management of patients has also been greatly improved over recent years with advances in the medical management of patients, and with a better understanding of the pathophysiology of eyelid retraction, restrictive myopathy, and compressive optic neuropathy (CON). The surgical approaches to orbital decompression continue to evolve.

PATHOGENESIS

Although precisely what triggers thyroid eye disease and why the disease is more severe in some patients than other is unknown, the orbitopathy and dysthyroid state appear to be associated with immunological abnormalities. It is generally believed that the orbitopathy may be a closely related but separate organ-specific autoimmune disorder with target auto antigens and circulating auto antibodies.

THYROID ORBIT RELATIONSHIP

Approximately 80% of thyroid eye disease cases occur in association with hyperthyroidism although not all of these coincide with the onset of hyperthyroid symptoms. Patients may present with thyroid eye disease well before the onset of thyroid dysfunction, at the same time as the onset of thyroid dysfunction, or when the patient has become euthyroid following treatment.

If patients, who are thought to have euthyroid thyroid eye disease, are evaluated more extensively, they are often found to have some features of thyroid disease, e.g., a positive family history, thyroid stimulating hormone (TSH)-receptor-stimulating antibodies, positive thyroid peroxidase (TPO) antibodies, or an abnormal response to thyrotropin-releasing hormone (TRH). Approximately 50% of the patients with thyroid eye disease who initially appear euthyroid will go on to develop hyperthyroidism within 18 months of presentation.

In addition, approximately 10% of patients with thyroid eye disease have primary autoimmune hypothyroidism. These patients are characterized by the presence of moderate-to-high titers of TPO antibodies. The orbitopathy in these patients can be as great, or occasionally greater, than that seen in patients with hyperthyroidism.

Men and older patients (over 50 years of age) tend to have much more aggressive disease. Older patients are also more likely to have unilateral or very asymmetrical disease and are more likely to appear euthyroid or hypothyroid at the time of presentation.

Pathology

The extraocular muscles show inflammatory cell infiltration with lymphocytes, plasma cells, and mast cells. Although the inferior and medial rectus muscles are more commonly affected clinically, orbital imaging demonstrates that most if not all the extraocular muscles, including the levator muscle, are involved in the disease process. The muscles undergo degenerative changes caused by the deposition of glycosaminoglycans and collagen formation, and demonstrate infiltration with fat. The muscle belly is mainly involved in the process with the muscle tendon showing minimal or no enlargement. This differentiates thyroid eye disease from orbital myositis. The enlarged muscles may reach two to three times their normal volume (Fig. 19.1A). In the majority of patients, the disease process becomes inactive after a period of 18 months to 2 years. The degenerated extraocular muscles become replaced by fat and fibrous tissue resulting in a restrictive myopathy in severe or untreated cases.

In most patients, the orbital fat does not undergo significant structural changes although in some patients the orbital fat shows marked volumetric alterations which can be responsible for marked proptosis, even in the absence of extraocular muscle enlargement as seen on orbital imaging (Fig. 19.1B).

Pathophysiology

A single extraocular muscle or multiple extraocular muscles may be affected by the disorder. The disorder may present symmetrically or asymmetrically for reasons that are so far unclear. The extraocular muscle enlargement and/or orbital fat hypertrophy cause a secondary mass effect within the confines of the bony orbit. The secondary effects depend on a number of variable and interacting factors that are responsible for the wide range of clinical presentation of thyroid eye disease. These include:

1. The volume of the orbital cavity
2. The axial length of the globe
3. The integrity of the orbital septum
4. The degree and rapidity of onset of the orbital inflammation
5. The degree of enlargement of the extraocular muscles
6. The degree of hypertrophy of the orbital fat
7. The absence of lymphatics from the posterior orbital tissues

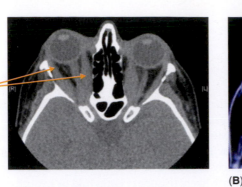
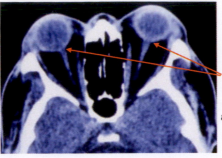

Massive enlargement of the medial and lateral recti

Marked proptosis with stretching of the optic nerves and tenting of the posterior poles of the globes in the absence of enlargement of the extraocular muscles

(A)   **(B)**

Figure 19.1 (**A**) An axial CT scan showing severe bilateral proptosis due to extra-ocular muscle enlargement with orbital apical crowding. (**B**) An axial CT scan showing marked bilateral proptosis in a patient with thyroid eye disease. The extra-ocular muscles are of normal size but the volume of orbital fat is increased. The optic nerves are stretched with tenting of the posterior poles of the globes. The patient had a severe dysthyroid optic neuropathy.

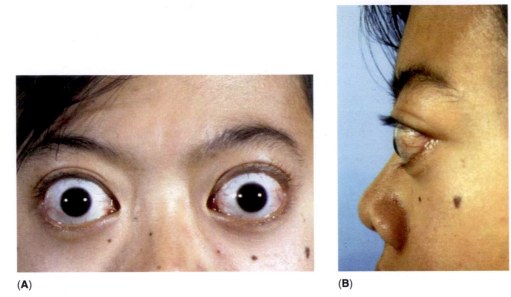

(A)   **(B)**

Figure 19.2 A young Malaysian patient with thyroid eye disease and marked symmetric proptosis. The patient has high axial myopia, malar hypoplasia, and shallow orbits.

If the orbital cavity is small, any mass effect can result in more severe degrees of proptosis and even in frank subluxation of the globe. Patients with axial myopia tend to experience a more severe cosmetic deformity resulting from proptosis (Fig. 19.2).

The degree of proptosis, which results from the orbital mass effect, is influenced by the tightness of the orbital septum. A lax orbital septum offers little resistance to the forward movement of the globe. The degree of resultant proptosis is governed by the size of the orbital cavity, the axial length of the globe, the degree of extraocular muscle and/or orbital fat swelling, the compliance of the extraocular muscles, and the length of the optic nerve. The resultant proptosis represents a spontaneous orbital decompression that may be severe enough to result in spontaneous subluxation of the globe. It may also be severe enough to cause a stretching of the optic nerve and deformation of the posterior aspect of the globe that may cause an optic neuropathy with visual loss.

In contrast, where the orbital septum is tight, as seen in the younger patient, the globe is prevented from moving forward and the pressure within the orbit rises. This rise in intraorbital pressure, in conjunction with swelling of the extraocular

muscles in the confined bony space of the orbital apex, can result in an insidious compressive optic neuropathy (CON). The degree of visual impairment may be out of proportion to the apparent clinical extent of the disease (Fig. 19.3).

The tightness of the orbital septum and the absence of deep orbital lymphatic vessels also influence the magnitude of secondary periorbital tissue edema. If the orbital inflammation progresses rapidly, the secondary congestive changes can be severe resulting in so-called "malignant exophthalmos" (Fig. 19.16).

Epidemiology

The estimated incidence of thyroid eye disease in the general population is 16 females and 3 men per 100,000 head of population per annum. The prevalence appears to have declined in most European countries over the last decade, a trend which may be related to earlier diagnosis and management of thyroid dysfunction by endocrinologists and a decreased prevalence of smoking. It is well recognized that smoking greatly increases the severity of the ophthalmopathy.

Patients with thyroid eye disease are older than patients with Graves' hyperthyroidism. The disease is more common in females than males but males tend to have a more severe

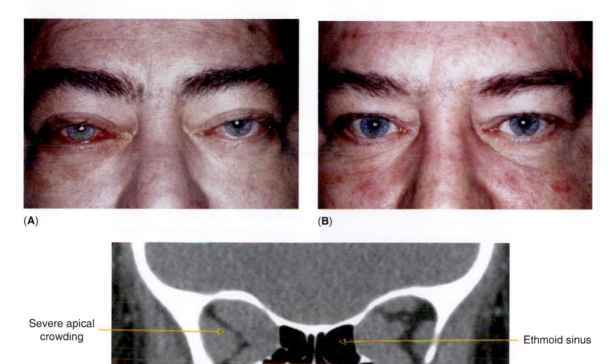

(A) (B)

(C)

Figure 19.3 (**A**) A patient with bilateral severe compressive optic neuropathy (CON) unresponsive to aggressive medical therapy. (**B**) The patient following bilateral 2 wall orbital decompression. (**C**) A coronal CT scan demonstrating orbital apical crowding from extra-ocular muscle enlargement.

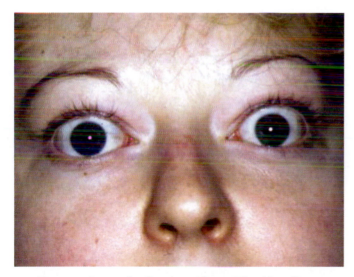

Figure 19.4 A young female patient with type 1 thyroid eye disease.

ophthalmopathy as do older patients. European patients have a far greater risk of developing thyroid eye disease than Asian patients.

A number of factors may increase the risk of developing thyroid eye disease in patients with Graves' disease. These include genetic predisposition, gender, radioactive iodine treatment, smoking, TSH receptor antibodies, drugs, age, and stress.

Patients often have a history or family history of other autoimmune disorders, e.g., diabetes mellitus, pernicious anemia, Addison's disease and myasthenia gravis. The prevalence of insulin-dependent diabetes mellitus is higher in patients with thyroid eye disease than in the normal population. Also, patients with thyroid eye disease and diabetes have a higher incidence of CON, and have a worse recovery of visual function following treatment of the neuropathy. These patients also pose a higher risk of intraoperative and postoperative bleeding.

Myasthenia is 50 times more common in patients with thyroid eye disease compared with the general population. Patients who develop ptosis or a changing pattern of ocular motility restriction should be investigated for myasthenia.

> **KEY POINT**
>
> Patients who develop ptosis or a changing pattern of ocular motility restriction should be investigated for myasthenia.

Clinical Presentation

The clinical manifestations of thyroid eye disease can be very variable and may be acute or insidious in onset. Patients can be divided into two subtypes.

Type 1

Patients with type 1 or "non-infiltrative" orbitopathy tend to be younger and usually present with symmetric proptosis, eyelid retraction, minimal inflammatory signs, and no extra-ocular muscle restrictions (Fig. 19.4). These clinical features tend to be manifestations of hyperthyroidism and may even regress once the hyperthyroidism has been controlled.

The diagnosis of thyroid eye disease in this subset of patients does not usually present a problem.

Type 2
Patients with type 2 or "infiltrative" orbitopathy are usually middle-aged and run a much more fulminant course. The orbitopathy is likely to be more asymmetric and the patient is likely to present with chemosis, diplopia, and CON (Fig. 19.5).

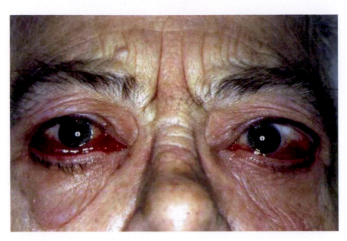

Figure 19.5 An older female patient with type 2 thyroid eye disease.

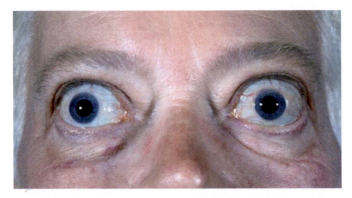

Figure 19.6 A female patient with bilateral proptosis and eyelid retraction.

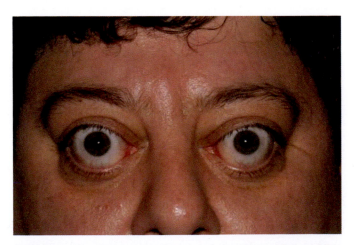

Figure 19.7 Marked bilateral lower lid retraction in a patient with severe bilateral proptosis.

Clinical Symptoms

The symptoms of thyroid eye disease are variable and may be non-specific. They include ocular irritation, a foreign body sensation, tearing, photophobia, diplopia, and visual impairment. Diplopia, when it develops, is usually first noticed either on waking, when tired, or on extremes of gaze. It is sometimes accompanied by aching, particularly on upgaze. Some patients with type 2 orbitopathy complain of a constant deep boring orbital pain unrelated to ocular movements.

Visual complaints such as blurring of vision, which may be patchy or generalized, or disturbances of color perception, occur in only 5% of patients. These complaints may, however, herald the onset of CON, and as the symptoms may not be volunteered by the patient, they should be specifically elicited in the history in all patients.

Patients are also greatly disturbed by changes in their appearance caused by the disease process. Subluxation of the globe is very rare but can be extremely alarming and upsetting for both the patient and witnesses to the event. It is more likely to affect patients with shallow orbits, e.g., black patients.

Clinical Signs

The physical signs are variable and it is very unusual for a patient to present with all of them. The physical signs include:

1. Proptosis
2. Eyelid retraction
3. Eyelid lag
4. Lagophthalmos
5. Periorbital edema
6. Conjunctival and caruncular edema
7. Eyelid erythema
8. Injection of the vessels along the horizontal recti
9. Limitation of ocular motility
10. Exposure keratopathy
11. Glabellar rhytids
12. Superior limbic keratoconjunctivitis
13. Optic disc edema/pallor with signs of optic nerve dysfunction
14. Raised intraocular pressure on attempted upgaze
15. Choroidal folds
16. Globe subluxation
17. Lacrimal gland enlargement/prolapse

It should be noted that these physical signs, with the exception of superior limbic keratoconjunctivitis and glabellar rhytids, may be observed, singly or in combination, in any orbital inflammatory disorder.

> **KEY POINT**
>
> The main physical signs seen in thyroid eye disease may be observed, singly or in combination, in any orbital inflammatory disorder.

The physical signs in thyroid eye disease can alter with subtle remissions and exacerbations.

Thyroid eye disease is the commonest cause of unilateral or bilateral proptosis in an adult (Fig. 19.6).

Proptosis correlates significantly with lower lid retraction (Fig. 19.7). It should be borne in mind, however, that proptosis in a patient with known thyroid dysfunction may have another cause. Patients may have more than one pathology.

The causes of eyelid retraction in thyroid eye disease are discussed in chapter 8. Eyelid retraction is the most frequent sign seen in thyroid eye disease and affects the vast majority of patients at some stage. It frequently varies with attentive gaze (Kocher's sign). If eyelid retraction is absent, it is wise to question the diagnosis. Eyelid retraction may often be accompanied by a lateral flare, an appearance that is almost pathognomonic for thyroid eye disease (Fig. 19.8).

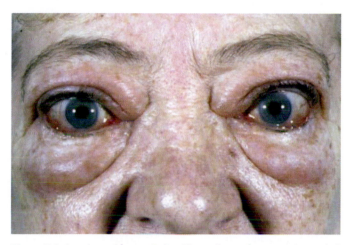

Figure 19.8 A patient with type 2 thyroid eye disease demonstrating typical periorbital edema and lid retraction with lateral flare.

The downward movement of the upper eyelid often lags behind the downward movement of the globe and remains high (lid lag or von Graefe's sign) (Fig. 19.9). Patients with marked proptosis and eyelid retraction are at risk of incomplete reflex or voluntary eyelid closure (lagophthalmos). This can lead to corneal exposure and sight-threatening corneal ulceration, particularly in patients with an absent Bell's phenomenon. The keratopathy can be exacerbated in some patients whose proptosis can also result in a lateral upper eyelid entropion (Fig. 19.10).

Although ptosis can develop in longstanding thyroid eye disease, usually due to a levator aponeurosis dehiscence secondary to marked upper eyelid edema, it is very unusual for patients to present with a ptosis. The presence of a ptosis should raise the suspicion that the patient has a concomitant ocular myasthenia or myasthenia gravis. Likewise, a divergent strabismus is unusual in thyroid eye disease and should again raise the suspicion of myasthenia (Fig. 19.6).

KEY POINT

If upper eyelid retraction is absent, the diagnosis of thyroid eye disease should be questioned.

Periorbital edema is an early sign of thyroid eye disease. The edema is variable and can be particularly prominent in the upper lids and tends to be maximal in the morning, diminishing throughout the day (Fig. 19.8).

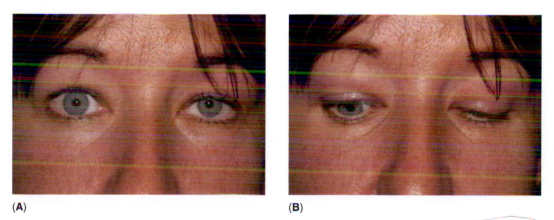

(A)   (B)

Figure 19.9 (A) A patient with right upper eyelid retraction. (B) The patient demonstrating eyelid lag on down gaze.

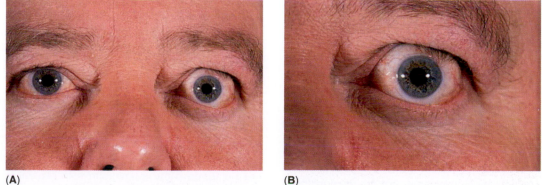

(A)   (B)

Figure 19.10 (A) A left upper eyelid entropion as a consequence of thyroid eye disease. (B) A close-up of the left side demonstrating the upper eyelid entropion with marked upper eyelid retraction, proptosis, and thickening of the sub-brow tissue.

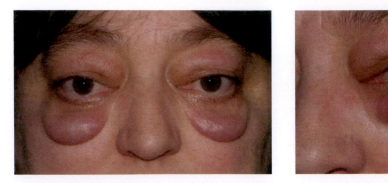

Figure 19.11 Bilateral periorbital edema with lower eyelid festoons.

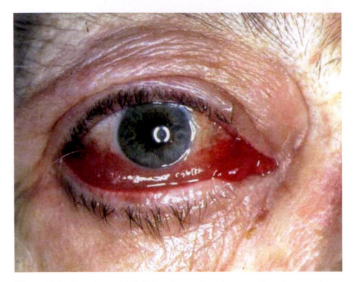

Figure 19.12 A patient with inferior chemosis and caruncular edema and erythema of the upper eyelid.

Periorbital edema should be differentiated from eyelid fat prolapses, which patients often refer to as eyelid swellings.

Subcutaneous fluid pouches, referred to as "festoons," may occur at the junction of the lower eyelids and cheek (Fig. 19.11). Occasionally these may persist for many years after the disease has become inactive.

Caruncular edema may be quite subtle. This, in conjunction with conjunctival chemosis, is a clinical measure of disease activity and response to medical therapy. Chemosis can be very marked in some patients and may interfere with the normal distribution of the tear film (Fig. 19.12). Erythema localized to the eyelids is not uncommon and may persist for many years.

Injection of episcleral vessels occurs along the course of the horizontal recti, which helps to differentiate thyroid eye disease from a local flow arterio-venous shunt (Fig. 19.13).

Ocular motility limitation is often variable and frequently asymmetric (Fig. 19.14). Symmetrical restriction may spare the patient from diplopia but frequently asymmetric progression results in diplopia. The inferior recti followed by the medial recti are the most frequently affected muscles (Figs. 19.14 and 19.15). Vertical diplopia with discomfort and pain that increases on upgaze is most frequently seen. Forced duction testing confirms restriction of motility. A rise in intraocular pressure may be noted on upgaze. It is important not to overlook the possibility of myasthenia gravis as a cause of a changing or unusual ocular deviation in a patient with thyroid eye disease.

Exposure keratopathy can occur due to:

1. Severe proptosis
2. Eyelid retraction with lagophthalmos
3. Conjunctival chemosis causing dellen formation

All corneal signs are secondary phenomena of thyroid eye disease. A widened palpebral aperture results in more rapid tear evaporation, which, in combination with incomplete eyelid closure, results in superficial punctuate erosions and the symptoms of superficial ocular irritation. These symptoms in turn cause the patient to overuse the corrugator supericilii and procerus muscles with the development of marked glabellar rhytids (Fig. 19.15). Corneal thinning, scarring or frank ulceration can occur resulting in severe visual morbidity (Fig. 19.16).

Superior limbic keratoconjunctivitis is a non-specific ocular lesion which has no known cause but is frequently associated with thyroid eye disease when present bilaterally (Fig. 19.17).

In patients with a restrictive myopathy, the intraocular pressure (IOP) may rise on attempted upgaze. The diagnosis of primary open angle glaucoma (POAG) in patients with thyroid eye disease should be made with caution as an increased IOP may simply be the result of a slight elevation of the eyes forced by the head posture required for applanation tonometry. The increase in IOP when looking upward is common in patients with thyroid eye disease, and it does not cause glaucoma more often than in the general population.

CON can occur as an insidious complication of thyroid eye disease, often occurring in patients without marked proptosis and often in the absence of any fundoscopic abnormalities. Only a small percentage of patients demonstrate optic disc edema. The incidence of optic neuropathy in patients with thyroid eye disease is approximately 4% to 5%. A high index of suspicion for its development should be maintained when examining patients with thyroid eye disease. In general patients with a more severe myopathy pose the greatest risk for the development of CON.

KEY POINT

Compressive optic neuropathy (CON) can occur as an insidious complication of thyroid eye disease, often occurring in patients without marked proptosis and often in the absence of any fundoscopic abnormalities. In general patients with a more severe myopathy pose the greatest risk for the development of CON.

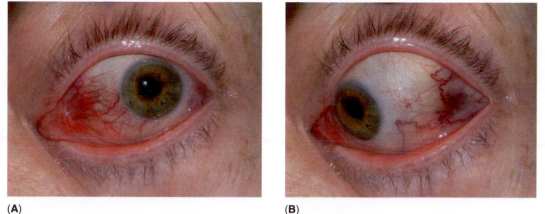

(A)   (B)

Figure 19.13 Injection limited to the horizontal recti.

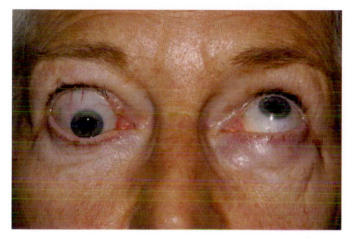

Figure 19.14 A patient with inactive thyroid eye disease showing marked restriction of upgaze of the right eye with secondary eyelid retraction.

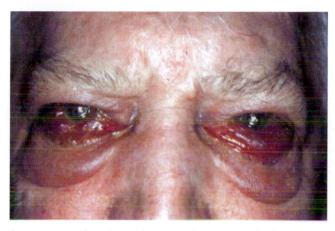

Figure 19.16 A male patient with severe infiltrative thyroid orbitopathy and a bilateral "malignant exophthalmos." He has severe lagophthalmos and exposure keratopathy.

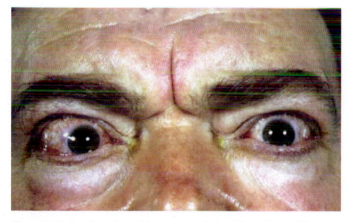

Figure 19.15 A male patient with severe type 2 thyroid eye disease. The severity of the myopathy should alert his clinicians to the possibility of an insidious compressive optic neuropathy. He also demonstrates a typical contraction of the procerus and corrugator supercilii muscles with marked glabellar rhytids creating a very aggressive appearance.

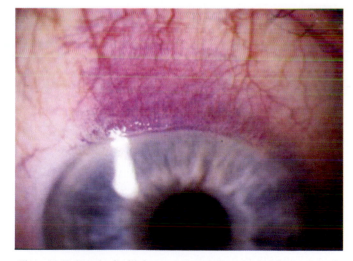

Figure 19.17 Superior limbic keratoconjunctivitis stained with Rose Bengal.

Choroidal folds are seen very rarely (Fig. 19.18). They are thought to develop when the globe is mechanically deformed by the secondary effects of extraocular muscle enlargement in a confined bony space.

Subluxation of the globe is a distressing situation for a patient where the eyes are so protrusive that they may prolapse out of the orbit especially on attempting to look up. The eyelids may close behind the eye (Fig. 19.19). Such patients are naturally reluctant to look up during examination of their ocular motility. Great care should be taken during the use of an exophthalmometer as this can

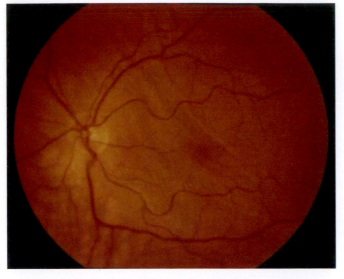

Figure 19.18 Choroidal folds in a patient with thyroid eye disease.

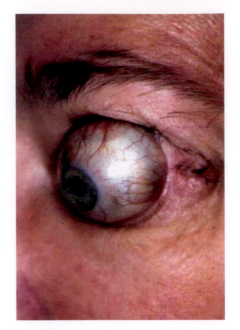

Figure 19.19 Subluxation of the globe in a patient who has previously undergone an inappropriate lateral tarsorrhaphy.

also provoke a globe subluxation. If subluxation should occur the globe should be manually repositioned immediately.

Lacrimal gland enlargement may also be seen in some patients, and, particularly in patients with shallow orbits and extreme degrees of proptosis, the glands may prolapse (Fig. 19.20).

Patient Evaluation

In the majority of patients with thyroid eye disease, there is no difficulty in establishing the diagnosis, as there is a prior history of thyroid dysfunction or characteristic clinical findings. In patients with no prior history of thyroid dysfunction, thyroid function tests are performed along with antibody studies. The diagnosis can be particularly difficult to establish in the small percentage of patients who present with no prior history of a thyroid disorder or who demonstrate no abnormality of thyroid function. The assistance of an endocrinologist should be sought in the evaluation and management of all patients with suspected thyroid eye disease.

When evaluating a patient referred with thyroid eye disease, it is important to address two initial questions.

1. Is the diagnosis of thyroid eye disease correct?
2. Does the patient show any evidence of sight-threatening disease?

A thorough and detailed clinical history should be taken. Patients should be examined repeatedly and thoroughly with a special emphasis on tests of optic nerve function:

- The patient's best corrected visual acuity should be measured and recorded in each eye along with any refractive error.
- The pupil responses should be carefully assessed looking for the presence of a relative afferent pupil defect.
- The patient's color vision should be tested. Testing in the blue/yellow axis is far more sensitive and more likely to detect early color vision defects associated with CON. Red/green pseudo-isochromatic charts, e.g., Ishihara color plates, are

more readily available in clinics and remain very useful. Each eye should be tested separately using good illumination. the patient should wear his/her reading glasses to undertake the test. This assumes that the patient does not suffer from color blindness. In such patients visual-evoked potentials (VEP) can be used. The pattern reversal VEP is very sensitive at detecting early CON and may also be a useful means of following patients after treatment.

- The patient should undergo automated perimetry. Characteristically, a central scotoma or an inferior altitudinal defect is seen in patients with CON. Other visual field defects include an enlarged blind spot, paracentral scotomata, nerve fiber bundle defects, or a generalized constriction.
- Careful fundoscopy should be undertaken looking for optic disc swelling or choroidal folds.
- The patient's proptosis should be measured using a Hertel exophthalmometer.
- The patient's palpebral apertures should be measured.
- The patient's levator function should be measured.
- The degree of lid lag on down gaze and the degree of lagophthalmos on passive eyelid closure should be recorded.
- An orthoptic evaluation should be undertaken, recording the patient's ocular motility restrictions, the field of binocular single vision and a Hess chart. A pre-existing strabismus will inevitably complicate this assessment.
- Pain on ocular motility should be documented.
- All inflammatory signs should be recorded.
- The corneas should be carefully examined for signs of exposure keratopathy.

Bilateral lacrimal gland
enlargement and prolapse

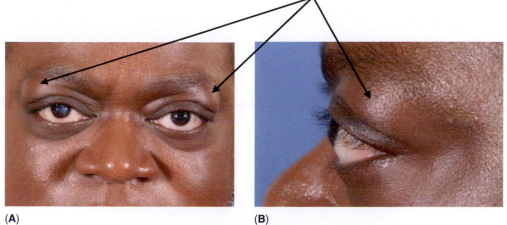

(A)   (B)

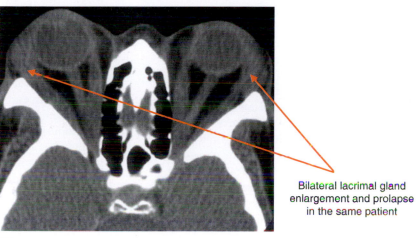

Bilateral lacrimal gland
enlargement and prolapse
in the same patient

(C)

Figure 19.20 (**A**) A black patient with thyroid eye disease. She shows right corneal scarring from a previous corneal hydrops and bilateral lacrimal gland enlargement and prolapse. (**B**) The patient is seen in profile showing marked proptosis. (**C**) The axial CT scan confirms marked bilateral proptosis, shallow orbits, moderate enlargement of the horizontal recti, and enlargement and prolapse of the lacrimal glands.

- The intraocular pressure should be measured, both in the primary position, down gaze and upgaze.
- Clinical photographs should be taken as a baseline assessment for later comparison.

In the evaluation of patients with thyroid eye disease two additional aspects should be considered:

1. The *activity* of the disease
2. The *severity* of the disease

During the course of thyroid eye disease, the disease process passes through several phases. The initial phase involves worsening symptoms and signs with orbital inflammation, followed by a plateau phase during which the symptoms and signs become stable. A phase of gradual spontaneous improvement follows until eventually no further change occurs, although permanent abnormalities of both ocular function and cosmetic appearance may remain. These phases, however, vary greatly in duration from patient to patient. The typical course of thyroid eye disease in patients receiving no specific treatment, except that to control thyroid dysfunction, was first described by Rundle in 1957.

Severity of thyroid eye disease

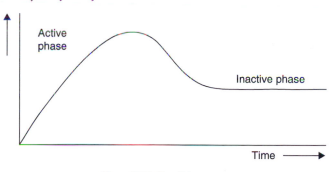
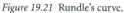

Figure 19.21 Rundle's curve.

He depicted this in a graph, which is known as Rundle's curve (Fig. 19.21).

The activity of the disease is determined clinically by the patient's soft tissue symptoms and signs. It can also be determined by a "STIR" sequence (short Tau inversion recovery) MRI scan that suppresses the normal bright signal form orbital fat on T-1 weighted images.

The severity of thyroid eye disease describes the degree to which ocular function or the patient's cosmetic appearance is affected. The severity is determined by assessing the effect of the disease on:

1. Optic nerve function
2. Ocular motility
3. The cornea
4. The position of the eyelids
5. The position of the globe
6. The patient's cosmetic appearance

Determining the activity and severity of thyroid eye disease at each clinical assessment is fundamental to formulating a management plan, which is tailored to the individual needs of the patient.

A number of classifications of the ophthalmic changes in thyroid eye disease have been described in an attempt to quantify the orbitopathy. The classification by Werner was frequently used because of the easily remembered mnemonic "NOSPECS." "NOSPECS" refers to: *No* physical signs or symptoms, *Only* signs, *Soft* tissue involvement, *Proptosis*, *Extraocular* muscle involvement, *Corneal* involvement, and *Sight* loss. Although widely used, there are many difficulties in applying this and other classifications. The preferred classification is that of Mourits et al. who devised the clinical activity score (CAS) in 1989 (Table 19.1). This scoring system allows patients to be classified as either active or inactive although some clinical features may reflect orbital congestion rather than inflammation. It indicates the position of the patient on Rundle's curve. Although no scoring system is perfect, "NOSPECS" remains a useful reminder of the clinical features which should be assessed.

Classification of Severity of Thyroid Eye Disease
It is useful to classify the severity of disease in an individual patient to assist in the decision as to whether or not the patient should be subjected to treatments which carry risks. Patient can be divided into three major categories:

1. Mild
2. Moderate
3. Severe

The High Risk Patient
The following patients are at an increased risk of developing severe orbitopathy and CON:

- Male patients
- Patients over 55 years of age
- Diabetic patients
- Smokers
- Patients treated with radioactive iodine

Orbital Imaging
Orbital CT
A computerized tomography (CT) scan of the orbit is a quick, readily available, and relatively cheap investigation. It is the initial orbital imaging technique of choice in the patient with thyroid eye disease but, because of concerns about radiation exposure, it should not be used repeatedly.

CT scanning of the orbit and paranasal sinuses should be performed in both axial and coronal planes. (Modern CT techniques now permit coronal sections without requiring the

Table 19.1 Clinical Activity Score (CAS)
1. Spontaneous orbital pain
2. Gaze evoked orbital pain
3. Eyelid swelling due to active disease
4. Eyelid erythema
5. Conjunctival injection due to active disease
6. Chemosis
7. Inflammation of caruncle or plica
8. Increase of 2 mm or more in proptosis
9. Decrease in uniocular excursion in any one direction of > 8°
10. Decrease in visual acuity equivalent to 1 Snellen line
One point is given for each feature.

patient to extend the neck.) It has an important role in the evaluation of the patient with thyroid eye disease.

a. It can assist in determining the cause of decreased visual function by demonstrating orbital apical muscle enlargement and a "and a crowded orbital apex."
b. It can assist in excluding other mimicking orbital disorders or dual pathology (Figs. 19.24 and 19.25).
c. It provides an evaluation of the size of the orbits and the size and status of the paranasal sinuses.
d. It demonstrates the true extent of the patient's proptosis.
e. It assesses the relative contributions of extraocular muscle enlargement versus orbital fat enlargement to the patient's proptosis.
f. A coronal view demonstrates the position of the cribriform plate and its relationship to the fronto-ethmoidal suture line (Fig. 19.22).

A crowded orbital apex is demonstrated well on coronal sections. The imaging assists in making the diagnosis of CON. The diagnosis is not, however, made from the imaging alone.

It is important to exclude an additional pathological process as a cause of proptosis, particularly with asymmetric disease.

An axial scan can demonstrate the true extent of the proptosis and the relationship of the globe to the anterior bony opening of the orbit. Extreme stretching of the optic nerve may be seen and can represent another mechanism for optic neuropathy (Fig. 19.1B).

If a patient requires an orbital decompression, a preoperative CT scan is essential and should be available for examination in the operating room during surgery. The type of orbital decompression required by the individual patient is largely determined by the CT scan appearances. It is important to be aware of the proximity of the cribriform plate to the fronto-ethmoidal suture line (Fig. 19.22). Patients with a low cribriform plate and a narrow fovea ethmoidalis are at greater risk of intraoperative damage to the cribriform plate and a subsequent cerebrospinal fluid (CSF) leak.

It is important to be aware that enlargement of the inferior rectus muscle in thyroid eye disease can be mistaken for an orbital apical mass on an axial CT scan, particularly in patients with unilateral proptosis (Fig. 19.23). The true cause of the patient's proptosis is readily seen on coronal views.

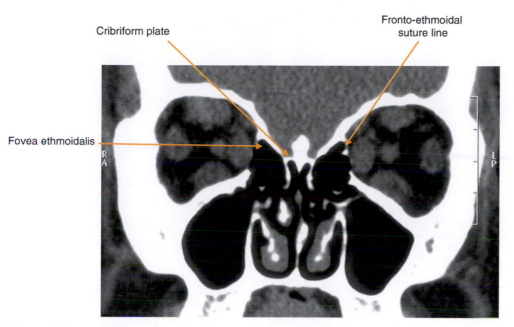

Figure 19.22 A coronal CT scan demonstrating extra-ocular muscle enlargement. The ethmoid sinuses are clear with plenty of room between the cribriform plate and the fronto-ethmoidal suture line but the very low position of the cribriform plate in this patient should be noted.

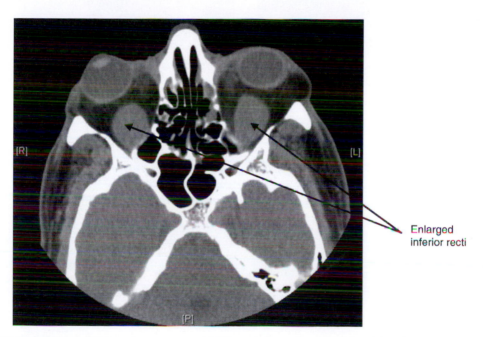

Figure 19.23 Bilateral orbital apical "masses." This appearance on an axial CT scan is due to the angle of the axial section cutting across enlarged inferior rectus muscles. The scan also demonstrates shallow orbits and the true extent of this patient's severe bilateral proptosis.

Patients at risk of developing CON may also show a dilated superior ophthalmic vein, and an anterior displacement of the lacrimal gland. A herniation of fat through the superior orbital fissure into the middle cranial fossa can sometimes be seen.

Orbital MRI

MRI gives a better resolution of orbital soft tissues and does not expose the patient to radiation risks. It is however costly, lengthy to perform and not as readily available. An MRI scan is useful to determine the activity of the disease by assessing the signal from the extraocular muscles prior to committing the patient to corticosteroids, radiotherapy or anti-metabolite agents. An "STIR" sequence with fat suppression is particularly useful.

Orbital Ultrasound

Ultrasound has the advantage of being non-invasive and easily repeatable but it has low inter-observer reproducibility and it does not allow visualization of the orbital apex. Its role in the assessment of the patient with thyroid eye disease is very limited.

DIFFERENTIAL DIAGNOSIS

Orbital disorders that may mimic thyroid eye disease in their clinical presentation produce inflammation and infiltration of the orbital muscles (Fig. 19.24). None of the eye signs are specific to thyroid eye disease. These disorders include:

1. Non-specific orbital inflammatory syndrome
2. Arterio-venous shunts

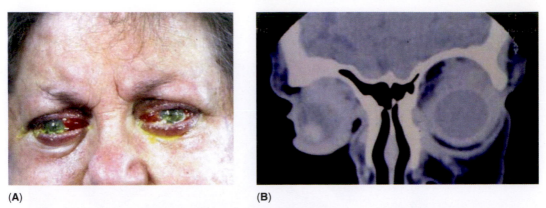

(A)   (B)

Figure 19.24 (**A**) A female patient with hyperthyroidism who presented with bilateral visual loss and diplopia. A diagnosis of severe thyroid orbitopathy had been made by her general ophthalmologist. She developed severe exposure keratopathy while undergoing orbital radiotherapy. (**B**) A coronal CT scan of the same patient demonstrated bilateral infiltrating orbital masses. A biopsy confirmed the diagnosis of metastatic breast carcinoma.

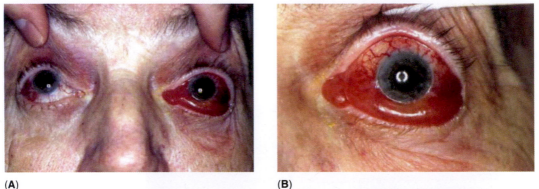

(A)   (B)

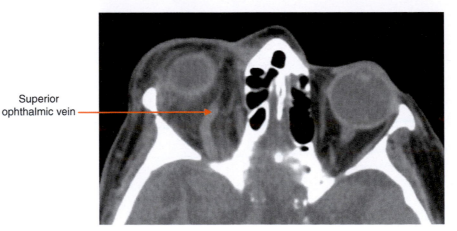

(C)

Figure 19.25 (**A**) A patient with a low flow arterio-venous shunt. (**B**) A close-up photograph of the left eye demonstrating chemosis and enlargement of the episcleral vessels. (**C**) An axial CT scan showing a grossly dilated superior ophthalmic vein.

3. Extraocular muscle metastases
4. Wegener's granulomatosis
5. Sarcoidosis
6. Amyloidosis
7. Collagen vascular diseases.

Most of these disorders should be readily differentiated on the basis of the history, clinical appearances, and imaging characteristics, e.g., an orbital myositis is usually painful, and does not spare the tendon of insertion of the extraocular muscle(s) on orbital imaging in contrast to the myopathy of thyroid eye disease.

A low flow arterio-venous shunt can, however, create diagnostic confusion as this can cause a diffuse enlargement of the extraocular muscles as seen on orbital imaging, along with conjunctival chemosis (Fig. 19.25A and B). Distension of the episcleral vessels is not, however, confined to those over the horizontal recti, and the superior ophthalmic vein, unless thrombosed, is dilated. This is best seen on axial CT scan images (Fig. 19.25C).

KEY POINT

It should be borne in mind that patients with thyroid dysfunction can develop other orbital disorders. An open mind should always be maintained and the diagnosis questioned.

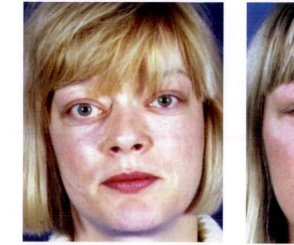
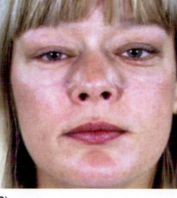

(A)

(B)

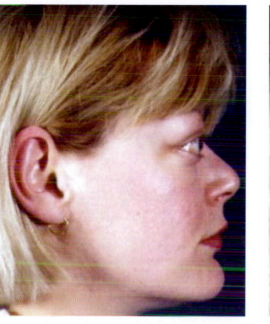
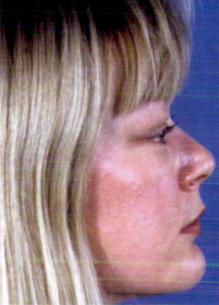

(C)

(D)

Figure 19.26 A patient before (**A,C**) and after (**B,D**) a bilateral 3 wall transeyelid orbital decompression procedure performed for cosmetic rehabilitation.

Management

The goals in the management of the patient with thyroid eye disease are to:

a. Resolve or control the orbital inflammation
b. Prevent visual loss
c. Re-establish ocular muscle balance
d. Provide cosmetic rehabilitation

In attempting to achieve these goals the patient should be placed at minimum risk of complications. It is important to identify and treat patients who are at particular risk of sight threatening complications as early as possible. It is important to involve an endocrinologist in the patient's management and to communicate effectively. Good control of thyroid function is imperative:

a. There is a relationship between the severity of hyperthyroidism and the severity of the orbitopathy.
b. The patient's thyroid disorder must be under good control prior to any surgery.

Many of the ophthalmic consequences of mild thyroid eye disease can be managed conservatively, e.g., the patient's head should be elevated when sleeping, topical lubricants should be prescribed and dark glasses used to improve photophobia. The patient should be kept under regular review to ensure that the disease does not progress to a more severe stage. The patient should be advised about the adverse effects of smoking. The majority of such patients will experience spontaneous improvement over the course of 3 to 6 months.

The management options for moderate or severe disease should be discussed carefully with the patient. Sight-threatening disease, however, should be treated urgently. In the absence of sight-threatening disease, treatment is not obligatory, but should be considered carefully, weighing up the pros and cons, risks, and potential complications of treatment. The decision to treat and the modality selected depends on an assessment of disease activity. During the active phase of thyroid eye disease, immune-suppression with steroids with the possible addition of an anti-metabolite agent, e.g., azathioprine, orbital irradiation, or the combination of the two, are likely to be beneficial.

If the disease process has entered the inactive phase, rehabilitative surgical intervention may be required. In more severe cases, multiple surgical interventions may be required over a long period of time.

Medical Management

The aim of medical management is to avoid surgery if at all possible or to minimize the orbital inflammation in order to optimize the outcome of surgery.

Medical treatment consists of

    a. Immuno-suppressive therapy-corticosteroids, anti-metabolites
    b. Radiotherapy

Immuno-suppressive therapy is used for two groups of patients:

    1. Patients with severe acute inflammatory orbital disease
    2. Patients with CON

The beneficial effect of both intravenous methylprednisolone therapy as well as high dose oral prednisolone in patients with active and moderately severe thyroid eye disease has been proven, and therefore systemic steroid treatment is evidence based.

Patients with acute inflammatory eye disease typically respond very quickly to steroids but maintenance doses frequently lead to steroid complications. Patients with chronic inactive disease do not respond to corticosteroids or alternative medical therapy.

The therapeutic threshold for CON is very high with some patients requiring corticosteroid doses in excess of 100 mg per day. Pulsed intravenous methylprednisolone acetate, 1.0 g daily for 3 days given on an in-patient basis, arrests the congestive orbital disease process more quickly. In some patients, the orbitopathy abates and the patient can be successfully weaned off steroids without the need for further treatment. In others, steroid will fail to control the optic neuropathy and orbital decompression surgery is required to prevent visual loss.

It should be borne in mind, however, that acute and severe liver damage has been reported during pulsed intravenous methylprednisolone treatment. This has resulted in a small number of deaths. Patients should be very carefully selected for this treatment and should be very carefully monitored during and after their treatment by their endocrinologist. They should be screened for any liver disease prior to the commencement of this treatment. The total cumulative dose of intravenous methylprednisolone should not exceed 6 g.

Although the retrobulbar injection of steroids has not been proven to be as effective as systemic steroid therapy, it has been used by some clinicians in an attempt to treat the orbital inflammation locally while minimizing systemic side effects. The treatment does, however, carry the added risk of orbital hemorrhage or direct injury to the globe.

Anti-metabolite drugs, e.g., azathioprine, may be used in conjunction with steroids as steroid sparing agents. This reduces the steroid side effects but exposes the patient to the risks of further immuno-suppression. Patients have to be closely and carefully monitored by their physician. These drugs should not be used on their own.

Radiotherapy also has been proven to improve ocular motility disturbance in patients with active disease. There is now good evidence that the combination of radiotherapy and steroid treatment in patients with early active thyroid eye disease is more beneficial than when these therapies are used alone. This combination exploits the more rapid action of steroids and the more persistent effects of radiotherapy. It has not been proven to have any beneficial effects in reducing proptosis or treating CON. Indeed, radiotherapy temporarily exacerbates orbital inflammation.

Radiotherapy is focused on the posterior orbit, sparing the globe and has a low morbidity. It should not be used, however, in patients with diabetes and severe hypertension, or in patients under the age of 35 (due to the long latency of radiation-induced tumors). Patients must be monitored very closely following radiotherapy treatment.

KEY POINT

It is extremely important to be aware of the potential serious systemic side effects of the use of corticosteroids and anti-metabolites, e.g., aseptic necrosis of the femoral head, osteoporosis, pathological fractures, duodenal ulceration with gastrointestinal hemorrhage, secondary diabetes mellitus, cataracts, glaucoma, and predisposition to opportunistic infection. Patients should be carefully warned about the risks. Patients must be monitored very closely and in conjunction with an endocrinologist who can monitor for and treat osteoporosis. Patients should also be warned about the potential for adrenocortical insufficiency associated with steroid treatment and the need for supplemental steroid treatment in the event of trauma, surgery or acquired infection.

Patients being treated with steroids should receive supplements to protect against osteoporosis and pathological fractures. They should have their weight, blood glucose, and blood pressure closely monitored.

Other agents, e.g., Rituximab, a chimeric monoclonal antibody against the protein CD20, which is primarily found on the surface of B cells, are being investigated for their potential role in the medical management of patients with acute thyroid eye disease. Selenium may also play a future role in the management of mild to moderate disease.

Surgical Management

Surgical intervention should be approached in a specific sequence. Decompressive surgery may alter ocular muscle balance, and ocular muscle surgery may alter eyelid position. Surgery is therefore performed in a sequence recognizing that not all patients require surgery of each stage but may omit various stages. The order of surgical intervention is therefore:

    1. Orbital decompression
    2. Strabismus surgery
    3. Eyelid repositioning surgery
    4. Blepharoplasty

In some cases, however, a lower eyelid blepharoplasty may be performed in conjunction with an orbital decompression depending on the surgical approach.

A patient with reduced orbital compliance, who demonstrates resistance to simple retropulsion of the globe, will gain much less effect from any orbital decompression procedure than a patient with the same degree of proptosis who has normal orbital compliance.

Strabismus and eyelid repositioning surgery should preferably be deferred until the clinical signs are stable. Surgical intervention may, however, have to be performed urgently for severe corneal exposure or for CON unresponsive to medical therapy.

Patients must understand the possible requirement for multiple surgical procedures, which may take some considerable time to complete. Such patients need to be counseled very carefully in order to ensure that their expectations are realistic.

Surgical Orbital Decompression

The cardinal indication for surgical decompression remains CON but, as decompressive surgery continues to evolve, the indications have become far less conservative.

Indications
1. CON unresponsive to medical treatment
2. Recurrent subluxation of the globe
3. Severe proptosis with exposure keratopathy
4. Cosmetic rehabilitation of unsightly proptosis
5. Constant boring orbital pain unresponsive to medical treatment
6. Reduction of proptosis prior to extraocular muscle recessions

Surgery may be urgent for the management of CON or severe exposure keratopathy or elective for the remaining indications. In general, surgery for the management of CON should be undertaken only after initial medical intervention.

Some patients have constant aching orbital pain due to congestion of the orbital tissues. This can be relieved by a decompression procedure in the majority of cases.

In some patients with marked proptosis, the degree of proptosis may worsen following extraocular muscle surgery undertaken to improve diplopia. In such patients, a decompression operation may be considered desirable prior to such extraocular muscle surgery.

Decompressive surgery is being requested more and more frequently to improve the aesthetic appearance of patients as the surgical results and safety of the surgery have improved considerably over recent years. Such surgery should be regarded as "rehabilitative" rather than "cosmetic" (Fig. 19.26). There is no doubt that the changes in appearance caused by thyroid eye disease can have a devastating psychological effect on patients and such surgery can achieve significant improvements. The goal is to restore the appearance to that which existed prior to the onset of this disease process. However, such goals are rarely achieved completely and patients must be counseled very carefully preoperatively to ensure that they have realistic expectations. They should also be warned about the risks and potential complications of such surgery.

Surgical Approaches

The orbit may be decompressed by:

1. Reducing the orbital contents (removal of orbital fat)
2. Expanding the orbital volume (removing orbital walls/advancing the lateral orbital wall).

These decompression procedures can be used in isolation or in combination.

Orbital Fat Removal

Removal of orbital fat may achieve a satisfactory reduction in proptosis in a patient without significant enlargement of the extraocular muscles who has no resistance to retropulsion of the globe clinically. This can be performed alone or it can be used to gain an additional decompressive effect in patients undergoing a bony decompression. The fat may be removed in combination with an upper and/or lower eyelid blepharoplasty. The surgical approach is transcutaneous in the upper eyelid. In the lower eyelid, it may be transcutaneous or transconjunctival. Better surgical exposure for removal of inferolateral orbital fat is achieved if a transconjunctival approach is combined with a lateral canthotomy and inferior cantholysis (a "swinging lower eyelid flap" approach).

The removal of orbital fat demands extreme care and patience to avoid inadvertent damage to other intraorbital structures. Respect must be paid to meticulous hemostasis. The fat is gently teased out with gentle dissection of the delicate orbital septa. The amount of fat which can be safely removed varies from 2 to 6 ml (Fig. 19.27).

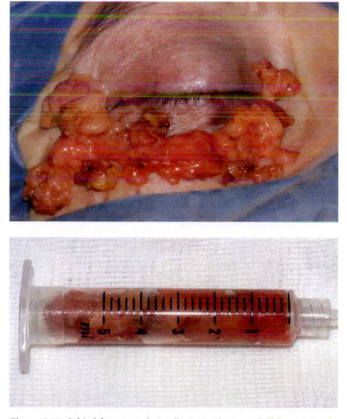

Figure 19.27 Orbital fat removed via a "swinging lower eyelid" flap approach.

Hemostasis is facilitated by the use of a Colorado needle used on constant coagulation mode. Bipolar cautery is applied to larger vessels as these appear, and before they bleed. Good retraction by an assistant is essential. The pupil should be monitored throughout the surgery and any pressure on the globe released at intervals. *The patient's vision must be monitored very closely postoperatively* if no bony orbital decompression has been performed as postoperative orbital bleeding may occur and cause a retrobulbar hematoma with optic nerve compression.

Advantages
1. This approach avoids the risk of inferior displacement of the globe
2. There is no risk of injury to structures external to the periorbita, e.g., the dura, the lacrimal sac, the infraorbital nerve
3. The surgical incisions are minimal
4. The postoperative recovery is rapid
5. It can further improve the reduction in proptosis achieved by surgery on the orbital walls

Disadvantages
1. The surgery is time consuming
2. It risks damage to delicate intraorbital structures
3. Postoperative bleeding can jeopardize vision when fat is removed alone

Increasing Orbital Volume
Over the years all four walls of the orbit have been resected, singly or in combination, for the purposes of orbital decompression. There is no longer any indication for surgery to be performed on the orbital roof. Patients should not be merely subjected to the surgeon's favorite operation for orbital decompression. The choice of decompressive procedure should be tailored to the individual patient's needs based on the following:

1. The indication(s) for the surgery
2. The patient's age and general health
3. The size and status of the paranasal sinuses
4. The size of the orbits
5. The size of the globe
6. The amount of proptosis
7. The relative contributions of extraocular muscle enlargement versus orbital fat swelling to proptosis
8. The orbital compliance

A medial orbital wall decompression may be performed in isolation in patients who have a CON but only a moderate degree of proptosis. Likewise a lateral orbital wall decompression may be performed in isolation in patients who require a modest improvement in proptosis. It is preferable to balance the medial wall decompression with a lateral wall decompression.

Unless a large decompression is required for severe proptosis, the orbital floor should be maintained intact to avoid the risk of a postoperative hypoglobus with potential worsening of any upper eyelid retraction, and postoperative anesthesia in the distribution of the infraorbital nerve. If the orbital floor needs to be decompressed a medial bony strut should be maintained between the medial orbital wall and the orbital floor decompression to reduce the risk of a postoperative esotropia or frank medial globe dystopia. Also, if removal of the orbital floor is required, this should be conservative leaving the central floor intact and avoiding any damage to the infraorbital neurovascular bundle.

KEY POINT
Surgery for compressive optic neuropathy (CON) should provide adequate relief of orbital apical compression.

The lateral orbital wall can be removed and advanced with the use of titanium plates and screws or the lateral wall can undergo a valgus rotation and be maintained in place with the placement of titanium screws. Such procedures are very rarely required.

It should be borne in mind that proptosis improves over the course of 12 to 18 months from the time of orbital decompression, particularly when the patient has active inflammation at the time of surgery. For this reason, overly aggressive orbital decompression should be avoided in such patients.

The bony walls can be accessed in a variety of ways. Each of these approaches has its advantages and disadvantages.

1. Via a nasal endoscopic approach
2. Via a lower eyelid transconjunctival incision ("swinging eyelid" flap approach)
3. Via a lower eyelid subciliary or skin crease incision
4. Via a transcaruncular approach
5. Via an inferior fornix approach
6. Via a medial canthal ("Lynch") skin incision
7. Via a lateral canthal/lateral orbitotomy/upper eyelid incision
8. Via a bicoronal flap approach
9. Via a transantral (Caldwell Luc) approach

APPLIED ANATOMY
It is important for any surgeon who wishes to undertake a bony orbital decompression to have a sound knowledge of the anatomy of the paranasal sinuses (see chap. 2).

Bony Orbital Decompression - Surgical Approaches
1. Nasal Endoscopic Approach
This approach is normally utilized by an ENT surgeon who has expertise in endoscopic sinus surgery. The approach may also be used by the orbital surgeon, in conjunction with an eyelid incision approach, to assist safe orbital apical bone removal in patients with a congested orbit and severe proptosis.

Advantages
1. There is no requirement for a skin or conjunctival incision
2. The operation can be performed quickly in experienced hands
3. An excellent view of the most posterior medial orbital wall can be obtained
4. It obviates the need for retraction on the globe intraoperatively

Disadvantages
1. The middle turbine may have to be sacrificed to proceed with the surgery losing its important physiological function
2. The infraorbital neurovascular bundle cannot be protected easily during removal of the medial part of the orbital floor
3. This approach alone cannot be combined with a lateral orbital wall decompression without resorting to a skin or conjunctival incision. If a balanced decompression is required to reduce the risks of postoperative diplopia, or to achieve a greater degree of orbital decompression, many of the advantages of an endoscopic approach are removed
4. This approach requires expensive equipment
5. This approach does not permit the safe removal of any orbital fat

The endoscopic approach avoids the need for any skin incisions and is excellent for access to the orbital apex in patients with CON. It offers a major advantage in the following group of patients

1. Those with severe proptosis and a "tight" orbit
2. Patients with high myopia
3. Patients with cardiovascular disease
4. Patients with peripheral corneal thinning

These patients pose problems with access to the medial orbital wall and the orbital apex. The view may be difficult. Retraction of the globe may temporarily close to the central retinal artery with the attendant risks in the patient with cardiovascular disease. Patients with peripheral corneal thinning from chronic exposure keratopathy, or scleral thinning from high myopia, pose a risk of globe rupture with aggressive retraction by a surgical assistant.

2. The Lower Eyelid Approach
The eyelid approach leaves a cosmetically excellent scar (or no visible scar with a transconjunctival incision) and permits access to the medial and lateral walls and the orbital floor. If necessary, it can be used in conjunction with an endoscope to gain an excellent view of the most posterior aspect of the medial orbital wall. Orbital fat can be safely removed via this approach. The surgery can be performed bilaterally or unilaterally depending on the patient's individual circumstances. Patients undergoing such surgery are usually in hospital for only one night.

Lower Eyelid Transconjunctival Approach
This approach, which obviates the need for a skin incision, is used by some surgeons and is analogous to the approach used for a transconjunctival blepharoplasty.

Advantages
1. There is no visible scar
2. The surgical approach is familiar to the oculoplastic surgeon who performs transconjunctival blepharoplasties
3. The approach permits access to three orbital walls through the same incision

4. The approach permits the removal of orbital fat to supplement the effect of the decompression
5. The approach can be combined with a lower eyelid blepharoplasty with removal of extraconal fat

Disadvantages
1. The surgical access is quite restricted and the view of the orbital apex is difficult

This approach is ideal for the patient who has plenty of extraconal fat, marked lower lid fat pad prolapses, and who requires a minimal bony decompression

Lower Eyelid Subciliary or Skin Crease Incision
This incision permits good access, in the majority of patients, to the medial orbital wall and its apex, to the floor of the orbit but does not permit as good a degree of access to the lateral wall of the orbit as the "swinging eyelid flap" approach.

Advantages
1. The surgical approach is familiar to the oculoplastic surgeon who performs transcutaneous blepharoplasties
2. The approach permits access to 3 orbital walls through the same incision
3. The approach permits the removal of orbital fat to supplement the effect of the bony decompression
4. The approach can be combined with a lower eyelid blepharoplasty with removal of excess skin and muscle as well as extraconal fat
5. For the younger female patient who does not require a lower eyelid blepharoplasty, the surgical scar is unobtrusive and does not extend into the lateral canthal skin

Disadvantages
1. The lower eyelid may retract postoperatively unless the patient complies with postoperative eyelid massage
2. The view of the orbital apex may be obscured if there is inadvertent premature opening of the periorbita
3. The view of the orbital apex can be difficult in the patient with a "tight" orbit or high axial myopia

Lower Eyelid Transconjunctival Incision with Lateral Canthotomy and Inferior Cantholysis ("swinging eyelid flap" approach)
This approach is commonly used by many orbital surgeons.

Advantages
1. A cutaneous scar is confined to the lateral canthus
2. The approach to the orbital walls can be achieved quickly
3. The approach permits access to the whole of three orbital walls through the same incision
4. The approach permits the removal of orbital fat to supplement the effect of the bony decompression
5. The approach can be combined with a lower eyelid blepharoplasty with removal of extraconal fat

Disadvantages
1. The approach is associated with more postoperative chemosis and discomfort particularly at the lateral canthus
2. The view of the orbital apex may be obscured if there is inadvertent premature opening of the periorbita
3. The view of the orbital apex can be difficult in the patient with a "tight" orbit or high myopia
4. A lateral canthal dystopia can occur if the lateral canthal repair is not undertaken meticulously

3. Medial Canthal ("Lynch") Skin Incision

This approach offers no advantages over alternative approaches and has significant disadvantages, e.g., a visible obtrusive scar prone to "bow stringing." It necessitates the removal of the medial canthal tendon with a risk of postoperative medial canthal dystopia, and the division of the ethmoidal arteries. Such manoeuvers are unnecessary in alternative approaches.

4. Lateral Canthal/Lateral Orbitotomy/Upper Eyelid Incision

These incisions permit access to the lateral orbital wall particularly in cases where a formal lateral orbitotomy and an advancement/valgus rotation of the lateral wall are required for more extreme degrees of proptosis. An extended upper eyelid crease incision can give good access to the lateral orbital wall and can be combined with a transcaruncular approach to the medial wall with good results for moderate degrees of proptosis.

5. Bicoronal Flap Approach

A bicoronal flap is a much more invasive operation that, in an era of small incision surgery, has very few indications.

Advantages
1. The approach affords good access to the medial wall, lateral wall and lateral portion of the floor of the orbit
2. It permits reduction of the procerus and corrugator supercilii muscles responsible for marked glabellar frown lines in patients with thyroid eye disease
3. The surgical scar is hidden behind the hairline

Disadvantages
1. It has to be combined with other incisions to afford good access to the whole of the orbital floor
2. It requires a greater amount of operating room time
3. It commits the surgeon to performing a bilateral operation which runs a risk, albeit small, of visual loss
4. It is associated with the risk of damage to the temporal branch of the facial nerve with a brow ptosis
5. It is commonly associated with a large area of loss of sensation in the forehead and scalp
6. It commonly results in temporal wasting with a secondary cosmetic defect
7. In male patients with hair loss, it leaves a large visible scar

6. Transantral (Caldwell Luc) Approach

This approach offers no advantages over alternative approaches and has significant disadvantages, e.g., a much higher risk of postoperative diplopia than alternative approaches. It is associated with significant postoperative discomfort.

7. Transcaruncular Approach

This approach allows quick and ready access to the medial orbital wall and orbital apex, and the conjunctival incision can be extended inferiorly to gain access to the medial aspect of the orbital floor. A separate incision, however, is required to gain access to the lateral orbital wall. This approach requires great care as the surface of the globe is exposed during the surgery. Some surgeons combine this approach with a lateral upper lid skin crease approach to the lateral orbital wall. Such an upper lid incision can provide access to the lateral and supero-lateral orbital wall permitting a deep burring to be undertaken but this approach does not provide as great a degree of exposure as the "swinging eyelid flap" approach. It does, however, provide excellent cosmesis and avoids the risk of a postoperative lateral canthal dystopia.

Surgical Approach

The "swinging eyelid flap" approach, which is the approach most commonly used in the author's practice, will be described in detail.

Preoperative Preparation

The patient should be reviewed in a pre-assessment clinic 2 to 3 weeks prior to admission. The patient's thyroid function should be well controlled and the thyroid function test results should be available to the anesthetist. A full blood count and platelet count should be performed. A history of excessive bleeding should be excluded. All anti-platelet agents should be discontinued 2 weeks prior to surgery. Patients on anticoagulants must be admitted and transferred to intravenous heparin under the supervision of a hematologist. The preoperative axial and coronal CT scans must be available in the operating room.

On induction of anesthesia the patient should be given Diamox 500 mg intravenously. This lowers intraocular pressure and permits easier subperiosteal retraction and an improved view of the posterior aspect of the medial orbital wall. In addition, dexamethasone 8 mg is given intravenously along with a broad spectrum antibiotic, e.g., Cefuroxime. In the absence of any contraindications, the anesthetist should be asked to induce a moderate degree of hypotension. A throat pack should be placed and its presence recorded. The patient is placed into a reverse Trendelenberg position to reduce venous pressure. A nasal epistaxis tampon is placed in the nose, advanced toward the medial canthus, and then moistened with 5% cocaine solution. A lateral canthal skin crease incision is marked using gentian violet. Two milliliters of 0.5% Bupivacaine with 1:200,000 units of adrenaline are injected into the lower eyelid immediately under the skin and a further 5 mls are injected into the temporal fossa. The eyelid is then compressed for 5 minutes.

A headlight and surgical loupes must be worn throughout this surgical procedure.

Surgical Technique
1. A 4/0 Silk traction suture is placed through the gray line of the lower eyelid.
2. A lateral canthal skin incision is made along the previously marked crease using a Colorado needle.

The incision is deepened to expose the periosteum of the lateral orbital margin.

3. Next a lateral canthotomy and an inferior cantholysis are performed using the Colorado needle or using blunt-tipped Westcott scissors.

4. Hemostasis is obtained using bipolar cautery.

5. The lower eyelid is then everted over a small Desmarres retractor. The silk suture is fixated to the face drapes using a small curved artery clip.

6. A conjunctival incision is made just below the inferior border of the tarsus extending from just below the inferior punctum to the lateral canthus using the Colorado needle.

7. Hemostasis is achieved using bipolar cautery when required.

8. A plane of dissection is created anterior to the orbital septum. The orbicularis muscle is clearly seen using the bloodless approach with a Colorado needle and the dissection is continued, keeping immediately posterior to this muscle.

9. This plane is dissected all the way to the inferior orbital margin.

10. A number of 4/0 silk traction sutures are placed through the medial and lateral aspects of the conjunctival/lower eyelid retractor complex. The sutures are then fixated to the forehead drapes using curved artery clips to protect the cornea during the rest of the surgery (Fig. 19.28). Care is taken to ensure that the sutures themselves do not abrade the cornea.

11. The orbital septum is then opened and any prolapsing fat is removed medially, centrally, and laterally. This facilitates easier access to the subsequent subperiosteal dissection (Fig. 19.28).

12. Great care is taken to identify the inferior oblique muscle lying between the medial and central preaponeurotic eyelid fat pads. Once the inferior oblique muscle has been clearly identified, the fat is gently removed avoiding any damage to the muscle. The septa with the fat are dissected using the Colorado needle until the fat has been freed sufficiently to allow a curved artery clip to be placed across the base of the fat. The fat is then resected using the Colorado needle and the stump of fat lying along the length of the artery clip is cauterized before the clip is released.

13. The arcuate expansion separating the central and lateral fat pads may be kept intact and the lateral fat pad is debulking in a similar fashion. The fat is kept in a moistened swab for re-implantation along the inferior orbital margin at the completion of the decompression surgery.

14. One or two Jaffe lid retractors are inserted into the wound and fixated to the drapes using a curved artery clip.

15. Using the Colorado needle the periosteum is incised 2 mm below the rim commencing medially carrying this incision to a slightly lower position laterally (Fig. 19.29).

16. The periosteum is elevated from the underlying bone using the sharp end of a Freer periosteal elevator (Fig. 19.30A).

17. The periorbita is then elevated from the orbital floor medially using the Freer periosteal elevator, taking great care not to rupture the periorbita.

18. The blade of a medium Sewall retractor is placed carefully into the subperiosteal space and the orbital contents are retracted.

19. A constant vessel is encountered along the centre of the orbital floor passing from the infraorbital neurovascular bundle to the orbit (Fig. 19.30B). This should be cauterized as it enters the periorbita and cut with Westcott scissors.

20. The periorbita is then elevated from the medial orbital wall as far as the anterior and posterior ethmoidal vessels, which can be seen to pass through the periorbita to the anterior and posterior ethmoidal foramina. This marks the superior limit of the medial wall dissection.

21. The dissection is continued posteriorly until the body of the sphenoid bone is encountered. This marks the posterior limit of the medial dissection (Fig. 19.31).

KEY POINT

Great care should be taken to ensure that the periorbita is maintained intact throughout this dissection. Inadvertent damage to the periorbita will result in an immediate prolapse of orbital fat, which will obscure any further dissection increasing the risk of complications.

22. The bone of the central aspect of the medial orbital wall is in-fractured using a Freer periosteal elevator (Fig. 19.32A).

23. The lamina papyracea is then removed anteriorly as far as the posterior lacrimal crest using a small Kerrison rongeur, taking care not to damage the lacrimal drainage apparatus, and posteriorly as far as the body of the sphenoid using Wilde Blakesley ethmoidectomy forceps (Fig. 19.32B). The body of the sphenoid is noted by the change of character of the bone from very thin and friable to solid. This bone lies just in front of the optic canal.

KEY POINT

It is essential to decompress the medial orbital wall to the body of the sphenoid in patients with compressive optic neuropathy (CON). In patients undergoing a decompression for any other reason, it is safer to be conservative and not extend the dissection this far posteriorly.

24. The ethmoid air cells and mucosa are very carefully removed using the ethmoidectomy forceps. Great care is taken to stay below the ethmoidal vessels. The mucosa bleeds but once the mucosa and air cells have been exenterated the bleeding ceases. Any bleeding which obscures the view can be controlled by the gentle insertion of small patties moistened with 1:1000 adrenaline that should be left in position for a few minutes.

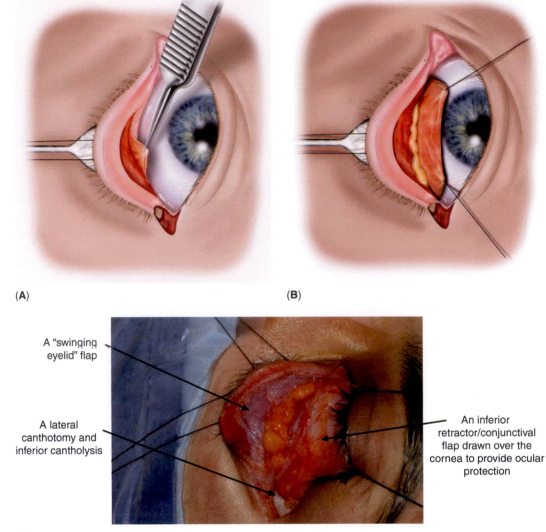

Figure 19.28 (**A**) A drawing showing a "swinging lower eyelid flap" being commenced. (**B**) A drawing showing the inferior retractor/conjunctival flap being drawn up over the cornea. The traction sutures are placed medially and laterally avoiding any contact with the cornea. (**C**) A "swinging lower eyelid flap" approach to an orbital decompression. The orbital septum should be opened at this stage and the fat which presents should be removed, as it can otherwise cause problems with surgical access to the orbital walls.

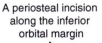

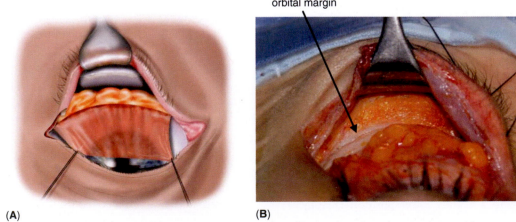

Figure 19.29 (**A**) A drawing showing the exposed inferior orbital margin from the surgeon's perspective. (**B**) A periosteal incision has been made just below the orbital margin.

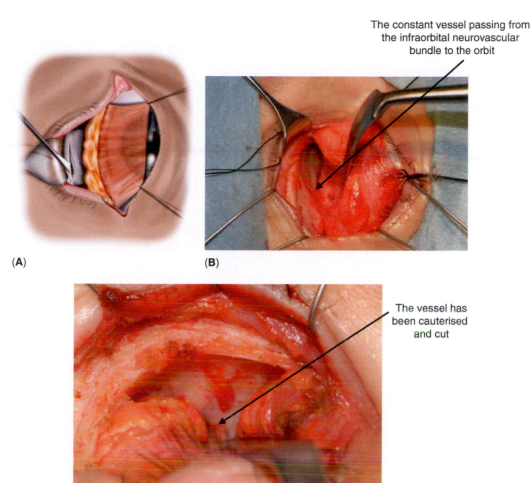

The constant vessel passing from the infraorbital neurovascular bundle to the orbit

(A)

(B)

The vessel has been cauterised and cut

(C)

Figure 19.30 (**A**) A drawing showing the commencement of the periosteal elevation from the inferior orbital margin. (**B**) The periorbita has been reflected from the floor of the orbit and a Sewell retractor is used to retract the orbital contents. A vessel can be seen arising from the infraorbital canal and passing into the orbit. (**C**) The surgeon's view of the orbital floor. The vessel has been cauterized and cut.

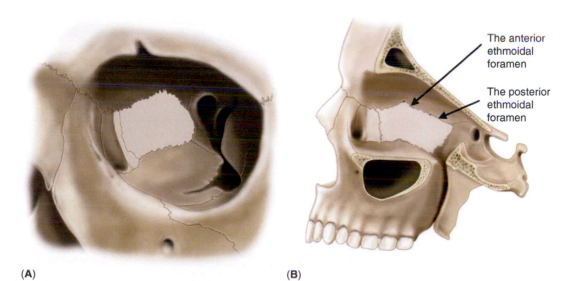

The anterior ethmoidal foramen

The posterior ethmoidal foramen

(A)

(B)

Figure 19.31 (**A**) The area of bone removal from the medial wall is illustrated. The posterior extent of the bone resection is limited by the body of the sphenoid anterior to the optic foramen. (**B**) A side view demonstrates that the anterior and posterior ethmoidal vessels lie at the superior aspect of the medial wall resection. The posterior lacrimal crest marks the anterior limit of the medial wall resection.

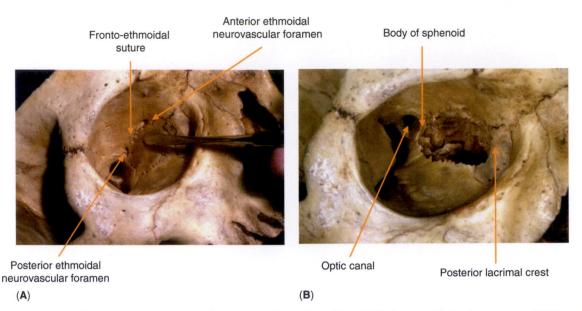

Fronto-ethmoidal
suture

Anterior ethmoidal
neurovascular foramen

Body of sphenoid

Posterior ethmoidal
neurovascular foramen

Optic canal

Posterior lacrimal crest

(A)   **(B)**

Figure 19.32 (**A**) The position of the tip of the Freer periosteal elevator marks the position of the initial in fracture of the lamina papyracea. (**B**) The medial orbital wall has been removed posteriorly as far as the body of the sphenoid and anteriorly as far as the posterior lacrimal crest. The anterior and posterior ethmoidal vessels lie at the superior aspect of the medial wall resection.

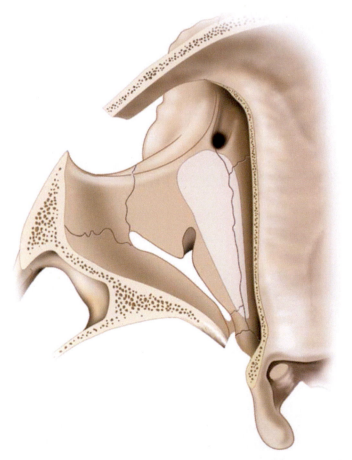

Figure 19.33 The area of bone removal from the medial aspect of the orbital floor is demonstrated.

25. The fovea ethmoidalis is seen to arch above the position of the fronto-ethmoidal suture line. More medially lies the cribriform plate. Great care should be taken to avoid any damage to these structures that could result in a CSF leak.

26. At the inferior aspect of the medial orbital wall, the bony dissection is discontinued if it is intended to

leave a medial strut between the medial wall and a decompression of the medial half of the orbital floor. Otherwise, if a medial wall decompression alone is being performed, or if this is being balanced with a lateral orbital decompression, the medial wall decompression can be extended to include the most medial aspect of the orbital floor.

27. If the orbital floor is to be decompressed, the bone of the orbital floor medial to the infraorbital canal is in-fractured using the Freer periosteal elevator, medial to the infraorbital nerve. Bone is then removed from the medial half of the orbital floor using Kerrison rongeurs (Fig. 19.33). Bone is removed to the posterior wall of the maxillary sinus. The maxillary sinus mucosa is removed from the roof of the maxillary sinus.

28. Damage to the infraorbital vessels should be avoided as these can bleed profusely.

29. The periorbita is now opened in a posterior to anterior direction along the medial orbital wall using a curved sharp blade. Great care is taken to avoid damage to the medial rectus muscle. The incisions are then extended using blunt-tipped Westcott scissors, and the periorbita is removed.

30. The periorbita is then elevated from the lateral aspect of the orbital floor and around the anterior aspect of the inferior orbital fissure to the lateral aspect of the orbital floor.

31. The zygomatico-facial and zygomatico-temporal neurovascular bundles are cauterised and divided. The periorbita is reflected deeply into the orbit exposing the greater wing of the sphenoid bone and as superiorly as possible along the lateral orbital wall (Fig. 19.34).

32. A piece of Supramid sheeting is cut to the shape of a guitar plectrum and is inserted into the subperiosteal space. A medium Sewall retractor is then inserted beneath this. This aids in retraction of the orbital

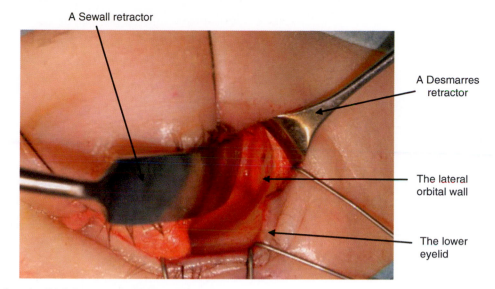

A Sewall retractor

A Desmarres retractor

The lateral orbital wall

The lower eyelid

Figure 19.34 The lateral wall is being exposed taking care to keep the periorbita intact to prevent a premature prolapse of orbital fat into surgical field.

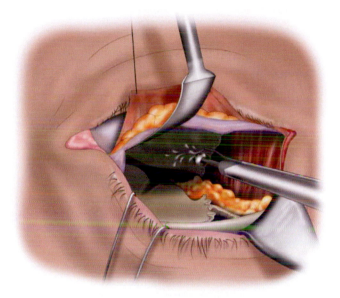

Figure 19.35 A drawing showing the bone of the lateral orbital wall being carefully burred using a rose head burr with an irrigation sleeve.

contents, particularly if there is any premature opening of the periorbita, with a prolapse of orbital fat.

33. The exposed bone of the lateral aspect of the orbital floor and the lateral orbital wall is burred away using a 4-mm rose-head burr (Fig. 19.35). The tip of the burr should be constantly irrigated using a sleeve irrigation apparatus attached to the drill head. The assistant should ensure that the tip of a sucker is placed below the drill.

34. The convexity of the bone deep within the orbit is first burred away down to the diploe. Great care should be taken not to expose the underlying dura.

35. The infero-temporal fat pad and the deep layer of the deep temporalis fascia are then gradually exposed anteriorly (Fig. 19.36).

36. Further bone is removed anteriorly, inferiorly, and superiorly using Kerrison rongeurs.

37. The lateral periorbita is now opened in a posterior to anterior direction along the medial orbital wall using a curved sharp blade. Great care is taken to avoid damage to the lateral rectus muscle. The incisions are then extended using blunt-tipped Westcott scissors and the periorbita is removed.

38. Orbital fat can be removed from the inferolateral orbit as required, depending on the degree of reduction in proptosis achieved.

39. The orbit is inspected for bleeding and bipolar cautery used as required.

40. The fat, which has been removed, is now divided into small pearls using Westcott scissors and then replaced along the inferior orbital margin to help to prevent adhesions.

41. The conjunctiva is closed with two or three interrupted 7/0 Vicryl sutures.

42. The lateral canthus is repaired with a 5/0 Vicryl suture, suturing the lateral tarsus to the periosteum of the lateral orbital margin. The skin is closed with interrupted 7/0 Vicryl sutures.

43. Topical antibiotic ointment is instilled into the eye and a compressive dressing is applied.

Postoperative Management
The compressive dressing is removed the following day. Systemic antibiotics and a rapidly tapering course of systemic steroids are prescribed for a week postoperatively. Topical antibiotic ointment is applied to the lower eyelid wound three times a day for 2 weeks. Topical lubricants are prescribed for comfort. Gentle upward massage to the lower eyelid is commenced 5 days postoperatively and continued for 6 weeks. The patient is instructed not to blow the nose or hold the nose if sneezing for a period of 6 weeks.

Potential Complications
Potential complications of orbital decompression surgery should be borne in mind when counseling patients about this surgical procedure and when taking informed consent from

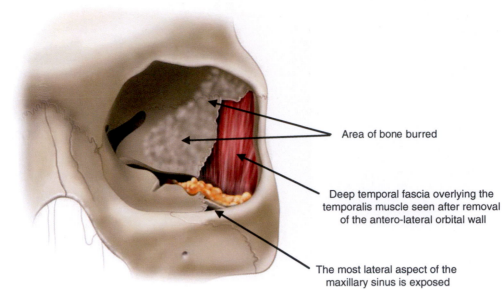

Area of bone burred

Deep temporal fascia overlying the
temporalis muscle seen after removal
of the antero-lateral orbital wall

The most lateral aspect of the
maxillary sinus is exposed

Figure 19.36 The area of bone which can be removed from the lateral wall and the most lateral part of the orbital floor is demonstrated, along with the area which can be burred down.

patients. The risks of general anesthesia should also be considered in patients with co-existent disease, e.g., diabetes mellitus, myasthenia, cardiovascular, and respiratory disease.

Diplopia

Strabismus is quoted as the most common potential complication of orbital decompression surgery but its incidence varies markedly from centre to centre. It is a common problem in patients with preoperative ocular motility restrictions. Approximately 30% of such patients have some degree of worsening of their diplopia. Approximately 10% of such patients require strabismus surgery. The results of strabismus surgery are generally very good with a very small percentage of patients experiencing permanent and disabling diplopia. Postoperative diplopia should be a very uncommon problem in patients without preoperative motility restrictions if the surgery is performed meticulously and appropriately.

The risk of postoperative motility disturbances can be minimized by:

a. Attempting to leave a bony strut between the medial wall and the orbital floor
b. Avoiding the removal of the orbital floor or an excessive removal of the orbital floor
c. Avoiding trauma to the extraocular muscles when opening the periorbita
d. Avoiding the origin of the inferior oblique muscle
e. Paying meticulous attention to hamostasis at all stages of the procedure

Blindness

Visual loss following orbital decompression surgery is a devastating complication but fortunately extremely rare. The risks can be minimized by:

a. Avoiding prolonged retraction on the globe
b. Paying meticulous attention to hemostasis at all stages of the procedure

c. Monitoring the pupil at intervals
d. Avoiding a compressive dressing when an orbital fat decompression alone has been performed
e. Monitoring the patient for pain, sudden proptosis, and visual disturbance every 30 minutes postoperatively for 12 hours when an orbital fat decompression alone has been performed
f. Avoiding orbital apical dissection if the view is suboptimal
g. Avoiding undue traction on orbital fat during orbital fat dissection

CSF Leak/Meningitis

A CSF leak is a rare complication and can be readily avoided by:

a. Ascertaining the position of the cribriform plate with respect to the fronto-ethmoidal suture line on a pre-operative coronal CT scan
b. Ensuring good visualization of the ethmoidal air cells by good hemostasis, by good retraction, and by avoiding damage to the periorbita with premature prolapse of orbital fat. If the view of the medial orbital wall is poor because of a "tight" orbit, the lateral orbital wall can be decompressed first allowing the orbital contents to shift laterally.

Hemorrhage

Blood loss from an orbital decompression should be minimal (less than 5 ml). The risk of bleeding can be minimized as discussed under "preoperative preparations." In addition, blood loss can be minimized by:

a. Ensuring the medial wall dissection remains below the ethmoidal arteries
b. Identifying and cauterizing the constant vessels coursing from the infraorbital neurovascular bundle to the inferior orbit

c. Avoiding the use of bone rongeurs close to the infraorbital neurovascular bundle

d. Identifying and cauterizing the zygomatic vessels

Infraorbital Anesthesia

Neurosensory defects in the distribution of the infraorbital nerve usually recover after a period of months. They are, however, disturbing to patients and can be avoided by meticulous bone removal using a diamond burr adjacent to the infraorbital neurovascular bundle. Excessive use of cautery adjacent to the nerve will cause postoperative neurosensory defects. Some degree of neurosensory deficit is inevitable if the whole of the orbital floor has to be removed in a patient with severe proptosis. In such patients, the nerve should be unroofed with great care.

Orbital Cellulitis

Postoperative infection is a potentially serious complication. The risk is minimized by the use of antibiotics postoperatively and by advising the patient to avoid blowing the nose for 6 weeks.

Hypoglobus

The risk of an inferior displacement of the globe and a secondary worsening of upper eyelid retraction is avoided by minimizing the degree of orbital floor decompression.

Enophthalmos

Enophthalmos can occur if too aggressive an orbital decompression is undertaken during the acute inflammatory phase of the disease. As the orbital edema subsides and the orbit remodels, a progressive enophthalmos can occur over the course of up to 2 years following the surgery. The stage of the disease must therefore be taken into consideration when proceeding with an orbital decompression.

Epiphora

The lacrimal sac is prone to injury if the medial wall dissection is carried too far anteriorly.

A number of additional complications are specific to other approaches, e.g., oro-antral fistula following a transantral approach.

In view of the risk, albeit small, of visual loss from an orbital decompression, the procedure should be performed on each orbit on separate occasions unless the patient poses unacceptable risks from separate general anaesthetics. Postoperative edema and ecchymosis is minimized by a compressive dressing that is well tolerated unilaterally but is distressing for the patient when applied bilaterally. The operating time is reduced, as is any blood loss. The effects of the surgery can be seen and the surgical management of the fellow orbit modified if necessary.

It is wise to be conservative with an orbital decompression procedure. It is much easier to perform additional decompressive surgery than it is to attempt to correct the problems encountered following overly-aggressive surgery, e.g., a hypoglobus.

Ocular Muscle Surgery

Muscle recession is the major surgical procedure performed in cases of thyroid myopathy. The use of adjustable sutures has improved surgical results but in many cases management may be very difficult, especially after surgical orbital decompression. It is rare to obtain single vision in all fields of gaze.

Eyelid Repositioning Surgery

Surgery to alleviate upper and lower lid retraction should be deferred until the eyelid position is stable and until other treatment modalities have been completed unless the patient has significant corneal exposure. The management of thyroid related eyelid retraction is discussed in detail in chapter 8.

It is important to emphasize to patients at the outset that the road to recovery from the disfiguring and disabling effects of thyroid eye disease may be quite long.

ADDITIONAL READING

1. Adenis JP, Robert PY, Lasudry JG, Dalloul Z. Treatment of proptosis with fat removal orbital decompression in Graves' ophthalmopathy. Euro J Ophthalmol 1998; 8(4): 246–52.
2. Bailey CC, Kabala J, Laitt R, at al. Magnetic resonance imaging in thyroid eye disease. Eye 1996; 10 (5): 617–19.
3. Char DH. Thyroid eye disease. Br J Ophthalmol 1996; 80 (10): 922–6.
4. Claridge KG, Ghabrial R, Davis G, et al. Combined radiotherapy and medical immunosuppression in the management of thyroid eye disease. Eye 1997; 11(Pt 5): 717–22.
5. Dutton JJ, Haik BG, eds. Thyroid Eye Disease. New York, NY: Marcel Dekker, 2002.
6. Dutton JJ. Atlas of Clinical and Surgical Orbital Anatomy, Philadelphia, PA: W.B. Saunders, 1994.
7. Wormald PJ. Endoscopic Sinus Surgery: Anatomy, 3-Dimensional Reconstruction, and Surgical Technique. New York, NY: Thieme, 2005. (ISBN: 1-58890-285-4).
8. Goldberg RA, Kim AJ, Kerivan KM. The lacrimal keyhole, orbital doorjamb, and basin of the inferior orbital fissure. Three areas of deep bone in the lateral orbit. Arch Ophthalmol 1998; 116(12): 1618–24.
9. Goldberg RA, Peny JD, Hortaleza V, Tong JT. Strabismus after balanced medial plus lateral wall versus lateral wall only orbital decompression for dysthyroid orbitopathy. Ophthal Plast Reconstr Surg 2000; 16(4): 2, 71–7.
10. Goldberg RA. The evolving paradigm of orbital decompression surgery. Arch Ophthalmol 1998; 116(l): 95–6.
11. Graham SM, Chee L, Alford MA, Carter KD. New techniques for surgical decompression of thyroid-related orbitopathy. Annal Acad Med, Singapore 1999; 28(4): 494–7.
12. Wiersinga WM, Kahaly GJ, eds. Graves' Orbitopathy: A Multidisciplinary Approach. Basel, Switzerland: S Karger, 2007 (ISBN: 978-3-8055-8342-8).
13. Khanna D, Chong KK, Afifiyan NF, et al. Rituximab treatment of patients with severe, corticosteroid-resistant thyroid-associated ophthalmopathy. Source Ophthalmol 2010; 117(1):133–9.e2.
14. Lazarus JH. Relation between thyroid eye disease and type of treatment of Graves' hyperthyroidism. Thyroid 1998; 8(5): 437.
15. Mourits MP, Prummel MF, Wiersinga WM, Koornneef L. Clinical activity score as a guide in the management of patients with Graves' ophthalmopathy. Clin Endocrinol 1997; 47(1): 9–14.
16. Paridaens DA, Verhoeff K, Bouwens D, van Den Bosch WA. Transconjunctival orbital decompression in Graves' ophthalmopathy: lateral wall approach ab intemo. Br J Ophthalmol 2000; 84(7): 775–81.
17. Perros P, Kendall-Taylor P. Natural history of thyroid eye disease. Thyroid 1998; 8(5): 423–5.
18. Scott IU, Siatkowski MR. Thyroid eye disease. Semin Ophthalmol 1999; 14(2): 52–61.
19. Shorr N, Baylis HI, Goldberg RA, Perry JD. Transcaruncular approach to the medial orbit and orbital apex. Ophthalmology 2000; 107(8): 1459–63.

20. The European Group on Graves' Orbitopathy (EUGOGO). Clinical assessment of patients with Graves' orbitopathy: the European Group on Graves' Orbitopathy recommendations to generalists, specialists and clinical researchers. Euro J Endocrinol 2006; 155: 387–9.

21. Ünal M, İleri F, Konuk O, Hasanreisoğlu B. Balanced orbital decompression combined with fat Removal in Graves ophthalmology. Ophthal Plast Reconstr Surg 2003; 19(2): 112–8.

22. Van Ruyven RL, Van Den Bosch WA, Mulder PG, Eijkenboom WM, Paridaens AD. The effect of retrobulbar irradiation on exophthalmos, ductions and soft tissue signs in Graves' ophthalmopathy: a retrospective analysis of 90 cases. Eye 2000; 14 Pt 5: 761–4.

23. Wright ED, Davidson J, Codere F, Desrosiers M. Endoscopic orbital decompression with preservation of an inferomedial bony strut: minimization of postoperative diplopia. J Otolaryngol 1999; 28(5): 252–6.

20 The diagnosis and management of epiphora

INTRODUCTION

The complaint of a watering eye is very common and may affect patients of any age. It is important to establish the true nature of the patient's complaint. The term *epiphora* refers to the overflow of tears onto the cheek. The complaint by a patient of a "watering" or "watery" eye, or "tearing" may not imply that tears actually overflow from the eye. There are many abnormalities that can lead the patient to seek attention for this complaint. It is important to establish the underlying cause by obtaining an accurate detailed history and by performing an appropriate clinical examination and, where indicated, supplementary investigations. It should not be assumed that this complaint automatically signifies a lacrimal drainage system obstruction.

APPLIED ANATOMY

The anatomy of the lacrimal drainage system and nose is described in detail in chapter 2. This anatomy should be carefully reviewed.

HISTORY

A history of irritation, foreign body sensation, or allergy should alert the clinician to the possibility of reflex hypersecretion of tears. Patients with a dry eye may paradoxically present with the complaint of epiphora due to increased reflex tear secretion. It is essential to exclude such an underlying etiology, as such patients will not benefit from any form of lacrimal drainage surgery however well performed. The use of topical medications, e.g., glaucoma drops, should raise the suspicion of allergy with an associated lower lid dermatitis or a cicatrizing conjunctivitis with punctal or canalicular obstruction. A history of previous dacryocystitis indicates the presence of a nasolacrimal duct obstruction.

A history of previous intranasal surgery or facial trauma should alert the clinician to the possibility of a nasolacrimal duct obstruction and may require more detailed preoperative investigations, e.g., a coronal computed tomography (CT) scan to determine the presence and location of microplates or bone grafts and the position of the cribriform plate. A history of bloody tears, nasal obstruction, or epistaxis should raise the suspicion of nasal, sinus, or lacrimal sac malignancy or Wegener's granulomatosis (Fig. 20.1). Such patients should be evaluated with the assistance of an ear, nose, and throat (ENT) colleague. A previous history of a facial palsy should alert the clinician to the possibility of "crocodile tears," a residual incomplete blink or frank lagophthalmos.

The history taking should be tailored to the patient's age, bearing in mind the common causes of epiphora in each age group:

- Infants and children
  - congenital nasolacrimal duct obstruction
  - congenital anomalies of the lacrimal drainage system
- Young patients
  - trauma—canalicular/lacrimal sac lacerations, nasoethmoidal fractures
  - canalicular scarring—herpes simplex canaliculitis
- Middle-aged patients
  - dacryoliths—actinomyces infection
  - cicatricial disorders of the lower eyelid anterior lamella
- Older patients
  - idiopathic primary acquired nasolacrimal duct obstruction
  - involutional eyelid malpositions

Dacryoliths (lacrimal sac stones) are found in 2% to 5% of dacryocystorhinostomies. Dacryoliths consist of dried mucus, lipid, and inflammatory debris, and are more often seen in patients with chronic dacryocystitis. They can be seen as small soft flakes, multiple small stones, or they can form an entire cast of the lacrimal sac (Fig. 20.2). They can sometime be seen as filling defects on dacryocystography.

The examination of infants and children with epiphora is considered separately under nasolacrimal duct probing and intubation below.

EXTERNAL EXAMINATION

A number of abnormalities of the eyelids may be responsible for the complaints of epiphora and can be overlooked with a cursory examination (Fig. 20.3).

1. Lower lid ectropion (Fig. 20.4)
2. Punctal stenosis/eversion/obstruction (Fig. 20.5)
3. Accessory puncta and/or fistulae (Fig. 20.6)
4. Lower lid/upper lid entropion
5. Trichiasis
6. Eyelid lesions, e.g., molluscum contagiosum
7. Conjunctivochalasis (Fig. 20.7)
8. An incomplete blink
9. Aberrant reinnervation of the facial nerve (crocodile tears)
10. "Kissing puncta" (Fig. 20.8)

The patient should be examined closely for the presence of conjunctivochalasis, a redundant fold of conjunctiva which can prevent the access of tears to the inferior puncta (Fig. 20.7).

Stenosis of the inferior punctum is commonly associated with an early punctal ectropion.

A lower eyelid ectropion should be carefully evaluated as described in chapter 6. It is important to exclude shortening of the anterior lamella or vertical eyelid tightness as causes of a cicatricial ectropion (Fig. 20.10). Subtle changes are easily overlooked and may be due to dry "weather beaten" skin or a mid-face ptosis.

The degree of laxity of the lower eyelid and the medial and lateral canthal tendons should be assessed. The degree of horizontal lower eyelid laxity is assessed by performing a "distraction" test, a "pinch" test and a "snap" test (see chap. 6)

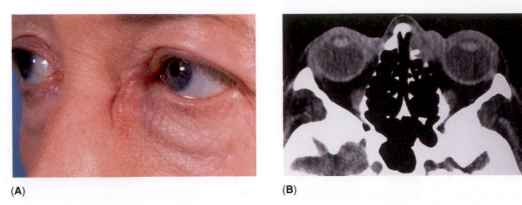

(A)   (B)

Figure 20.1 (**A**) A patient who presented with a history of painless epiphora who was thought to have a nasolacrimal duct obstruction and a secondary mucocele. She was referred following a biopsy performed during an attempted external DCR. The biopsy revealed a lacrimal sac carcinoma. (**B**) An axial CT scan of the patient demonstrating a mass in the region of the lacrimal sac.

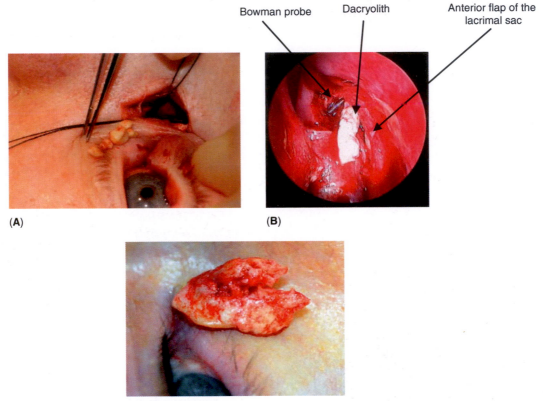

(A)   (B)

(C)

Figure 20.2 (**A**) Multiple small dacryoliths removed at an external DCR. (**B**) An endoscopic view of a large dacryolith seen after opening the lacrimal sac during an endonsasal DCR. (**C**) A large lobulated dacryolith removed during an endonasal DCR.

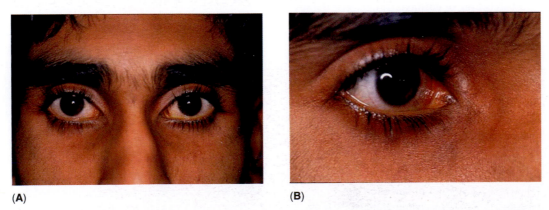

(A)   (B)

Figure 20.3 (**A**) A patient referred with a long-standing history of constant epiphora. (**B**) A side view revealed an antero-displacement of the anterior limbs of the medial canthal tendons, drawing the puncta away from the globe. The patient has a prominent nose. The diagnosis is "Centurion syndrome". The treatment is a repositioning of the medial canthal tendons. Failure to recognize the true cause of the epiphora can lead to inappropriate surgical procedures.

A lower eyelid entropion may be intermittent. The patient should be asked to look down and to forcibly close the eyes to ascertain whether or not an entropion can be provoked. This also enables an assessment of orbicularis function. The medial canthus should be palpated for any intrinsic lacrimal sac lesions, e.g., a lacrimal sac mucocele or tumor (Fig. 20.11), or an extrinsic lesion compressing the lacrimal sac, e.g., an ethmoid sinus tumor (Fig. 20.12).

Slit Lamp Examination

Biomicroscopy should be used to exclude causes of reflex hypersecretion of tears and tear film abnormalities, e.g., blepharitis or a dry eye. The vertical height of the tear meniscus should be noted prior to the instillation of any drops. The puncta should be examined carefully to ensure normal position and exclude an early eversion, stenosis, or obstruction by cilia or other lesions (Fig. 20.13). The puncta should

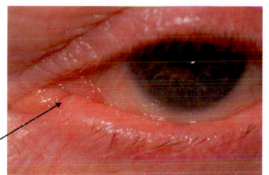

Figure 20.4 A lower eyelid punctal ectopion.

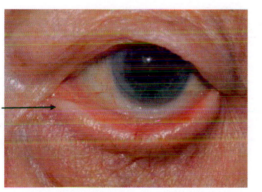

Figure 20.5 Inferior punctal stenosis in the presence of a chronic lower lid involutional ectropion.

not normally be visible on slit lamp examination without digital manipulation to evert them. The puncta should face slightly posteriorly towards the lacus lacrimalis. All four puncta should be carefully examined to assess their presence and patency. The puncta should be examined for discharge with and without digital pressure applied to the lacrimal sac. A chronic inflammatory swelling of the eyelid medial to the puncta may indicate a canaliculitis due to an actinomyces infection (Fig. 20.14). Such a swelling should not be confused with a chalazion or meibomian cyst, which would be located within the tarsus lateral to the puncta. Pressure applied to the canaliculi may cause a cheesy material to be expressed.

The lacrimal sac should be massaged and the puncta observed for any discharge. Reflux of mucoid material is pathognomonic for a lower lacrimal drainage system obstruction.

CLINICAL EVALUATION OF THE LACRIMAL DRAINAGE SYSTEM

The following simple clinical tests should be performed:

- Fluorescein dye disappearance test
- Syringing of the lacrimal drainage system
- Probing of the canaliculi
- Endoscopic nasal examination

Fluorescein Dye Disappearance Test

This is a very simple physiological method for assessing the lacrimal drainage system and can be used in children. A drop of 2% fluorescein is instilled into the inferior fornix of each eye. Complete disappearance of the dye after a period of 4 to 5 min excludes any significant lacrimal drainage system obstruction. A delayed or asymmetrical dye disappearance is an indication to progress with further clinical tests of the lacrimal drainage system. (The Jones dye tests are not used by the author, who does not find them practical to perform or useful in clinical practice.)

Syringing of the Lacrimal Drainage System

KEY POINT

The patient should be advised that this is not a therapeutic but a diagnostic procedure. It should be performed by the surgeon and never delegated to a nurse. The details of the findings should be carefully recorded.

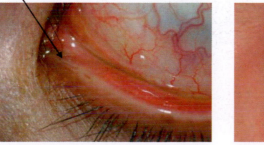
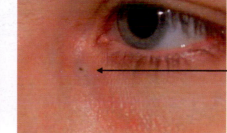

(A)   (B)

Figure 20.6 (A) An accessory inferior punctum. (B) A congenital lacrimal fistula leaking tears.

A local anesthetic drop is instilled into the conjunctival sac and the residual fluorescein dye is washed from the conjunctival sac. The patient should be placed in a semi-recumbent position on an examination couch and an illuminated magnifier should be used. The surgeon should always stand on the side which is being syringed. Dilatation of the puncta should only be required where the puncta are stenosed. If this is necessary it should be done with great care using a very fine Nettleship dilator in order to avoid creating a false passage. A fine lacrimal cannula on a 2-ml syringe of sterile saline is gently manipulated through the inferior punctum and along the inferior canaliculus with the eyelid pulled laterally. The cannula should be advanced following the correct anatomical line of the canaliculus and taking great care not to concertina the canaliculus, which creates a false impression of a canalicular or common canalicular obstruction (a common mistake).

Very gentle pressure should be applied to the syringe. Normal patency of the system will allow easy passage of saline to the nasopharynx with no regurgitation. It should be noted, however, that irrigation is applied at a far higher hydrostatic pressure than normal tear outflow. Patients with epiphora due to relative stenosis of the nasolacrimal duct may have apparently normal findings on irrigation. This is an indication for the use of lacrimal scintilligraphy. Passage of saline to the nasopharynx after applying more pressure to the syringe suggests a partial obstruction of the lacrimal drainage system or the presence of a dacryolith.

Regurgitation of saline stained with fluorescein through the opposite punctum indicates patent canaliculi but suggests a distal obstruction. It excludes lacrimal pump failure as a cause of epiphora as the fluorescein reached the lacrimal sac. The procedure should be repeated via the upper punctum if the lower punctum is absent or if there is an inferior canalicular obstruction. Regurgitation of mucoid or mucopurulent material suggests a nasolacrimal duct obstruction. Regurgitation of blood is an indication to exclude the possibility of a lacrimal sac malignancy.

Probing of the Canaliculi

If syringing of the lacrimal drainage system has suggested a canalicular obstruction, careful probing of the canaliculi using a 00 Bowman probe is undertaken. The probe should not be forced through any obstructions. If concretions are present, e.g., following chronic actinomyces infection, the surgeon may feel a gritty sensation with the probe.

If the probe enters the lacrimal sac a "hard stop" is felt as the probe abuts bone (Fig. 20.15). The presence of a "soft stop" suggests a canalicular or common canalicular obstruction as long as the probe has not been inadvertently pushed into the side wall of the canaliculus, which creates a false impression of a "soft stop" (Figs. 20.16 and 20.17).

The site of any obstruction is determined by withdrawing the probe after grasping it by the punctum with forceps and measuring the length of the probe that is withdrawn. By using this maneuver a canalicular or common canalicular obstruction may be diagnosed.

KEY POINT

Be careful to avoid the false impression of a soft stop, which can occur if the canaliculus is allowed to kink during probing. Avoid this by ensuring that the eyelid is stretched laterally during the examination. Under no circumstances should the nasolacrimal duct be probed as a diagnostic procedure in an adult.

Endoscopic Nasal Examination

It is essential to perform a nasal examination before embarking on lacrimal drainage surgery. This should be performed using a rigid nasal endoscope and is undertaken to exclude intranasal pathology, e.g., allergic rhinitis, polyps, or tumors which may contribute to obstruction of the lacrimal drainage system, and to exclude anatomical variations which may adversely interfere with lacrimal drainage surgery, e.g., a deviated nasal septum or concha bullosa. Although the nose can be

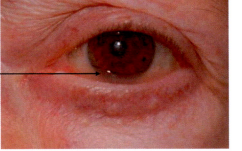

Conjunctivochalasis

Figure 20.7 Conjunctivochalasis.

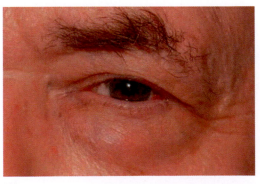

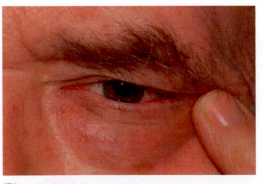

(A)   (B)

Figure 20.8 (**A**) "Kissing puncta." The eyelids meet medially preventing access of the tears to the puncta. (**B**) The effect of a lateral tarsal strip procedure is being mimicked by drawing the eyelid laterally. The puncta have now separated. A lateral tarsal strip procedure is the treatment of choice for this problem.

examined using a headlight and a nasal speculum, an endoscope provides a far superior view of the intranasal structures.

A rigid 4-mm 0° endoscope is ideal for most patients. Other viewing angles, e.g., 30° are not required for routine nasal endoscopy in a clinic. A rigid 2.7-mm endoscope has the advantage that it can be used routinely for adult nasal examination without the need for nasal decongestion but it has the disadvantage that it is relatively fragile. Sterilization of endoscopes in between patients is another practical problem that requires special attention for clinic organization.

Nasal Preparation
The nasal mucosa can be decongested in clinic using a simple decongestant spray, e.g., oxymetazoline (Otrivine) or a combined decongestant and local anesthetic spray, e.g., Cophenylcaine. If a local anesthetic is used the patient should be warned to avoid any hot drinks for an hour after the application. In children who are sufficiently co-operative, a simple pediatric decongestant drop, e.g., oxymetazoline (pediatric Otrivine) should be used only.

Technique of Nasal Endoscopy
Patient Preparation
The patient should be reclined at 45° and should be asked to breathe gently through the mouth. If the examiner is right handed he/she should stand to the right side of the patient to examine both right and left nasal cavities.

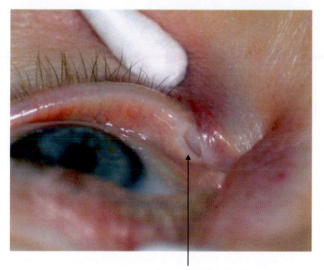

An enlarged inferior punctum

Figure 20.9 An enlarged inferior punctum following a previous three-snip punctoplasty (surgeon's view from above).

Patient Examination
The tip of the endoscope should be gently wiped with cotton wool soaked in warm sterile water. The examiner should insert the tip of the endoscope very carefully into the nasal vestibule taking great care not to touch any intranasal structures. Only after the tip of the scope has been inserted into the nose should the examiner look through the endoscope. The endoscope can then be gently advanced.

The floor of the nose can be inspected along with the lower part of the nasal septum but it is difficult to examine the inferior meatus with a 4-mm endoscope and if it is necessary to do so a 2.7-mm endoscope should be used. The endoscope should then be directed above the inferior turbinate where the maxillary line is seen on the lateral nasal wall extending up to the root of the middle turbinate, the anterior part of the middle turbinate, and the middle meatus. The endoscope should not be directed to a higher position as this is likely to induce sneezing.

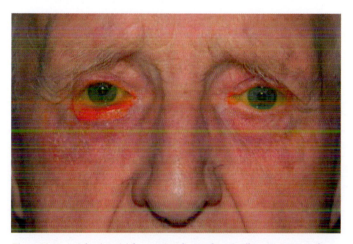

Figure 20.10 A right cicatricial ectropion due to chronic allergy to Betagan drops.

ANATOMICAL VARIATIONS OF THE MIDDLE TURBINATE
The middle turbinate normally curves away from the lateral wall of the nose and has a slightly curved lateral surface (Fig. 20.18). There are a number of variations in the anatomy of the middle turbinate, which should be recognized as these will otherwise confuse the inexperienced examiner. These variations can also have implications for the surgical management of lacrimal drainage system obstructions.

- Paradoxical (convex laterally rather than medially)
- Concha bullosa (a pneumatized anterior portion of the middle turbinate continuous with the ethmoid air cells)
- Bifid
- Duplicated
- Lateralized

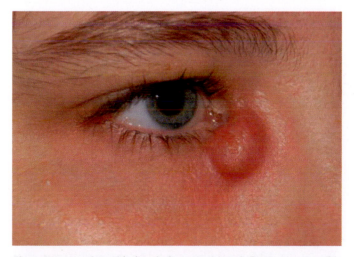

Figure 20.11 A patient with chronic dacryocystitis and a large non-expressible lacrimal sac mucocele.

Mass

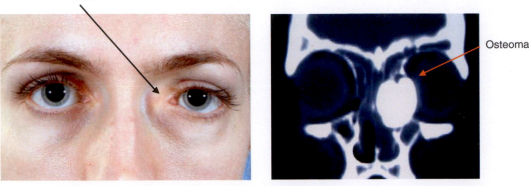

Osteoma

(A)   **(B)**

Figure 20.12 (**A**) A patient presenting with left epiphora and firm palpable mas at the medial canthus extending above the medial canthal tendon. (**B**) A coronal CT scan of the same patient showing a large ethmoidal osteoma.

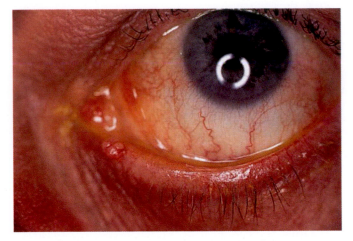

Figure 20.13 A papillomatous lesion obstructing the inferior punctum.

A large middle turbinate that extends anteriorly can cause problems with the correct placement of a Lester Jones (LJ) tube. A partial middle turbinectomy may have to be performed to address the problem. Great care should be taken, however, bearing in mind that the middle turbinate is attached to the skull base at the level of the cribriform plate. A twisting action should be avoided. Such a surgical procedure should only be undertaken if it is deemed necessary.

If the lateral surface of the middle turbinate is in very close proximity to or in direct contact with the lateral wall of the nose, there is an increased risk of the development of postoperative adhesions following lacrimal drainage system surgery. Such adhesions can be responsible for the occlusion of the drainage ostium following a dacryocystorhinostomy (DCR).

The inferior turbinate is also prone to some anatomic variations. The casual observer must also be wary of not mistaking a hypertrophied inferior turbinate for a nasal mass or polyp.

Nasal Septum
A significantly deviated nasal septum may make lacrimal drainage surgery particularly difficult and may adversely affect the success of lacrimal bypass surgery using an LJ tube. A decision can be made following nasal endoscopy in clinic about

the likely requirement for a submucosal resection (SMR) of the septum. The patient can then be counseled and consented appropriately prior to surgery and appropriate adjustments made to the anticipated time allocated for the surgery.

IMAGING
In the vast majority of patients presenting with epiphora, a good history followed by a meticulous clinical evaluation alone will suffice in enabling the surgeon to make a correct diagnosis and to determine the appropriate therapeutic option for the patient, e.g., a patient with a long history of epiphora who has a lacrimal sac mucocele with no prior history of nasal surgery or trauma and a normal endoscopic nasal examination does not require further investigations. In a small proportion of patients (depending on the specialist nature of the service and the referrals) further investigations may be required. More than one investigation, from the following list, may be required to help to establish the cause of the patient's epiphora:

- Dacryocystography (DCG)
- Dacryoscintigraphy
- Computed tomography (CT)

Dacryocystography
This investigation, which involves the injection of a radio-opaque dye into the lower or the upper canaliculi followed by the taking of magnified radiological images, provides an anatomical assessment of the lacrimal drainage system.

Indications
1. Suspected lacrimal sac tumor
2. Abnormal anatomy—previous trauma, craniofacial surgery, congenital anomalies
3. Suspected dacryoliths in a patient patent to syringing
4. Partial or functional obstruction of the nasolacrimal duct

Superior images of the lacrimal drainage system are obtained using computerized digital subtraction dacryocystography (Fig. 20.19). Additional films should be obtained 10 min after injection of dye to evaluate dye retention.

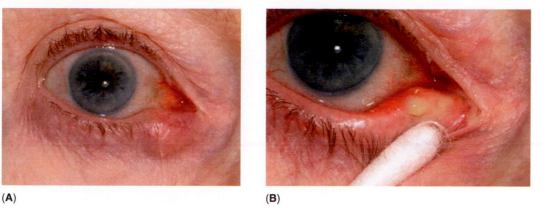

(A)   **(B)**

Figure 20.14 (**A**) A patient with a swelling of the medial aspect of the lower eyelid and a history of chronic epiphora. (**B**) Pressure applied to the lesion caused a regurgitation of a mucopurulent discharge from the inferior punctum.

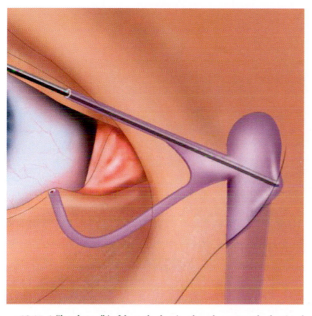

Figure 20.15 A "hard stop" is felt as the lacrimal probe enters the lacrimal sac and strikes the bone on the medial aspect of the lacrimal sac.

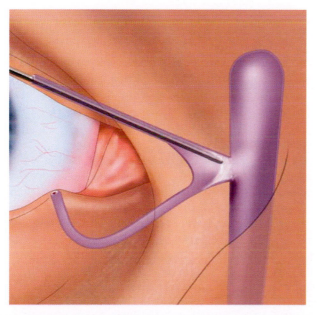

Figure 20.16 A "soft stop" is felt in the presence of a canalicular or common canalicular obstruction.

Dacryoscintigraphy

This investigation provides a physiological assessment of the lacrimal drainage system. The investigation involves the instillation of a radionuclide tracer into the conjunctival sac. The lacrimal system is then imaged with a gammagram. It is a more sensitive for the diagnosis of incomplete obstructions, particularly of the more proximal system. It is very rarely required.

Computed Tomography

CT is required in the following situations:

1. Following trauma
2. To evaluate a patient with a suspected lacrimal sac malignancy (see Fig. 20.1)
3. To evaluate the infant with a medial canthal mass

SURGICAL MANAGEMENT − INFANTS AND CHILDREN
Nasolacrimal Duct Probing and Intubation

Congenital lacrimal drainage system obstruction is present in approximately 3% to 6% of newborns. Of these, approximately 0.3% are bilateral. The most common cause is a membranous obstruction of the distal end of the nasolacrimal duct, although there is a variety of rarer anatomical variations that can also cause obstruction of the duct, e.g., nasolacrimal duct atresia, a complete bony obstruction of the duct, impaction of the inferior turbinate, a duct ending within the inferior turbinate, and nasolacrimal duct diverticula. There are a number of other congenital anomalies that must be excluded as a cause of epiphora, including punctal atresia, supernumerary puncta, congenital absence of the canaliculi, duplication of the canaliculi, and lacrimal sac fistula (see Fig. 20.20). There are also anomalies associated with facial clefts, e.g., in Goldenhar's syndrome.

Other ocular or eyelid abnormalities which can cause tearing must be excluded, e.g., buphthalmos, or distichiasis.

Most infants present with epiphora and a recurrently sticky eye, which has failed to respond to topical antibiotic treatment. Pressure applied over the lacrimal sac may produce a regurgitation of mucopurulent material. A frank mucocele may be present. Dacryocystitis is unusual.

A much rarer condition of newborn infants is an amniocoele. This appears as a soft bluish mass at the medial canthus below the level of the medial canthal tendon. This may simply

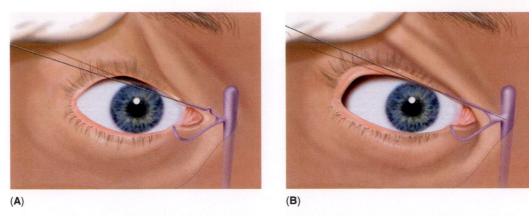

(A)   **(B)**

Figure 20.17 (**A**) A false impression of a "soft stop" has been caused by inadvertently pushing the end of the probe against the side wall of the canaliculus. (**B**) Care should be taken to ensure that the eyelid is drawn laterally and that the probe is advanced respecting the anatomical configuration of the canaliculus.

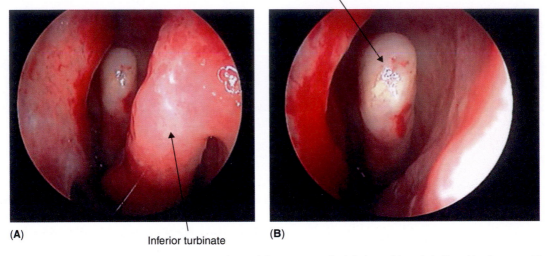

(A)   **(B)**

Figure 20.18 (**A**) An endoscopic view of the nose following the use of a nasal decongestant. The inferior turbinate is indicated by the arrow. The inferior meatus and the opening of the nasolacrimal duct lies under the inferior meatus. (**B**) The middle turbinate is indicated by the arrow. The middle meatus lies beneath this.

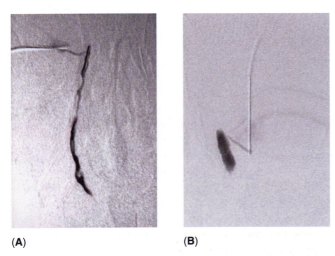

(A)   **(B)**

Figure 20.19 (**A**) Computerized digital subtraction dacryocystography (DCG) demonstrating normal right lacrimal drainage system. (**B**) A computerized digital subtraction DCG demonstrating a complete left nasolacrimal duct obstruction and a dilated lacrimal sac.

respond to firm pressure applied to the mass if the associated membranous obstruction of the nasolacrimal duct gives way. It is important to differentiate the lesion from a meningocoele or a capillary hemangioma as these can have very similar appearances.

Patient Assessment

In the majority of cases the diagnosis can be established from a good history and careful clinical examination. A dye disappearance test is easy to perform and causes the patient no pain or discomfort. It may demonstrate leakage through a dimple in the eyelid skin, indicating a congenital fistula. Syringing and probing can only be performed under general anesthesia. A dacryocystogram and a CT scan may be required for patients with craniofacial anomalies. Dacryocystography is not required for the vast majority of pediatric patients with a congenital nasolacrimal duct obstruction, but this can be performed in the operating room prior to any intervention in selected cases if the facility to do so is available.

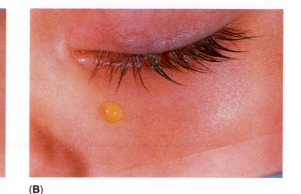

(A)   (B)

Figure 20.20 (**A**) A lacrimal sac fistula seen as a small dimple below the medial canthus. (**B**) Leakage of fluorescein from the fistula.

Management of Congenital Nasolacrimal Duct Obstruction
This should be conservative initially. The parents should be instructed to apply firm massage to the lacrimal sac in a downward direction after feeding. They must understand how to do this properly. This increases hydrostatic pressure in the lacrimal drainage system and may accelerate opening of the lower end of the nasolacrimal duct. Topical antibiotics can be prescribed intermittently. Over 90% of congenital nasolacrimal duct obstructions resolve spontaneously within the first year, with the figure increasing further by the age of 24 months. Surgical intervention should therefore be deferred until this age unless the patient is experiencing recurrent severe infections, or there is an amniocoele or dacryocystitis.

Probing should not, however, be deferred beyond the age of 2 years as the effectiveness of probing decreases with age.

KEY POINT

Over 90% of congenital nasolacrimal duct obstructions resolve spontaneously within the first year, with the figure increasing further by the age of 24 months. Surgical intervention should therefore be deferred until this age unless the patient is experiencing recurrent severe infections, or there is an amniocoele or dacryocystitis.

Nasolacrimal Duct Probing
This is performed under general anesthesia with the patient's airway protected with a laryngeal mask. Oxymetazoline (Afrazine) is sprayed into the patient's nostril immediately after the induction of anesthesia. The nose is packed beneath the inferior turbinate with small neurosurgical patties moistened with oxymetazoline. The superior canaliculus is dilated, taking great care to avoid creating a false passage. Next, a lacrimal cannula is inserted into the mid-canaliculus and a gentle irrigation of saline is performed. If there is reflux of saline, note which canaliculus the saline refluxes from. The cannula should then be gently advanced into the lacrimal sac and further irrigation should be performed. The patency of the lower canaliculus should then be similarly checked.

A no. 00 Bowman probe is then passed along the canaliculus while drawing the upper lid laterally, remembering the anatomical configuration of the canaliculus. Once a hard stop is felt, the probe is withdrawn minimally into the lacrimal sac and rotated 90° into a vertical position and then passed

inferiorly, laterally, and posteriorly, respecting the anatomical configuration of the nasolacrimal duct and without any force. The probe should lie against the infant's brow. It is often necessary to bend the probe slightly, particularly in the presence of a prominent brow (Fig. 20.21B).

Usually the membranous obstruction is felt to give way. The probe can be visualized beneath the inferior turbinate with a small endoscope (2.7 mm, 0°). This allows confirmation that a false passage has not been created through the nasal mucosa of the lateral nasal wall or inferior turbinate, a common cause of failure (Fig. 20.22).

A second syringing is then performed using saline stained with fluorescein. Patency is confirmed by means of a simultaneous endoscopic examination. If the inferior turbinate is found to be abnormally positioned or impacted, it can be gently infractured using the blunt end of a Freer periosteal elevator placed under the turbinate (Fig. 20.23). The turbinate is pushed towards the nasal septum. No postoperative ocular medications are required.

Management of a Failed Nasolacrimal Duct Probing
If a single probing has failed, the next step is to repeat the probing with placement of a silicone stent. The nose is packed beneath the inferior turbinate with small neurosurgical patties soaked in oxymetazoline. If necessary the nasal mucosa around the turbinate can be injected with 0.25% Bupivacaine with 1:200,000 units of adrenaline. The patties are left for 5 min and removed. After probing the nasolacrimal duct, a Crawford silicone stent is placed, again confirming that the stent wire has passed to the correct anatomical location beneath the inferior turbinate. The olive tip of the Crawford stent is easily engaged in the end of an Anderson–Hwang grooved director or with a Crawford retrieval hook and withdrawn from the nose (Fig. 20.24). This can be achieved in a blind fashion by the feel of metal on metal or with the use of a 2.7-mm 0° endoscope.

A Ritleng stent is even simpler to remove by using a small blunt hook along the floor of the nose and hooking the nylon suture which precedes the silicone stent (Fig. 20.25). The author prefers the less rigid Crawford stent introducer.

The stents are grasped with a locking Castroviejo needle holder at the tip of the inferior turbinate after spreading apart the eyelids to ensure that the stent in not under tension. A single surgeon's knot is tied tightly. The stent is released and the ends trimmed below the knot, leaving the cut ends

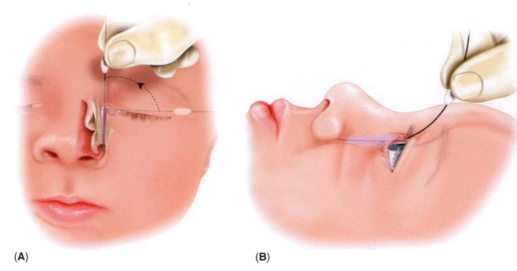

Figure 20.21 The technique of nasolacrimal duct probing.

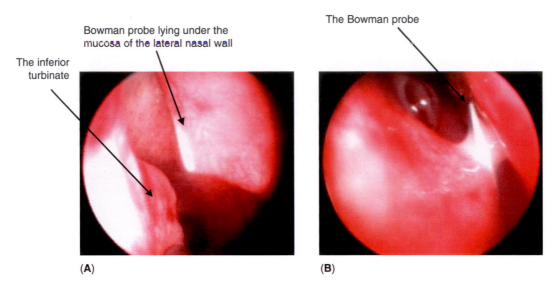

Figure 20.22 (**A**) An endoscopic view of a Bowman probe lying in a submucosal position in the lateral wall of the nose. (**B**) The appearance after the mucosa has been divided with a myringotomy blade with mucus appearing.

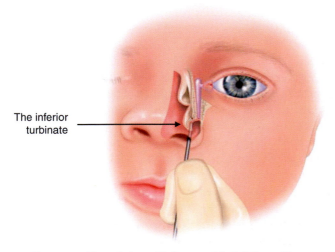

Figure 20.23 The technique of infracture of the inferior turbinate.

just visible beneath the turbinate (Fig. 20.26). It is unnecessary to secure the stent using any other device. The position of the stent at the medial canthus is again checked. An overly tightened stent will cause cheese-wiring of the puncta. The stent is left in place for at least 6 months and removed under a very short general anesthetic. If the patient has only one patent canaliculus a monocanalicular Crawford style stent is used. No postoperative ocular medications are required. The use of drops or ointments is more likely to lead to a stent prolapse.

If this procedure fails or if the patient develops a dacryocystitis, an external DCR is indicated. The operation is performed in precisely the same manner as in an adult (see below) and can be performed relatively easily in infants. It is the author's preference to avoid endoscopic DCRs in the majority of infants in whom the nasal space in too narrow to safely manipulate the instrumentation. In addition, the patient is not able to

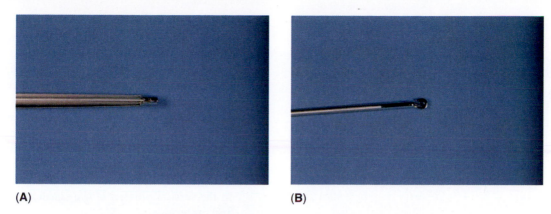

(A)   **(B)**

Figure 20.24 (**A**) Anderson-Hwang grooved director. (**B**) Crawford retrieval hook.

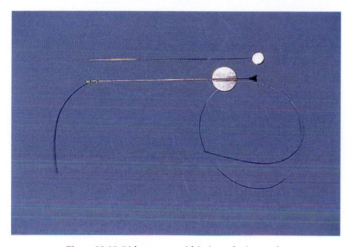

Figure 20.25 Ritleng stent within introducing probe.

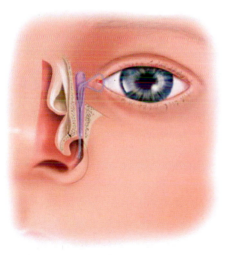

Figure 20.26 A stent has been placed through the lacrimal drainage system and has been tied with the knot and ends of the stent lying in the inferior meatus.

undertake the postoperative nasal douching which is required to aid the success of endoscopic surgery.

If a patient presents with a completely prolapsed bicanalicular silicone stent, this can be removed by rotating the knot via the inferior canaliculus before cutting the stent. It is for this reason that a single surgeon's knot is used when tying the stent

in the nose. The parents should be warned of this possibility and instructed to tape the stent to the side of the nose before making arrangements to be seen. The parents should be instructed not to cut or to pull on the stent.

Dacryocystocoele

This unusual lesion forms in utero when there is a combination of a congenital nasolacrimal duct obstruction and a competent valve of Rosenmüller. The lacrimal sac expands, as the mucus produced within the sac is unable to escape. A medial canthal mass is visible at birth and may become infected if not treated with a degree of urgency (Fig. 20.27).

The dacryocystocoele is managed by simple probing under a short general anesthetic. It is unwise to attempt to perform the probing without general anesthesia as this is painful and may act as a powerful stimulant to the oculocardiac reflex.

Lacrimal Sac Fistula

A lacrimal sac fistula is a rare congenital abnormality, which is easily overlooked; it usually occurs in conjunction with a congenital nasolacrimal duct obstruction. The fistula may connect to the common canaliculus, the lacrimal sac, or to the nasolacrimal duct. Tears may be seen emanating from a tiny hole in the inferior aspect of the medial canthus. This is more easily demonstrated with a fluorescein dye disappearance test (Fig. 20.20). The nasolacrimal duct obstruction is managed as described above, with placement of a silicone stent and the fistula is completely excised.

Punctal Atresia

This is a rare congenital abnormality in which one or more puncta are absent. An examination under general anesthesia can be performed to ascertain whether or not the puncta are merely occluded by a surface membrane with an underlying intact canalicular system. This can be managed by a simple dilatation of the punctum using a sharp Nettleship punctal dilator. The position of the punctum can usually be identified by the position of the lacrimal papilla, which is usually visible using the operating microscope. If a single punctum is completely absent no treatment is usually required, as the patient is usually only symptomatic in cold and windy conditions. If there is a single punctal agenesis with symptoms, however, it should be assumed that the patient has an associated nasolacrimal duct obstruction and a probing via the

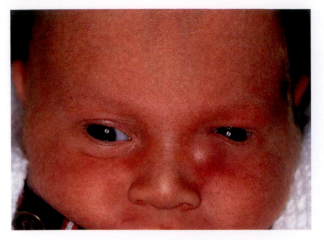

Figure 20.27 A congenital dacryocystocele.

intact punctum should be undertaken. A very careful retro-grade exploration of the affected canaliculus can be attempted, however, using a pigtail probe to ascertain whether or not the rest of the canalicular system distal to the absent punctum is intact if a complete nasolacrimal duct obstruction is found and a DCR is deemed necessary. If both puncta are absent along with the canalicular system the only remaining option is to perform a conjunctivo-dacryocystorhinostomy with placement of a LJ tube as soon as the patient is old enough to cooperate with aftercare of the tube (not usually prior to the age of 7 years).

SURGICAL MANAGEMENT—ADULTS
Eyelid Surgery
Eyelid malpositions and trichiasis are managed according to the principles outlined in chapters 3–6.

Punctoplasty
It is rarely necessary to perform surgical procedures on the inferior punctum. Simple punctal dilatation using a Nettle-ship dilator usually suffices when this is combined with a pro-cedure to correct a lower eyelid medial ectropion, e.g., a medial spindle procedure. If the effect of simple punctal dila-tation is found to be temporary this can be repeated and a silicone stent placed for a few weeks. It is the author's prefer-ence to place a bicanalicular Crawford silicone stent, particu-larly if the superior punctum is also stenosed. The use of perforated punctal plugs is an option but such plugs have a tendency to extrude. This is particularly useful if stenosis of the canaliculi is also present. This can avoid the need for a punctoplasty procedure, which can interfere with the effec-tiveness of the normal lacrimal pump mechanism and is irre-versible. If necessary a three-snip punctoplasty can be used for severe punctal stenosis unresponsive to more simple mea-sures. One- or two-snip punctoplasty procedures are not par-ticularly effective. If available, a Kelly punch is a much more effective tool to use to enlarge puncta. The punctum is first dilated sufficiently to permit the tip of the punch to be inserted into the punctum. The punch mechanism is then activated and the punctum enlarged with one or more bites as required.

Three-Snip Punctoplasty
1. A drop of proxymethacaine is instilled into the conjunctival sac.
2. One milliliter of 2% Lidocaine with 1:80,000 units of adrenaline is injected subconjunctivally just beneath the inferior punctum.
3. The inferior punctum is approached from above, with the surgeon seated at the head of the patient.
4. The punctum is dilated with a very fine tipped Nettleship dilator.
5. Using a sharp-tipped Westcott scissors, a cut is made in the vertical portion of the canaliculus inferiorly and posteriorly.
6. The scissors are turned 90° and a second cut is made just posterior and parallel to the eyelid margin.
7. Holding the tissue posterior to this cut with a 0.12 Castroviejo forceps, a third cut is made, removing a triangle of canaliculus.

Kelly Punch Punctoplasty
1. A drop of proxymethacaine is instilled into the conjunctival sac.
2. One milliliter of 2% Lidocaine with 1:80,000 units of adrenaline is injected subconjunctivally just beneath the inferior punctum.
3. The inferior punctum is approached from above, with the surgeon seated at the head of the patient.
4. The punctum is dilated with a very fine-tipped Nettleship dilator.
5. The tip of the Kelly punch is then inserted vertically into the inferior punctum.
6. The punch mechanism is then activated and the punctum enlarged with one or more bites as required.

CANALICULOTOMY
A canaliculotomy is usually performed to manage canalicular obstructions and infections caused by actinomyces (strepto-thrix). Actinomyces is a facultative anaerobe or a strictly anaerobic Gram-positive bacillus. This should be suspected in a patient who shows a unilateral upper or lower canaliculitis associated with conjunctivitis, a discharge from a pouting punctum with or without applied pressure, inflammation medial to the punctum, and a lacrimal drainage system which may be freely patent to syringing.

The punctum should be dilated and the affected canalicu-lus slit open for a distance of 4 to 5 mm using a pair of sharp tipped Westcott scissors (Fig. 20.28). The canaliculus should then be thoroughly curetted using a small curette. Topical Penicillin drops or Tobradex drops should then be prescribed for 3 to 4 weeks postoperatively. The edges of the slit canaliculus usually heal quite well without the develop-ment of secondary scarring.

DACRYOCYSTOSTOMY
This procedure is performed for the management of a lacrimal sac abscess complicating an acute dacryocystitis. This can be performed under local or general anesthesia. It should be borne in mind, however, that tissues affected by an abscess have an altered pH and can be resistant to the effects of local anesthetic solutions.

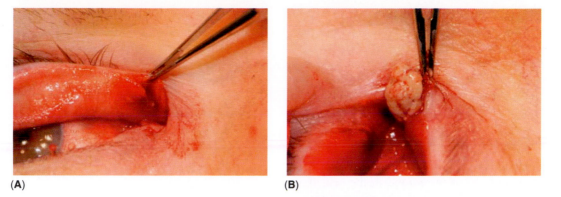

(A)   (B)

Figure 20.28 (**A**) A canaliculotomy has been performed. (**B**) Cheesy canalicular debris is being curetted from the canaliculus.

The abscess should be incised with a no. 15 Bard Parker blade and the wound opened using blunt-tipped Stevens tenotomy scissors. A sucker can be used to aspirate the pus. The abscess cavity should then be packed using a proflavin gauze leaving 2 cm protruding. The gauze is then gradually shortened and removed over the course of the next few days. Arrangements are then made for the patient to undergo a DCR within 2 to 3 weeks. In selected cases an endoscopic DCR can be performed to manage an acute dacryocystitis (Fig. 20.29), as this does not expose the patient to the risk of the spread of infection.

DACRYOCYSTORHINOSTOMY

Dacryocystorhinostomy (DCR) is a lacrimal drainage operation in which a fistula is created between the lacrimal sac and the nasal cavity in order to bypass an obstruction in the nasolacrimal duct. Such an obstruction may be partial or complete. The procedure can be performed via an external skin incision (external DCR) or through the nose (endoscopic DCR), either under local anesthesia, with or without intravenous sedation, or under general anesthesia. The surgical approach will depend on the requirements of the patient but will also depend on the relative expertise and experience of the surgeon.

Indications
1. Chronic epiphora due to a nasolacrimal duct obstruction
2. Recurrent or chronic dacryocystitis
3. Failed probings and silicone intubations in a child
4. Proposed intraocular surgery in the presence of nasolacrimal duct obstruction

Contraindications
1. Acute dacryocystitis
2. Malignant lacrimal sac tumor

The procedure should not be performed on most patients with acute dacryocystitis, although in selected patients it may be reasonable to undertake an endoscopic DCR. The infection should first be cleared with systemic antibiotics and any abscess drained via a small skin incision over the lacrimal sac.

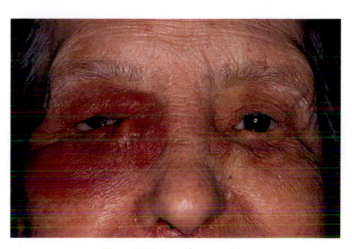

Figure 20.29 Acute dacryocystitis.

Dacryocystitis may be acute, sub-acute, or chronic. The differential diagnoses which should be considered in such patients are:

1. Acute skin infection
2. Acute ethmoiditis
3. Infected ethmoid sinus mucocele
4. A ruptured dermoid or epidermoid cyst
5. A lacrimal sac tumor

Causes of chronic dacryocystits which should be considered include Wegener's granulomatosis and sarcoidosis. If these are suspected, incisional biopsies should be undertaken at the time of a DCR.

> **KEY POINT**
>
> Any patient in whom a lacrimal sac malignancy is suspected, e.g., a history of bloody tears, should not undergo a DCR but should undergo a CT scan and an incisional biopsy.

The procedure is normally performed on a patient who has patent superior and inferior canaliculi although it may be successfully performed for a patient with a single patent canaliculus. Monocanalicular Crawford style silicone stents with an olive-tipped wire introducer are now available for use in such patients.

Goals and Risks of the Operation

Prior to scheduling a patient for a DCR, the goals and risks of the operation should be discussed with the patient and the relative merits of an external DCR versus an endoscopic DCR should be discussed. A diagram outlining the anatomical defects which need correction is presented to the patient. Pertinent features of the discussion should include:

1. The success/failure rate of the operation (the procedure should be successful in >95% of cases)
2. The location and size of the wound in the case of an external DCR (which may interfere with wearing glasses comfortably for 2 to 3 weeks postoperatively)
3. The likelihood of postoperative pain (usually minimal)
4. The need to refrain from using aspirin and anti-inflammatory drugs (and any other drugs which inhibit platelet function) for 2 weeks prior to the operation
5. The possibility of postoperative epistaxis
6. The need to refrain from blowing the nose after surgery/rubbing the eye
7. The possibility of stent prolapse, its prevention, and its management
8. The risk of CSF leak (<0.01%)
9. The type of anesthesia to be recommended

Many patients, and indeed other clinicians, perceive this procedure as a relatively minor surgical intervention. It is important to dispel such misconceptions. It is not appropriate to perform such surgery on elderly patients with cardiovascular disease who are merely inconvenienced by chronic epiphora.

> **KEY POINT**
>
> It is essential to ensure that the patient does not have undiagnosed, untreated, or poorly controlled hypertension.

External DCR

The majority of patients in the United Kingdom undergo an external DCR under general anesthesia although the operation can easily be performed under local anesthesia, with or without intravenous sedation, in suitably selected patients. General anesthesia has the advantage that both the airway and the patient's blood pressure can be controlled. The anesthetist should be asked to place a throat pack, which must be recorded and removed at the completion of surgery. The anesthetist must be informed prior to the use of any topical or subcutaneous agents to aid hemostasis. The majority of patients in the United Kingdom undergo this surgery on an in-patient basis because of the small risk of postoperative epistaxis within the first 12 hours following surgery. This surgery can, however, be performed on an out-patient basis if the patient lives within a few miles of the hospital and can return without difficulty in the event of any postoperative problems.

If local anesthesia is selected for the patient, the nostril should be sprayed with local anesthetic solution first followed by the subcutaneous injection of local anesthetic solution in the infratrochlear region and along the incision line. The patient may be sedated by an anesthetist using a combination of Midazolam and Propofol. The sedation must be safe conscious sedation, however, as the airway may be compromised by any intraoperative bleeding. The patient is then prepared for the surgery.

Patient Preparation

> **KEY POINT**
>
> Performing a successful DCR is greatly facilitated by a bloodless field.

Appropriate identification of surgical landmarks and a respect for the integrity of the nasal mucosa are essential. The patient should be placed in 15° to 20° of reverse Trendelenburg position. The first step in performing a successful DCR is correct packing of the nose. The middle turbinate must be identified and the nose packed with an epistaxis tampon lightly coated with Lacrilube ointment, which is then moistened with 5% cocaine solution (or oxymetazoline in patients with cardiovascular disease) (Fig. 20.30). The epistaxis tampon is gently inserted with its superior end abutting the anterior the tip of the middle turbinate. The cocaine or oxymetazoline solution is then dripped onto the epistaxis tampon, which gradually enlarges to fill the nasal cavity. This ensures an even delivery of the cocaine to the nasal mucosa. The epistaxis tampon is soft, non-abrasive, and easily removed. It soaks up any bleeding from the cut mucosal edges, facilitating posterior flap suturing (Fig. 20.31).

A straight diagonal incision line is drawn with gentian violet applied with a cocktail stick (Fig. 20.32). Degreasing the skin with an alcohol wipe prior to marking allows injection and prepping without losing the skin incision mark when the patient is prepped and draped. The line of the incision is marked halfway between the bridge of the nose and the medial canthus, starting at the level of the medial canthal tendon, and directed down toward the lateral ala of the nose extending for 1 to 1.5 cm (Fig. 20.33A). The incision line lies on the nasal skin and not the eyelid skin. It should not extend above the medial canthal tendon to avoid a "bow-string" scar (Fig. 20.34).

Two milliliters of 0.5% Bupivacaine with 1:200,000 units of adrenaline mixed 50:50 with 2% Lidocaine with 1:80,000 units of adrenaline is injected into the subcutaneous tissue and periosteum under the skin incision (Fig. 20.33B).

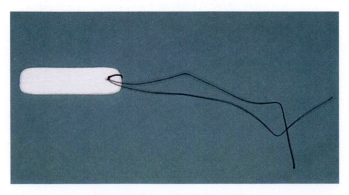

Figure 20.30 A nasal epistaxis tampon.

The surgeon should wait 10 min prior to starting the operation to allow the adrenaline to take effect.

The surgeon should wear a headlight and operating loupes.

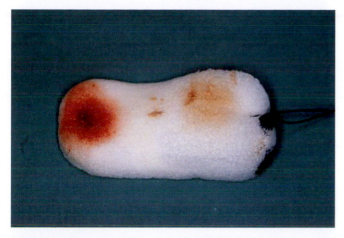

Figure 20.31 The appearance of the nasal epistaxis tampon after removal at the completion of the DCR.

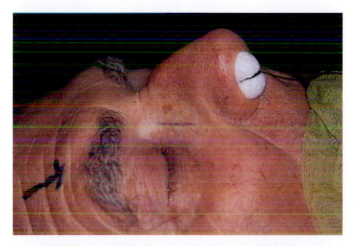

Figure 20.32 The correct side for surgery has been identified and marked. A diagonal incision has been marked with a cocktail stick and gentian violet. A nasal epistaxis tampon has been placed and moistened with cocaine solution. A throat pack has been placed.

Surgical Procedure

The operation consists of four parts:

1. Skin incision, retraction of the wound, and exposure of the lacrimal fossa
2. The osteotomy
3. The mucosal flaps and stent placement
4. The wound closure

Incision, Retraction and Exposure

1. The surgeon sits or stands at the patient's side.
2. The skin incision is made using a no. 15 Bard Parker blade.
3. Blunt-tipped Stevens tenotomy scissors are then inserted into the center of the wound and spread open along the line of the wound. These are used to dissect bluntly and bloodlessly through the orbicularis muscle down to the underlying periosteum. Alternatively, a Colorado needle can be used (Fig. 20.35).
4. The angular vessels can be seen easily and cauterized with bipolar cautery wherever necessary to prevent bleeding.
5. The periosteum is then incised to the bone with the no. 15 Bard Parker blade or Colorado needle.
6. The periosteum is then elevated off the frontal process of the maxilla and nasal bone using blunt dissection with a Freer periosteal elevator.
7. Next, 4/0 black silk traction sutures are used for retraction of the wound edges. The needle is passed deeply into the wound through the orbicularis and brought out just under the skin. Generally, four silk sutures are used (Fig. 20.36). The sutures are clamped to the drapes. Use of the sutures greatly enhances visibility and hemostasis throughout the operation, particularly if a surgical assistant is not available to hold retractors.
8. Next, the periosteum is elevated toward the anterior lacrimal crest. The sutura notha is located 1 to 2 mm anterior to the anterior lacrimal crest (Figs. 20.37 and 20.38). This is an important and consistent landmark, which should be recognized. Often, bleeding from a branch of the infraorbital artery, which travels in the groove, will occur.

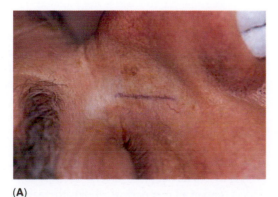

(A)

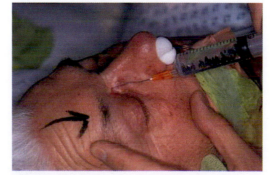

(B)

Figure 20.33 (**A**) The DCR incision has been marked. (**B**) A subcutaneous injection is given along the incision line.

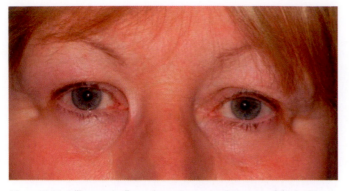

Figure 20.34 A "bow-string" scar due to incorrect placement of the incision.

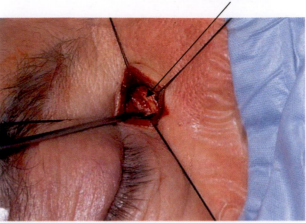

Figure 20.37 The sutura notha is identified (arrowed).

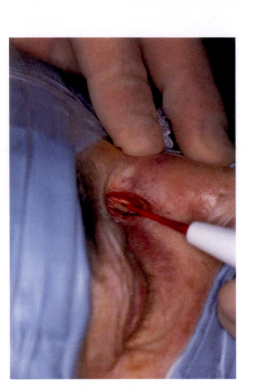

Figure 20.35 The skin incision and dissection to the periosteum can be performed with a Colorado needle.

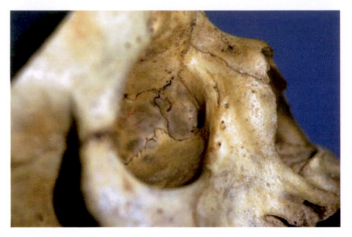

Figure 20.38 A skull viewed from the side in the position of the surgeon undertaking an external DCR.

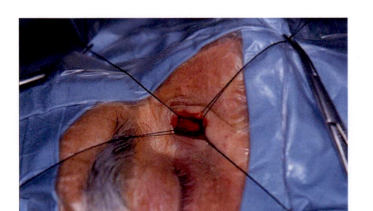

Figure 20.36 4/0 Silk traction sutures are placed to aid hemostasis and to improve exposure. These avoid the necessity for an assistant and avoid the use of rake retractors close to the globe.

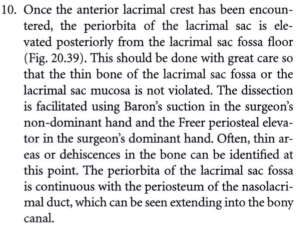

9. Bone wax should be applied to the sutura notha for hemostasis.
10. Once the anterior lacrimal crest has been encountered, the periorbita of the lacrimal sac is elevated posteriorly from the lacrimal sac fossa floor (Fig. 20.39). This should be done with great care so that the thin bone of the lacrimal sac fossa or the lacrimal sac mucosa is not violated. The dissection is facilitated using Baron's suction in the surgeon's non-dominant hand and the Freer periosteal elevator in the surgeon's dominant hand. Often, thin areas or dehiscences in the bone can be identified at this point. The periorbita of the lacrimal sac fossa is continuous with the periosteum of the nasolacrimal duct, which can be seen extending into the bony canal.

The Osteotomy

11. A small curved artery forceps or the blunt end of a Freer periosteal elevator is used to carefully puncture through the floor of the lacrimal fossa (Fig. 20.40A). Care must be taken not to disrupt

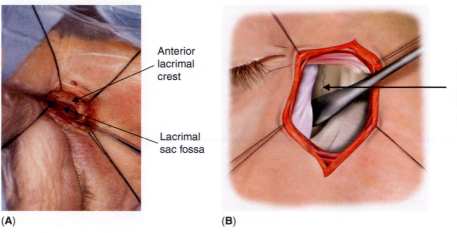

Figure 20.39 (**A**) The lacrimal sac is elevated from the lacrimal sac fossa floor. The anterior lacrimal crest is seen (solid arrow). The suture lying between the lacrimal bone and the maxillary bone is seen. (**B**) A diagram showing the exposure of the lacrimal fossa using a Freer periosteal elevator.

the underlying nasal mucosa. If a thin area cannot be identified, it is often possible to break through the suture line between the lacrimal and maxillary bones (lacrimo-maxillary suture) just anterior to the posterior lacrimal crest. In some patients with very thick bone, a diamond burr will be required to thin down the bone before proceeding further.

12. Once the artery forceps have broken through the bone, the jaws of the forceps are spread, enlarging the hole (Fig. 20.40B).

13. The osteum is then enlarged using a 90° Hardy sella or similar punch (Fig. 20.41). This punch is small and easily fits in the osteum. Occasionally, anterior ethmoidal air cells may be encountered in the posterior aspect of the osteotomy. The mucosa of the ethmoidal air cells is thin, relatively avascular, and gray in contrast to the thick well-vascularized pinkish nasal mucosa. If an anterior ethmoidal air cell is encountered, the osteotomy is placed anterior to the air cell and the air cell can be removed.

14. The Hardy sella punch is used until the osteotomy is large enough to permit the introduction of a small Kerrison rongeur. The osteotomy into the nose is then enlarged with increasing sizes of the Kerrison rongeurs. These bone-crunching instruments must be used delicately to avoid damage to the underlying nasal mucosa. Damage to the nasal mucosa at this point will cause a bloody surgical field for the remainder of the case and will make flap formation difficult. The blunt tip of the rongeur should be placed against the nasal mucosa and rotated 90°. This allows the cutting edge of the rongeur to slip behind the bone without disturbing the underlying nasal mucosa.

15. The osteotomy is carried anteriorly removing 3 to 4 mm of the anterior lacrimal crest. Inferiorly, the osteotomy can be completed using a curved Belz lacrimal rongeur or a diamond burr to remove a spine of bone between the nasal mucosa and the nasolacrimal duct.

16. The anterior limb of the medial canthal tendon crosses over the superior one-third of the sac. Some surgeons cut the tendon to offer better exposure of the sac. Generally, this is not necessary and the medial canthal tendon forms the superior extent of the osteotomy. Care must be taken to cut, not crack, bone in this area, thereby avoiding the risk of fractures that could involve the cribriform plate and lead to a CSF leak. The limits of the osteotomy are slightly different in each case. The surgeon removes only the bone that is necessary to facilitate flap formation (Fig. 20.42).

17. At this point additional local anesthetic solution is injected into the nasal mucosa. The hydrostatic effects of the local injection cause the mucosa to blanch and swell and help to stop any bleeding. Later, the effect of the adrenaline will also help to control bleeding. If these measures do not work, it may be necessary to pack the wound with gelfoam soaked in thrombin solution or with Surgicel. Bleeding from any of the bone edges is controlled by applying bone wax with the Freer periosteal elevator or cotton-tipped applicators.

Flaps

18. The lacrimal sac flaps are formed by incising the lacrimal sac mucosa vertically from the fundus of the sac down into the commencement of the nasolacrimal duct. The position of the incision is best defined by placing a no. 1 Bowman probe through the canalicular system into the sac. The tip of the probe can be seen tenting the sac towards the nasal mucosa. Generally, the position of the internal opening of the common canaliculus is in the superior aspect of the wound just below the medial canthal tendon. The incision through the lacrimal sac is made using a no. 66 Beaver blade (Fig. 20.43).

19. The sac and the superior aspect of the nasolacrimal duct should be inspected for the presence of any dacryoliths, which, if present, should be

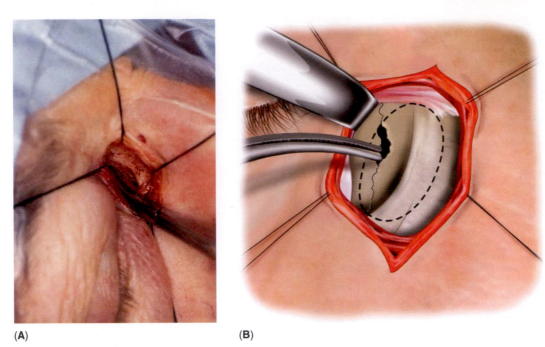

(A)   (B)

Figure 20.40 (**A**) The floor of the lacrimal sac fossa is punctured with the tip of a curved artery clip. (**B**) The tips of the artery clip are gently opened to create sufficient room for the end of a rongeur.

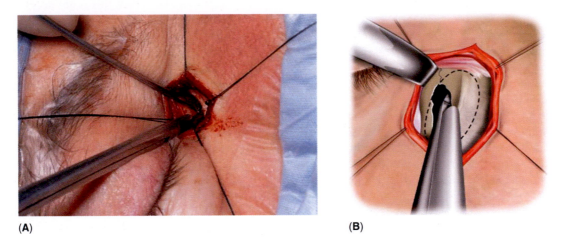

(A)   (B)

Figure 20.41 (**A**) A Hardy sella punch is used to begin the osteotomy. (**B**) The use of the punch is demonstrated diagrammatically.

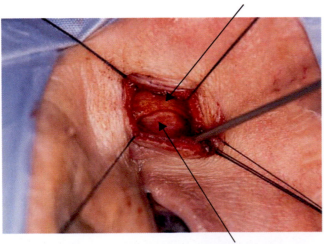

Anterior edge of
bone resection

Nasal mucosa

Figure 20.42 The osteotomy completed with nasal mucosa intact.

carefully removed. An alternative is to make a horizontal incision at the junction of the sac and the nasolacrimal duct and to make the vertical incision with Werb's angled scissors. The overlying periorbita of the lacrimal sac as well as the lacrimal sac mucosa must be incised to enter the sac. Incisions perpendicular to the vertical incision placed at the superior and inferior aspects of the lacrimal sac allow the lacrimal sac mucosa to open anteriorly and posteriorly creating anterior and posterior lacrimal mucosal flaps. The interior of the sac may now be visualized. The lacrimal probe can be seen entering the sac through the common internal punctum.

20. The probe may be pushed medially touching the nasal mucosa. Generally, the point where the probe touches the nasal mucosa is chosen as the point of incision in the nasal mucosa. In some cases a membrane may cover the internal punctum, blocking

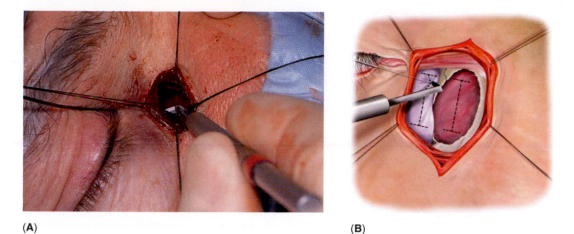

(A)   (B)

Figure 20.43 (**A**) A no. 66 Beaver blade is used to open the lacrimal sac. (**B**) A no. 1 Bowman probe is used to "tent" the lateral wall of the lacrimal sac.

the progress of the probe. This may be broken with a pointed Bowman probe (used carefully).

21. Forming the anterior and posterior flaps of the nasal mucosa is similar to forming the flaps of the lacrimal sac. The nasal mucosa is, however, much thicker than the lacrimal sac. Using a no. 66 Beaver blade, an incision is made from the most superior aspect of the osteotomy to the most inferior aspect of the osteotomy (Fig. 20.44). Again, perpendicular cuts allow the flaps to be opened anteriorly and posteriorly.

22. Additional bone may be removed anteriorly to lengthen the anterior nasal flap if necessary.

23. Rarely, the tip of the middle turbinate is seen to obstruct the osteum. In this case the turbinate should be injected with Bupivacaine and adrenaline solution and the tip resected using a Kerrison rongeur. This should be done very carefully to avoid postoperative intranasal adhesions, and to avoid causing damage to the cribriform plate with a CSF leak.

24. Next, the flaps are sutured together. A 5/0 Vicryl suture is coated with bone wax for lubrication. This aids passage of the suture and reduces the risk of cheese-wiring. The 5/0 Vicryl suture on a short 1/2-circle needle is passed from the posterior nasal mucosal flap through the posterior lacrimal sac flap (Fig. 20.45). This suture is carefully tied. Single throws of these sutures are used, as these sutures will bear no tension. The surgeon should avoid pulling the suture up when tying the knot. Generally, two sutures are placed in the posterior mucosal flaps.

25. The nasal epistaxis tampon should now be removed from the nose.

26. Crawford silicone stents are passed through the canalicular system into the nose. The stent is passed through the canalicular system, through the lacrimal sac, and into the osteotomy. The stent wire is retrieved using a grooved director placed into the nose via the nares (Figs. 20.46 and 20.47). The stent is then pushed out through the nose. The stent wire is removed and the stent is tied with a single tight knot.

27. The anterior flaps are then closed in a fashion similar to the posterior flaps (Fig. 20.48).

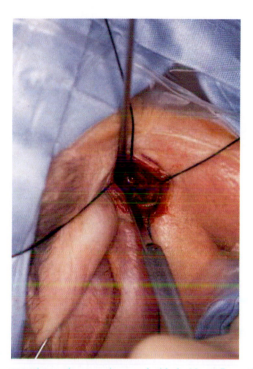

Figure 20.44 The nasal mucosa is opened with the No. 66 Beaver blade.

KEY POINT

It is important to ensure that the stent is not tight at the medial canthus by gently parting the eyelids to avoid cheese-wiring of the puncta and canaliculi (Fig. 20.49).

Wound Closure

28. The skin should be closed with interrupted 7/0 Vicryl sutures placed in a vertical mattress fashion. These sutures can be removed after 7 to 10 days or left to dissolve. It is preferable to avoid the use of subcutaneous sutures, which can predispose to thickening of the wound or infection.

29. A nasal epistaxis tampon is then cut in half and coated with antibiotic ointment, This is gently inserted into the nasal cavity to lie below the flaps and is soaked with saline until it expands.

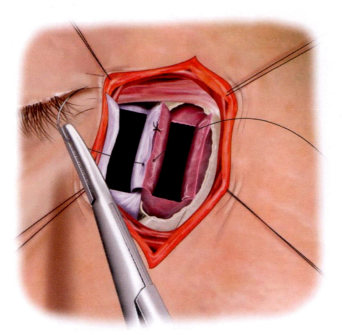

Figure 20.45 The posterior flaps are sutured.

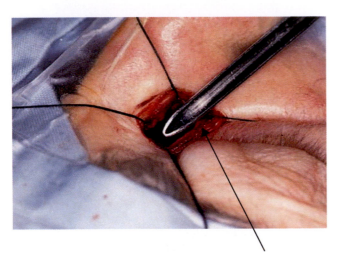

Anterior flap of
lacrimal sac mucosa

Figure 20.46 A Quickert grooved director.

Postoperative Care

The nasal epistaxis tampon is very gently removed a few hours later after soaking it with saline. Topical antibiotic ointment alone is used along the wound postoperatively unless the patient has had previous dacryocystitis or has a predisposition to infection, e.g., diabetes mellitus, in which case the patient should be prescribed a 1-week course of oral antibiotics. The patient should be instructed to perform wound massage along the line of the wound for at least 3 min three to four times per day commencing 2 weeks postoperatively after applying Lacrilube ointment. This should be continued for a period of approximately 6 weeks. The patient should be instructed to avoid any vigorous nose blowing until the stent has been removed.

The patient should also be instructed to place two fingers over the stent at the medial canthus when sneezing to avoid

causing a stent prolapse. The patient should also be instructed not to pull or cut the stent should it prolapse but to tape it to the side of the nose before contacting the hospital. The stent can usually be repositioned easily with the aid of an endoscope and a pair of "crocodile" forceps. The stent should be removed in clinic with the aid of an endoscope 6 to 8 weeks postoperatively. This is very simple. The stent is cut between the eyelids with a pair of blunt tipped scissors, and the stent is withdrawn from the nose with a pair of "crocodile" forceps.

The patient should be reviewed in clinic 1 to 2 weeks postoperatively and the nose should be examined with an endoscope. Any debris or early synechiae between the lateral nasal wall and the septum or middle turbinate can be removed with the aid of a pair of small Blakesley forceps.

Redo External DCR

A repeat DCR may be required for the management of a failed DCR or a "sump syndrome". A "sump syndrome" is characterized by a patent but high anastomosis with a residual dilated lacrimal sac, which fills with stagnant tears and mucus. A preoperative DCG can be useful in this situation to demonstrate the abnormality responsible for the patient's symptoms and clinical signs, particularly when the initial surgery has been performed elsewhere.

Surgical Procedure

1. A skin incision is made as for a standard DCR.
2. Skin–muscle flaps are fashioned and 4/0 silk traction sutures are placed.
3. A Freer periosteal elevator is used to bluntly dissect down to bone anterior to the previous osteotomy.
4. Periosteum is then elevated off the bone and the rhinostomy is enlarged. It is not uncommon to find that the original rhinostomy has not been of the correct size and is not in the correct position.
5. The nasal mucosa and scarred anastomosis are incised vertically (Fig. 20.50).
6. Bowman probes are placed into the canaliculi and scar tissue is dissected away with Westcott scissors until the ends of the probes are located.
7. Any residual lacrimal sac is opened fully (Fig. 20.51).
8. If any flaps can be fashioned, these should be sutured as for a standard DCR. Crawford-style lacrimal stents are placed before the anterior flaps are sutured.
9. The wound is closed as for a standard external DCR and the stents are left in place for a minimum period of 6 months.

Postoperative Care

This is as described for an external DCR.

If a DCR fails after it was performed appropriately by the original surgeon, it is usually preferable to dissect any scar tissue endoscopically using a sharp sickle knife, a crescent blade, or small Blakesley–Wilde through-cutting forceps. The endoscopic approach is much simpler both for the surgeon and the patient. The stents can also be placed endoscopically. In selected cases, Mitomycin may be applied to the ostium to help to prevent re-stenosis.

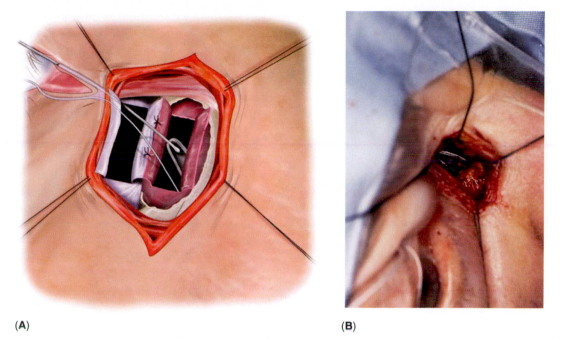

(A)   **(B)**

Figure 20.47 (**A**) Diagram demonstrating insertion of stent into grooved director. (**B**) Stent being inserted into grooved director.

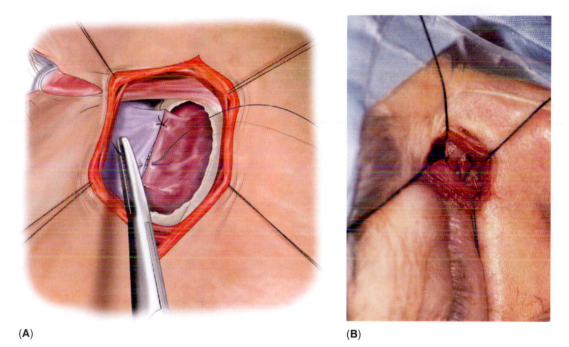

(A)   **(B)**

Figure 20.48 (**A**) A diagram showing the suturing of the anterior flaps. (**B**) The anterior flaps have been sutured.

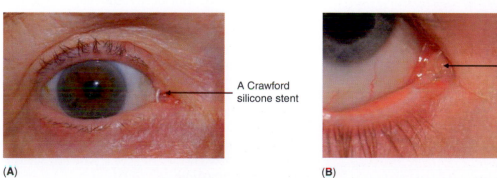

A Crawford
silicone stent

A "cheese-wired"
Crawford silicone
stent

(A)   **(B)**

Figure 20.49 (**A**) A correctly positioned stent. (**B**) An over-tightened stent has resulted in "cheese-wiring" of the inferior punctum and canaliculus.

Endoscopic Non-laser Assisted DCR

This operative approach requires skill with the use of the endoscope and good intraoperative hemostasis. It requires enthusiasm and commitment on the part of the oculoplastic surgeon if he/she wishes to undertake this procedure and consistently achieve results which are comparable with those achieved with a standard external DCR. It offers the patient the advantage of having no medial canthal wound and no cutaneous scar. It also offers the advantage that the patient's reflex blink is undisturbed, in contrast to an external DCR.

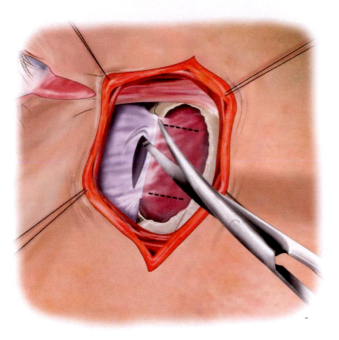

Figure 20.50 The nasal mucosa and scarred area of the anastomosis are incised.

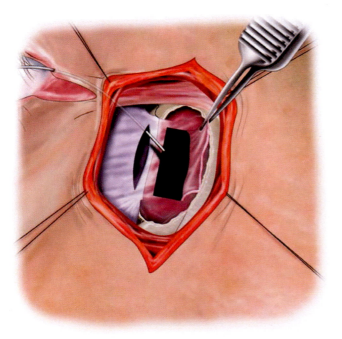

Figure 20.51 Scar tissue is resected with probes in the canaliculi.

This is a frequently overlooked cause of persistent postoperative epiphora, particularly in the cold and wind, following an otherwise successful external DCR. The cosmetic deformity associated with the scar is, however, frequently overstated. With appropriate placement of the incision and postoperative wound care and massage, the cutaneous scar is barely visible in the vast majority of patients, particularly those over 50 years of age.

Young patients, particularly female patients and those at risk of hypertrophic or keloid scars, may, however, prefer to opt for an endoscopic approach. It has generally been accepted that the success rate of this approach is slightly inferior to that of a standard external DCR, which has long been held as the "gold standard," but with improvements in instrumentation and surgical techniques, the success rate of an endoscopic non-laser assisted DCR in appropriately selected patients should not differ significantly from that of an external DCR.

It is essential that the patient has undergone an endoscopic nasal examination in clinic to ensure that the procedure is technically feasible. Some patients may require other nasal procedures to enable this approach to be used, e.g., a submucosal resection of the nasal septum if this is grossly deviated. Patient selection is important, e.g., an elderly, infirm patient with a nasolacrimal duct obstruction who has suffered acute dacryocystitis should be offered an external DCR under local anesthesia and not a endoscopic DCR.

Most patients prefer to undergo this procedure under general anesthesia, although it can be performed under local anesthesia, with or without sedation. Sedation must not compromise the airway. The operation consists of four parts:

1. The fashioning of a nasal mucosal flap
2. The osteotomy
3. The opening of the lacrimal sac and the creation of anterior and posterior flaps
4. The manipulation and replacement of the nasal mucosal flap and placement of the silicone stent

> **KEY POINT**
>
> It is very important to gain practice inserting sharp instruments atraumatically under endoscopic control before undertaking this surgical procedure.

Patient Preparation

After the induction of general anesthesia the patient should be placed in 15° to 20° of reverse Trendelenburg position. The first step in performing a successful endoscopic DCR is correct packing of the nose. The middle turbinate must be identified and the nose packed with an epistaxis tampon lightly coated with antibiotic ointment, which is then moistened with 5% cocaine solution (or oxymetazoline in patients with cardiovascular disease) (Fig. 20.30). The epistaxis tampon is gently inserted with its superior end abutting the anterior the tip of the middle turbinate. The cocaine or oxymetazoline solution is then dripped onto the epistaxis tampon, which gradually enlarges to fill the nasal cavity. This ensures an even delivery of the cocaine to the nasal mucosa. The patient is prepped and draped and the endoscopic equipment set up. The epistaxis tampon is removed once the surgeon is scrubbed and ready to commence the procedure.

Surgical Procedure

1. One to two milliliters of 2% Lidocaine with 1:80,000 units of adrenaline are injected at several points into the tip of the middle turbinate, the lateral wall of the nose above the inferior turbinate, and just below the root of the middle turbinate and into the nasal septum using a dental syringe.

2. The nose is then repacked with neurosurgical patties gently moistened with 1:1,000 adrenaline solution to the tip of the middle turbinate. The surgeon should wait 5 min prior to starting the operation to allow the adrenaline to take effect.

3. The surgeon positions himself/herself on the right side of the operating table (or left side if left-handed) ensuring that he/she has an unobstructed view of the visual display unit.

4. The patient's head should be tilted slightly towards the surgeon,

5. A 4-mm 0° endoscope is used unless the nasal cavity is small (e.g., in a child), in which case a 2.7-mm 0° endoscope is used.

6. The nasal patties are removed. The endoscope should be held comfortably balanced in the fingers of the left hand at the junction of the light source and should be inserted superiorly into the nose inserted below the endoscope with the right hand. Care should be taken to avoid touching any mucosal surface with the endoscope. An anti-fog device, e.g., ELVIS® or FRED® should be placed by the patient's head and the tip of the endoscope wiped gently across the surface each time the endoscope is removed from the nasal cavity.

The Fashioning of a Nasal Mucosal Flap

7. The use of a canalicular light pipe is not required for a standard endoscopic non-laser

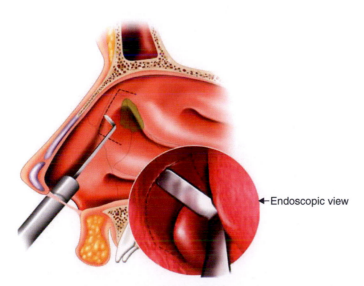

←Endoscopic view

Figure 20.52 The nasal mucosa is incised using a crescent blade so that the mucosa can be flapped back to cover the middle turbinate, keeping it out of the way of instruments and the sucker.

assisted DCR. The blunt end of a Freer periosteal elevator can be used to gently flatten the nasal mucosa of the lateral nasal wall and can be used to gently push the tip of the middle turbinate medially.

8. A phacoemulsification crescent blade is then inserted into the nose and used to make a nasal mucosal incision commencing from a point 7 to 10 mm anterior to the root of the middle turbinate continuing inferiorly along a line approximately 7 to 10 mm anterior to the anterior lacrimal crest (Fig. 20.52) and finishing a few millimeters above the inferior turbinate.

9. Using the crescent blade additional incisions are made superiorly and inferiorly at 90° to the vertical incision in a posterior direction. (Fig. 20.52).

10. This nasal mucosal flap is then raised with the Freer periosteal elevator and pushed posteriorly. The middle turbinate is now covered and protected by the nasal mucosal flap. The flap is now kept out of the way of the instruments used for the osteotomy.

The Osteotomy

11. A 45° long-handled up-biting laminectomy punch is now inserted into the nasal cavity and used to take bites of bone anteriorly into the frontal process of the maxilla, commencing at the midpoint of the mucosal incision (Fig. 20.53). The punch can be easily rotated and inserted under the anterior lacrimal crest to commence this bone removal. The inferior aspect of the lacrimal sac is thereby exposed. Once this part of the lacrimal sac has been clearly identified the bone removal can be continued until the whole of the lacrimal sac has been exposed. Care should be taken not to remove too much bone anteriorly as this will expose orbicularis muscle.

12. The thin lacrimal bone lying posterior to the lacrimal sac can be removed using small Blakesley-Wilde forceps. Occasionally some anterior ethmoid air cells will be exposed and may also be removed with the Blakesley forceps.

13. Bone removal with the punch is continued as far superiorly as possible until the bone becomes too thick for the punch to engage. At this point the punch is exchanged for a 15° curved 2.9-mm rough diamond burr (Medtronic Xomed, Jacksonville, Florida, USA), which is attached to a microdebrider with irrigation and suction. This is then used to remove the rest of the bone as far as the superior extent of the nasal mucosal incision Fig. 20.54A). It can also be used to smooth off the anterior aspect of the bone edges inferiorly.

14. A 00 Bowman probe is inserted into the superior canaliculus and the lacrimal sac is tented. The bone removal is continued superiorly until the probe no longer abuts bone when inserted horizontally.

The Opening of the Lacrimal Sac and the Creation of Anterior and Posterior Flaps

15. The lacrimal sac is then opened with the crescent blade. The sac is first tented with the Bowman probe. A vertical incision is then made over the most tented position of the sac mid-way between the most anterior and posterior aspects of the sac (Fig. 20.54B). The crescent blade is move superiorly and inferiorly opening the whole vertical extent of the sac.

16. The blade is then used to make anterior relieving cuts at the most superior and inferior aspects of the sac creating an anterior flap. Posterior flaps are created using endoscopic scissors (Fig. 20.55A).

17. Using the Freer elevator the anterior lacrimal sac flap is then moved forward over the exposed bone. If the flap so created is too short and does

not lie passively in this position the anterior flap can instead be removed using pediatric Blakesley–Wilde through-biting forceps.

The Manipulation and Replacement of the Nasal Mucosal Flap and Placement of the Silicone Stent

18. A curved window is now cut from the original nasal mucosal flap with the same through-biting forceps. A C-shaped flap is fashioned which is then repositioned with the Freer elevator so that the nasal mucosa above and below the "C" is in contact with the posterior lacrimal sac mucosal flap (Fig. 20.55B).

19. A Crawford silicone stent is then passed in the same way as with an external DCR using a grooved director. This is tied in the same way and care taken to ensure that the stent is not under tension at the medial canthus (Fig. 20.55C).

20. A nasal epistaxis tampon is then cut in half and coated with antibiotic ointment, This is gently inserted into the nasal cavity to lie below the flaps and is soaked with saline until it expands.

Postoperative Care

The postoperative appearance is shown in Figure 20.56. The patient is asked to irrigate the nose at least twice a day with Sinurinse® to remove dried clots and debris for a minimum period of 2 weeks postoperatively. A steroid nasal spray and a decongestant nasal spray nasal are prescribed for 5 days. A gentle syringing of the lacrimal drainage system is undertaken at the first postoperative visit 1 week following the surgery. An endoscopic examination should be performed and any excessive intranasal debris removed. The stent should be removed in clinic endoscopically 6 to 8weeks postoperatively. Topical or systemic antibiotics are only used in patients who have had previous dacryocystitis or who are diabetic or immuno-compromised. They are not otherwise used routinely.

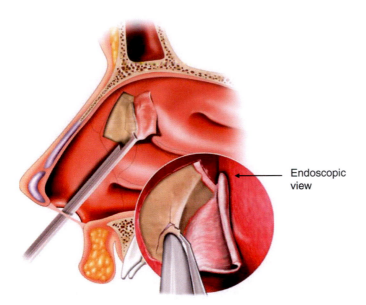

Endoscopic view

Figure 20.53 A 45° laminectomy punch is inserted into the nose and positioned behind the anterior lacrimal crest before bone is nibbled away.

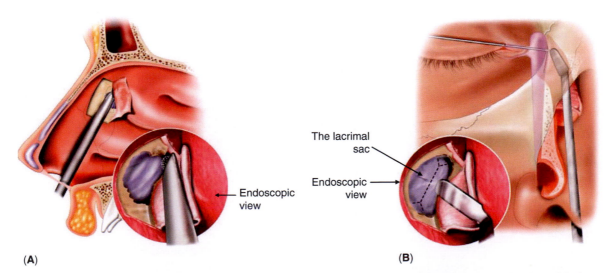

Endoscopic view

The lacrimal sac

Endoscopic view

(A)   **(B)**

Figure 20.54 (**A**) A guarded diamond burr is used to remove bone adjacent to the fundus of the lacrimal sac and to smooth the edges of the bone around the osteotomy. (**B**) The lateral wall of the lacrimal sac is "tented" using a Bowman probe and incised using a crescent blade.

The endoscopic approach is also particularly advantageous for the failed DCR where the ostium has simply stenosed or scarred over completely. This can be reopened with a sharp sickle blade, a crescent blade or scar tissue can be removed using a Blakesley–Wilde through-cutting forceps, and a stent passed relatively easily in a short operative procedure.

Endonasal Laser-Assisted DCR

Advocates of endoscopic laser-assisted DCR point to a number of potential advantages of this technique.

Advantages

1. Local anesthetic day case procedure
2. Short operating time (15 to 30 min)
3. Minimal postoperative morbidity
4. Minimal disruption of adjacent structures
5. No cutaneous scarring
6. High patient acceptance
7. Easy revisionary surgery
8. Ideal for the patient with a bleeding diathesis or who is using anti-coagulants

There are, however, a number of disadvantages of the procedure.

Disadvantages

1. Low long-term success rate (less than 60%)
2. Potential risk of laser complications
3. High cost of equipment
4. Some cases require combined skills of an ophthalmologist and an ENT surgeon
5. Potential morbidity in not recognizing a lacrimal sac tumor intraoperatively

Surgical Procedure

1. The patient is prepared as described above.
2. A 20-gauge retinal light pipe is inserted via the upper canaliculus and positioned in the lower part of the

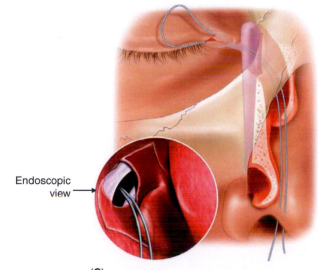

(A)

(B)

(C)

Figure 20.55 (**A**) The posterior flap of the lacrimal sac is created using endoscopic scissors. (**B**) The silicone stents have been passed into the nose. (**C**) A "C"-shaped resection of the nasal mucosa has been undertaken and the nasal mucosa has been repositioned against the lateral wall of the nose.

lacrimal sac, and the area is visualized endoscopically (See Fig. 20.57).

3. The holmium–YAG laser probe is directed at the area of transillumination and, initially, a 7/8-mm diameter area of mucosa is ablated with the laser.
4. The underlying bone is then lasered at a higher energy setting.
5. The lacrimal mucosa adjacent to the area of the rhinostomy is ablated and an opening into the sac is created.
6. The silicone stent is then placed.

This procedure has not achieved the same status as the external DCR, which has very little morbidity in the hands of the experienced oculoplastic surgeon but a very high success rate. The external DCR remains the gold standard operation by which all other procedures have to be judged.

Postoperative Care
This is the same as described for a non-laser assisted endoscopic DCR.

CANALICULO-DACRYOCYSTORHINOSTOMY

A canaliculo-DCR is a lacrimal drainage operation in which a small section of obstructed canaliculus just lateral to the lacrimal sac is resected and the patent canaliculus anastomosed to the nasal mucosa using the lacrimal sac as a soft tissue bridge. The procedure can only be performed via an external skin incision, either under local anesthesia, with or without sedation, or general anesthesia. It cannot be performed endoscopically. For patients with a distal membranous obstruction overlying the common canaliculus, which can be overcome with a probe, the lacrimal drainage system should be simply intubated for a period of 3 to 6 months.

Indications

Obstruction of the common canaliculus or of the individual canaliculi just lateral to the sac with a minimum of 8 mm of patent canaliculus present.

Surgical Procedure

The patient is prepared as for a standard DCR.

1. A skin incision is made as for an external DCR
2. The superficial part of the medial canthal tendon is identified and divided with a no. 15 blade just lateral to its insertion on the nasal bone.
3. The tendon is reflected laterally, exposing the anterior surface of the fundus of the lacrimal sac (Fig. 20.58). The relationship of the canaliculi to the medial canthal tendon is demonstrated in Figure 20.59.
4. No. 1 Bowman's probes are placed into the superior and inferior canaliculi. The medial canthal tendon is dissected on its deep surface laterally, superiorly, and inferiorly using a Freer periosteal elevator until the probes are just visible.
5. The periosteum is incised over the anterior lacrimal crest and reflected laterally.
6. Next, a large rhinostomy is created.
7. The lacrimal sac is opened anteriorly adjacent to the Bowman probes from the fundus of the sac

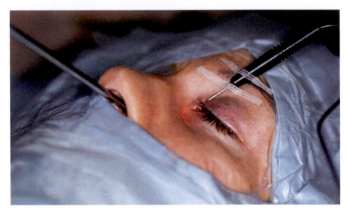

Figure 20.57 With the endoscope turned off the retinal light pipe can be seen transilluminating the lacrimal sac fossa.

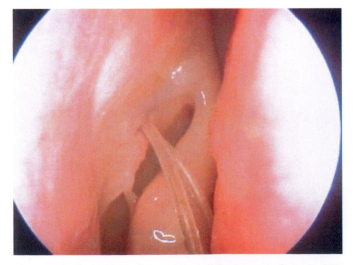

Figure 20.56 The postoperative appearance following an endoscopic DCR with the silicone stent in place.

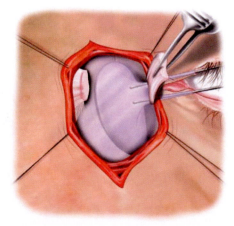

Figure 20.58 The anterior limb of the medial canthal tendon is disinserted from the nasal bone and reflected laterally with probes in the canaliculi helping to identify the position of the canaliculi.

to the commencement of the nasolacrimal duct (Fig. 20.60).

8. The canaliculi are incised and a silicone stent passed and used to draw the canaliculi laterally. The whole of the lacrimal sac is now rotated posteriorly to form the posterior flap of the anastomosis and a large nasal mucosal flap is formed and rotated anteriorly to form the anterior flap.

9. The lateral margins of the canaliculi are sutured to the adjacent lacrimal sac mucosa using 8/0 Vicryl sutures (Fig. 20.61).

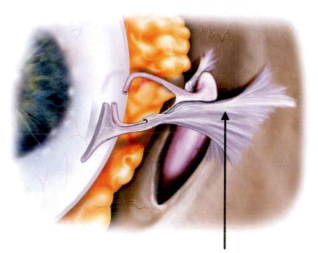

The anterior limb of the medial canthal tendon

Figure 20.59 A drawing showing the relationship of the canaliculi and the lacrimal sac to the medial canthal tendon.

10. The posterior flaps are then sutured and the anterior flaps sutured after the stent has been passed into the nose (Fig. 20.62).

11. The medial canthal tendon is sutured back to its stump using a 5/0 Vicryl suture.

12. The wound is closed as for a DCR.

Postoperative Care

This is as described for an external DCR. The stent is not removed for at least 6 months.

CONJUNCTIVO-DACRYOCYSTORHINOSTOMY (CDCR)

This surgical procedure is an extension of a DCR with the addition of several steps involved in the placement of a pyrex glass LJ tube. This procedure creates a lacrimal drainage pathway from the conjunctiva into the nasal space, bypassing the canaliculi and the lacrimal sac. The proximal end of the tube lies at the medial commissure and the distal end lies within the middle meatus of the nose. The procedure has a high degree of success in experienced hands but such success requires good postoperative cooperation from the patient.

Indications

1. Symptomatic epiphora secondary to extensive scarring of both upper and lower canaliculi
2. Congenital atresia or complete absence of the canaliculi with epiphora
3. Symptomatic epiphora secondary to lacrimal pump failure, e.g., chronic facial palsy
4. Failed canaliculoDCR
5. Failed redo DCR
6. Chronic epiphora due to eyelid malpositions which eyelid surgery has failed to or is unable to control, e.g., Centurion syndrome, ichthyosis, severe chronic eczema

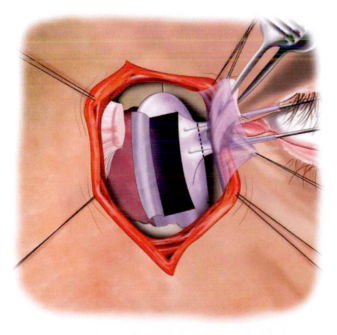

Figure 20.60 The lacrimal sac is opened very anteriorly creating a large posterior flap. The anterior flap is created from nasal mucosa after fashioning a large rhinostomy.

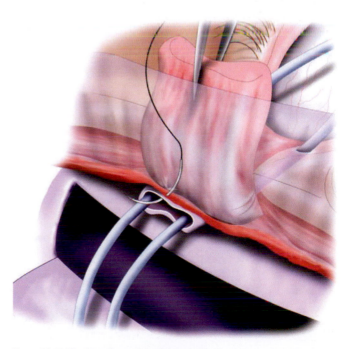

Figure 20.61 The lateral margins of the canaliculi are sutured to the adjacent lacrimal sac mucosa using 8/0 Vicryl sutures.

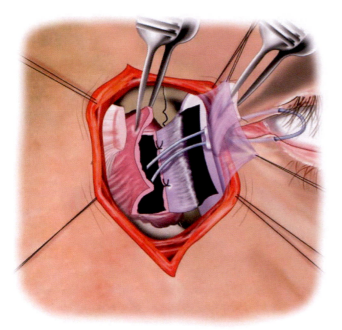

Figure 20.62 The posterior flaps have been sutured and the stent has been passed before the anterior flaps are sutured and the anterior limb of the medial canthal tendon repaired.

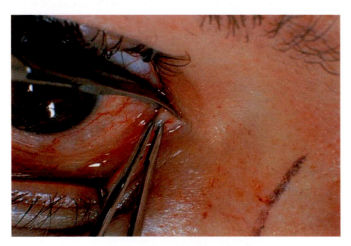

Figure 20.63 Resection of the caruncle.

Patient Evaluation

Each patient must be counseled about the pros, cons, risks, and potential complications of this operative procedure. In particular, the patient must understand that the LJ tube is a device which is permanently implanted, committing the patient to lifelong maintenance of the tube and follow-up. Careful patient selection is essential. Only patients whose lifestyle is adversely affected by constant epiphora and who are willing to comply with aftercare should be offered such surgery.

The patient should be carefully examined to determine whether or not additional surgical procedures may be required. Any significant eyelid malposition or medial canthal dystopia will need to be addressed. An endoscopic nasal examination must be performed to exclude intranasal abnormalities and to confirm that there is adequate space for placement of the LJ tube. Some abnormalities, e.g., an elongated middle turbinate or a nasal septal deviation, can be managed at the time of the CDCR. Occasionally such abnormalities may need to be addressed by an ENT surgeon prior to the patient undergoing a CDCR. Occasionally a coronal CT scan will be required to evaluate the medial canthal anatomy if the patient has undergone previous craniofacial surgery, trauma, or bone grafting. It is important in such patients to ascertain the position of the cribriform plate or the position of micro or miniplates. The operation itself can be performed externally or endoscopically, under general or local anesthesia. It is now much more frequent for such surgery to be performed endoscopically.

EXTERNAL CDCR AND LJ TUBE
Surgical Procedure

The patient is prepared as for a standard external DCR. A DCR is performed to the point at which flaps of nasal and lacrimal sac mucosa are made taking care not to disrupt the medial canthal tendon. The osteotomy is made no more than 4 to 5 mm inferior to the lower border of the medial canthal tendon to prevent too inferior an angulation of the LJ tube. The osteotomy is made respecting an approximate 5-mm radius centered on the position of the common canaliculus. The posterior flaps are sutured.

1. Next, the caruncle is resected with Westcott scissors (Fig. 20.63).

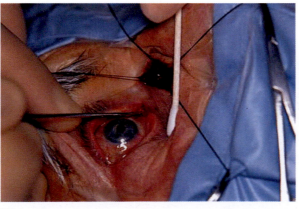

(A)

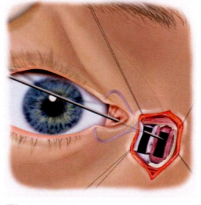

(B)

Figure 20.64 (**A**) A Kirschner wire is passed through the bed of the resected caruncle. (**B**) The Kirschner wire is then directed through the lateral wall of the lacrimal sac in the region of the common canaliculus.

2. An 18-gauge sharp-tipped Kirschner wire is then pushed from the bed of the caruncle to the lacrimal sac in the region of the common canaliculus to lie just anterior to the tip of the middle turbinate (Fig. 20.64). If the middle turbinate interferes with the desired placement of the wire the tip can be resected with care using Blakesley-Wilde forceps, avoiding twisting motions, which can damage the cribriform plate and lead to a CSF leak (Fig. 20.65).

3. Next, the track is enlarged using a series of standard gold dilators (Fig. 20.70) or, if necessary, a small Elliot's trephine (Fig. 20.66A). Care should be taken not to overdilate the track, which could otherwise lead to instability of the LJ tube. The track should grip the tube firmly.

4. The length of LJ tube required is then estimated by passing a Putterman probe along the fistulous track to lie 2 to 3 mm from the nasal septum. The measurement of the length of tube required is provided on a scale on the probe (Fig. 20.67). The tube is checked for the length and collar size (usually 3.5 or 4 mm).

5. An LJ tube is then slipped over a fine blunt-tipped guidewire and pushed into position using the surgeon's thumbnails until the neck lies in the caruncular bed (Fig. 20.68). It is preferable to avoid the use of metal instruments to push the tube into place as these can easily break or scratch the tube.

6. The guidewire is removed.

7. The position of the LJ tube in the nose should be checked using a nasal speculum and headlight or using an endoscope if this is available. If the tube is found to be too long or too short, the guidewire is replaced and the tube removed. It is replaced with an alternative size and rechecked. Occasionally, an angulated tube will be required if the middle turbinate or nasal septum cause problems with satisfactory placement.

8. Next, the anterior flaps are sutured together and the tube irrigated to clear any blood clots.

9. A 7/0 Vicryl suture is wrapped around the tube and passed through the lower eyelid emerging a few millimeters below the eyelid margin, and tied (Fig. 20.69). This is to prevent migration of the tube towards the nose.

10. The wound is closed as for an external DCR.

11. A firm compressive dressing is placed overnight.

Postoperative Care

The wound care is the same as in the case of an external DCR. There is no need to prescribe topical antibiotic or steroid drops. There is no requirement for the routine use of systemic antibiotics in the absence of specific indications for their use. The patient is also instructed to instill Hypromellose drops into the eye morning and evening and, while occluding the opposite nostril with a finger, to sniff vigorously. This is undertaken at least twice a day on a permanent basis. The patient is instructed to place two fingers over the LJ tube when sneezing and is warned about the sensation of air passing across the eye when blowing the nose. The patient is instructed to report any

A straight Lester Jones tube

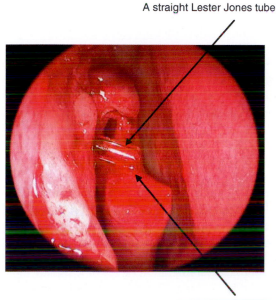

A partially resected middle turbinate

Figure 20.65 An intraoperative endoscopic view of a partial middle turbinectomy performed endoscopically with a straight LJ tube lying in a satisfactory position.

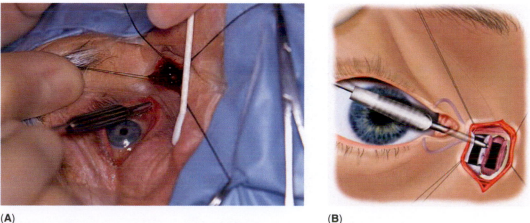

(A)   (B)

Figure 20.66 (**A**) An Elliott's trephine is slipped over the Kirschner wire. (**B**) The trephine is pushed through the lateral wall of the lacrimal sac.

problems with the tube immediately as adjustments to the tube or replacement of the tube are much easier at this stage than if the patient presents some time after losing the tube, when the fistulous track has usually fibrosed. Occasionally, blocked tubes may need to be flushed through with saline using a syringe and lacrimal cannula in the clinic.

Endoscopic CDCR and LJ Tube

The endoscopic CDCR has a number of advantages, which should be weighed against the disadvantages. The individual patient should be carefully assessed preoperatively to determine which approach is most suitable and to determine whether or not an ENT colleague is required to assist with any additional intranasal procedures that may be required. This approach is now undertaken far more frequently than an external approach in the author's practice.

Advantages
1. This approach avoids a cutaneous scar.
2. The surgery is minimally invasive.
3. This approach permits the correction of common intranasal abnormalities simultaneously.
4. This approach permits an easier and quicker approach to reoperations.

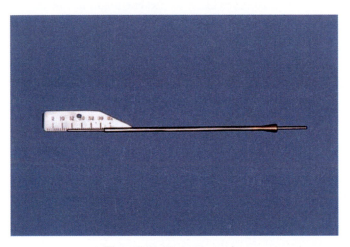

Figure 20.67 A Putterman probe.

Disadvantages
1. Meticulous intraoperative hemostasis is required to maintain good visualization.
2. Expensive equipment is required.
3. This approach is unsuitable for patients with severe bony deformities of the medial canthus.

Surgical Procedure

The operation is performed as for a non-laser assisted endoscopic DCR. The osteotomy required, however, is much smaller and there is no need to expose the whole of the lacrimal sac. Too large an osteotomy is associated with less stability of the LJ tube. Once the internal rhinostomy has been completed the lacrimal sac is opened and the LJ tube is placed as described above while visualizing its position endoscopically. If a patient has previously undergone DCRs, which have failed or a previous CDCR with loss of the LJ tube, the endoscopic approach is relatively simple. The bony rhinostomy has already been performed and placement of the LJ tube is performed as described above and the intranasal position of the tube observed endoscopically (Fig. 20.70). An example of the postoperative appearance of a typical patient is shown in Figure 20.71.

Postoperative Care

This is as described above with the exception of the use of a topical antibiotic ointment. In addition the patient should be instructed to undertake nasal douching using Sinurinse® at least twice a day for 2 weeks.

Complications

Although there are a multitude of complications that can occur following placement of an LJ tube, the most frequently encountered problem is that of tube displacement. This needs to be managed early to avoid additional secondary ocular complications, e.g., a scleritis from local scleral indentation and irritation. Lateral migration of the tube usually indicates that the tube is too long. The tube should be removed and replaced with a more appropriately sized tube. The nose should be examined endoscopically to determine whether or not intranasal abnormalities are also responsible for the migration.

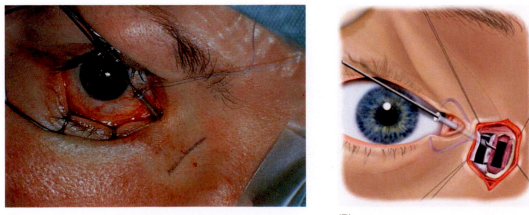

(A)   **(B)**

Figure 20.68 (**A**) The Lester Jones tube is passed along a blunt-tipped guidewire. (**B**) The Lester Jones tube is then passed over the guidewire into the nose.

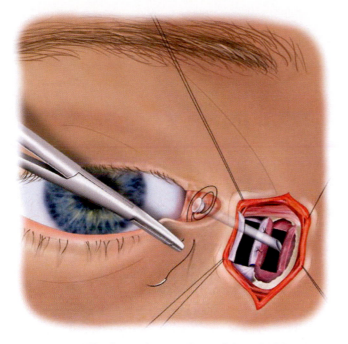

Figure 20.69 A 7/0 Vicryl suture is wrapped around the neck of the tube. The suture is brought through the full thickness of the lower eyelid and tied on the skin to prevent inward migration of the tube while postoperative edema is subsiding.

Medial migration can lead to the tube becoming invisible at the medial canthus. This should be removed endoscopically and replaced with a tube with a larger diameter neck. Granulation tissue around the tube should be removed with Westcott scissors and the base cauterized with bipolar cautery.

Most long-term complications associated with the use of a LJ tube, e.g., occlusion of the tube, can be avoided by good compliance on the part of the patient with aftercare instructions and long-term follow-up.

Endoscopic Nasal Septoplasty

Not infrequently patients requiring a LJ tube will be found to have a deviated nasal septum which prevents adequate endoscopic surgical access to create the nasal osteotomy and to place a LJ tube satisfactorily. Such patients require a submucosal resection of the nasal septum (SMR). This can be undertaken endoscopically at the same time as an endoscopic CDCR. An oculoplastic surgeon who has gained skill and experience undertaking endoscopic lacrimal drainage surgery should also be able to acquire the relevant surgical skills to perform an endoscopic SMR.

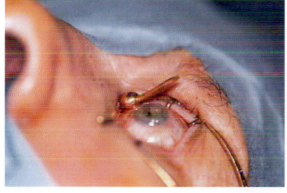

(A)

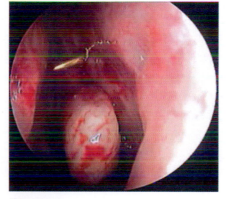

(B)

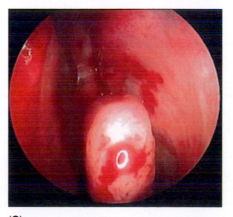

(C)

Figure 20.70 (**A**) A gold dilator is passed via the caruncular bed. (**B**) The position of the dilator is observed endoscopically. In this patient the dilator is entering the nasal cavity just in front of the middle turbinate. (**C**) This Lester Jones tube was positioned at a higher level than normal but functioned well.

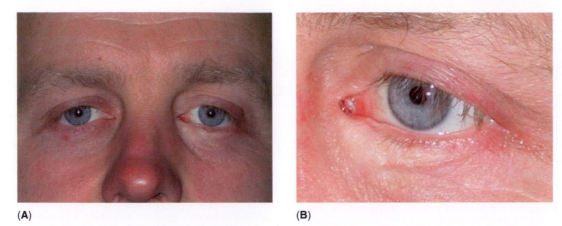

(A)   **(B)**

Figure 20.71 (**A**) A patient who was referred with a lower eyelid medial cicatricial extropion and extensive canalicular scarring following trauma. A lower eyelid skin graft has been placed to reposition the eyelid and a Lester Jones (LJ) tube has been placed endoscopically. (**B**) A side view of the LJ tube position.

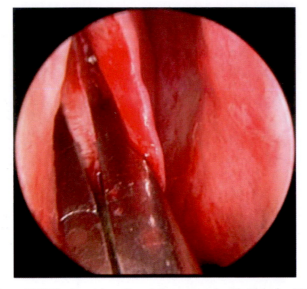

Figure 20.72 Nasal septal cartilage being removed with Blakesley–Wilde through biting forceps.

Surgical Procedure

1. Two to three milliliters of 2% lidocaine with 1:80,000 units of adrenaline are injected submucosally on each side of the nasal septum using a dental syringe and a local anesthetic cartridge and a 4-mm 0° nasal endoscope.
2. Each nasal cavity is then packed gently with soft neurosurgical patties moistened with 1:1,000 adrenaline. A few minutes are allowed for the adrenaline to take effect.
3. Next a straight incision is made horizontally through the nasal mucosa approximately 10 mm above the columella on the side on which the CDCR is to be performed using a crescent blade.
4. The nasal mucosa is then elevated from the nasal septal cartilage using a Freer periosteal elevator.
5. The sharp end of the Freer periosteal elevator is then used to cut through the nasal cartilage a few millimeters above the mucosal incision taking care not to cut through the nasal septal mucosa on the other side of the cartilage.

6. The Freer periosteal elevator is then used to elevate the nasal mucosa from the cartilage on the other side. The submucosal position of the elevator can be observed endoscopically from the opposite nostril.
7. Next, medium Blakesley-Wilde through biting forceps are used to remove the deviated nasal septal cartilage piecemeal (Fig. 20.72).
8. Alternatively, a diamond burr can be used to thin the cartilage. It is important to leave approximately 8 mm of cartilage anteriorly to avoid collapse of the nasal strut.
9. The middle meatus is then inspected at intervals and as soon as sufficient room has been created to permit the placement of a LJ tube the nasal septal mucosa is laid back in its original position. No sutures are required.

Postoperative Care

The postoperative care is as described above with the additional prescription of a topical antibiotic, which is gently smeared along the nasal septal mucosal wound three times per day for a week. The mucosal wound heals spontaneously.

DACRYOCYSTECTOMY

A dacryocystectomy is indicated for the following groups of patients:

1. Patients with malignant epithelial lacrimal sac tumors
2. Elderly patients with dacryocystitis but without epiphora

In patients with malignant epithelial cell tumors of the lacrimal sac, the entire lacrimal sac should be widely excised along with the canaliculi and the nasolacrimal duct. This is usually combined with a lateral rhinostomy and postoperative radiotherapy should also be considered.

A dacryocystectomy is a relatively short operative procedure which is well tolerated under local anesthesia, with or without sedation in the elderly. It has a short recovery period. It is preferable to a DCR for dacryocystitis in the absence of epiphora or in the presence of a dry eye problem.

Surgical Procedure

1. A standard external DCR incision is marked with a gentian violet.
2. Two to three milliliters of 2% lidocaine with 1:80,000 units of adrenaline are injected subcutaneously around the lacrimal sac and along the medial aspect of the upper and lower eyelids. An infratrochlear nerve block can also be used.
3. The surgeon sits or stands at the patient's side.
4. The skin incision is made using a no. 15 Bard Parker blade.
5. Blunt-tipped Stevens tenotomy scissors are then inserted into the center of the wound and spread open along the line of the wound. These are used to dissect bluntly and bloodlessly through the orbicularis muscle down to the underlying periosteum.
6. The medial canthal tendon is exposed.
7. The angular vessels can be seen easily and cauterized with bipolar cautery wherever necessary to prevent bleeding.
8. The periosteum is then incised to the bone with the no. 15 Bard Parker blade.
9. The periosteum is then elevated off the frontal process of the maxilla and nasal bone using blunt dissection with a Freer periosteal elevator.
10. Next, 4/0 black silk traction sutures are used for retraction of the wound edges. The needle is passed deeply into the wound through the orbicularis and brought out just under the skin. Generally, four silk sutures are used. The sutures are clamped to the drapes.
11. Next, the periosteum is elevated toward the anterior lacrimal crest. The sutura notha is located 1 to 2 mm anterior to the anterior lacrimal crest. Often, bleeding from a branch of the infraorbital artery, which travels in the groove, will occur.
12. Bone wax should be applied to the sutura notha for hemostasis.
13. Once the anterior lacrimal crest has been encountered, the periorbita of the lacrimal sac is elevated posteriorly from the lacrimal sac fossa floor. This should be done with great care so that the thin bone of the lacrimal sac fossa or the lacrimal sac mucosa is not violated. The dissection is facilitated using Baron's suction in the surgeon's non-dominant hand and the Freer periosteal elevator in the surgeon's dominant hand. Often, thin areas or dehiscences in the bone can be identified at this point. The periorbita of the lacrimal sac fossa is continuous with the periosteum of the nasolacrimal duct, which can be seen extending into the bony canal.
14. The anterior limb of the medial canthal tendon is severed at its attachment to the bone and reflected medially to expose the fundus of the sac.
15. Next, subcutaneous tissue attachments to the sac are dissected with blunt-tipped Westcott scissors, including fibers adjacent to the origin of the inferior oblique muscle, taking great care not to damage the muscle.
16. Subcutaneous tissue attachments to the superior and inferior preseptal orbicularis oculi muscle and also dissected in order to mobilize the entire body and fundus of the lacrimal sac.
17. The Westcott scissors are then used to excise the lacrimal sac at the level of the common canaliculus superiorly and inferiorly at the junction of the membranous nasolacrimal duct with the bony nasolacrimal canal. This is adequate for the management of the elderly patient with dacryocystitis.
18. The skin should be closed with interrupted 7/0 Vicryl sutures placed in a vertical mattress fashion. These sutures can be removed after 10 to 14 days or left to dissolve. It is preferable to avoid the use of subcutaneous sutures, which can predispose to thickening of the wound or infection.

Postoperative Care

Topical antibiotic ointment alone is used along the wound postoperatively and the patient is prescribed a 1-week course of oral antibiotics. The patient should be instructed to perform wound massage along the line of the wound for at least 3 min three to four times per day commencing 2 weeks postoperatively after applying Lacrilube ointment. This should be continued for a period of approximately 6 weeks.

If a tumor is suspected, an incisional biopsy of the lacrimal sac should be performed and the results of a formalin-fixed, paraffin-embedded histopathological examination should be reviewed in a multi-disciplinary team meeting before proceeding with further surgery. If a malignant epithelial tumor is diagnosed, the dacryocystectomy should be combined with a lateral rhinostomy performed by an ENT surgeon, with the removal of the entire nasolacrimal duct and canal along with a partial inferior turbinectomy. Postoperative radiotherapy may also be required. Postoperatively the patient should be kept under review in clinic at regular intervals with nasal endoscopy and an examination of the regional lymph nodes.

FURTHER READING

1. Albert DM, Lucarelli MJ. Lacrimal surgery. In: Clinical Atlas of Procedures in Ophthalmic Surgery. Chicago, IL: AMA P, 2004: 320–39.
2. Ceaser RH, McNab AA. A brief history of punctoplasty: the 3-snip revisited. Eye 2005; 19: 16–18.
3. Codère F, Gonnering R, Wobig JL, Dailey RA. Surgery of the tear sac. In: Wobig JL, Dailey RA, eds., Oculofacial Plastic Surgery: Face, Lacrimal System, and Orbit. New York, NY: Thieme, 2004: 167–89.
4. Collin JRO. Lacrimal surgery. In: Manual of Systematic Eyelid Surgery, 3rd edn. Philadelphia, PA: Butterworth-Heinemann Elsevier, 2006: 165–76.
5. Olver J. Colour Atlas of Lacrimal Surgery. Oxford: Butterworth-Heinemann, 2002 (ISBN: 0-7506-4486-9).
6. Dale DL. Embryology, anatomy and physiology of the lacrimal system. In: Stephenson CM, ed., Ophthalmic Plastic, Reconstructive and Orbital Surgery. Boston, MA: Butterworth-Heinemann, 1997: 19–30.
7. Detorakis ET, Zissimopoulos A, Katernellis G, et al. Lower eyelid laxity on functional acquired epiphora: evaluation with quantitative scintigraphy. Ophthal Plast Reconstr Surg 2006; 22(1): 25–9.
8. Wormald PJ. Endoscopic Sinus Surgery: Anatomy, Three-Dimensional Reconstruction, and Surgical Technique. New York, NY: Thieme, 2005 (ISBN: 1-58890-285-4).
9. Kallman JE, Foster JA, Wulc AE, et al. Computer tomography in lacrimal outflow obstruction. Ophthalmology 1997; 104: 676–82.
10. Levine MR. Dacryocystorhinostomy. In: Levine MR, ed., Manual of Oculoplastic Surgery, 3rd edn. Boston, MA: Butterworth-Heinemann, 2003: 51–9.

11. Linberg JV. Surgical anatomy of the lacrimal system. In: Linberg JV, ed., Lacrimal Surgery. Contemporary Issues in Ophthalmology. New York, NY: Churchill Livingstone, 1988: 5: 1–18.

12. McEwen CJ, Young JDH. Epiphora during the first year of life. Eye 1991; 5: 596–600.

13. MFCllner K. Ritleng intubation set: a new system for lacrimal pathway intubation. Ophthalmologica 2000; 214: 237–9.

14. Nowinski TS. Anatomy and physiology of lacrimal system. In: Bosniak S, ed. Principles and Practice of Ophthalmic Plastic and Reconstructive Surgery, vol. 2. Philadelphia, PA: WB Saunders, 1996: 731–47.

15. Pediatric Eye Disease Investigator Group. Primary treatment of nasolacrimal duct obstruction with probing in children less than four years old. Ophthalmology 2008; 115(3): 577–83.

16. Stefanyszyn MA, Hidayat AA, Pe'er JJ, Flanagan JC. Lacrimal sac tumours. Ophthal Plast Reconstr Surg 1994; 10(3): 169–84.

17. Watkins LM, Janfaza P, Rubin PAD. The evolution of endonasal dacryocystorhinostomy. Surv Ophthalmol 2003; 48(1): 73–84.

18. Weber AL, Rodriguez-DeVelasquez A, Lucarelli MJ, Cheng HM. Normal anatomy and lesions of the lacrimal sac and duct: evaluated by dacryocystography, computed tomography, and MR imaging. [Review] [122 refs] Neuroimag Clin North Am 1996; 6(1): 199–217.

19. Werne, MJ, Pitts J, Frank J, Rose GE. Comparison of dacryocystography and lacrimal scintigraphy in the diagnosis of functional nasolacrimal duct obstruction. Br J Ophthalmol 1999; 83: 1032–551.

20. Woog JJ, Kennedy RH, Custer PL, et al. Endonasal dacryocystorhinostomy. Ophthalmology 2001; 108: 2369–77.

21. Wormald PJ. Powered endoscopic dacryocystorhinostomy. The Larygoscope 2002; 112: 69–72.

22. Yagci A, Karci B, Ergezen F. Probing and bicanalicular silicone tube intubation under nasal endoscopy in congenital nasolacrimal duct obstruction. Ophthal Plast Reconstr Surg 2000; 16: 58–61.

21 Enucleation and evisceration

INTRODUCTION

The removal of an eye and the subsequent management of the anophthalmic socket still pose a considerable challenge for the ophthalmic surgeon in spite of many recent advances in orbital implant materials. Good results from such surgery are not easy to achieve consistently and a poor result can have profound psychological implications for the patient for the rest of his/her life. The preoperative counseling of a patient who requires an enucleation demands time and considerable compassion on the part of the ophthalmic surgeon. Close collaboration between the ophthalmic surgeon and the ocularist is essential and should commence preoperatively whenever possible.

The goals of an enucleation or an evisceration are to achieve the following:

- A healthy and comfortable socket free of discharge which can be fitted with a stable ocular prosthesis that mimics the fellow eye in appearance and movement
- A symmetric appearance without enophthalmos or an upper eyelid sulcus deformity
- An absence of an upper or a lower eyelid malposition
- Normal eyelid closure over the ocular prosthesis

To achieve these goals, the enucleation must be approached in the same manner as any intraocular procedure and must be performed meticulously.

INDICATIONS FOR ENUCLEATION

There are a number of indications for enucleation:

1. A blind painful eye, e.g., following failed retinal reattachment surgery, rubeotic glaucoma
2. A blind unsightly eye
3. An intraocular tumor, e.g., a large choroidal melanoma
4. Severe irreparable ocular trauma and a high risk of sympathetic ophthalmia

It is important to consider alternatives to enucleation. The movement of a blind (or partially sighted) eye, or of a microphthalmic or phthisical eye can be more natural than that of an orbital implant and such an eye may tolerate a cosmetic shell or cosmetic contact lens. A painful eye may respond to simple surgery to relieve the pain, e.g., cyclo-destructive procedures or a conjunctival flap, and may also then tolerate a cosmetic shell or contact lens.

PREOPERATIVE PREPARATION

The majority of patients undergo an enucleation as an elective procedure. The operation is rarely performed as an emergency. The patient should be advised about:

1. The advantages, disadvantages, risks, and potential complications of an enucleation procedure
2. The advantages, disadvantages, risks, and potential complications of the use of any orbital implant
3. The implant options
4. The options regarding implant wrapping materials
5. The choice of anesthesia
6. Postoperative pain and its management
7. The use of a postoperative compressive dressing
8. The use of a temporary suture tarsorrhaphy
9. The use of a postoperative conformer
10. The likelihood of a temporary postoperative ptosis
11. The role of the ocularist and the timing of the fitting of the ocular prosthesis

Informed consent should be obtained after the patient has had time to consider the options.

The patient should discontinue aspirin and any other antiplatelet drugs, if medically permissible, at least 2 weeks preoperatively. Likewise, anticoagulants should only be altered or discontinued after discussion with the patient's hematologist. Any bacterial conjunctivitis should be treated preoperatively and topical steroids used to reduce any conjunctival inflammation.

KEY POINT

A computed tomography (CT) scan of the orbits and paranasal sinuses should be performed if a patient has previously suffered orbital trauma to exclude the possibility of a missed orbital wall blowout fracture. If a fracture is present of a significant size, this should be repaired at the time of the enucleation and prior to the placement of the orbital implant.

ORBITAL IMPLANT MATERIALS

Enucleation (or evisceration) of an eye creates an orbital volume deficit which varies from patient to patient. This necessitates the replacement of the equivalent spherical volume of approximately 6 to 7 ml (depending on the size of the globe). This can be partially compensated for by the placement of an orbital implant. An 18-mm spherical implant has a volume of only 3.1 ml. The average ocular prosthesis (artificial eye) must then be over 2 ml to make up the difference. The advantage of using a larger orbital implant is to keep the ocular prosthesis as light as possible. This will reduce the incidence of inferior displacement of the lower eyelid by gravitational force on the ocular prosthesis. This advantage, however, must be balanced against the disadvantages of the use of a larger implant:

- Increased pressure on the conjunctival wound with a risk of dehiscence and implant exposure or extrusion
- A longer period of time required for vascularization of a porous implant
- Insufficient room for placement of a motility peg in the case of a porous implant

- Insufficient room for the ocularist to fit an ocular prosthesis with sufficient thickness to adequately mimic the presence of an anterior chamber

If no orbital implant is placed, or if the implant is of insufficient size, the ocular prosthesis will have to be made larger than is desirable in an attempt to reduce the volume deficit, which manifests itself by an enophthalmic appearance and an upper eyelid sulcus deformity. The lower lid eventually becomes stretched, the ocular prosthesis becomes inferiorly and posteriorly displaced, the levator palpebrae superioris muscle loses its fulcrum of action, and the upper eyelid sulcus deformity becomes more exaggerated. The patient then exhibits features referred to as the post-enucleation socket syndrome (PESS) (Fig. 21.1). In the absence of an orbital implant, a posterior rotation of the levator muscle and superior rectus complex and the superior orbital fat occurs, with an anterior rotation of the inferior rectus muscle and the inferior orbital fat. This may result in a retraction of the upper lid in some patients. It is also responsible for the backward tilt seen with the ocular prosthesis.

Primary Orbital Implant

The ideal time for orbital implantation is at the time of enucleation/evisceration unless primary implantation is contraindicated, e.g., in the case of severe ocular and orbital trauma or infection. The overall results of primary enucleation/evisceration are superior and there is a much-reduced need for subsequent surgical procedures.

Controversy has raged about the use of evisceration versus enucleation. Some ophthalmologists prefer evisceration to enucleation because, in the hands of the general ophthalmologist, it may offer a more functional and cosmetically acceptable orbit compared with enucleation. Evisceration tends to produce less disruption of the orbital tissues and the physiological dynamics of muscle function, and the orbital volume can be maintained very close to its original state. It has the advantage that it can be performed very quickly under local anesthesia with sedation and it is therefore ideal for elderly patients with blind painful eyes. It should be noted, however, that evisceration, although a faster and simpler surgical procedure, has the following potential disadvantages:

- The possible dissemination of an unsuspected intraocular tumor (all globes with opaque media should be subjected to an ultrasound examination prior to surgery)
- An inadequate pathological specimen is provided
- A phthisical globe will not accept an adequately sized implant
- There is concern about the possible risk, albeit small, of sympathetic ophthalmia

> **KEY POINT**
>
> All globes with opaque media should be subjected to an ultrasound examination prior to undergoing an evisceration.

Secondary Orbital Implant

An implant can be inserted secondarily into the anophthalmic socket but the surgical procedure is more difficult and the results are less predictable. Patients undergoing secondary orbital implantation are more likely to require additional surgical procedures to address a residual volume deficit, conjunctival adhesions/cysts and eyelid malpositions. Similarly, the removal of an extruding, exposed or migrated implant with an implant exchange can be difficult.

Choices of Orbital Implant

Over the years, many different implant materials have been used, the first being glass. Many materials have followed, including cartilage, fat, bone, cork, aluminum, wood, silk, ivory, and paraffin! Many of these orbital implants were associated with numerous problems and have been abandoned. Until the arrival of hydroxyapatite, bio-ceramic, and porous polyethylene, the most commonly used materials were acrylic and silicone, with the most common configuration being spherical.

Orbital implants can be classified as non-integrated or integrated.

Non-Integrated Implants

Non-integrated implants have no direct attachments to the extraocular muscles and are usually single spheres of inert material (silicone or acrylic) buried beneath the conjunctiva and Tenon's capsule in the muscle cone. The rectus muscles may or may not be incorporated into the soft tissue closure anterior to the implant. Such implants may be inserted behind the posterior layer of Tenon's capsule within the intraconal fat space. Such implants commonly migrate within the orbit, causing secondary problems with fitting and stability of the ocular prosthesis. They have largely been abandoned for use after enucleation but are still useful for elderly patients undergoing an evisceration (Fig. 21.2).

Integrated Implants

Integrated orbital implants may be further classified as buried or exposed.

Buried Integrated Implants

These may have either a spherical or an irregular shape. The spherical implants may be wrapped in donor sclera, fascia lata, temporalis fascia, Alloderm, bovine pericardium or Vicryl or Mersilene mesh to which the extraocular muscles can be sutured. Some spherical implants may be left unwrapped, and

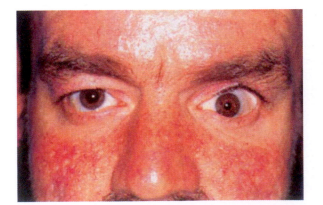

Figure 21.1 A patient exhibiting features of a post-enucleation socket syndrome.

the muscles sutured directly to the implant material, such as the porous polyethylene (Medpor) implant. In buried integrated orbital implants with an irregular surface, muscle attachment is achieved by passing the muscles through tunnels in the implant (Allen, Castroviejo implants—Fig. 21.3) or through grooves in the implant created by mounds on the anterior aspect (Iowa and Universal implants). The Roper Hall implant has a magnetic strip incorporated into the centre of the implant to enable a magnetic coupling to occur with a metallic strip inserted into the prosthesis (Fig. 21.4). Although this implant is no longer used, patients are still seen in clinic who received this implant in the 1970s and 1980s.

Exposed Integrated Implants

These have the muscles directly attached to the implant and a portion of the implant is exposed to the outside environment (an Arruga implant). The exposed portion is in the form of a projection or an indentation, which permits the implant to be directly coupled to a prosthetic eye with its posterior projection (Fig. 21.5).

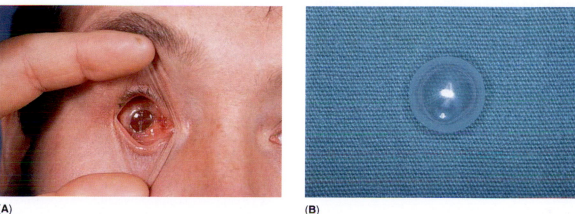

(A)   (B)

Figure 21.2 (**A**) A simple acrylic spherical orbital implant extruding. (**B**) The implant following removal.

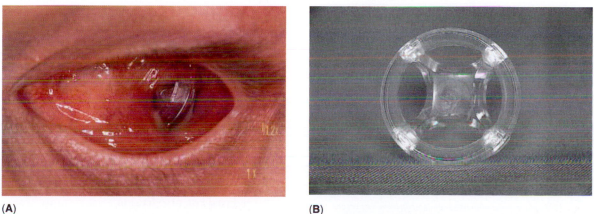

(A)   (B)

Figure 21.3 (**A**) An extruding Castroviejo orbital implant. (**B**) The implant following removal.

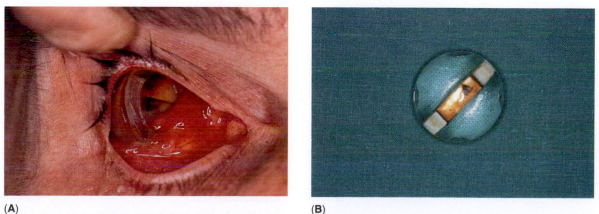

(A)   (B)

Figure 21.4 (**A**) An extruding magnetic orbital implant. (**B**) The implant following removal.

Although these implants provided excellent motility, this benefit was outweighed by their disadvantage of chronic infections and extrusion. Such implants have been abandoned.

Current Orbital Implants
The orbital implants currently used are:

1. Hydroxyapatite implant
2. Porous polyethylene implant (Medpor)
3. Bioceramic implant
4. "Baseball" implant
5. Simple acrylic sphere implant
6. Simple silicone sphere implant
7. Universal implant
8. Dermis fat graft

The most popular orbital implants available today are the hydroxyapatite implant, the porous polyethylene (Medpor) implant, and the aluminum oxide (Bioceramic) implant. Hydroxyapatite is an inorganic salt of calcium phosphate similar to the inorganic portion of normal human bone. The hydroxyapatite implant gained enormous popularity following its introduction in the 1990s and rapidly became the implant of choice among many leading oculoplastic surgeons in many countries (Fig. 21.6).

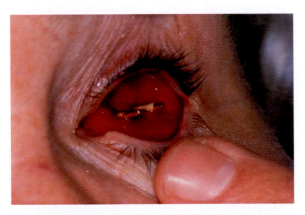

Figure 21.5 An Arruga orbital implant.

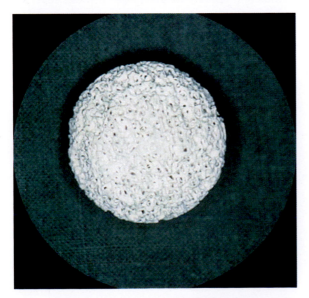

Figure 21.6 The hydroxyapatite orbital implant.

A synthetic form of hydroxyapatite is also available. Medpor has likewise gained in popularity along with the synthetic bioceramic implant (aluminum oxide—Al_2O_3), which is also purported to offer yet further advantages over other porous implants, with even better biocompatability. These implants are all available in 14 to 22 mm sizes.

These materials have the capacity to develop complete fibrovascular ingrowth. The time taken for this to occur depends on a number of following factors:

- The size of the implant
- The use of the implant—as a primary, secondary, or exchange implant
- The wrapping material used

The porous hydroxyapatite and bioceramic implants can be directly coupled with the ocular prosthesis to improve movement by means of a small methylmethacrylate peg, which fits into a hole drilled into the buried implant. The conjunctiva will grow down the sides of this drilled hole only if the implant is fully vascularized. Alternatively, a titanium-sleeved peg can now be screwed into the implant after creating a central guide hole with a series of free needles of increasing size. Likewise, a titanium motility peg system is available for the Medpor implant. The use of motility pegs has decreased dramatically over recent years as most surgeons have experienced problems with their use, e.g., foreign body granulomas, recurrent inflammation, and discharge.

The time to complete vascularization varies from 4 to 12 months. The vascularization of the implant may be determined by a computed tomography (CT) scan with contrast, a magnetic resonance imaging (MRI) scan with gadolinium or a technetium-99 m bone scan. These are not accurate, however, and it is preferable to observe a minimum safe waiting period before proceeding with the insertion of a motility peg: i.e., 6 months for primary implants and 12 months for secondary implants.

These implants have been heavily marketed on the basis of a number of purported advantages over other implants.

Advantages

1. Once the implant has become vascularized, it has a reduced risk of extrusion
2. The risk of migration of the implant within the orbit is reduced
3. The implant permits better movement of the ocular prosthesis
4. The motility peg allows the weight of the ocular prosthesis to be borne by the implant rather than by the lower eyelid, reducing the chances of instability of the artificial eye and the need for lower eyelid tightening procedures later
5. The implant is quickly and easily inserted and has a low complication rate in the hands of an experienced surgeon

These purported advantages are not, however, completely borne out in clinical practice.

Disadvantages
The implant has a number of disadvantages. These include the additional costs involved: the cost of the implant, the

requirement and expense of the second stage procedure to place a motility peg, and the required modifications to the ocular prosthesis. Additional expense may also be incurred if scans are used to determine whether or not the implant is vascularized and safe to drill. A small proportion of patients will require management of minor complications, e.g., removal of foreign body granulomas associated with the motility peg.

Results

The results of primary implantation tend to be very good, and an implant exposure rate of less than 1% can be achieved with meticulous surgery. The results of secondary implantation are less predictable as the socket anatomy has been disrupted and the eye muscles are retracted, scarred and difficult to locate at the time of surgery. The results of implant exchange surgery vary depending on the type of implant that has to be removed, and whether or not this has become exposed. In experienced hands, however, the results are usually good but the degree of movement is very variable from patient to patient.

Rationale for Implant Use

Hydroxyapatite is a relatively expensive implant material. The successful use of this material in most surgeons' hands appears to require the use of a wrapping material (unless used in conjunction with an evisceration) that:

- Adds expense (Vicryl mesh)
- Carries a risk for viral disease transmission (donor sclera)
- Incurs further surgical morbidity (autologous fascia)

The same applies to the bioceramic implant.

The early complication rate of hydroxyapatite implants was higher than that of other materials. Particular problems with implant exposure have been the subject of a number of publications and the potential advantages with regard to late complications, such as migration and extrusion, await the test of time. Its main advantage lies in its ability to accept a motility peg to enhance movement of the ocular prosthesis. It is now clear that the use of a motility peg has greatly diminished because of a high incidence of complications. The assumption is, therefore, that the majority of patients are satisfied with the initial motility achieved. Nonetheless, there is no evidence that when similar techniques are used, unpegged hydroxyapatite implants have superior motility to solid sphere implants. Further, there is no anatomical basis for this to be so. Although the superior motility of the pegged hydroxyapatite implant is continually alluded to, there has yet to be a double-blind study to confirm this. There is little evidence to support the use of this more expensive implant in patients who do not wish to undergo the extra time and expense required to fit a motility peg. It seems reasonable to reserve the use of the hydroxyapatite implant or other porous implants for patients who desire the enhanced motility the peg offers (in full knowledge of what is involved—including the increased incidence of severe postoperative pain).

Concern has also been raised as to whether the hydroxyapatite system of motility enhancement will stand the test of time, and we can only wait and see whether such a system is sustainable over a lifetime.

Similar criticism can be leveled at the Medpor implant, although this implant does offer the advantage that it can readily accept direct suturing, which obviates the need for a wrapping material. The implant is smooth, in contrast to the rough brittle surface of the hydroxyapatite implant, although the hydroxyapatite implant is now available with a smooth surface coating. Synthetic hydroxyapatite implants have also been developed with a smooth anterior surface, with preformed drill holes and suture posts to enable direct suturing, and synthetic hydroxyapatite implants are also available prewrapped in Vicryl mesh.

The ability of the Medpor implant to accept direct suturing without the necessity for a wrapping material is certainly an attractive quality. Long-term results of the placement of motility pegs in Medpor implants are not yet available, however, and concerns have been raised about the implant's pore size and completely porous nature as well as its hydrophobic surface characteristics. There are reports of implant exposure requiring further surgery, which therefore raises concerns about the wisdom of utilizing the implant without a wrapping material as a preventative measure. Modifications of the implant shape have been described to reduce the problems of residual upper lid sulcus deformity. Some surgeons have placed this implant with a motility peg already inserted. This is then "externalized" later. This fails to recognize, however, that the implant can alter position postoperatively and that the peg placement should be determined by the ocularist and not by the surgeon.

Alternative Implants

1. *"Baseball" implant.* This remains a simple, inexpensive but effective primary implant. The acrylic sphere is wrapped in donor sclera (or autogenous fascia, or Mersilene mesh) and buried behind posterior Tenon's fascia (Figs. 21.7 and 21.8). It is of particular use in older patients who do not wish to take advantage of the second stage motility peg placement of porous implants.
2. *Simple acrylic sphere implant.* This is easy to place at the time of an evisceration in the elderly, although the use of a subconjunctival patch of sclera or autogenous fascia will reduce the risk of implant exposure and/or extrusion.
3. *Simple silicone sphere implant.* Silicone has achieved a certain notoriety with patients and is used infrequently. It is used in the same way as a simple acrylic sphere implant.
4. *Universal implant.* This remains a primary implant of choice in many centres in the United States. It has a good track record, with few complications, although its placement is not as simple to perform as a spherical porous implant.
5. *Castroviejo implant.* This implant is still used in a small number of centres in the United Kingdom but is associated with long-term problems with posterior tilting and extrusion of the implant. Its use is not to be recommended.
6. *Dermis fat graft.* This autogenous implant is still useful for the surgical rehabilitation of sockets which have a conjunctival lining problem in addition to a volume deficit, although some surgeons

use such implants for primary cases where other implants would pose a higher risk of exposure or extrusion, e.g. in acute severe trauma. It is more commonly used as an exchange implant for one which has extruded.

The search for the ideal implant material and design will continue. The surgeon faced with the patient requiring an enucleation or evisceration, or a secondary or exchange implant reconstruction of an anophthalmic socket, currently has a number of implants to choose from and should select the implant most appropriate to the individual patient. The choice will be influenced by a number of factors:

- The age and general health of the patient
- Consideration of cost
- The motivation of the patient to undergo a second-stage motility peg procedure
- The relative expertise of the surgeon
- The risk factors for implant extrusion

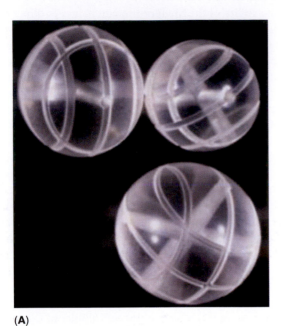

(A)

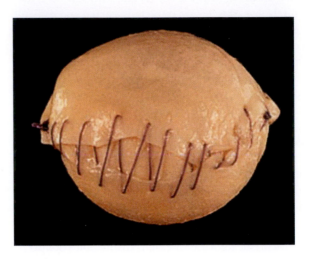

(B)

Figure 21.7 (**A**) Acrylic spheres. (**B**) A "baseball" orbital implant.

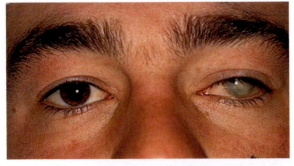

(A)

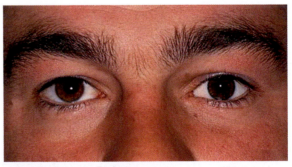

(B)

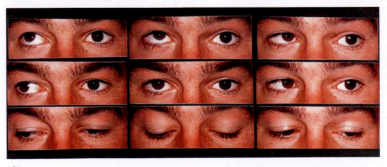

(C)

Figure 21.8 (**A**) A patient with a blind painful unsightly eye. (**B**) The patient following an enucleation with placement of a primary "baseball" orbital implant. (**C**) The patient demonstrating a fair range of motility of the artificial eye.

suture so that this can be readily identified following the enucleation.

21. Next, the superior oblique tendon is identified and hooked using a muscle hook. The tendon is cut using Westcott scissors. No sutures are used and the tendon is allowed to retract.

22. The silk sutures are attached to artery clips which are used to apply forward traction on the globe.

23. Any residual Tenon's fascia is carefully dissected from the globe using Westcott scissors.

24. Enucleation scissors are used to cut the optic nerve. These are inserted infero-laterally and the optic nerve palpated with the ends of the scissors first to establish its position. The nerve can first be crushed with a curved artery clip prior to the use of the scissors to reduce bleeding. Alternatively, a snare may be used (Fig. 21.14). Its use is, however, contraindicated in the presence of a soft globe (the snare may transect the globe), if a large corneal section or penetrating keratoplasty has been performed (the globe may rupture), or if a long length of optic nerve is required (enucleation for a retinoblastoma).

25. The globe is removed carefully cutting any residual Tenon's fibers still adherent to the globe.

26. The socket is then packed tightly with two small swabs moistened with saline.

27. Firm pressure is applied for 5 minutes.

28. The enucleated globe is inspected thoroughly before being sent for histopathological examination. Any autologous sclera to be used for a patch graft should be removed at this stage before the globe is placed into a specimen pot containing formalin.

29. The swabs are then removed and the site inspected for any bleeding.

30. Any residual bleeding vessels are cauterized using bipolar cautery.

31. If the patient is deemed unsuitable for an orbital implant, the horizontal and vertical recti are simply tied to each other in a cruciate fashion.

32. The conjunctiva is closed with interrupted 7/0 Vicryl sutures.

33. A sterile surgical conformer of appropriate size and shape is inserted into the conjunctival sac. Topical antibiotic ointment is instilled into the conjunctival sac and a pressure dressing is applied supported by a bandage. This is removed 2 to 3 days postoperatively.

34. If a spherical orbital implant is to be inserted, the appropriate size is determined with the use of sizing spheres (Fig. 21.15). The most frequently used size is 20 mm. (Great care should be taken when using a larger implant ensuring that this is not too large for the patient's socket.)

35. First, posterior Tenon's fascia is identified (Fig. 21.16A) and then opened by blunt dissection using Stevens scissors in a spreading fashion, exposing the intraconal fat space.

36. 4/0 silk traction sutures are placed through the edges of the posterior Tenon's fascia (Fig. 21.16B). If posterior Tenon's fascia cannot be closed over the surface of the sizing sphere without undue tension, a smaller sphere should be substituted (Fig. 21.16C).

37. The implant of an appropriate size is then wrapped in the material that has been selected, e.g., Vicryl mesh, for an hydroxyapatite implant, Mersilene mesh or donor sclera for a "baseball" implant.

38. The implant is then inserted into the intraconal fat space behind posterior Tenon's fascia using a Carter sphere injector (Fig. 21.17). This can be aided by the use of Wright's orbital retractors to help to prevent any tissue drag. If a Medpor implant is used, this is inserted using the plastic inserted device which has been especially designed for use with this implant (Fig. 20.18).

39. The posterior Tenon's fascia is then closed with interrupted 5/0 Vicryl sutures (Fig. 21.19).

40. The recti and the inferior oblique muscle are attached to the implant by passing the needles through posterior Tenon's and through the implant wrapping material as anteriorly as possible. This is preferable to placing the muscles first and then trying to close the posterior Tenon's. The precise

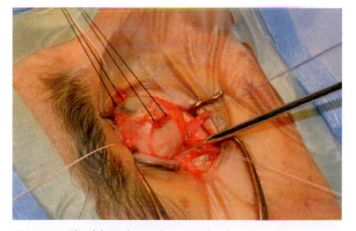

Figure 21.14 The globe is about to be removed with a snare. All four recti and the inferior oblique have been tagged with Vicryl sutures and placed on gentle traction. The silk sutures placed through the stumps of the medial and lateral recti are being used to apply forward traction to the globe.

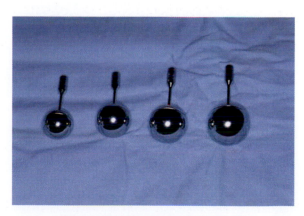

Figure 21.15 Orbital implant sizing spheres.

Severed optic nerve

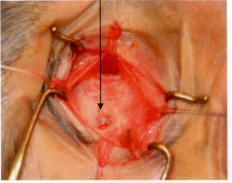

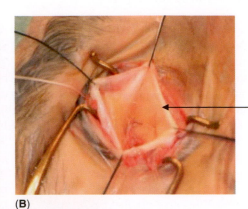

Posterior Tenons's

(A)   **(B)**

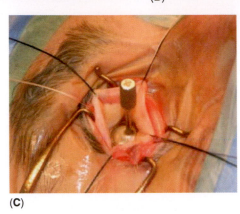

(C)

Figure 21.16 (**A**) The appearance of the socket following an enucleation. The extraocular muscles can be seen to exit between anterior and posterior Tenon's fascia. A hole is seen in the posterior Tenon's fascia where the severed optic nerve is shown. (**B**) The posterior Tenon's fascia has been opened, exposing the intraconal fat space. (**C**) A 20-mm sizing sphere has been inserted into the socket. Posterior Tenon's fascia can be closed easily over the sizing sphere.

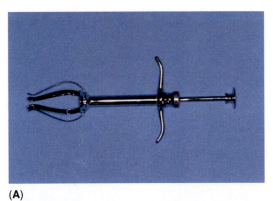

(A)

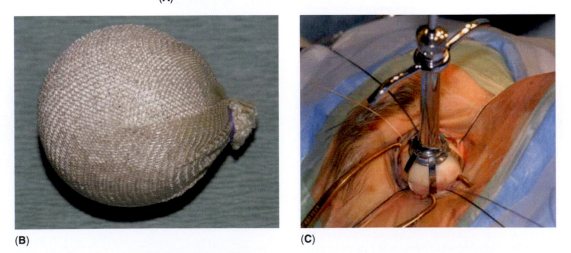

(B)   **(C)**

Figure 21.17 (**A**) A Carter sphere injector. (**B**) An hydroxyapatite orbital implant wrapped in Vicryl mesh. (**C**) The orbital implant is injected into the intraconal fat space using the Carter sphere injector.

closure of posterior Tenon's is key to long-term success in this surgery.

41. In those patients at increased risk of conjunctival wound dehiscence and implant exposure, e.g. following previous failed retinal reattachment surgery, glaucoma surgery, or severe trauma, a patch graft of autogenous temporalis fascia or donor sclera is then placed over the suture line to reduce the risk of postoperative implant exposure. Next, the conjunctiva with anterior Tenon's fascia is closed with interrupted 7/0 Vicryl sutures (Fig. 21.20).

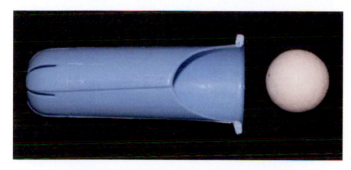

Figure 21.18 A Medpor implant with its inserter.

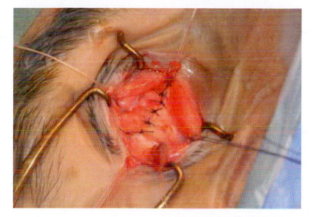

Figure 21.19 Posterior Tenon's fascia has been closed completely over the implant with interrupted 5/0 Vicryl sutures.

42. A sterile surgical conformer of appropriate size and shape is inserted into the conjunctival sac, ensuring that the eyelids will close passively over the conformer without creating tension on the conjunctival suture line.

43. A temporary suture tarsorrhaphy should be undertaken using a central 4/0 nylon suture passed through tarsorrhaphy tubing (Fig. 21.21).

44. A retrobulbar injection of 3 to 5 ml of 0.5% Bupivacaine with 1:200,000 units of adrenaline is given to aid postoperative analgesia.

45. Injections of an anti-inflammatory agent and an opiate analgesic are given by the anesthetist.

46. Topical antibiotic ointment is instilled into the conjunctival sac either side of the tarsorrhaphy.

47. Jelonet is placed over the eyelids along with two eye pads and Micropore tape, and a bandage is applied before the patient's anesthesia is reversed.

KEY POINT

The meticulous closure of posterior Tenon's fascia is crucial to the prevention of postoperative implant exposure.

Postoperative Care

The patient will usually experience postoperative nausea and pain and is not usually discharged until the second postoperative day. It is extremely important not to under-estimate the degree of pain that can be associated with an enucleation or evisceration with placement of an orbital implant and adequate analgesia must be provided as soon as the effects of local anesthesia wear off.

Postoperative analgesia is provided using intraoperative intravenous paracetamol and an intravenous non-steroidal anti-inflammatory agent (such as paracoxib or diclofenac) provided neither is contraindicated (the only contraindication to paracetamol is allergy or intolerance). Contraindications to non-steroidal anti-inflammatory drug (NSAID) therapy are:

• A history of wheezing with aspirin in an asthmatic (probably 5% of asthmatics)

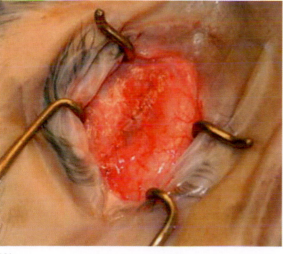

(A)

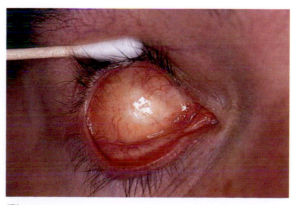

(B)

Figure 21.20 (**A**) The appearance of the socket at the completion of surgery. (**B**) A patient in whom a subconjunctival patch graft has been placed seen 3 years following surgery. The socket is quiet and the patch graft clearly visible.

- Known renal insufficiency
- Hiatus hernia
- Duodenal ulceration
- Other bleeding disorder
- Unstable angina

The NSAID has the additional advantage of providing an anti-inflammatory action.

There is a relatively high incidence of postoperative nausea and vomiting (PONV) after socket surgery with the placement of an implant, possibly as a result of the oculo-emetic reflex. It is therefore best to avoid the use of potent opioids in the immediate postoperative period, although once the local anesthetic has worn off, morphine may be required. A combination of intraoperative intravenous dexamethasone 8 mg and ondansetron 4 mg is used to prevent PONV. Regular paracetamol and NSAIDs are continued (unless contra-indicated) postoperatively for 2 weeks. A proton-pump inhibitor (omeprazole) may be required during the NSAID therapy to reduce dyspepsia. The patient should be discharged home on regular analgesics, e.g., paracetamol and codeine combination therapy.

The patient is also discharged on a week's course of a broad-spectrum oral antibiotic. The patient is instructed to remove the bandage and the dressing 3 days after surgery, and to clean the eyelids and tarsorrhaphy tubing with cotton wool and sterile saline or cooled boiled water. Topical antibiotic ointment is then smeared across the eyelid margins for 2 weeks. The temporary suture tarsorrhaphy is removed in clinic 2 to 3 weeks postoperatively and the topical antibiotic ointment is changed to topical antibiotic drops. These are continued for a further 2 weeks.

KEY POINT

It is extremely important not to underestimate the degree of pain that can be associated with an enucleation or evisceration with placement of an orbital implant and adequate analgesia must be provided as soon as the effects of local anesthesia wear off.

The patient's conformer is then checked, cleaned, and replaced or changed for a different size and shape if required. The patient should not be fitted with an ocular prosthesis until a minimum of 8 weeks have elapsed to allow sufficient wound healing and complete resolution of postoperative edema. If the ocular prosthesis is fitted too soon after surgery the risk of implant exposure is increased. In addition, the ocular prosthesis will not fit the socket properly once complete resolution of postoperative orbital edema has occurred increasing the likelihood of postoperative socket inflammation and discharge.

The patient should remain under the care of the ocularist, who will ensure that the ocular prosthesis is checked and polished at least on an annual basis. If the patient has an incomplete blink or lagophthalmos, the ocular prosthesis should be polished more frequently (Fig. 21.22). Topical lubricants should be prescribed, e.g., Systane® drops, particularly for a patient who has an incomplete blink. The socket should be examined to exclude implantation cysts, papillary conjunctivitis, and impending or actual implant exposure. Failure to maintain the artificial eye will risk conjunctival inflammation, discharge, conjunctival breakdown, and implant exposure.

KEY POINT

The regular long-term postoperative care of the ocular prosthesis by an ocularist is crucial to the success of orbital implant surgery.

Complications
Implant Exposure
A small area of exposure of any orbital implant can usually be managed successfully in the absence of infection. The conjunctiva and anterior Tenon's tissue should be undermined and a patch graft placed, e.g., autogenous temporalis fascia,

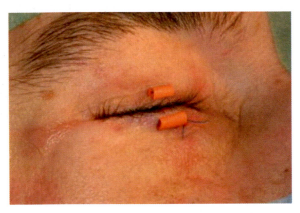

Figure 21.21 A temporary suture tarsorrhaphy.

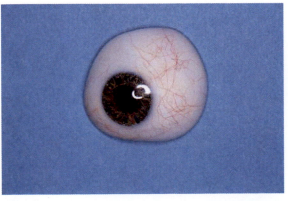 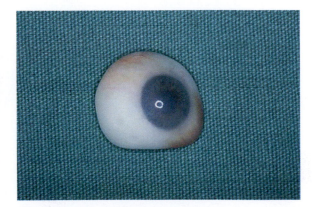

(A)  **(B)**

Figure 21.22 **(A)** A recently polished artificial eye. **(B)** A neglected artificial eye with a poor appearance and a rough surface. The patient had a chronically discharging socket.

a dermal graft, or a hard palate graft. If a large area is exposed or if there is evidence of infection the implant should be removed and replaced with a dermis fat graft (Figs. 21.23 and 21.24). The management of orbital implant exposure is outlined in more detail in chapter 22.

Over-Sized Implant
If the implant size was correctly selected at surgery, the situation may improve spontaneously with resolution of socket edema. If, however, there is insufficient room for a comfortable and aesthetically satisfactory artificial eye, the implant can be explored and debulked with a diamond burr, or the lateral wall of the orbit may be decompressed using a rose head burr via a lateral canthal skin incision. Alternatively, the implant will have to be removed and exchanged for a smaller sized implant. This is, however, more traumatic to the socket tissues and the recovery period will be more prolonged.

Orbital Hematoma
A postoperative orbital hematoma can seriously compromise a patient's outcome following an enucleation (Fig. 21.25). This can predispose to a wound dehiscence, implant exposure and infection, and socket contracture. Precautions should be taken to ensure that such an occurrence is prevented by strict attention to detail: the discontinuation of preoperative medications which predispose to bleeding, the preoperative management

of hypertension, a meticulous surgical technique with strict attention to intraoperative haemostasis, and the use of a compressive dressing postoperatively.

Conjunctival Prolapse
A conjunctival prolapse should never be seen following an enucleation if a temporary suture tarsorrhaphy is used routinely. The occurrence of a conjunctival prolapse can be managed by the placement of a temporary suture tarsorrhaphy.

MOTILITY PEG PLACEMENT (HYDROXYAPATITE IMPLANT)
If the movement of the patient's artificial eye is unsatisfactory in spite of good movement of the orbital implant, a motility peg can be placed. This should be done in consultation with an ocularist who is best placed to determine the appropriate location for the peg. It is unwise to place a motility peg in any patient who has socket inflammation and excessive discharge, papillary conjunctivitis, lagophthalmos, or an implant which is lying in an eccentric position in the socket. Some synthetic implants may also be prone to cracking during the placement of a motility peg.

Preoperatively, a wax drilling template is made by the ocularist. This is placed in the socket, with the patient in a sitting position. A mark is made on the conjunctival surface with gentian violet through the hole in the template, which is then removed (Fig. 21.26).

The patient is warned that the eye will not fit correctly until it has been modified at the next appointment with the ocularist 2 weeks later, when the permanent round-headed peg is placed and the posterior surface of the artificial eye is hollowed out to accept it.

KEY POINT
It is unwise to place a motility peg in any patient who has socket inflammation and excessive discharge, papillary conjunctivitis, lagophthalmos, or an implant which is lying in an eccentric position in the socket.

Surgical Procedure
1. The patient's artificial eye is soaked in iodine.
2. A peri-implant injection of 5 to 7 ml of 0.5% Bupivacaine with 1:200,000 units of adrenaline

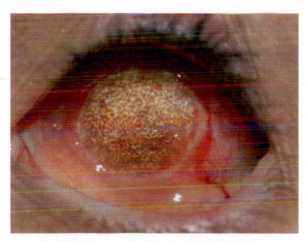
Figure 21.23 A large area of exposure of an hydroxyapatite orbital implant.

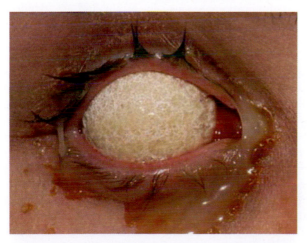
Figure 21.24 An infected extruding hydroxyapatite orbital implant.

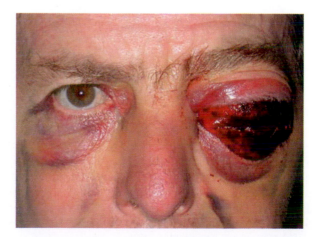
Figure 21.25 A massive orbital hematoma following an enucleation in a patient taking anticoagulants which were not discontinued preoperatively.

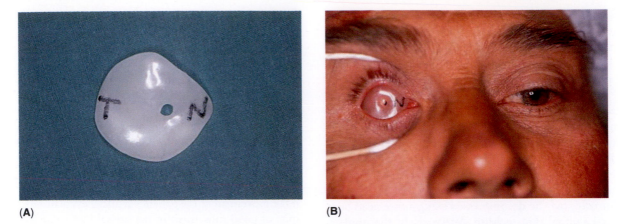

Figure 21.26 (**A**) A wax drilling template marked N for nasal and T for temporal orientation. (**B**) The wax template has been placed in the socket and a mark on the conjunctiva made with gentian violet.

mixed with Hyalase (hyaluronidase) is given. It is important to avoid causing conjunctival edema from an excessive volume of local anesthetic.

3. The face, eyelids, and conjunctival sac should be thoroughly prepared with an antiseptic agent, e.g., diluted aqueous Betadine solution, and a cataract drape is applied.

4. A Clarke's eyelid speculum is placed to exclude the eyelashes from the surgical field.

5. The conjunctiva is cauterized at the position indicated by the gentian violet using a disposable cautery.

6. Next, a hole is made in the implant using a series of needles of gradually increasing size (Fig. 21.27).

7. These are mounted on a holder (with the exception of the largest needle whose handle is sufficiently large to manipulate) and are screwed into the implant in a vertical orientation to a depth of 10 mm only, aiming towards the apex of the orbit (Fig. 21.28).

8. Once the hole is of sufficient size and depth, the titanium-sleeved peg is screwed into the implant with a small screwdriver to lie flush with the conjunctiva.

9. A temporary flat-headed titanium peg is inserted into the sleeved peg.

10. All deposits of hydroxyapatite dust are then removed from the conjunctival sac with careful irrigation.

11. The patient's artificial eye is replaced. If this does not fit comfortably, a surgical conformer is placed instead.

12. A pressure dressing is applied.

If the titanium pegging system is deemed too expensive, the alternative is to use an acrylic peg, which is placed after drilling the implant. A 2.5-mm diamond burr is used to create a hole (Fig. 21.29). It is extremely important to ensure that the burr is orientated correctly before the drilling procedure is commenced. A 3-mm burr is then used to enlarge the hole, which is drilled to a depth of 10 mm. A temporary flat-headed peg is placed, which is replaced with a permanent round-headed peg 2 weeks later when the drilling hole has become lined with conjunctiva (Figs. 21.29 and 21.30).

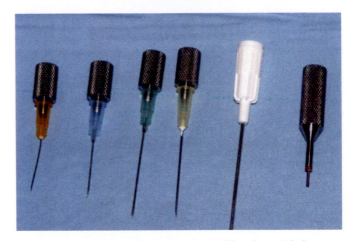

Figure 21.27 A series of needles mounted on holders along with the screwdriver used to place the titanium sleeve.

Postoperative Care
The pressure dressing is removed by the patient the following day. Topical antibiotic drops are prescribed three times per day for 2 weeks.

The posterior aspect of the artificial eye is modified by the ocularist to accept the head of the permanent motility peg 2 weeks postoperatively (Figs. 21.31 and 21.32).

Complications
Most complications are usually minor and are avoided by attention to detail both in selecting the appropriate patients for the procedure and in the surgery itself (Fig. 21.33). A peg should not be placed until the implant is fully vascularized. Imaging techniques are not entirely reliable. It is preferable to delay the procedure for a sufficient length of time (a minimum period of 6 months following implantation for primary implants and 12 months for secondary implants).

Foreign body granulomas can occur and are more likely to be seen where the adjacent implant has become exposed. The granuloma should be excised, and any exposed area of implant will need to be burred down with a diamond burr. A small patch graft using temporalis fascia or a piece dermis (a dermis fat graft with the attached fat removed) may be required (see chap. 13).

The motility peg or the titanium sleeve may become overgrown with conjunctiva requiring a local conjunctival

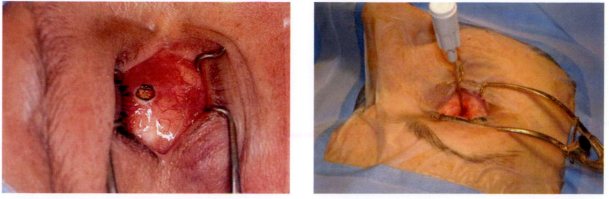

(A)   **(B)**

Figure 21.28 (**A**) The conjunctiva has been cauterized over the marked area using a disposable thermal cautery. (**B**) A needle is being used to create a hole in the hydroxyapatite orbital implant.

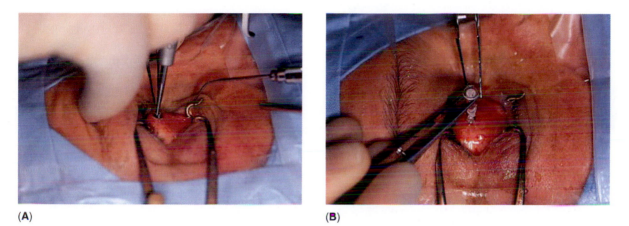

(A)   **(B)**

Figure 21.29 (**A**) A burr is being used to drill a hole into a hydroxyapatite orbital implant. Correct orientation of the burr is essential. (**B**) A flat-headed temporary peg is placed into the hole in the implant.

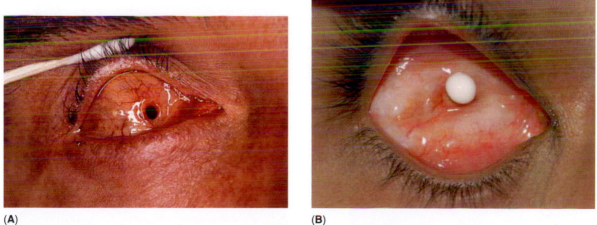

(A)   **(B)**

Figure 21.30 (**A**) The appearance of the hole 2 weeks after drilling. (**B**) A permanent round-headed motility peg.

resection. Chronic inflammation and discharge may necessitate the removal and abandonment of the motility peg.

Dermis Fat Graft
Surgical Procedure

1. A standard enucleation is performed as described above.

2. The dermis fat graft is harvested from the upper outer quadrant of the buttock or from the left lower lateral non-hair bearing abdominal wall and trimmed to size (Fig. 21.34). The graft is compressed with a dry swab to dehydrate it. This reduces the size of the graft making its insertion into the socket easier.

3. The graft, with the dermis uppermost, is inserted into the intraconal fat space and the extraocular muscles are sutured onto the anterior surface of the dermis (Fig. 21.35).

4. If there is a conjunctival lining deficit the sutures are positioned closer to the edge of the graft in order to leave a central bare area of graft exposed. This epithelializes gradually and spontaneously.

5. As the sutures are tied the fat is reduced into the intraconal fat space.

6. The conjunctiva is sutured to the front surface of the graft with interrupted 7/0 Vicryl sutures leaving an area of the graft bare in the presence of socket contracture. In the absence of a lining deficit the conjunctiva is closed over the dermis fat graft.

7. A sterile surgical conformer of appropriate size and shape is inserted into the conjunctival sac, ensuring that the eyelids will close passively over the conformer without creating tension on the conjunctival suture line.

8. A temporary suture tarsorrhaphy should be undertaken using a central 4/0 nylon suture passed through tarsorrhaphy tubing.

9. A retrobulbar injection of 3 to 5 ml of 0.5% Bupivacaine with 1:200,000 units of adrenaline is given to aid postoperative analgesia.

10. Injections of an anti-inflammatory agent and an opiate analgesic are given by the anesthetist.

11. Topical antibiotic ointment is instilled into the conjunctival sac either side of the tarsorrhaphy.

12. Jelonet is placed over the eyelids along with two eye pads and Micropore tape, and a bandage is applied before the patient's anesthesia is reversed.

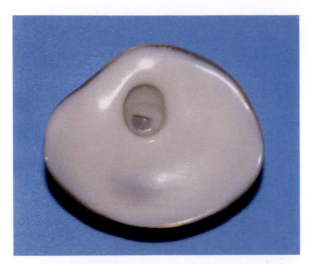

Figure 21.31 A modified posterior surface of an artificial eye.

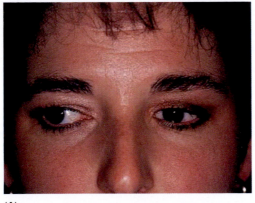
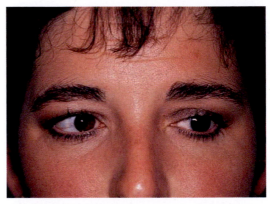

(A) (B)

Figure 21.32 A patient with a secondary pegged hydroxyapatite orbital implant placed following removal of an extruding Castroviejo orbital implant.

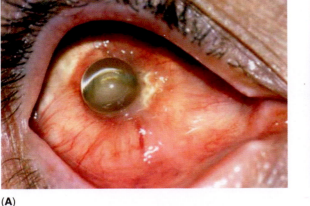
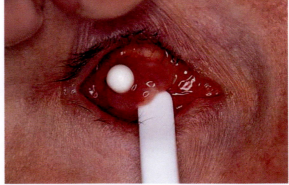

(A) (B)

Figure 21.33 (A) Exposure of an hydroxyapatite implant adjacent to an acrylic motility peg with chronic discharge. (B) A foreign body granuloma lying beneath the head of a motility peg.

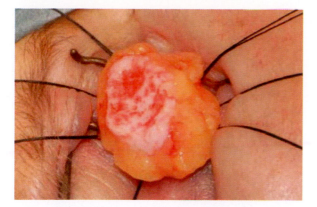

Figure 21.34 A dermis fat graft prepared and ready for implantation in the socket.

Postoperative Care

This is as described above for a spherical implant. The ocular prosthesis is not fitted until the dermis has completely epithelialized. This is usually 6 to 8 weeks postoperatively although in some cases this can take longer.

EVISCERATION

There are different approaches to this procedure which depend on the age of the patient and the indications for the procedure. If the indication for the evisceration is infection, the procedure is very quick and simple and should take no more that a few minutes. If the procedure is being undertaken in an elderly patient for a blind painful eye, e.g., severe rubeotic glaucoma following a central retinal vein occlusion, the procedure can be

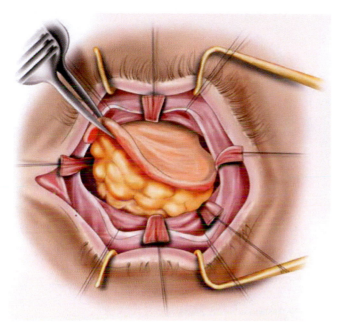

(A)

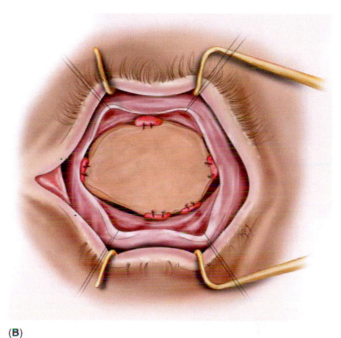

(B)

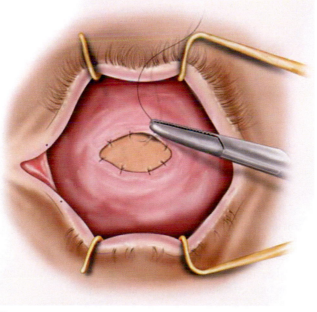

(C)

Figure 21.35 (A) The dermis fat graft is inserted into the socket. (B) The extraocular muscles attached to the dermis. (C) The conjunctival edges are sutured to the anterior surface of the dermis.

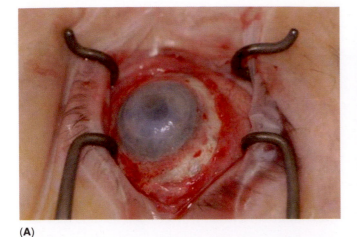

(A)

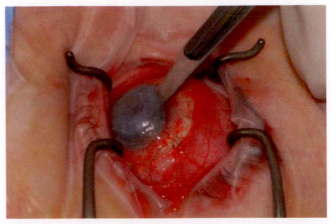

(B)

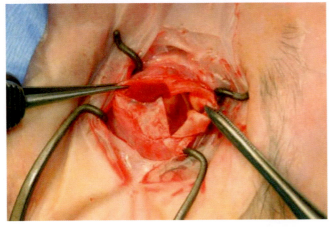

(C)

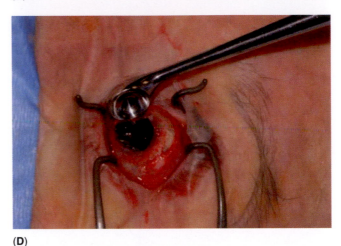

(D)

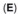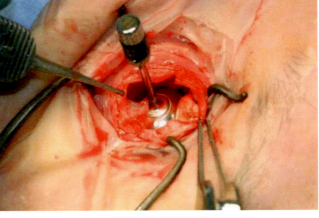

(E)

(F)

Figure 21.36 (**A**) A conjunctival peritomy has been performed. (**B**) A corneal section is performed with a no. 15 Bard Parker blade. (**C**) A keratectomy is performed. (**D**) The intraocular contents are removed with an evisceration spoon. (**E**) Relieving incisions have been made in the sclera medially and laterally. (**F**) A sizing sphere is used to ensure that the scleral edges can be closed over the implant without any tension.

performed under local anesthesia with sedation along with the use of a simple acrylic sphere implant and a subconjunctival patch graft. If the procedure is to be used in a younger healthy patient in preference to an enucleation with placement of a porous implant, the procedure is modified to include cruciate incisions in the posterior sclera in between the recti with a removal of the central posterior sclera and optic nerve to enable a larger implant to be placed than can be accommodated within an intact scleral coat.

Surgical Procedure

1. The face, eyelids, and conjunctival sac should be thoroughly prepared with an antiseptic agent, e.g., diluted aqueous Betadine solution and a cataract drape applied.
2. A Clarke's eyelid speculum is placed to exclude the eyelashes from the surgical field.
3. Using a Moorfield's forceps and blunt-tipped Westcott scissors, a 360° peritomy is performed

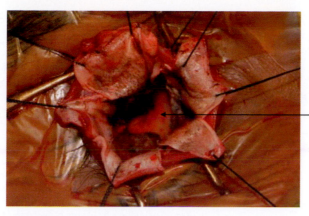

— The intraconal fat space

Figure 21.37 The radial incisions have been made in the sclera in the quadrants between the recti, the optic disc has been excised exposing the intraconal fat space and traction sutures have been placed through the edges of the sclera and the conjunctiva in preparation for the insertion of a porous spherical implant.

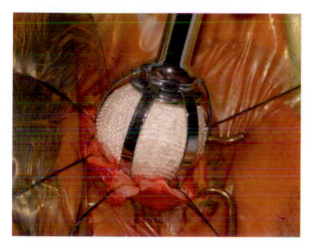

Figure 21.38 An hydroxyapatite orbital implant wrapped in Vicryl mesh is being inserted into the intraconal fat space using a Carter sphere injector.

taking care to preserve as much conjunctiva as possible (Fig. 21.36A). This may be difficult following previous failed retinal reattachment surgery. (This step is omitted in the presence of infection.)

4. A small full-thickness peripheral corneal incision is made with a no. 15 Bard Parker blade (Fig. 21.36B).
5. The cornea is then removed using Westcott scissors with one blade inserted into the anterior chamber (Fig. 21.36C).
6. The intraocular contents are removed with an evisceration spoon (Fig. 21.36D). These contents and the cornea are sent for histopathological examination.
7. The scleral shell is thoroughly cleaned out with cotton-tipped applicators soaked in absolute alcohol followed by repeated thorough saline rinses.
8. The interior of the scleral shell is inspected to ensure all uveal remnants have been removed. Bipolar cautery is used to seal any bleeding vessels.
9. Horizontal relieving incisions are made in the scleral rim medially and laterally (Fig. 21.36E). If the patient is deemed unsuitable for placement of an orbital implant no further surgical intervention is required.

10. A surgical conformer of appropriate size and shape is inserted and a compressive dressing applied.
11. The dressing is maintained in place for 2 days. The patient is discharged on oral and topical antibiotics and is not fitted with an ocular prosthesis until the socket has healed completely. The scleral shell collapses and shrinks and is gradually covered by conjunctiva.
12. If a simple acrylic sphere implant is to be inserted into the intact scleral coat, the appropriate size is determined with the use of sizing spheres (Fig. 21.36F).
13. A spherical implant (usually a size of 15 or 16 mm) is inserted into the scleral coat ensuring that the scleral edges can be easily approximated over the implant, covering this completely.
14. The sclera is closed over the implant using interrupted 5/0 Vicryl sutures with the scleral edges overlapping each other.
15. Any "dog ears" of sclera removed to effect the closure are then used as patch grafts over the suture line. Alternatively a patch graft of donor sclera (with appropriate informed consent) or autogenous temporalis fascia is then placed over the suture line to reduce any risk of implant exposure.
16. Next, the anterior Tenon's fascia and conjunctiva are closed with interrupted 7/0 Vicryl sutures.
17. A sterile surgical conformer of appropriate size and shape is inserted into the conjunctival sac, ensuring that the eyelids will close passively over the conformer without creating tension on the conjunctival suture line.
18. A temporary suture tarsorrhaphy is then undertaken using a central 4/0 nylon suture passed through tarsorrhaphy tubing.
19. A retrobulbar injection of 5ml of 0.5% Bupivacaine with 1:200,000 units of adrenaline is given to aid postoperative analgesia.
20. Injections of an anti-inflammatory agent and an opiate analgesic are given by the anesthetist.
21. Topical antibiotic ointment is instilled into the conjunctival sac either side of the tarsorrhaphy.

22. Jelonet is placed over the eyelids along with two eye pads and Micropore tape, and a bandage is applied before the patient's anesthesia is reversed.

If a porous implant is to be placed the procedure is modified.

1. Incisions are made through the sclera in the quadrants between the recti with a no. 15 Bard Parker blade and completed with iris scissors (Fig. 21.37).
2. A circular incision is then made through the sclera with the no. 15 Bard Parker blade around the optic disc.
3. The optic disc and a length of adjacent optic nerve are removed with Stevens scissors.
4. 4/0 silk traction sutures are placed through the edges of the sclera and conjunctiva and placed on traction with artery clips (Fig. 21.37).
5. The porous implant is inserted into the intraconal fat space with a Carter sphere injector (Fig. 21.38).
6. The remainder of the operation is as described above.

Postoperative Care
This is the same as following an enucleation.

FURTHER READING

1. Cepela M, Teske S. Orbital implants (Review article). Curr Opin Ophthalmol 1996; 7: 38–42.
2. Edelstein C, Shields CL, De Potter P, Shields JA. Complications of motility peg placement for the hydroxyapatite orbital implant. Ophthalmology 1997; 104: 1616–21.
3. Codere F. Hydroxyapatite implants: a rational approach (editorial). Can J Ophthalmol 1995; 30: 235–7.
4. Rubin PA, Popham JK, Bilyk JR, Shore JW. Comparison of fibrovascular ingrowth into hydroxyapatite and porous polyethylene orbital implants. Ophthal Plast Reconstr Surg 1994, 10: 96–103.
5. McNab A. Hydroxyapatite orbital implants. Experience with 100 cases. Aust N Z J Ophthalmol 1995; 23: 117–23.
6. Shields CL, Shields JA, De Potter P, Singh AD. Lack of complications of the hydroxyapatite orbital implant in 250 consecutive cases. Trans Am Ophthalmol Soc 1993; 91: 177–89.
7. Karesh JW, Dresner SC. High-density porous polyethylene (Medpor) as a successful anophthalmic socket implant. Ophthalmology 1994, 10: 1688–95.
8. Edelstein C, Shields CL, De Potter P, Shields JA. Complications of motility peg placement for the hydroxyapatite orbital implant. Ophthalmology 1997; 104: 1616–21.
9. Migliori ME, Putterman AM. The domed dermis-fat graft orbital implant. Ophthal Plast Reconstr Surg 1991; 7: 23–30.
10. Jordan DR, Anderson RL. The universal implant for evisceration surgery. Ophthal Plast Reconstr Surg 1997; 13: 1–7.
11. Levine MR, Pou CR, Lash RH. Evisceration: is sympathetic ophthalmia a concern in the new millenium? Ophthal Plast Reconstr Surg 1999; 15: 4–8.
12. Dutton JJ. Coralline hydroxyapatite as an ocular implant. Ophthalmology 1991; 98: 370–7.
13. Flanders AE, De Potter P, Rao VM, et al. MRI of orbital implants. Neuroradiology 1996; 38: 273–7.
14. Goldberg RA, Holds JB, Ebrahimpour J. Exposed hydroxyapatite orbital implants. Report of six cases. Ophthalmology 1992; 99: 831–6.
15. Nunery WR, Heinz GW, Bonnin JM, Martin RT, Cepela MA. Exposure rate of hydroxyapatite spheres in the anophthalmic socket: histopathologic correlation and comparison with silicone sphere implants. Ophthal Plast Reconstr Surg 1993; 9: 96–104.
16. Buettner H, Bartley GB. Tissue breakdown and exposure associated with hydroxyapatite orbital implants. Am J Ophthalmol 1992; 113: 669–73.
17. Dortzbach RK Holds JB. Theoretical considerations in the placement of hydroxyapatite orbital implants (letter). Ophthal Plast Reconstr Surg 1997; 13: 147–51.
18. Ashworth JL, Brammar R, Leatherbarrow B. A clinical study of the hydroxyapatite orbital implant. Eur J Ophthalmol 1997; 7: 1–8.
19. Ashworth JL, Brammar R, Inkster C, Leatherbarrow B. A study of the hydroxyapatite orbital implant drilling procedure. Eye 1998; 12: 37–42.
20. Smit TJ, Koornneef L, Zonneveld FW, Groet E, Otto AJ. Computed tomography in the assessment of the post enucleation socket syndrome. Ophthalmology 1990; 97: 1347–51.
21. Kim YD, Goldberg RA, Shorr N, Steinsapir KD. Management of exposed hydroxyapatite orbital implants. Ophthalmology 1994; 101: 1709–15.
22. Shields JA, Shields CL, De Potter P. Hydroxyapatite orbital implant after enucleation—experience with 200 cases. Mayo Clin Proc 1993; 68: 1191–5.
23. Kaltreider SA, Newman SA. Prevention and management of complications associated with the hydroxyapatite implant. Ophthal Plast Reconstr Surg 1996; 12: 18–31.
24. Goldberg RA. Who should have hydroxyapatite orbital implants? (editorial). Arch Ophthalmol 1995; 113: 566–7.
25. Ashworth JL, Rhatigan M, Sampath R, et al. The hydroxyapatite orbital implant: a prospective study. Eye 1996; 10: 29–37.
26. De Potter P, Shields CL, Shields JA, Flanders AE, Rao VM. Role of magnetic resonance imaging in the evaluation of the hydroxyapatite orbital implant. Ophthalmology 1992; 99: 824–30.
27. Jordan DR, Allen LH, Ells A, et al. The use of Vicryl mesh (polyglactin 910) for implantation of hydroxyapatite orbital implants. Ophthal Plast Reconstr Surg 1995; 11: 95–9.
28. American Academy of Ophthalmology. Basic and Clinical Science Course: Orbit, Eyelids, and Lacrimal System, section 7. San Francisco, CA: The American Academy of Ophthalmology, 2006/7: 119–29.
29. Chalasani R, Poole-Warren L, Conway RM, Ben-Nissan B. Porous orbital implants in enucleation: a systematic review. Surv Ophthalmol 2007; 52(2): 145–55.
30. Chen TC, Yuen SJA, Sangalang MA, Fernando RE, Leuenberger EU. Retrobulbar chlorpromazine injections for the management of blind and seeing painful eyes. J Glauco 2002; 11: 209–13.
31. Custer PL, Kennedy RH, Woog JJ, Kaltreider SA, Meyer DR. Orbital Implants in enucleation surgery. Ophthalmology 2003; 110: 2054–61.
32. Custer PL, Trinkaus KM. Porous implant exposure: incidence, Management and morbidity. Ophthal Plast Reconstr Surg 2007; 23(1): 1–7.
33. Griepentrog GJ, Lucarelli MJ, Albert DM, Nork TM. Sympathetic ophthalmia following evisceration: a rare case. Ophthal Plast Reconstr Surg 2005; 21(4): 316–8.
34. Nerad JA, Carter KD, Alford MA. Disorders of the orbit: anophthalmic socket. In: Rapid Diagnosis in Ophthalmology: Oculoplastic & Reconstructive Surgery. Philadelphia, PA: Mosby Elsevier, 2008: 260–7.
35. Nunery WR, Hetzler KJ. Dermal-fat graft as a primary enucleation technique. Ophthalmology 1985; 92: 1256.
36. O'Donnell BA, Kersten R, McNab A, Rose G, Rosser P. Enucleation versus evisceration. Clin Exp Ophthalmol 2005; 33: 5–9.
37. Sami D, Young S, Peterson R. Perspective on orbital enucleation implants. Surv Ophthalmol 2007; 52(3): 244–65.
38. Tanenbaum M. Enucleation, evisceration and exenteration. In: Yanoff M, Duker J, eds. Ophthalmology. Philadelphia, PA: Mosby, 2004: 752–60.
39. Tarantini A. Hintschich C. Primary dermis-fat grafting in children. Orbit 2008; 27(5): 363–9.
40. Wobig JL, Dailey RA. Enucleation and exenteration, In: Wobig JL, Dailey RA, eds. Oculofacial Plastic Surgery: Face, Lacrimal System, and Orbit. New York, NY: Thieme, 2004: 255–66.

22 Secondary anophthalmic socket reconstruction

INTRODUCTION

The optimal time to achieve the best functional and cosmetic result for the anophthalmic patient is at the time of enucleation or evisceration. Preoperative planning and a meticulous surgical approach will minimize the risks of complications and reduce the need for secondary surgical reconstruction. Nevertheless, secondary socket surgery represents a significant workload for the oculoplastic surgeon and can be extremely challenging.

Most socket reconstructive surgeries are required to address the following problems:

1. A volume deficit following loss of the globe
2. Contracture of the socket
3. Orbital implant exposure, extrusion, and malposition

Many patients have additional eyelid malpositions which also require surgery. The patient must be carefully assessed and counseled about the nature of any proposed surgery, its risks, and potential complications. The surgery may have to be carried out in stages. The patient may have to accept a lengthy period of time without an ocular prosthesis (artificial eye). Such surgery can have profound effects on a patient professionally, socially, and emotionally. It is important to ensure that the patient has realistic expectations of the surgery.

PATIENT EVALUATION
History

The patient's current complaints must be documented, e.g., pain, discomfort, discharge, instability of the ocular prosthesis, poor movement of the ocular prosthesis, and poor cosmetic appearance. The following details should be obtained:

1. The date of the enucleation/evisceration
2. The indication for the enucleation/evisceration
3. The type and size of any orbital implant used
4. The nature of any previous socket or eyelid surgery
5. A history of prior radiotherapy treatment
6. A history of previous trauma

Examination

The patient should be examined initially with the ocular prosthesis in place. Any features of the post-enucleation socket syndrome (PESS) are noted. These features are:

- Enophthalmos
- An upper eyelid sulcus deformity
- Ptosis or eyelid retraction
- Laxity of the lower eyelid
- A backward tilt of the ocular prosthesis (Fig. 22.1).

Any eyelid malpositions or lagophthalmos are noted (Fig. 22.2). The degree of movement of the ocular prosthesis is ascertained. The prosthesis is then removed noting any instability.

The prosthesis is examined for scratches, surface deposits, or other blemishes. Its size and shape are noted.

The socket and the conjunctival fornices are examined carefully. Any discharge, bleeding, conjunctival inflammation, implant exposure, granulomas, cysts, sinuses, adhesions, or fornix contracture are noted (Figs. 22.2–22.4).

The upper eyelid is everted to exclude the presence of papillae (Fig. 22.5). The socket is gently palpated with a gloved finger to confirm the presence or absence of an orbital implant. The patient is asked to look in all directions as the socket is observed to ascertain the positions of the ocular muscles and the degree of movement of the socket. In particular, the position of the inferior rectus muscle is determined. These positions are documented. If the patient has an upper lid ptosis, the patient should be examined thoroughly to determine the underlying cause. A patient who complains of tearing and discharge should be examined to exclude the possibility of an associated obstruction of the lacrimal drainage system.

CORRECTION OF AN ORBITAL VOLUME DEFICIENCY

Patients who present with a typical PESS may benefit from secondary orbital implant surgery, but the surgical procedure is more difficult and the results are less predictable than primary orbital implantation. Patients undergoing secondary orbital implantation are more likely to require additional surgical procedures. Although the volume deficiency improves following surgery, there is commonly a variable recurrence of the upper lid sulcus defect some months following surgery once postoperative orbital edema has completely resolved.

The type of orbital implant to be used needs to be determined taking a number of factors into consideration:

1. The age and general health of the patient
2. The condition of the socket
3. The size, nature, and complications of any orbital implant already present
4. The degree of movement of the extraocular muscles
5. The condition of the ocular adnexae
6. The cost

The orbital implants of choice for secondary orbital implantation are:

1. The "baseball implant"
2. Hydroxyapatite implant
3. Porous polyethylene (Medpor) implant
4. Bioceramic implant
5. Dermis fat graft implant

1. The "baseball implant" is of use in older patients who do not wish to take advantage of the second stage placement of a motility peg. The implant can improve a volume deficiency but the motility results are unpredictable. If the degree of movement of

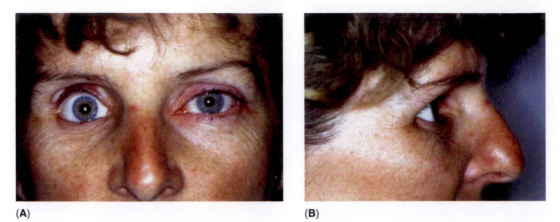

Figure 22.1 (**A**) A young female patient who has the typical features of a right post-enucleation socket syndrome (PESS). No orbital implant was placed in this patient following an enucleation. (**B**) A lateral view of the patient demonstrating a typical backward tilt to the prosthesis.

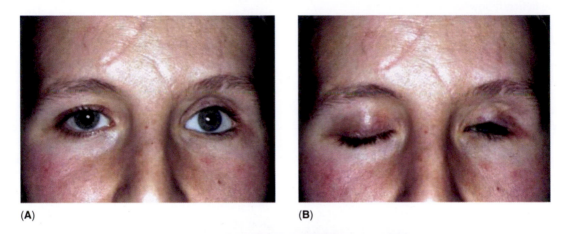

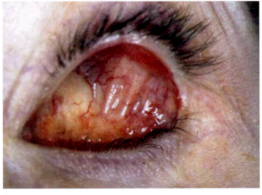

Figure 22.2 (**A**) An anophthalmic patient with left upper eyelid retraction and an upper eyelid sulcus defect. (**B**) The same patient demonstrating lagophthalmos. (**C**) An examination of the socket reveals that superior fornix contracture is the cause of her lagophthalmos.

the implant is good but that of the overlying ocular prosthesis poor, this has to be accepted as it cannot be improved surgically.

2. One of the modern porous implants is ideally reserved for a patient who would wish to undergo a second-stage placement of a motility peg if the movement of the artificial eye were poor in spite of acceptable movement of the implant itself. This type of implant is ideal for the patient who has an old extruding/tilted implant. An implant exchange is performed in the absence of any socket infection. The use of this type of implant is ill advised, however, following prior radiotherapy, in the presence of conjunctival inflammation or socket contracture, or for the reconstruction of a badly disorganized socket.

3. The dermis fat graft is preferred for the reconstruction of the socket that has mild to moderate contracture in addition to a volume deficiency. It is the implant of choice for the reconstruction of badly disorganized sockets, and when complications have necessitated the removal of a porous implant or an infected/extruding synthetic implant.

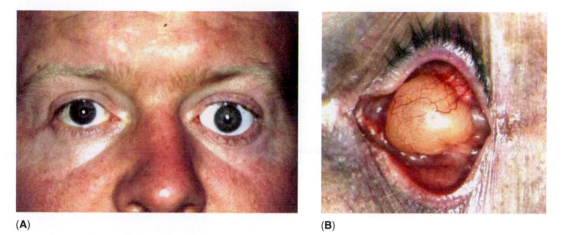

(A)   **(B)**

Figure 22.3 (**A**) This patient complained of poor cosmesis and instability of his artificial eye. (**B**) Examination of his socket revealed a large conjunctival inclusion cyst.

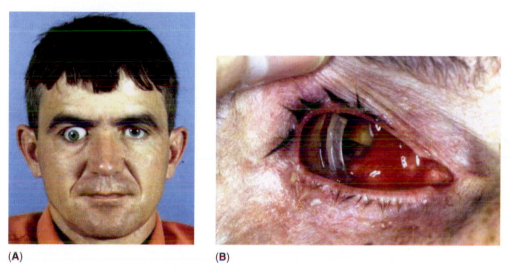

(A)   **(B)**

Figure 22.4 (**A**) This patient also complained of poor cosmesis and instability of his artificial eye. (**B**) An examination of his socket revealed an extruding Castroviejo orbital implant.

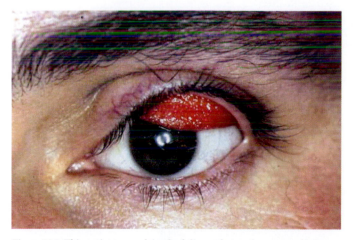

Figure 22.5 This patient complained of discomfort and a mucus discharge. His artificial eye had not been polished for a number of years. Eversion of the upper eyelid revealed a papillary conjunctivitis.

Preoperative Preparation

The patient should be advised about:

1. The advantages, disadvantages, risks, and potential complications of a secondary implant procedure

2. The implant options
3. The options regarding implant wrapping materials
4. Postoperative pain and its management
5. The use of a postoperative compressive dressing
6. The use of a temporary suture tarsorrhaphy
7. The use of a postoperative conformer
8. The likelihood of a temporary postoperative ptosis
9. The role of the ocularist and the timing of the fitting of the ocular prosthesis

It is extremely important that the patient remains under the long-term care of an ocularist, who will ensure that the artificial eye is polished at least on an annual basis. Topical lubricants should be prescribed e.g. Systane® or Hylo®-Forte, particularly for a patient who has an incomplete blink. The socket is examined by the ocularist to exclude implantation cysts, papillary conjunctivitis, and implant exposure. Failure to maintain the artificial eye will risk conjunctival inflammation, discharge, conjunctival breakdown, and implant exposure.

The risks associated with such surgery include: infection which might necessitate removal of the implant, malposition of the implant which might lead to instability or a poor fit of the ocular prosthesis, exposure which will require further surgery, e.g., a patch graft, socket cyst formation requiring further surgery, and chronic inflammation, pain or chemosis. Informed consent should be obtained after the patient has had time to consider the options.

The patient should discontinue aspirin and any other antiplatelet drugs if medically permissible at least 2 weeks preoperatively. Likewise anticoagulants should only be altered or discontinued after discussion with the patient's hematologist. Any bacterial conjunctivitis should be treated preoperatively and topical steroid drops used 2 hourly for 2 weeks prior to surgery to reduce any conjunctival inflammation. In addition, it is preferable for the patient to refrain from wearing an old ocular prosthesis and to wear a well-fitting surgical conformer for at least 2 weeks prior to surgery.

> **KEY POINT**
>
> A CT scan of the orbits and paranasal sinuses should be performed if a patient has previously suffered orbital trauma to exclude the possibility of a missed orbital wall blowout fracture (Figs. 22.6–22.8). If a significant fracture is discovered, this should be repaired before undertaking the secondary orbital implant procedure in order that the ideal orbital implant size can be selected and placed in the correct anatomical location in the socket.

Secondary Orbital Implant Procedure

The anesthetist should be warned that the dissection of the socket could provoke the oculocardiac reflex inducing a severe bradycardia and occasionally asystole. The anesthetist may wish to use intravenous glycopyrolate or atropine prior to the dissection. Prior to the induction of general anesthesia it is very important that the surgeon examines the patient's socket while asking the patient to look up and down. The position of the inferior rectus muscle is marked on the conjunctiva using gentian violet. This is to reduce the risk of inadvertently placing the orbital implant beneath the inferior rectus muscle.

> **KEY POINT**
>
> The surgeon must also ensure that the fellow eye is instilled with Lacrilube ointment, and is taped closed and fully protected from inadvertent injury during the course of the surgery.

SURGICAL TECHNIQUE
Spherical Implant

1. An intravenous injection of a broad-spectrum antibiotic is given by the anesthetist.

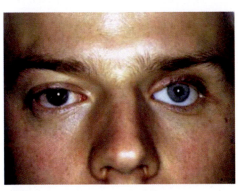

(A)

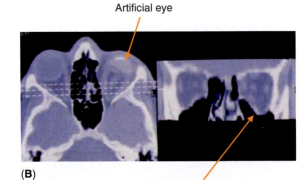

Artificial eye

Orbital floor blowout fracture

(B)

Orbital floor blowout fracture

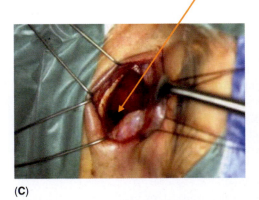

(C)

(D)

Figure 22.6 (**A**) A patient with a post enucleation socket syndrome referred for a secondary orbital implant procedure. He had undergone an enucleation of a badly ruptured globe following blunt trauma without the placement of an orbital implant. (**B**) A preoperative CT scan revealed a previously overlooked orbital floor and a minor anterior medial wall blowout fracture. (**C**) The appearance of the orbital floor fracture seen intraoperatively. The orbital floor fracture was approached via a sub-ciliary skin incision rather than via a swinging eyelid flap approach. (**D**) The postoperative appearance of the patient following repair of the orbital floor blowout fracture with placement of an orbital floor Medpor implant, the secondary implantation of a hydroxyapatite orbital implant and the fitting of a custom made ocular prosthesis.

2. The face, eyelids, and conjunctival sac should be thoroughly prepared with an antiseptic agent and a cataract drape applied.
3. A Clarke's eyelid speculum is placed to exclude the eyelashes from the surgical field.
4. Three to five milliliters of 0.5% Bupivacaine with 1:200,000 units of adrenaline mixed with Hyalase 500 units are injected subconjunctivally and deeper into the orbit to try to prevent the oculo-cardiac reflex.
5. A horizontal incision is made through the conjunctiva above the inferior rectus muscle using a no. 15 Bard Parker blade.
6. The conjunctiva is dissected into the inferior fornix and then 8 to 10 mm into the superior fornix using blunt tipped Westcott scissors taking great care not to damage the underlying levator aponeurosis.
7. 4/0 silk traction sutures are then placed through the superior and inferior edges of the conjunctiva using a double pass and fixated to the drapes with curved artery clips.
8. The central Tenon's fascia is then incised centrally with sharp straight scissors and then blunt-tipped straight scissors are opened repeatedly to expose the intraconal fat.
9. A finger is inserted into the socket to ascertain whether any intraorbital adhesions are present (Fig. 22.9). Any adhesions found are dissected bluntly in order to minimize any trauma to the motor nerves supplying the extraocular muscles.

10. Four 4/0 silk traction sutures are placed through the Tenon's fascia and fixated to the drapes with artery clips (Fig. 22.10).
11. A double-armed 5/0 Vicryl suture is placed through the approximate anterior positions of all four recti muscles. The muscles themselves are not formally dissected to avoid further trauma.
12. If an implant is present, this must be very carefully dissected from the surrounding tissues. A Castroviejo/Roper Hall type of implant is relatively easy to remove and an implant exchange yields very good results as the recti are easily identified and preserved. The implant capsule should be carefully dissected from the socket (Fig. 22.11). Other types of implant are not as straightforward to remove.
13. The appropriate size of orbital implant is determined with the use of sizing spheres. If the Tenon's fascia cannot be closed over the surface of the sizing sphere without undue tension, a smaller sphere should be substituted.
14. The implant of appropriate size is then wrapped in the material which has been selected by the patient during the preoperative consultation, e.g., donor sclera, vicryl mesh, autogenous fascia lata, or Alloderm.
15. The implant is then inserted into the intraconal fat space using a Carter sphere injector.
16. The vicryl sutures are attached to the implant as far anteriorly as possible, and further interrupted 5/0 Vicryl sutures are placed as required to ensure

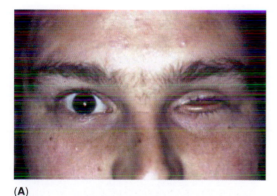 (A)

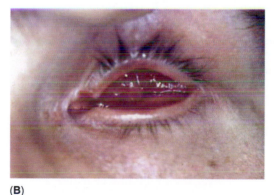 (B)

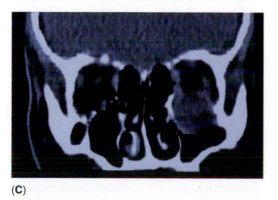 (C)

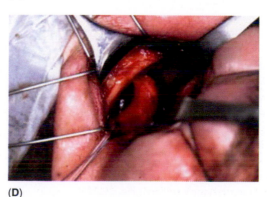 (D)

Figure 22.7 (**A**) A patient referred for the management of a post enucleation socket syndrome following a history of blunt trauma. (**B**) The appearance of his contracted anophthalmic socket. (**C**) His preoperative CT scan revealed the presence of an extensive orbital floor blowout fracture with the left globe subluxated into the maxillary sinus. (**D**) The intraoperative appearance of the globe seen below the inferior orbital margin.

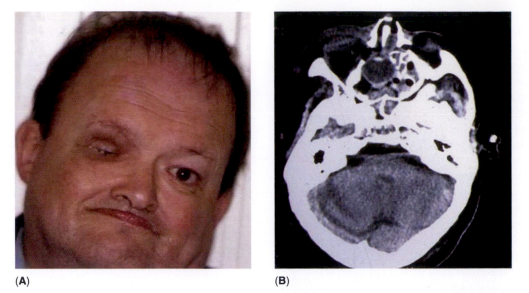

(A)   **(B)**

Figure 22.8 (**A**) A patient with severe learning difficulties referred following blunt trauma to his right orbit with an apparent anophthalmos. (**B**) A CT scan revealed that the right globe was completely subluxated into the adjacent ethmoid sinus.

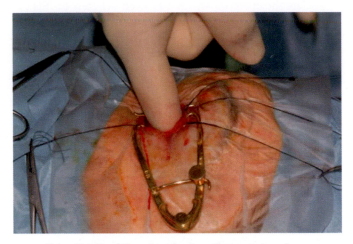

Figure 22.9 Blunt dissection of socket adhesions using a finger.

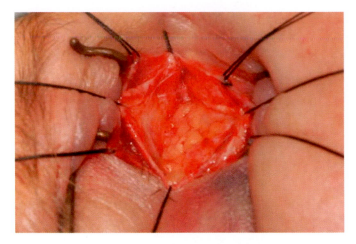

Figure 22.10 A socket dissected and prepared for placement of a secondary implant.

that the posterior Tenon's fascia is completely closed over the implant.

17. A patch graft of donor sclera or autogenous fascia is then placed over the suture line to reduce any risk of implant exposure.

18. Anterior Tenon's fascia is then closed with interrupted 7/0 Vicryl sutures and finally the conjunctiva is closed likewise taking great care to ensure that the inferior fornix is not inadvertently shallowed.

19. A sterile surgical conformer of appropriate size and shape is inserted into the conjunctival sac ensuring that the eyelids will close passively over the conformer without creating tension on the conjunctival suture line.

20. A temporary suture tarsorrhaphy should be undertaken using a central 4/0 nylon suture passed through tarsorrhaphy tubing (Fig. 22.12).

21. A retrobulbar injection of 5 ml of 0.5% Bupivacaine with 1:200,000 units of adrenaline is given to aid postoperative analgesia.

22. Injections of an anti-inflammatory agent and an opiate analgesic are given by the anesthetist. An intravenous injection of steroid also acts as an anti-emetic as well as helps to reduce postoperative swelling.

23. Topical antibiotic ointment is instilled into the conjunctival sac on either side of the tarsorrhaphy.

24. Jelonet is placed over the eyelids along with two eye pads and Micropore tape, and a bandage is applied before the patient's anesthesia is reversed.

Postoperative Management

The patient will usually experience postoperative nausea and pain and is not usually discharged until the second postoperative day. It is extremely important not to underestimate the degree of pain that can be associated with an enucleation or evisceration with placement of an orbital implant and adequate analgesia must be provided as soon as the effects of local anesthesia wear off.

The patient is discharged on a week's course of a broad-spectrum oral antibiotic, a 2-week course of an oral

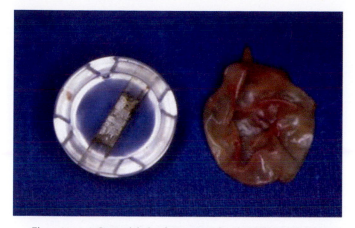

Figure 22.11 A Castroviejo implant removed with its fibrous capsule.

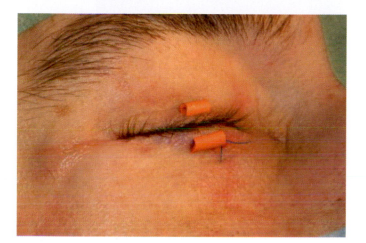

Figure 22.12 A temporary suture tarsorrhaphy.

anti-inflammatory agent, and analgesics (usually a combination of paracetamol and codeine). The patient is instructed to remove the bandage and the dressing 3 days after surgery, and to clean the eyelids and tarsorrhaphy tubing with cotton wool and sterile saline or cooled boiled water. Topical antibiotic ointment is then smeared across the eyelid margins for 2 weeks. The temporary suture tarsorrhaphy is removed in clinic 2 to 3 weeks postoperatively and the topical antibiotic ointment is changed to topical antibiotic drops. These are continued for a further 2 weeks.

KEY POINT

It is extremely important not to underestimate the degree of pain that can be associated with an enucleation or evisceration with placement of an orbital implant and adequate analgesia must be provided as soon as the effects of local anesthesia wear off.

The patient's conformer is then checked, cleaned, and replaced or changed for a different size and shape if required. The patient should not be fitted with an ocular prosthesis until a minimum of 8 weeks have elapsed to allow sufficient wound healing and complete resolution of postoperative edema. If the ocular prosthesis is fitted too soon after surgery the risk of implant exposure is increased. In addition, the ocular prosthesis will not fit the socket properly once complete resolution of postoperative orbital edema has occurred increasing the likelihood of postoperative socket inflammation and discharge.

The patient should remain under the care of the ocularist, who will ensure that the ocular prosthesis is checked and polished at least on an annual basis. If the patient has an incomplete blink or lagophthalmos, the ocular prosthesis should be polished more frequently. Topical lubricants should be prescribed, e.g., Systane® drops, particularly for a patient who has an incomplete blink. The socket should be examined to exclude implantation cysts, papillary conjunctivitis, and impending or actual implant exposure. Failure to maintain the artificial eye will risk conjunctival inflammation, discharge, conjunctival breakdown, and implant exposure.

KEY POINT

The regular long-term postoperative care of the ocular prosthesis by an ocularist is crucial to the success of orbital implant surgery.

The degree of movement of the implant may be poor initially as a consequence of neuropraxia or direct trauma to the extraocular muscles. This frequently improves over the course of the next few months.

The improvement in the features of a PESS following placement of a secondary orbital implant is demonstrated in Figure 22.13. The improvement gained by the exchange of a Castroviejo for a hydroxyapatite orbital implant is demonstrated in Figure 22.14.

Dermis Fat Graft
Surgical Procedure

1. A 25-mm circle is outlined on the inferior quadrant of the abdomen or on the upper outer quadrant of the buttock. The circle is extended to form an ellipse to facilitate wound closure.
2. Three milliliters of 0.5% Bupivacaine with 1:200,000 units of adrenaline are injected subconjunctivally in the socket and a further 10 ml are injected intradermally in the anterior abdominal wall at the proposed site of the graft excision to create a "peau d'orange" appearance (Fig. 22.15).
3. Next, a skin incision is made along the marks and the epidermis carefully shaved off the proposed graft in a single sheet using a no. 15 Bard Parker blade (Fig. 22.16). The pale dermis should now show multiple fine bleeding points and ideally very little of any fat should be visible (Fig. 22.16).
4. An incision is made through one edge of the dermis and the dermis fat graft is removed using Stevens scissors (Fig. 22.17).
5. The wound is closed using interrupted subcutaneous 4/0 Vicryl sutures and interrupted 4/0 nylon sutures for the skin.
6. The graft is subsequently cut to the desired shape required for a socket implant (Fig. 22.18).
7. The socket is prepared and dissected as for a secondary spherical implant.

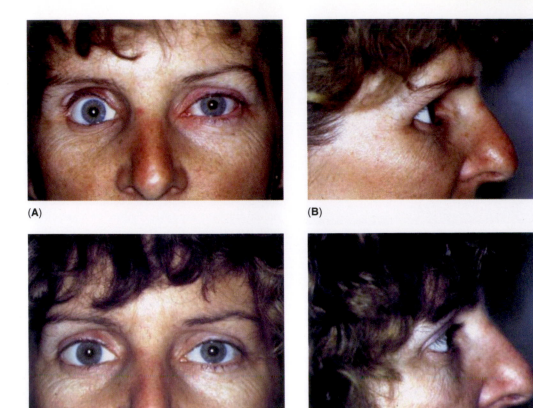

(A)   (B)

(C)   (D)

Figure 22.13 (**A**) A patient without an orbital implant who has a typical post enucleation socket syndrome. (**B**) A lateral view of the patient reveals a typical backward tilt of the artificial eye. (**C**) The same patient following the placement of a secondary orbital implant. (**D**) A lateral view of the same patient demonstrates that the artificial eye now lies in the correct plane.

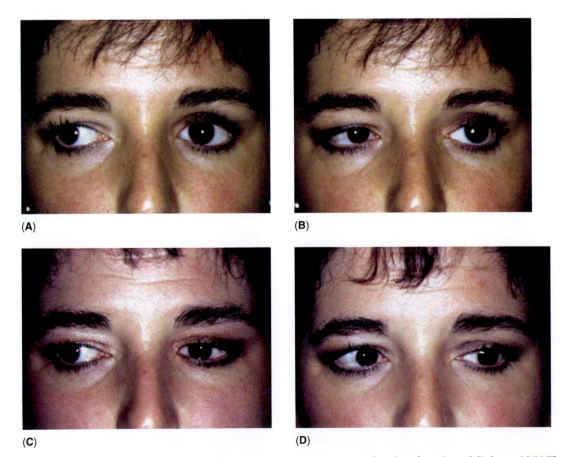

(A)   (B)

(C)   (D)

Figure 22.14 (**A,B**) A patient with a Castroviejo orbital implant who complained of a poor cosmesis, chronic socket pain, and discharge. (**C,D**) The patient following removal of the Castroviejo orbital implant which was exchanged for a hydroxyapatite orbital implant. The patient is seen following placement of a motility peg 12 months following implantation. This patient has remained trouble free for 15 years.

8. The dermis fat graft is then inserted into the socket and the vicryl sutures are attached to the anterior surface of the graft (Fig. 22.18).

9. If there is a conjunctival lining deficit the sutures are positioned closer to the edge of the graft in order to leave a central bare area of graft exposed. This epithelializes gradually. As the sutures are tied the fat is reduced into the intraconal fat space. The conjunctiva is sutured to the front surface of the graft with interrupted 7/0 Vicryl sutures leaving an area of the graft bare in the presence of socket contracture. In the absence of a lining deficit the conjunctiva is closed over the dermis fat graft.

10. A surgical conformer of appropriate size and shape is placed ensuring that the eyelids close passively.

The rest of the procedure is completed as done for a secondary spherical orbital implant procedure.

Postoperative Management
This is as described above for a spherical implant. The ocular prosthesis is not fitted until the dermis has completely

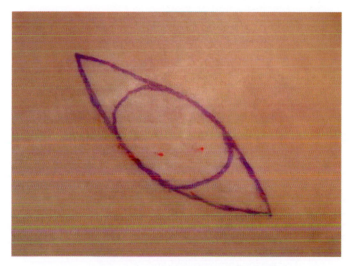

Figure 22.15 An outline of a dermis fat graft to be harvested with a "peau d'orange" appearance of the skin created by an intradermal injection of local anesthetic solution.

epithelialized. This usually takes 6 to 8 weeks postoperatively although in some cases this can take longer.

Correction of a Residual Orbital Volume Deficiency
If the patient has a residual orbital volume deficiency in spite of the insertion of a secondary orbital implant of adequate size, the next options are:

- Placement of a subperiosteal implant
- Structural fat grafting to the orbital apex
- Intermittent injection of a hyaluronic acid filler into the orbital apex
- The injection of small hydrogel implants into the orbital apex

Although there are a number of implant options, e.g., autogenous bone (e.g., a calvarial bone graft), acrylic, homologous cartilage, silicone blocks, porous polyethylene (Medpor) is the author's implant of choice. This synthetic implant is porous allowing fibrovascular ingrowth. It is malleable, and easy to shape and insert along the lateral and infero-lateral orbital wall through a small lateral canthal skin incision. It is well tolerated with excellent long-term results. The placement of a subperiosteal implant can be combined with a lateral tarsal strip procedure where there is lower lid laxity. This procedure can be performed under general anesthesia or under local anesthesia with or without intravenous sedation. This procedure can be undertaken on a day-case basis as long as the patient is provided with appropriate postoperative analgesia.

Structural fat grafting is an alternative approach to orbital volume enhancement but is associated with an unpredictable degree of postoperative fat atrophy and the procedure may have to be repeated to achieve the desired result. The risks associated with this technique in this location also have to be taken into consideration, i.e., inadvertent fat embolization and inadvertent penetration of the superior orbital fissure. The procedure should be used to provide volume enhancement in a socket which already has an orbital implant in place. If it is used for a purely anophthalmic socket, the rotational defects of such a socket may be exacerbated with fat migrating into an antero-inferior location with shallowing of the inferior fornix and instability of the artificial eye.

If the orbital volume deficit is to be addressed with the use of a subperiosteal implant or with structural fat grafting, the

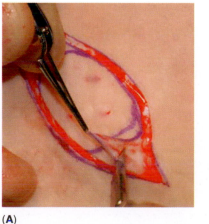

(A)

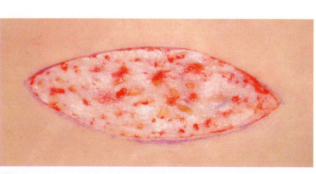

(B)

Figure 22.16 (A) The epidermis being removed with no. 15 Bard Parker blade. (B) The appearance of dermis following removal of epidermis.

patient must be made aware that a new ocular prosthesis may be needed.

The intermittent injection of a hyaluronic acid dermal filler (Restylane Sub-Q) into the orbital apex is a quick and simple procedure. It should be undertaken with safety precautions in case the injection stimulates the oculocardiac reflex. The dermal filler is simply injected along the posterolateral orbital wall and the effect of the injection on the upper lid sulcus is observed. The treatment is, however, expensive and lasts only for 9 to 12 months before a repeat injection is required. For this reason, it is not a practical solution for most anophthalmic patients.

The injection of small self-expanding hydrogel implants into the orbital apex offers another minimally invasive option for permanent socket volume enhancement for carefully selected patients. The implants are injected using a trochar and cannula. Great care should be exercised to ensure that the cannula is not inserted too far into the orbit with the risk of intracranial trauma. There is a risk that such implants might migrate within the socket.

Alternative or additional options are:

1. A contralateral camouflage blepharoplasty
2. A dermis fat graft insertion into the upper eyelid sulcus
3. The placement of fat pearls into the upper eyelid sulcus

A contralateral blepharoplasty may be performed on the opposite upper eyelid to provide a more symmetrical appearance in a patient who has an upper lid sulcus deformity but who does not wish to undergo a subperiosteal implant procedure or Coleman fat injections. The patient must appreciate the small risks involved in such surgery performed around an only eye. Great care must be exercised when undertaking this surgery.

A small dermis fat graft can be inserted into the upper lid sulcus after exposing the orbital roof via a skin crease incision. The dermis is sutured to the periosteum of the orbital roof while the fat is placed in such a position as to mimic the preaponeurotic fat. The dermis fat graft is oversized to allow for some postoperative atrophy. If the graft remains oversized, it can be debulked. This does tend to create a rather bulky appearance to the upper eyelid.

Individual fat pearls can be harvested from the peri-umbilical area and placed directly into the pre-aponeurotic space via an upper lid skin crease incision (Fig. 22.19). This can yield a good result, but the degree of postoperative fat atrophy is unpredictable.

Subperiosteal Orbital Implant
Surgical Procedure

1. An intravenous injection of a broad-spectrum antibiotic is given by the anesthetist.
2. A lateral canthal incision is marked along a skin crease using gentian violet.
3. Three milliliters of 0.5% Bupivacaine with 1:200,000 units of adrenaline are injected subcutaneously. (If the procedure is performed under local anesthesia with intravenous sedation a lateral peribulbar injection of the same solution is given.)
4. A lateral canthal skin incision is made using a Colorado needle leaving the lateral commissure intact.
5. The soft tissues are dissected down to the periosteum using the Colorado needle.
6. The periosteum of the lateral orbital margin is exposed by blunt dissection with a Freer periosteal elevator and a 2 to 3 cm vertical incision is made through the periosteum along the lateral orbital margin with the Colorado needle.
7. The periosteum is raised and reflected widely from the lateral orbital wall using a Freer periosteal elevator taking care to avoid the inferior orbital fissure.
8. The zygomatic vessels are cauterized using bipolar cautery.

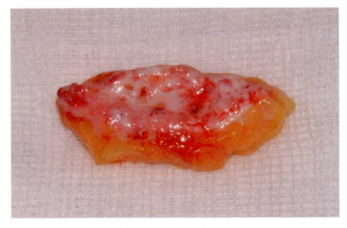

Figure 22.17 The appearance of a dermis fat graft.

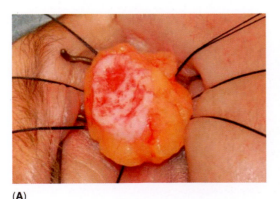 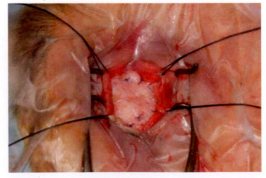

(A)   (B)

Figure 22.18 (**A**) A dermis fat graft prepared and ready for implantation. (**B**) The dermis fat graft has been sutured to Tenon's tissue with interrupted Vicryl sutures.

9. Next, a Medpor sheet implant is cut into small (approximately 1 cm in diameter) discs (Fig. 22.20).

10. The discs are then inserted deep into the subperiosteal space along the inferolateral orbital wall one by one with the aid of illumination from a headlight and a medium Sewall retractor (Fig. 22.20). The effect on the upper lid sulcus and the conjunctival sac is observed. It is important not to overcorrect the volume replacement. The implant discs should not be placed along the anterior aspect of the orbital floor where they can cause a shallowing of the inferior fornix and they should remain posterior to the lateral orbital margin. They should not be palpable through the lateral aspect of the upper or lower eyelids. If necessary a small T-bar titanium microplate can be screwed to the lateral orbital margin to secure the implants and prevent them from migrating forward.

11. The periosteum is then closed firmly using interrupted 5/0 Vicryl sutures.

12. The orbicularis muscle is closed with interrupted 5/0 Vicryl sutures.

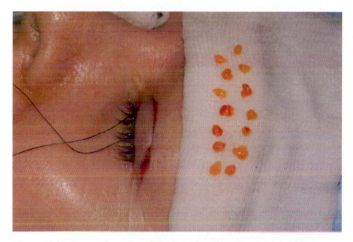

Figure 22.19 Fat pearls prepared for insertion into the upper eyelid preaponeurotic space via an upper eyelid skin crease incision (this is not an anophthalmic patient).

13. The skin is closed with interrupted 7/0 Vicryl sutures.

14. A sterile surgical conformer of appropriate size and shape is inserted into the conjunctival sac ensuring that the eyelids will close passively over the conformer. If the patient shows significant lower eyelid laxity, a lateral tarsal strip procedure can now be performed.

15. A topical antibiotic ointment is applied to the skin wound.

16. Jelonet is placed over the eyelids along with two eye pads and Micropore tape, and a bandage is applied before the patient's anesthesia is reversed.

Postoperative Management

The patient is discharged on a week's course of a broad-spectrum oral antibiotic, a 2-week course of an oral anti-inflammatory agent, and an oral analgesic. The dressing is removed 3 days postoperatively and topical antibiotic is applied to the wound for 2 weeks. The patient should not be fitted with an ocular prosthesis (the patient may require a new ocular prosthesis to be made or the previous ocular prosthesis may need to be modified by the ocularist to ensure a precise fit) until a minimum of 4 weeks have elapsed to allow sufficient wound healing and complete resolution of postoperative orbital edema (Fig. 22.21).

Structural Fat Grafting

This can be performed under general anesthesia, or under local anesthesia with intravenous sedation. It can be undertaken on a day-case basis as long as the patient is provided with adequate postoperative analgesic agents.

Surgical Procedure

The fat is harvested as described in chapter 13.

1. Three milliliters of 0.5% Bupivacaine with 1:200,000 units of adrenaline mixed with Hyalase 500 units are injected subconjunctivally and deeper into the orbit to try to prevent the oculocardiac reflex.

2. A small incision is made in the inferotemporal conjunctival fornix with a no. 15 Bard Parker blade.

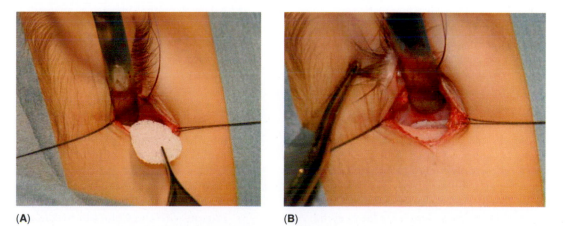

(A) (B)

Figure 22.20 (A) A piece of Medpor is being inserted into the subperiosteal space along the lateral wall of the orbit via a lateral canthal skin incision. (B) The Medpor implant is shown in the subperiosteal space. The implant is shown too anteriorly for the purpose of illustration. The implant will be positioned more deeply in the orbit before additional pieces of Medpor are laid over this.

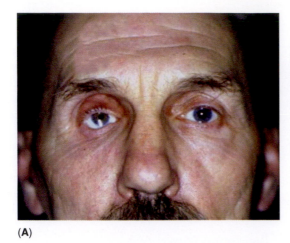
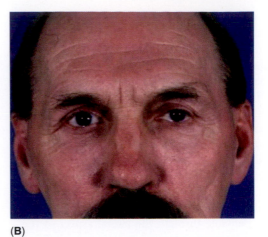

(A)   (B)

Figure 22.21 (**A**) A patient with a severe right post enucleation socket syndrome. (**B**) The same patient following the placement of a secondary "baseball" orbital implant and then a subperiosteal orbital implant combined with a lateral tarsal strip procedure.

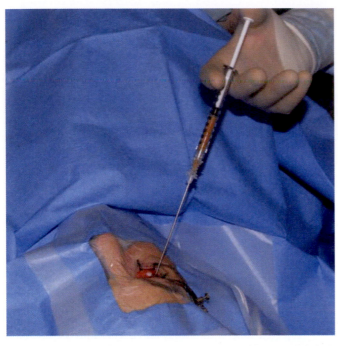

Figure 22.22 Coleman fat being injected into the apex of an anophthalmic socket via a small incision in the inferior conjunctival fornix.

3. A blunt-tipped Coleman injection cannula is attached to a 1-ml Luer lock syringe containing fat cells.
4. The injection cannula is advanced carefully towards the orbital apex ensuring that this is not advanced too far with the risk of penetrating the superior orbital fissure (Fig. 22.22).
5. The fat is injected slowly observing the effects on the superior sulcus and on the conjunctival fornices. Usually no more than 3 cm^3 are injected.
6. The small conjunctival wound is closed with one or two 7/0 Vicryl sutures.
7. A sterile surgical conformer of appropriate size and shape is inserted into the conjunctival sac ensuring that the eyelids will close passively over the conformer. If the patient shows significant lower eyelid laxity, the operation can be combined with a lateral tarsal strip procedure.
8. A topical antibiotic ointment is applied to the socket.

9. Jelonet is placed over the eyelids along with two eye pads and Micropore tape, and a bandage is applied before the patient's anesthesia is reversed.

Postoperative Management
The patient is discharged on topical antibiotic drops which are commenced following removal of the dressings 3 days postoperatively, and analgesics. The patient's conformer is checked, cleaned, and replaced or changed for a different size and shape if required. The patient should not be fitted with a new ocular prosthesis until a minimum of 6 weeks have elapsed to allow sufficient wound healing and complete resolution of postoperative edema.

Lower Eyelid Laxity
Lower eyelid laxity in the anophthalmic patient can be managed with a lateral tarsal strip procedure in most cases. A surgical conformer of an appropriate size and shape should be placed and the ocular prosthesis should not be worn for at least 4 weeks following the surgery. If the medial canthal tendon is very lax it is preferable to place a lower eyelid fascial sling using autogenous fascia lata.

Lower Lid Fascial Sling
Surgical Procedure
1. A lateral canthal incision is marked along a skin crease using gentian violet (Fig. 22.23A).
2. A small horizontal incision is also marked over the medial canthal tendon and three 2-mm subciliary incisions are marked in the lower eyelid (Fig. 22.23A).
3. Two to three milliliters of 0.5% Bupivacaine with 1:200,000 units of adrenaline are injected subcutaneously along the whole of the lower eyelid and medial and lateral canthi.
4. A lateral canthal skin incision is made using a Colorado needle or a no. 15 Bard Parker blade.
5. The soft tissues are dissected down to the periosteum with the Colorado needle or with Westcott scissors. The periosteum of the lateral orbital margin is exposed by blunt dissection using a Freer periosteal elevator and a 2 to 3 cm vertical

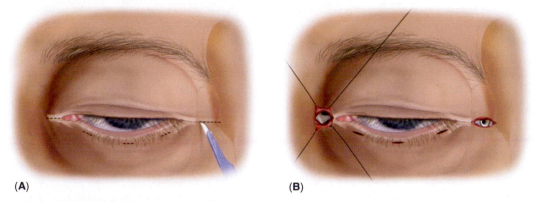

Figure 22.23 (**A**) The medial canthal tendon is exposed via a small horizontal skin incision and further small horizontal incisions are made in the lower eyelid just beneath the lash line. A slightly larger incision is made at the lateral canthus. (**B**) 4/0 silk traction sutures are placed to assist the exposure of the medial canthal tendon. A small drill hole is made through the lateral orbital margin.

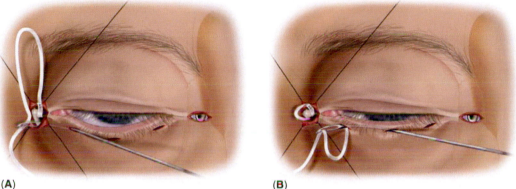

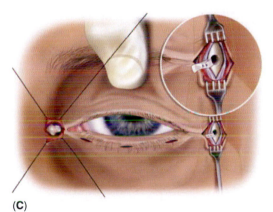

Figure 22.24 (**A**) The fascia is wrapped around the medial canthal tendon adjacent to its insertion and tied to itself and sutured to the medial canthal tendon. (**B**) The fascia is threaded along the eyelid using a paediatric Wright's fascial needle. (**C**) The fascia is threaded through a small drill hole in the lateral orbital margin and sutured to itself.

incision is made through the periosteum with the Colorado needle or no. 15 blade.

6. The periosteum is raised and reflected from the anterior portion of lateral orbital wall and from the internal aspect of the lateral orbital wall for a few millimeters.

7. A 2-mm hole is drilled through the bone at the level of insertion of the lateral canthal tendon (Fig. 22.23B). A small malleable retractor is placed into the subperiosteal space to protect the orbital contents while making the drill hole.

8. A small horizontal incision is made at the medial canthus in line with the medial commissure using the Colorado or no. 15 blade, and the medial canthal tendon is carefully exposed.

9. A 2 to 3 mm strip of autogenous fascia lata is threaded around the anterior limb of the medial canthal tendon close to its insertion on the bone taking great care not to damage the canaliculi (Fig. 22.24A).

10. The fascia is sutured firmly to itself and to the medial canthal tendon using a 5/0 Ethibond suture.

11. The fascia is threaded along the lower eyelid in front of the tarsal plate close to the eyelid margin via a series of small skin incisions using a pediatric Wright's ptosis needle (Fig. 22.24B). The fascia is then threaded through the hole in the lateral orbital margin from the internal to the external aspect of the hole, and, if possible, through a hole made in the periosteum. The fascia is then sutured to itself with a 5/0 Ethibond suture (Fig. 22.24C).

12. The lateral canthal wound is closed using interrupted 5/0 Vicryl sutures for the subcutaneous layer and interrupted 7/0 Vicryl sutures for the skin. The other skin wounds are closed with interrupted 7/0 Vicryl sutures.

13. A sterile surgical conformer of appropriate size and shape is inserted into the conjunctival sac ensuring that no undue pressure is exerted on the lower eyelid.

14. A topical antibiotic ointment is applied to the skin wounds.

15. Jelonet is placed over the eyelids along with two eye pads and Micropore tape, and a bandage is applied.

Postoperative Management
The dressing is removed 4 to 5 days postoperatively and topical antibiotic is applied to the wounds for 2 weeks. The ocular prosthesis is not replaced for at least 6 weeks.

Ptosis
A ptosis in an anophthalmic patient should be evaluated after the orbital volume deficit has been corrected, any lower eyelid tightening has been performed, and a new ocular prosthesis has been fitted. A temporary ptosis is common following any socket surgery and time should be allowed for spontaneous recovery. The oculist may be able to correct small degrees of ptosis by making adjustments to the ocular prosthesis but the use of an oversized prosthesis should be avoided.

Any residual ptosis is then evaluated and classified in a similar manner to that of a ptosis existing in a non-anophthalmic patient (chap. 7). Some aspects of the evaluation will differ, e.g., the patient cannot be evaluated for the presence or absence of a Bell's phenomenon. The decision about the type of ptosis procedure required still very much depends on a measurement of the patient's levator function. For patients with a levator function of 4 mm or less a frontalis suspension procedure will be required. The lagophthalmos induced by this procedure will, however, lead to a rapid degradation of the surface of the ocular prosthesis unless this is lubricated with artificial tears, e.g., Systane® drops, frequently each day and unless the prosthesis is polished every 3 months.

For patients with better levator function and 2 to 3mm of ptosis, a Müller's muscle resection procedure is much preferred to an anterior approach levator advancement as long as the conjunctiva is healthy and non-inflamed (chap. 7). This procedure yields very good cosmetic results in such patients without significantly compromising the patient's reflex blink (Fig. 22.25). The patient's ocular prosthesis is removed prior to the surgery. The patient should wear a well-fitting surgical conformer and should not be fitted with the ocular prosthesis until a minimum of 4 weeks have elapsed to allow sufficient wound healing and complete resolution of postoperative edema. The prosthesis may need to be adjusted by the oculist to achieve the best cosmetic result.

For patients with greater degrees of ptosis an anterior approach levator advancement should be performed (chap. 7). In contrast to a Müller's muscle resection procedure, the patient's ocular prosthesis should be left in place during the surgery to allow intraoperative adjustments to be made to the height and contour of the eyelid with a planned 1mm overcorrection on the table. The socket and the prosthesis should first be prepped with diluted iodine prior to the commencement of surgery.

Good cosmetic results can be achieved but any remaining overcorrection will tend to leave a rather "starey" appearance, which should be avoided if possible (see Fig. 22.26). The patient must appreciate that an anterior approach levator advancement procedure will inevitably compromise the patient's reflex blink necessitating the long-term use of topical lubricants and the requirement for more frequent polishing of the artificial eye.

Shallowing of the Inferior Fornix
The inferior fornix may shallow and cause instability of ocular prosthesis for the following three reasons:

1. The suspensory ligament of the inferior fornix has been damaged
2. There is contracture of the conjunctiva of the inferior fornix
3. An orbital or subperiosteal implant has been placed incorrectly or has migrated (Fig. 22.27)

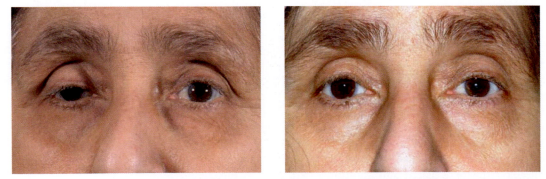

(A)   (B)

Figure 22.25 (**A**) An anophthalmic patient with a moderate right ptosis. (**B**) The patient following a right posterior approach Müller's muscle resection procedure.

Management

If the suspensory ligament is damaged but the conjunctival lining is normal, the inferior fornix can be reformed using fornix-deepening sutures in conjunction with a silicone explant. This is usually combined with a lateral tarsal strip procedure. It is important to ascertain that there is sufficient conjunctival lining present by holding the eyelid forward. The fornix will automatically reform if there is no shortage of conjunctiva (Fig. 22.28).

If there is conjunctival contracture, a mucous membrane graft will be required. An incorrectly placed implant will usually have to be removed and repositioned or exchanged for a dermis fat graft.

Fornix Deepening Sutures

Surgical Procedure

This procedure can be performed under either local anesthesia with or without sedation or under general anesthesia.

1. Three milliliters of 0.5% Bupivacaine with 1:200,000 units of adrenaline are injected subconjunctivally into the inferior fornix and subcutaneously around the infraorbital foramen.
2. If a lateral tarsal strip procedure is to be performed, the initial dissection is undertaken at this stage, making it easier to place the fornix deepening sutures.
3. A silicone explant (e.g., a 240 retinal explant) is shaped and two to three 4/0 nylon fornix-deepening sutures are passed (Fig. 22.29). The needle is carefully passed through the silicone explant, through the inferior fornix conjunctiva, through the full thickness of the eyelid catching the periosteum of the inferior orbital margin, exiting through a stab incision in the cheek just below the lower eyelid. The needle is then returned via the same stab incision, again taking a bite of the periosteum, through the eyelid, through the inferior fornix conjunctiva, and the explant, and then tied (Fig. 22.29).
4. The lateral tarsal strip procedure is now completed.
5. A sterile surgical conformer is placed. It is essential that the conformer selected is of the correct size and shape.
6. Antibiotic ointment is instilled into the socket.
7. A compressive dressing is applied.

Postoperative Management

The fornix-deepening sutures should not be removed for at least 6 weeks. Topical antibiotic drops are used three times a day for 4 weeks. The conformer must be left in place. The ocular prosthesis is fitted once the sutures and silicone explant have been removed.

Management of Orbital Implant Complications

Orbital Implant Exposure

The risk of exposure of an orbital implant should be minimized by:

1. Careful patient selection
2. Avoiding the placement of an oversized implant
3. The use of a suitable implant wrapping material
4. The use of a subconjunctival patch graft
5. Meticulous intraoperative hemostasis
6. Meticulous surgical technique
7. Strict attention to asepsis
8. The placement of a surgical conformer of the appropriate size and shape
9. The use of a temporary suture tarsorrhaphy,
10. The use of a compressive dressing postoperatively
11. Ensuring good quality ocular prosthetic aftercare at the appropriate time postoperatively

Implant exposure should be a rare problem. It can be classified into early and late exposures.

Early Exposure

If the orbital implant becomes exposed it is important to correct the defect as soon as possible to prevent further exposure and infection. The patient's ocular prosthesis should be removed and replaced with a surgical conformer, which is vaulted anteriorly ensuring no contact with the area of exposure. A topical antibiotic/steroid drop is prescribed.

Surgical Procedure

1. The face, eyelids, and conjunctival sac should be thoroughly prepared with an antiseptic agent and a cataract drape applied.
2. A Clarke's eyelid speculum is placed to exclude the eyelashes from the surgical field.

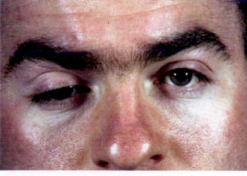
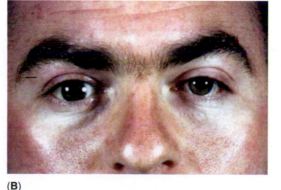

(A) **(B)**

Figure 22.26 (**A**) An anophthalmic patient with a marked right ptosis. (**B**) The patient following a right anterior approach levator aponeurosis advancement procedure with a slight overcorrection.

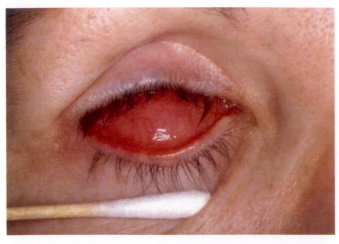

Figure 22.27 Marked shallowing of the inferior fornix due to the presence of an orbital implant placed too low within the socket.

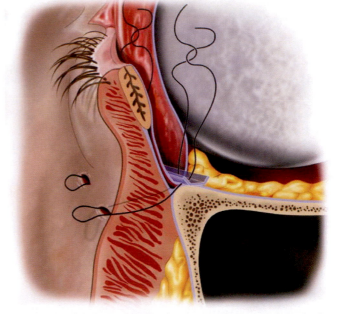

Figure 22.29 The silicone retinal explant is sutured into the inferior fornix.

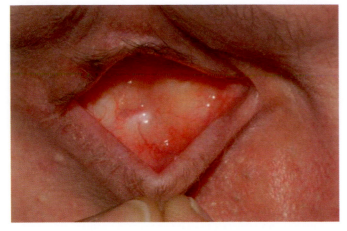

Figure 22.28 A patient with loss of the suspensory ligament of the inferior fornix. The inferior fornix reforms on pulling the eyelid forward.

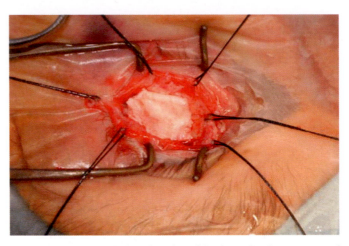

Figure 22.30 A temporalis fascial patch graft has been placed over an area of implant exposure.

3. Two to three milliliters of 0.5% Bupivacaine with 1:200,000 units of adrenaline are injected subconjunctivally in the socket.
4. The conjunctiva is gently undermined around the area of implant exposure and the edges trimmed with Westcott scissors.
5. If the implant is an hydroxyapatite or a bioceramic orbital implant, the area of exposed implant can be gently burred down using a diamond tipped burr with plenty of irrigation to prevent heating.
6. A temporalis fascial patch graft is harvested (chap. 13) and two circular pieces are shaped. These are inserted to lie over the exposed implant with the peripheral margins of the grafts lying beneath the conjunctiva, one on top of the other (Fig. 22.30). (A dermal graft or thinned dermis fat graft can also be used if preferred. Donor sclera is more convenient to use but its use is now rarely acceptable to patients because of the risk of transmissible disease.)
7. The conjunctival edges are then sutured to the graft with interrupted 8/0 Vicryl sutures. The graft is left to epithelialize spontaneously.
8. A well-fitting conformer is placed which is vaulted forward to ensure that there is no contact with the graft.

9. A temporary suture tarsorrhaphy should be undertaken using a central 4/0 nylon suture passed through tarsorrhaphy tubing.
10. A retrobulbar injection of 5 ml of 0.5% Bupivacaine with 1:200,000 units of adrenaline is given to aid postoperative analgesia.
11. Topical antibiotic ointment is instilled into the conjunctival sac either side of the tarsorrhaphy.
12. Jelonet is placed over the eyelids along with two eye pads and Micropore tape, and a bandage is applied before the patient's anesthesia is reversed.

Postoperative Management

This is as described above for secondary spherical orbital implant procedure. The ocular prosthesis is not replaced until the graft has epithelialized fully. This usually takes 6 to 8 weeks postoperatively.

Exposed hydroxyapatite implant

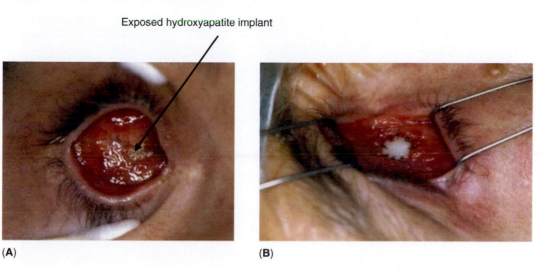

(A)   (B)

Figure 22.31 (**A**) A small area of exposure of a hydroxyapatite orbital implant. (**B**) The exposed area has been covered with a small hard palate mucosal graft.

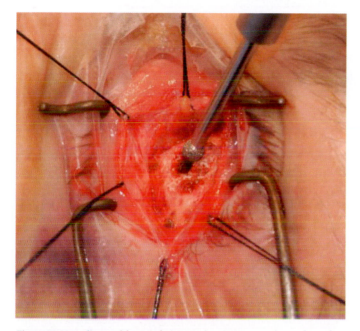

Figure 22.32 A diamond burr is being used to burr away the surface of an exposed hydroxyapatite orbital implant. Traction sutures have been placed through the edges of the conjunctiva and Tenon's fascia.

Late Exposure

The management of late implant exposure depends on the area of exposure and the health of the adjacent conjunctiva. A relatively small area of exposure can be managed with a temporalis fascial patch graft, a small hard palate mucosal graft (Fig. 22.31), or a small dermal graft. The exposed surface of an hydroxyapatite implant should first be burred away using a small diamond burr with plenty of irrigation before placing the graft (Fig. 22.32).

An alternative solution is to remove the implant and place a new implant deeper within the socket if this was not done at the time of the initial implantation. Procedures that involve the use of local tarsoconjunctival flaps should be avoided as these can cause secondary eyelid problems or socket contracture.

If there is a large area of implant exposure with unhealthy, friable adjacent conjunctiva or evidence of chronic infection,

the implant should be removed and exchanged for a dermis fat graft.

Implant Malposition

An orbital implant placed secondarily may become malpositioned in the socket and cause shallowing of a fornix. The ocularist may then have difficulty fitting the ocular prosthesis. A CT scan should be performed to demonstrate the relationship of the implant to the extraocular muscles (Fig. 22.33). The implant should then be removed and repositioned or exchanged for a dermis fat graft

Oversized Orbital Implant

Occasionally the ocularist will find that there is an apparent overcorrection of the orbital volume deficit when he/she comes to fit the ocular prosthesis. It is wise to defer fitting of the ocular prosthesis for a few more weeks to allow further resolution of postoperative edema. If the implant position remains too anterior leaving insufficient room for the ocular prosthesis, there are three options:

1. Remove the implant and replace it with smaller implant
2. Burr down the surface of the implant
3. Decompress the lateral orbital wall

Of these options a lateral orbital decompression is preferred. This causes the least disruption of the socket with a faster postoperative recovery and does not risk implant exposure. The lateral orbital wall is approached as described for a subperiosteal implant procedure. A 3-mm rose head burr is used to burr down the internal aspect of the lateral orbital wall creating more space in the conjunctival sac for the ocularist. This procedure can also be used to create more space for the ocularist if there is insufficient depth to an artificial eye to accommodate a motility peg. An orbital CT scan should be performed before such a procedure is undertaken.

Management of Socket Contracture

A contracted socket may be congenital or acquired. The management of congenital socket contracture is particularly

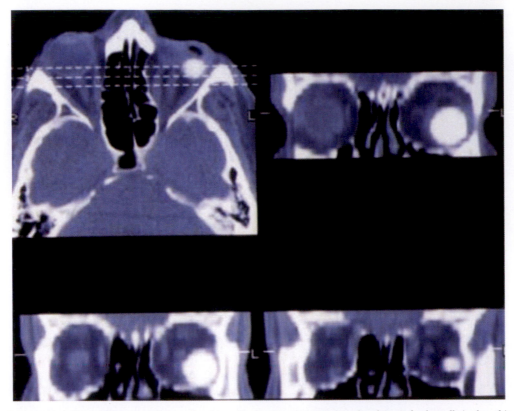

Figure 22.33 A CT scan demonstrating a malpositioned hydroxyapatite orbital implant lying inferolaterally in the orbit.

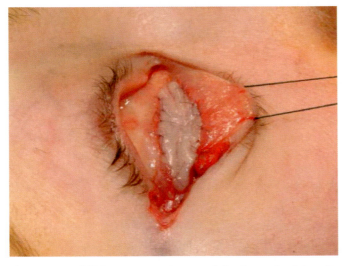

Figure 22.34 A labial mucous membrane graft has been placed into the inferior fornix. In addition a lateral tarsal strip has been prepared.

Figure 22.35 This patient has both a socket contracture and a volume deficit. The inferior fornix has contracted leading to a lower eyelid cicatricial entropion. This patient would be best managed with the use of a dermis fat graft as well as a labial mucous membrane reconstruction of the inferior fornix.

difficult and is beyond the scope of this book. This usually requires serial expansion of the socket from a very early age with the use of acrylic conformers placed by an ocularist in clinic or in the operating room under general anesthesia or with the use of self-expanding conformers. Rarely a soft tissue expander has to be placed into the socket via a bicoronal flap approach and the socket and eyelids gradually expanded with the weekly injection of saline into the remote port of the soft tissue expander placed behind the ear. When the expander is removed, the socket is reconstructed with an autogenous dermis fat graft, which, in an infant, can gradually grow in size providing additional expansion of the socket

and eyelids in conjunction with conformers, which are changed regularly.

Acquired socket contracture may be classified as mild, moderate, or severe. If possible, it is important to attempt to remedy the underlying cause before proceeding with surgical reconstruction. There are many factors which may contribute to the development of socket contracture:

1. Burns —chemical, thermal, irradiation
2. Trauma
3. Chronic infections
4. Previous socket surgery, e.g., implant extrusion

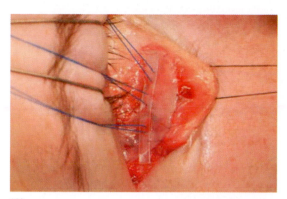

(A)

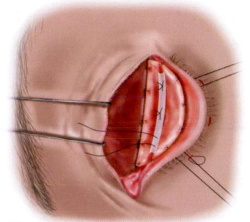

(B)

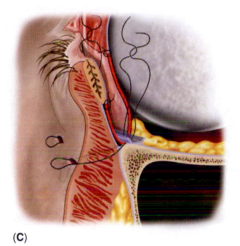

(C)

Figure 22.36 (A) The silicone retinal explant is placed and fornix deepening sutures are passed through the explant and the mucous membrane graft. (B) A drawing showing the placement of the explant and the sutures. (C) A drawing showing the placement of the sutures through the eyelid and the periosteum at the arcus marginalis.

5. Socket inflammation/infection
6. Poor maintenance of the ocular prosthesis
7. Cicatrizing conjunctival disease, e.g., pemphigoid

Mild Socket Contracture

A patient with a mild degree of socket contracture may have lagophthalmos with discomfort and socket discharge. The patient should be encouraged to lubricate the ocular prosthesis regularly. The ocular prosthesis should be polished every 6 months. Any associated papillary conjunctivitis should be treated with topical steroids. A mild degree of upper eyelid entropion can be managed with an anterior lamellar reposition procedure (chap. 4). A small linear conjunctival scar can be managed with a z-plasty or with a small labial mucous membrane graft.

Moderate Socket Contracture

More severe degrees of socket contracture require the use of mucous membrane grafts (Fig. 22.34). These are harvested from the lower lip and, if required, the upper lip. If there is insufficient mucous membrane available at these sites, buccal mucosa can be used taking care not to damage the parotid duct which opens just lateral to the second maxillary molar tooth.

If a contracted socket is also volume deficient, a dermis fat graft may be placed with the dermis left exposed. This gradually becomes epithelialized, thereby replacing both volume and conjunctival lining.

These patients will often have a cicatricial entropion, which may require additional eyelid surgery at the same time. If the tarsal plate in the upper eyelid has been markedly foreshortened, it may be necessary to place an auricular cartilage graft at the same time that mucous membrane grafts are placed (chap. 4). The upper eyelid retractors must be recessed. In some patients the anterior lamella of the upper eyelid will be chronically foreshortened and may require a skin graft or local skin-muscle transposition flap to lengthen it.

Fornix-deepening Sutures and Mucous Membrane Graft

The procedure is described for reconstruction of the inferior fornix. It can equally be applied to the superior fornix but great care must be taken not to damage the levator aponeurosis or the levator muscle centrally. It is usually combined with a lateral tarsal strip procedure.

The procedure is usually performed under general anesthesia although it can be performed under local anesthesia with intravenous sedation.

Surgical Procedure

1. A throat pack is placed and the anesthetist is asked to position the endotracheal tube to one corner of the mouth.
2. Three to five milliliters of 0.5% Bupivacaine with 1:200,000 units of adrenaline is injected subcutaneously into the lower eyelid and subconjunctivally into the inferior conjunctival fornix.
3. A 4/0 silk traction suture is inserted through the gray line of the lower eyelid and the eyelid is everted over a Desmarres retractor.
4. A horizontal incision is made through the conjunctiva along the whole length of the lower eyelid 3 to 4 mm below the inferior border of the tarsus with a no. 15 Bard Parker blade.
5. The margins of the conjunctiva are freed from the lid retractors, the orbital septum, and any associated scar tissue.

6. Next, a template is taken of the conjunctival defect using a piece of Steridrape and a sterile gentian violet marker pen.
7. Atraumatic bowel clamps are placed over a damp gauze swab over the lip margin and used to evert the lower lip.
8. The lower lip is dried with a swab.
9. The template is transferred to the lower lip mucosa avoiding the vermillion border, and outlined with gentian violet.
10. The lip is incised with a no. 15 blade and the graft is harvested free hand using blunt-tipped Westcott scissors. The scissors are gently opened and closed superficially underneath the lip mucosa keeping the tips clearly in view. This prevents inadvertent button-holing of the graft and prevents too deep a dissection, which can cause postoperative sensory loss.
11. The bowel clamps are removed and the graft donor site is treated with topical 1:1,000 adrenaline on a swab. Hemostasis is achieved with bipolar cautery. The lip mucosa does not require any sutures and is left to heal by secondary intention. If the buccal site is used instead of the lip this should be sutured with interrupted 6/0 Vicryl sutures.
12. The graft is shaped and any submucosal tissue carefully removed with Westcott scissors. The graft is then sutured into place with interrupted 7/0 Vicryl sutures.
13. A silicone explant (e.g., a 240 retinal explant) is shaped and two to three 4/0 nylon fornix-deepening sutures are passed (Fig. 22.36). The needle is carefully passed through the silicone explant, through the center of the graft, through the full thickness of the eyelid catching the periosteum of the inferior orbital margin, exiting through a stab incision in the cheek just below the lower eyelid. The needle is then

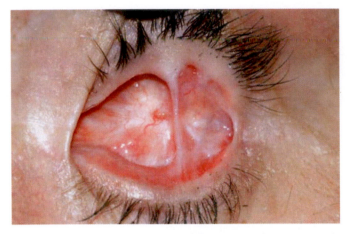

Figure 22.37 Severe socket contracture following a previous caustic soda injury. The patient has a poor prognosis for the achievement of a satisfactory result from the use of mucous membrane grafts.

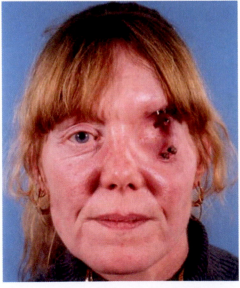

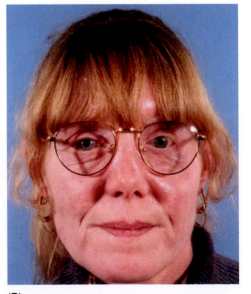

(A)   (B)

Figure 22.38 (**A**) A patient who had severe socket contracture following subtotal exenteration and placement of osseo-integrated implants. (**B**) The patient wearing her orbital prosthesis.

returned via the stab incision, again taking a bite of the periosteum, through the eyelid, through the mucosal graft and the explant, and tied (Fig. 22.36).

14. A sterile surgical conformer is placed. It is essential that the conformer selected is of the correct size and shape.
15. Topical antibiotic ointment is applied to the socket.
16. A compressive dressing is applied for 5 days.

Postoperative Management

The fornix-deepening sutures should not be removed for at least 8 weeks. Topical antibiotic drops are used for 8 weeks. The conformer must be left in place. The ocular prosthesis is fitted once the sutures and silicone explant have been removed. The patient is instructed to take a soft diet for 2 weeks and to avoid any hot drinks. An antiseptic mouthwash is prescribed and should be used three times a day for 5 days postoperatively.

Severe Socket Contracture

The patient should be carefully counseled about the surgical difficulties posed by severe socket contracture, particularly following previous trauma involving an alkali (Fig. 22.37). It may not be possible to achieve a result, which will be satisfactory to the patient, with the use of mucosal grafts. The admixture of skin and mucous membrane grafts in a socket should be avoided. This combination leads to a foul-smelling chronic discharge. It is possible to remove all residual mucosa and to line the socket with skin grafts instead but the aesthetic results achieved are rarely very good.

Alternative options should be considered taking into account the patient's age, general health, occupation, social interests, motivation, and the procedure costs. It may be more appropriate to consider the option of performing a conservative subtotal exenteration with the use of an orbital prosthesis. The patient may also be a suitable candidate for osseo-integrated orbital implants, which may yield a far superior cosmetic result (Fig. 22.38), but at far greater financial cost and inconvenience to the patient.

FURTHER READING

1. Ataullah S, Whitehouse RW, Stelmach M, Shah S, Leatherbarrow B. Missed orbital wall blow-out fracture as a cause of post-enucleation socket syndrome. Eye 1999; 13(Pt 4): 541–4.
2. Beaver HA, Patrinely JR, Holds JB, Soper MP. Periocular autografts in socket reconstruction. Ophthalmology 1996; 103(9): 1498–502.
3. Hintschich C, Zonneveld F, Baldeschi L, Bunce C, Koornneef L. Bony orbital development after early enucleation in humans. Br J Ophthalmol 2001; 85(2): 205–8.
4. Mazzoli RA, Raymond WR, Ainbinder DJ, Hansen EA. Use of self-expanding, hydrophilic osmotic expanders (hydrogel) in the reconstruction of congenital clinical anophthalmos. Cur Op Ophthalmol 2004; 15: 426–31.
5. Nerad JA, Carter KD, Alford MA. Disorders of the orbit: anophthalmic socket. In: Rapid Diagnosis in Ophthalmology-Oculoplastic & Reconstructive Surgery., Philadelphia, PA: Mosby Elsevier, 2008: 260–7.
6. Nerad JA, Carter KD, LaVelle WE, Fyler A, Branemark PI. The osseointegration technique for the rehabilitation of the exenterated orbit. Arch Ophthalmol 1991; 109: 1032.
7. Quaranta-Leoni FM. Treatment of the anophthalmic socket. Cur Opin Ophthalmol 2008; 19: 422–7.
8. Ragge NK, Subak-Sharpe ID, Collin JRO. A practical guide to the management of anophthalmia and microphthalmia. Eye 2007; 21: 1290–300.
9. Smit TJ, Koornneef L, Zonneveld FW, Groet E, Otto AJ. Computed tomography in the assessment of the post enucleation socket syndrome. Ophthalmology 1990; 97(10): 1347–51.
10. Tanenbaum M. Enucleation, evisceration and exenteration. In: Yanoff M, Duker J, eds., Ophthalmology. London: Mosby, 2004: 752–60.
11. Wobig JL, Dailey RA. Enucleation and exenteration. In: Wobig JL, Dailey RA, eds. Oculofacial Plastic Surgery: Face, Lacrimal System and Orbit. New York, NY: Thieme, 2004: 255–66.

23 Orbital exenteration

INTRODUCTION

Orbital exenteration is a surgical procedure that involves the removal of all the soft tissue contents of the orbit. An exenteration is classified as:

- Total
- Subtotal
- Extended

In a total exenteration all of the soft tissues of the orbit and periocular adnexa are removed. In a subtotal exenteration the eyelid skin is preserved. An extended exenteration involves resection of adjacent structures, e.g., the paranasal sinuses for the management of a sino-orbital malignant tumor. The extent of the surgical resection is dictated by the extent of the disease process.

This mutilating procedure is used for the management of a number of benign as well as malignant conditions which are not amenable to other treatment modalities.

Malignant Disorders

1. Malignant eyelid tumors with orbital involvement, e.g., basal cell or squamous cell carcinoma
2. Malignant eyelid tumors beyond simple surgical excision, e.g., sebaceous carcinoma with extensive conjunctival involvement
3. Malignant conjunctival lesions, e.g., extensive conjunctival melanoma
4. Orbital invasion by malignant paranasal sinus tumors
5. Primary malignant orbital tumors, e.g., lacrimal gland carcinomas

Non-malignant Disorders

1. Benign orbital tumors, e.g., aggressive orbital meningioma
2. Life-threatening infection, e.g., sino-orbital mucormycosis
3. Severe nonspecific orbital inflammatory disease with intractable pain and blindness
4. Severe orbital deformity, e.g., neurofibromatosis (Fig. 23.1)
5. End-stage socket contracture

Patients who are to undergo an orbital exenteration for malignant disease should be managed by a multidisciplinary team, which may include:

1. Orbital surgeon
2. Ear, nose, and throat (ENT) surgeon
3. Plastic surgeon
4. Neurosurgeon
5. Radiologist
6. Radiotherapist
7. Oncologist
8. Anesthetist
9. Mohs micrographic surgeon
10. Pathologist
11. Ocularist
12. Psychologist
13. Oculoplastic nurse practitioner

PREOPERATIVE EVALUATION

The preoperative evaluation comprises:

- A review of paraffin fixed histological sections
- A thorough ophthalmic examination of both eyes
- A general physical examination of the patient
- A review of radiological imaging

Mohs' micrographic surgery may be warranted to gain clearance of the skin margins in basal cell carcinomas (BCCs) and squamous cell carcinomas (SCCs).

As the operation may be associated with significant blood loss, typed and cross-matched blood should be made available. The patient should have a full blood count, platelet count, and coagulation profile performed preoperatively. All antiplatelet agents should be discontinued 2 weeks prior to surgery. The assistance of a hematologist should be sought for the management of any patient who takes anticoagulants.

PREOPERATIVE PATIENT PREPARATION

Most orbital exenterations are performed as elective procedures. The patient should receive appropriate counseling by senior, experienced members of the oculoplastic team about the diagnosis, prognosis, nature of the surgery, its goals, risks, and potential complications. The patient should be warned about inevitable and permanent anesthesia of the forehead, temple, and lateral canthus postoperatively. The options for surgical reconstruction of the exenterated socket should be discussed and determined according to the patient's wishes as well as the patient's age and general health. In determining the method of orbital reconstruction in the case of patients with a malignancy, the likelihood of recurrent disease must be taken into consideration.

The patient must be carefully prepared for the ensuing cosmetic deformity. Photographs of other patients who have undergone a similar exenteration may be helpful to use along with samples of typical orbital prostheses or methods of cosmetic camouflage.

The oculoplastic nurse practitioner should be on hand to explain his/her role in postoperative wound care and in coordinating aftercare in the community following discharge from hospital.

The pathologist should be consulted well in advance preoperatively and the possible need for frozen-section control of the resection margins discussed and organized.

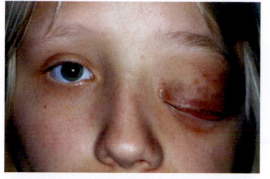

(A)

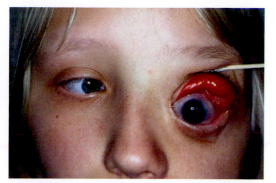

(B)

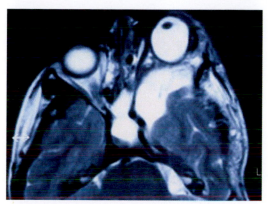

(C)

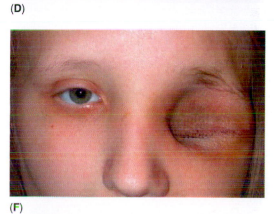

(D)

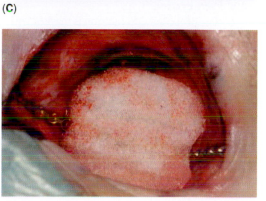

(E)

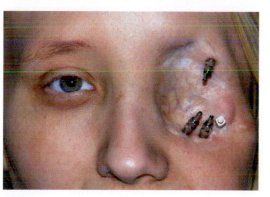

(F)

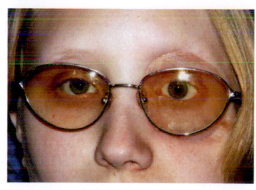

(G)

(H)

Figure 23.1 (**A**) A young female patient with Type 1 neurofibromatosis, a complete ptosis and orbital dystopia. She had a pulsatile proptosis. (**B**) The same patient demonstrating buphthalmos, proptosis, hypoglobus, and a grossly distorted upper eyelid from a plexiform neurofibroma. (**C**) An MRI scan confirmed an absence of the sphenoid wing with a large meningoencephalocoele extending into the orbit. (**D**) A channelled Medpor implant was shaped to act as an obturator in the exenterated orbit. (**E**) The patient underwent a sub-total orbital exenteration. The meningoencephalocoele was gently reposited into the cranial cavity and the channelled Medpor implant was fixated to the medial and lateral orbital margins with titanium screws. (**F**) The stretched skin of the eyelids was closed directly. The patient is shown 1 week postoperatively. (**G**) The patient underwent a first-stage osseointegration procedure 6 months postoperatively and the second stage after a further 6 months. She is seen here with guide pins and impression copings in position ready for the impression stage of her orbital prosthesis to commence. (**H**) The patient is seen wearing her orbital prosthesis.

ANESTHESIA

General anesthesia is preferable for this procedure although local anesthesia with intravenous sedation can be used for the patient who is medically unfit. For local anesthesia, 5 ml of 0.5% Bupivacaine with 1:200,000 units of adrenaline are given with Hyalase (hyaluronidase) as a retrobulbar injection. In addition, a further 10 to 12 ml of 0.5% Bupivacaine with 1:200,000 units of adrenaline are given as a series of subcutaneous injections around the orbital margin and as specific nerve blocks around the supratrochlear, supraorbital, infratrochlear, anterior ethmoidal, infraorbital, zygomatico-facial, and zygomatico-temporal nerves (Fig. 23.2). If the patient is under general anesthesia 10 to 12 ml of 0.5% Bupivacaine with 1:200,000 units of adrenaline are given with Haylase as a series of subcutaneous injections around the orbital margin and the same retrobulbar injection is given to try to block the oculocardiac reflex.

The anesthetist should be warned that the dissection of the socket can provoke the oculocardiac reflex, inducing a severe bradycardia and occasionally asystole. The anesthetist may wish to use glycopyrrolate or atropine prior to the dissection.

APPLIED SURGICAL ANATOMY

The surgeon must have a thorough knowledge of orbital anatomy in order to facilitate an expeditious exenteration that avoids excessive hemorrhage and other potentially serious complications. In particular, the surgeon should be aware of the following:

1. The anatomical position of all the major orbital blood vessels (Figs. 23.3 and 23.4).
2. The points of increased periosteal attachment within the orbit.
3. The potential weak areas in the bony orbital walls, e.g., the orbital roof in the elderly (Fig. 23.5).
4. The position of the superior and inferior orbital fissures.

For more detail chapter 2 "Applied Anatomy" should be reviewed.

EXENTERATION
Surgical Technique

The patient's computed tomography (CT) and/or magnetic resonance imaging (MRI) scans should be placed on the viewing screen in the operating room to be referred to if necessary during the course of the surgery.

> **KEY POINT**
>
> The surgeon must identify the correct side to be exenterated prior to the induction of general anesthesia. The surgeon must mark the correct side and be personally responsible for the prepping and draping of the patient. The surgeon must also ensure that the fellow eye is instilled with Lacrilube ointment and is taped closed and fully protected from inadvertent injury during the course of the surgery.

Total Exenteration

1. The proposed skin incision is marked with gentian violet around the orbital margin. The eyebrow is normally preserved unless involved in the malignant tumor.
2. The eyelids are sutured together with two 2/0 silk sutures and the sutures held with an artery clip.
3. Next, the skin and superficial subcutaneous tissues are incised with a Colorado needle.
4. The skin edges are firmly retracted and the dissection is carried down to the periosteum of the orbital rim using the Colorado needle. Careful attention is paid to hemostasis with additional use of bipolar cautery.
5. The periosteum at the orbital margin is then incised with the Colorado needle.
6. The periosteum is elevated from the margins of the orbit and into the orbit with a Freer periosteal elevator.
7. Jaffe retractors are placed around the orbit to retract the soft tissues (Fig. 23.6).
8. The periosteum is elevated from the orbital walls, beginning superotemporally. Care is taken to keep the periosteum intact to avoid a prolapse of orbital fat.
9. The Freer elevator should be used with great care along the orbital roof as dehiscences in the bone are frequent in the elderly. *This dissection must not be performed blind as this risks damage to the dura mater with a subsequent cerebrospinal fluid (CSF) leak. It is important to avoid the use of monopolar cautery along the orbital roof as this also risks causing a CSF leak in the presence of any bony defects.*
10. The dissection is continued inferotemporally.
11. The lateral canthal tendon is incised with the Colorado needle.

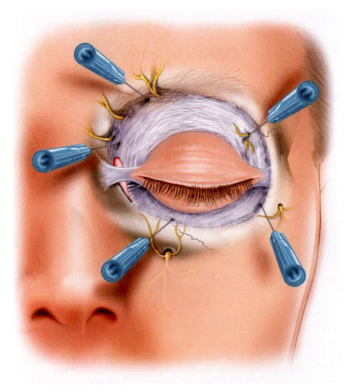

Figure 23.2 The series of regional blocks used to anesthetize an orbit prior to undertaking an orbital exenteration under local anesthesia.

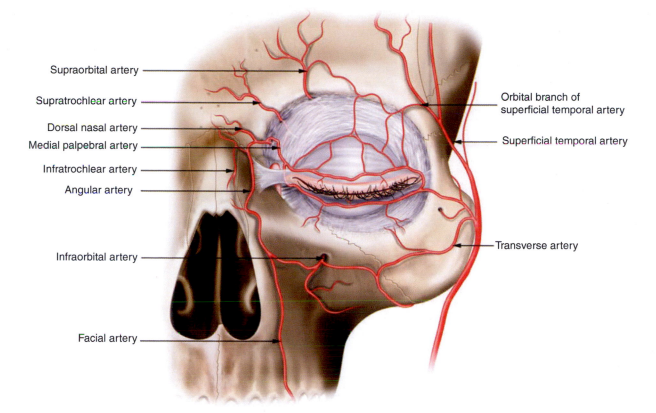

Supraorbital artery

Supratrochlear artery

Dorsal nasal artery

Medial palpebral artery

Infratrochlear artery

Angular artery

Infraorbital artery

Facial artery

Orbital branch of superficial temporal artery

Superficial temporal artery

Transverse artery

Figure 23.3 A coronal view of the vascular anatomy of the eyelids and periorbital region.

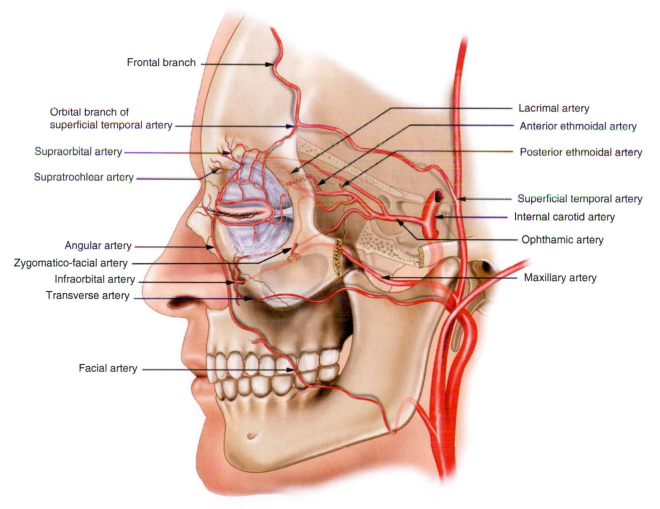

Frontal branch

Orbital branch of superficial temporal artery

Supraorbital artery

Supratrochlear artery

Angular artery

Zygomatico-facial artery

Infraorbital artery

Transverse artery

Facial artery

Lacrimal artery

Anterior ethmoidal artery

Posterior ethmoidal artery

Superficial temporal artery

Internal carotid artery

Ophthamic artery

Maxillary artery

Figure 23.4 A sagittal view of the vascular anatomy of the eyelids and periorbital region.

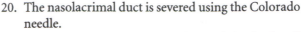

12. The zygomatico-temporal and zygomatico-facial vessels are cauterized as they are encountered using bipolar cautery. Any bleeding from the bone is managed with bone wax.

13. The dissection is then continued across the floor of the orbit. A constant vessel is encountered approximately 8 mm posterior to the inferior orbital margin. This is cauterized.

14. Great care is taken to avoid inadvertent injury to the infraorbital neurovascular bundle. The infraorbital nerve may lie exposed along the floor of the orbit.

15. The Colorado needle is used to dissect tissue across the anterior portion of the inferior orbital fissure.

16. The dissection then continues from the superolateral orbit to the superomedial orbit. The supraorbital and supratrochlear vessels are cauterized using bipolar cautery and transected.

17. As the dissection approaches the medial canthus, the angular vessels are cauterized using bipolar cautery.

18. The anterior limb of the medial canthal tendon is incised with the Colorado needle and reflected off the underlying bone with a Freer periosteal elevator.

19. The lacrimal sac is rotated posteriorly and laterally and the posterior limb of the medial canthal tendon is incised with the sharp end of the Freer periosteal elevator.

20. The nasolacrimal duct is severed using the Colorado needle.

21. The periorbita is raised from the medial orbital wall with the Freer elevator taking great care not to fracture the lamina papyracea.

22. The anterior and posterior ethmoidal vessels are identified as they pass through the periosteum to their respective foramina and are cauterized.

23. Superomedially, the trochlea is elevated along with the periosteum.

24. Once the dissection has approached the apex of the orbit, the periosteum is incised with the Colorado needle medially and laterally.

25. Two large curved artery clips are applied across the apical orbital tissues, one medially and one laterally.

26. Curved enucleation scissors are used to excise the tissues anterior to the clips while pulling anteriorly on the traction sutures. Alternatively, a snare may be used (Fig. 23.7).

27. The extent of the exenteration performed is dictated by the clinical requirements. The exenteration can be modified to a less extensive procedure or to a more radical resection that involves the removal of orbital walls and paranasal sinuses.

28. Bipolar cautery is applied to the stump of tissue at the orbital apex (Fig. 23.8B).

29. Bone wax may be required for any bleeding vessels that perforate the orbital walls.

30. Gelfoam soaked with thrombin is applied to the socket and swabs moistened with 1:1,000 adrenaline are placed over this. Pressure is applied for 5 min. In cases where there is excessive bleeding, Floseal®, a very effective hemostatic sealant, may be applied to the apex of the orbit. (Its use must, however, be avoided in patients who have a known allergy to materials of bovine origin.)

31. In cases where the indication for exenteration is a malignancy, the socket is carefully inspected for any residual tumor tissue. The adequacy of resection may be judged with the aid of frozen-section control. The resection of additional orbital apical tissue may be required.

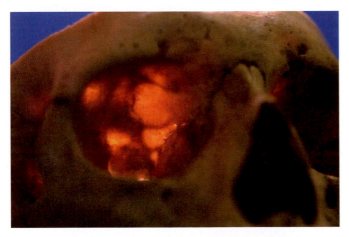

Figure 23.5 Transillumination of a skull demonstrating how thin the roof of the orbit (floor of the anterior cranial fossa) can be in some patients.

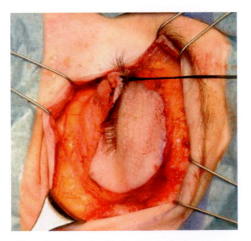

Figure 23.6 A total orbital exenteration in progress.

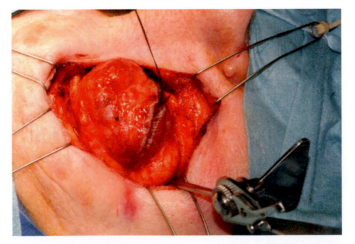

Figure 23.7 A snare is being used to complete an orbital exenteration (in this case a subtotal exenteration).

32. The stump of the nasolacrimal duct is over sewn with interrupted 5/0 Vicryl sutures if possible. Alternatively, the stump is thoroughly cauterized.

33. If the socket is to be left to heal by secondary intention or if a split-thickness skin graft is used (see below), antibiotic ointment is instilled and either an Aquacel® dressing (ConvaTec Ltd), or an Allevyn Cavity® dressing (Smith and Nephew), is placed into the socket and an occlusive secondary dressing comprising sterile eye pads and Opsite Flexifix® (Smith & Nephew) is applied along with a pressure bandage.

KEY POINT

The subperiosteal dissection along the orbital roof must not be performed blind as this risks damage to the dura mater with a subsequent cerebrospinal fluid (CSF) leak. It is important to avoid the use of monopolar cautery along the orbital roof as this also risks causing a CSF leak in the presence of any bony defects.

Postoperative Care

Many of the wound dressing products that are commercially available are manufactured for use in other types of wounds, and in practice very few are suitable for use in exenterated sockets. Dressings used in cavity wounds such as Aquacel® and Allevyn Cavity® need to be held in place by a secondary dressing, and Opsite Flexifix® is suitable for this purpose.

Aquacel® is a soft, sterile, hydrophilic non-woven ribbon dressing composed entirely of hydrocolloid fibers (sodium carboxymethylcellulose). The characteristics of the fibers are such that they absorb when they come into contact with liquid, and the absorbed fluid is retained within the structure of the fibers, even under compression. The dressing is applied dry, and as it absorbs exudate it is rapidly converted from a dry dressing to a soft coherent gel. It maintains a moist environment for optimal wound healing, aids autolytic debridement, and is easily removed with little or no damage to newly formed tissue. Aquacel® is therefore excellent for exuding wounds. It can be left in the wound for up to 7 days but it is better to remove this 3 to 4 days postoperatively as it can become over saturated and transform into a gel-like material which can be more difficult to remove. The dressing is also available impregnated with silver (Aquacel Ag®) which has anti-bacterial properties for use in the infected socket.

Allevyn Cavity® is a non-adhesive hydrocellular cavity dressing. It is 5 cm in diameter and is a biconvex hydrophilic polyurethane foam dressing, which is covered in a non-adhesive polymeric wrapping. Its flexible structure allows it to be manipulated easily into the socket cavity and it is able to absorb a moderate amount of exudate. It conforms very well to the shape of the socket and can bolster split-thickness skin grafts and retained skin from skin-sparing exenteration lids against the walls of the orbit (Fig. 23.9). This product is particularly recommended for use in the initial healing phase (the first 2 to 3 weeks) of post-operative exenteration wounds.

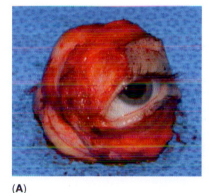

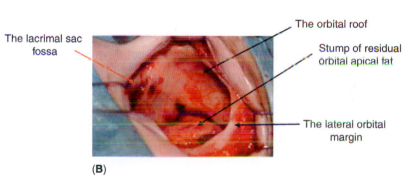

The lacrimal sac fossa

The orbital roof

Stump of residual orbital apical fat

The lateral orbital margin

(A) (B)

Figure 23.8 (**A**) An exenteration specimen. (**B**) The exenterated orbit at the completion of surgery.

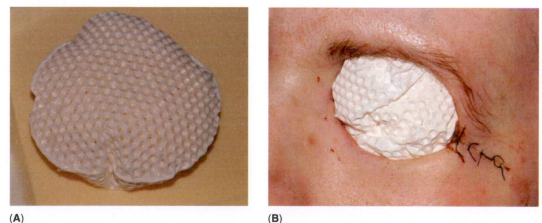

(A) (B)

Figure 23.9 (**A**) An Allevyn Cavity® cavity dressing. (**B**) The dressing in place in an exenterated socket.

The dressing is removed 5 to 6 days postoperatively (Fig. 23.10). The socket is cleaned daily for 2 weeks and an Allevyn Cavity® dressing gently reapplied. The frequency of the wound care is gradually reduced over the course of the next month. The wound can be left exposed and camouflaged with a Cartella shield once the discharge has ceased. The patient and the carers are encouraged to become actively involved in the care of the socket with the help and guidance of a specialist oculoplastic/wound care nurse wherever possible. Complete healing of the socket may take some months. An orbital prosthesis should not be fitted until the socket has completely healed.

Medihoney® (Comvita UK Ltd) is an antibacterial wound gel that contains 80% antibacterial honey (800 mg/g). It consists of honey derived from the group of plants Leptospernum (and several other plant species), and has been found to have a powerful antibacterial action. In addition, Medihoney has a high osmotic potential to clean wounds, deodorise malodorous wounds, promote autolytic debridement, and provides a protective layer, which allows for easy dressing removal. It can be used to aid the healing of difficult sockets.

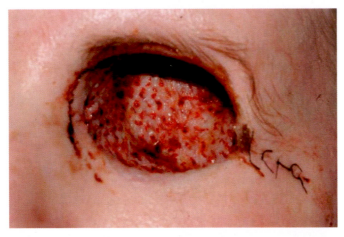

Figure 23.10 The appearance of the grafted socket using a meshed split-thickness skin graft 5 days postoperatively.

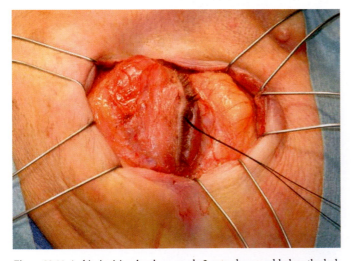

Figure 23.11 A skin incision has been made 2 mm above and below the lash line. The skin and orbicularis muscle have been dissected from the underlying orbital septum. Multiple Jaffe eyelid retractors have been placed to aid exposure of the orbital margins.

Subtotal Exenteration

In a subtotal exenteration the eyelid skin is preserved. The skin incision is placed 2 mm behind the lash line and a skin-orbicularis flap is undermined to the arcus marginalis of the orbit (Fig. 23.11). The exenteration is completed as for a total exenteration and the skin is then draped into the exenterated socket. If there is sufficient skin available, the edges are simply reapproximated with interrupted 7/0 Vicryl sutures. Antibiotic ointment is instilled. An Allevyn Cavity® dressing is placed into the socket and Opsite Flexifix® is applied along with a pressure bandage.

Postoperative Care

The dressing is removed after 5 to 7 days. The socket is then kept clean with sterile gauze swabs and sterile saline. The socket usually heals quickly over the course of 3 to 6 weeks (Fig. 23.12).

Extended Exenteration

In an extended exenteration, adjacent structures, such as paranasal sinuses, orbital bones, and intracranial structures, may be resected, depending on the extent of the patient's disease process. Such a procedure is performed by a multidisciplinary team and is beyond the scope of this text.

Orbital Reconstruction

There are a number of reconstructive options for the management of the exenterated socket. The suitability of these options must be determined for each individual patient.

Laissez Faire

Healing by secondary intention can yield good results, particularly in the case of elderly patients for whom more lengthy operative procedures are unsuitable (Figs. 23.13 and 23.14).

Advantages

This approach is simple and facilitates easy examination of the socket where the possibility of tumor recurrence exists. It reduces the operating time. It avoids potential morbidity at the site of flaps or skin grafts. Once completely healed, the socket does not tend to exhibit problems with skin desquamation in contrast to a skin-grafted socket. The socket cavity can then be

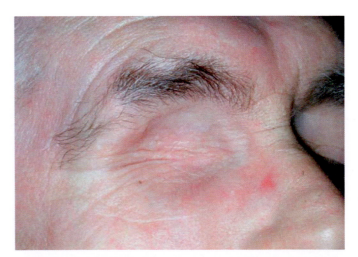

Figure 23.12 A patient who has undergone a subtotal exenteration with a completely skin lined socket and no fistulae.

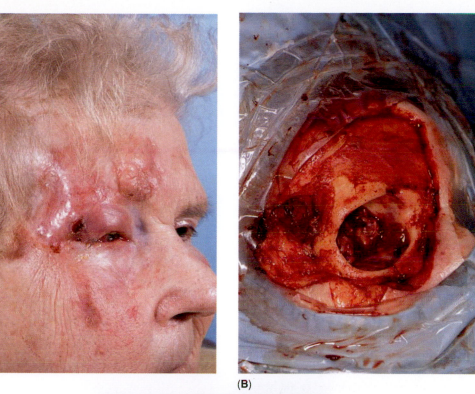

(A)   (B)

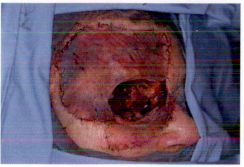

(C)

Figure 23.13 (**A**) An elderly female patient with a neglected squamous cell carcinoma of the periorbital region with orbital invasion. (**B**) An extensive resection of the tumor and a total exenteration. (**C**) A split-thickness skin graft has been placed over the forehead, temple and cheek wounds. The socket has been left to granulate.

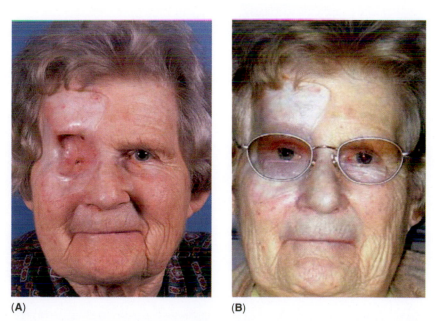

(A)   (B)

Figure 23.14 (**A**) The appearance of the socket 2 months postoperatively. (**B**) The appearance of the patient fitted with an orbital prosthesis.

covered with a patch or fitted with a silicone prosthesis, which is held in position either by a spectacle mount or by a tissue adhesive (Fig. 23.14).

Disadvantages
The healing period can be very prolonged and requires frequent dressing changes. Spontaneous fistulae communicating with the ethmoid sinus can occur. The eyebrow can be drawn inferiorly by wound contracture.

SPLIT-THICKNESS SKIN GRAFT
A split-thickness skin graft will take well on exposed and healthy orbital bone. The graft is harvested from the thigh with a dermatome set to 1/16 inch. The width of the required graft is determined and the appropriate blade chosen for the dermatome. The thigh is prepped and draped. Glycerine is used to lubricate the skin. The skin is then flattened with the edge of a small skin graft board in front of the dermatome (Fig. 23.15). The skin graft is then harvested. The thigh wound is covered with an Allevyn Non-Adhesive® (Smith and Nephew) foam dressing and attached using adhesive Opsite Flexifix® (Smith and Nephew) transparent film covering. A piece of Gamgee® (3M), a highly absorbent cotton roll padding with a non-woven cover, and a bandage is also applied to aid hemostasis and to reduce the amount of exudate. This dressing

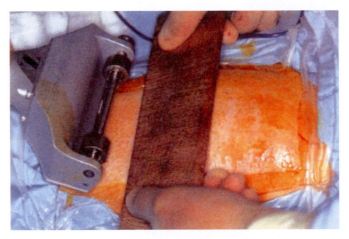

Figure 23.15 An assistant is flattening the skin of the thigh ahead of the dermatome.

should be changed if any exudate leaks from it. As the wound continues to heal a less absorbent dressing may be considered and an Allevyn Thin® or Compression® (Smith and Nephew) dressing can be used to protect the area from clothing and allow the wound to completely heal. Once healed the area should be then be massaged with Vaseline.

The skin graft is passed through a meshing device, which expands the graft and assists the egress of serosanguinous fluid (see chap. 13). The graft is inserted into the socket and the edges of the graft are sutured to the skin edges around the socket (Fig. 23.16A). Any excess is trimmed away and any remaining skin graft can be returned to the donor site to aid the speed of recovery. The socket cavity is packed with an Allevyn Cavity® dressing.

This is as described above. Any adherent debris can be removed with hydrogen peroxide.

Advantages
The use of a skin graft shortens the healing period. It prevents undue wound contracture and helps to maintain the depth of the socket, enabling suitable fitting of an orbital prosthesis. It also facilitates easy examination of the socket where the possibility of tumor recurrence exists.

Disadvantages
This approach requires a separate donor site and is associated with pain and potential morbidity (Fig. 23.17).

The skin graft may fail in patients who are at risk of poor healing, e.g., diabetic patients, following previous radiotherapy.

Local Flaps
A local flap, e.g., a temporalis muscle transposition flap, may be used in patients who do not pose a risk of tumor recurrence. This is covered with a split-thickness skin graft.

Advantages
The flap can be used to make the socket deformity shallower in a patient who does not want to wear a prosthesis. It can be combined with a split-thickness skin graft.

Disadvantages
The procedure leaves a secondary depression in the temple. The temporal branch of the facial nerve may be damaged, resulting in a brow ptosis.

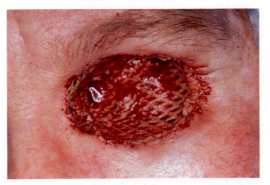

(A)

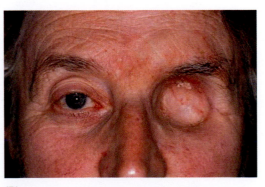

(B)

Figure 23.16 (**A**) A meshed split-thickness skin graft placed into the socket and sutured to the skin at the orbital margin. (**B**) The appearance of the healed socket 1 month postoperatively.

Other local flaps, e.g., a pericranial flap and a full-thickness skin graft may be used to cover a sino-orbital fistula.

Free Flaps

A free flap, e.g., a radial forearm free flap, is particularly useful for the reconstruction of the defects from an extended exenteration.

Advantages

The free flap can prevent the severe cosmetic disfigurement of an extended exenteration with exposed sinus cavities.

Disadvantages

These procedures are difficult to perform and extremely time-consuming. There is a risk of flap failure and donor site morbidity. If the flap is too bulky, it may prevent the successful wearing of an orbital prosthesis (Fig. 23.18).

Osseointegration Technique

Osseointegrated titanium implants permit direct coupling of an orbitofacial prosthesis to the bony orbital margins. This is a two-stage procedure. In the first stage titanium screws are implanted into the superior, lateral, and inferior orbital bony

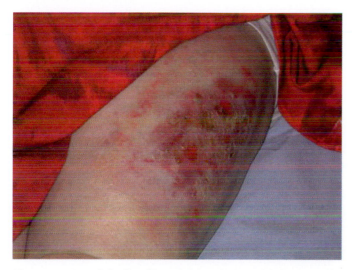

Figure 23.17 A poorly healing skin graft donor site in an elderly patient. The wound took 3 months to heal.

margins. These are covered by soft tissue and left to integrate with the bone. At the second stage, performed approximately 6 months later, the implants are exposed and titanium cylinders (abutments) are attached to the implants. A series of bars or magnetic devices are attached to the abutments. These allow firm fixation of the prosthesis (Fig. 23.1). Spectacles offer additional camouflage and protection to the remaining eye.

Advantages

This technique allows reliable alignment of the prosthesis and good retention. Removal and reattachment of the prosthesis by the patient are relatively easy. The prosthesis can be made lighter in weight. The edge of the prosthesis can also be made to blend with the surrounding skin more easily. The cosmetic results can be excellent for the carefully selected patient. The ideal patient is relatively young and highly motivated, with good hygiene, and will comply with long-term aftercare of the implants and will attend long-term follow-up appointments. The patient will usually require the additional use of tinted spectacles as additional camouflage.

Disadvantages

The technique is time-consuming and expensive. The implants must be kept meticulously clean to avoid inflammation or infection and ultimately loss of the implants. Extra implants may be placed as "sleepers" and used if implants are lost.

PROSTHETIC OPTIONS

Many patients abandon orbital and orbitofacial prostheses for a number of reasons.

- An unnatural appearance with an absence of blinking and ocular movements.
- Intolerance to local tissue adhesives.
- Difficulty camouflaging the edges of the prosthesis.
- Rapid degradation of the prosthesis.
- Expense.

A simple alternative is the use of a standard black patch. For female patients individual customized patches can be obtained (Fig. 23.18B). Spectacles with an opaque lens and a side shield may also be preferred by some patients.

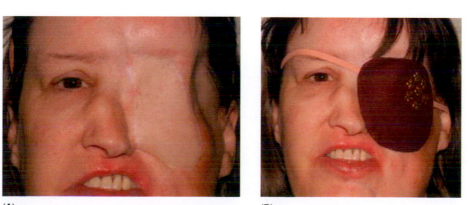

(A)						(B)

Figure 23.18 (**A**) A patient showing a free-flap reconstruction of an extended orbital exenteration. The patient had no room for an orbital prosthesis. (**B**) The patient instead resorted to the use of a customized occlusive patch.

FURTHER READING

1. Cooper J. Wound management following orbital exenteration surgery. [Review] [16 refs] Bri J Nurs 2009; 18(6): S4, S6, S8, passim.

2. Dutton JJ. Atlas of clinical and surgical orbital anatomy. Philadelphia, PA: W.B. Saunders, 1994.

3. Nerad JA. Techniques in Opthalmic Plastic Surgery – A Personal Tutorial. Saunders Elsevier Inc., 2010: 479–84. (ISBN: 978-1-4377-0008-4).

4. Melicher Larson JS, Nerad JA. The use of osseointegration and rare earth magnetic coupling for oculofacial prosthesis retention in the exenterated orbit. [Review] [18 refs] Curr Opin Ophthalmol 2009; 20(5): 412–16.

5. Nerad JA, Carter KD, LaVelle WE, Fyler A, Branemark PI. The osseointegration technique for the rehabilitation of the exenterated orbit. Arch Ophthalmol 1991; 109: 1032–8.

6. Nerad JA. Osseointegration for the exenterated orbit. In: Bosniak S, ed., Principles and Practice of Ophthalmic Plastic and Reconstructive Surgery. Philadelphia, PA: WB Saunders, 1996: 1150–60.

8. Rahman I, Maino A, Cook AE, Leatherbarrow B. Mortality following exenteration for malignant tumours of the orbit. Br J Ophthalmol 2005; 89: 1445–8.

9. Tanenbaum M. Enucleation, evisceration and exenteration. In: Yanoff M, Duker J, eds., Ophthalmology. Philadelphia, PA: Mosby, 2004: 752–60.

10. Wobig JL, Dailey RA. Enucleation and exenteration. In: Wobig JL, Dailey RA, eds., Oculofacial Plastic Surgery: Face, Lacrimal System and Orbit. New York: Thieme, 2004: 255–66.

24 The management of eyelid and lacrimal trauma

INTRODUCTION

Many ophthalmologists, regardless of the type of practice they have, may be called upon to assist in the management of patients who have sustained acute eyelid, lacrimal, or orbital trauma. A systematic approach to the evaluation and management of such patients by the ophthalmologist is essential and will:

- Maximize the results of primary treatment
- Minimize the need for secondary reconstruction
- Lessen the exposure of the ophthalmologist to medicolegal risks

When called upon to manage a patient who has sustained acute eyelid, lacrimal, or orbital trauma, it is useful to apply a set of cardinal principles (Table 24.1).

Most patients who suffer acute eyelid, lacrimal, or orbital trauma present to a general Accident and Emergency (A&E) department. There, initial triage and stabilization begin. Although the diagnosis of associated injuries is usually made independently of the ophthalmologist's examination, a certain redundancy in evaluation is necessary for trauma to be treated appropriately and expeditiously.

> **KEY POINT**
>
> It is imperative that the patient is examined thoroughly so that additional injuries are not overlooked.

The ophthalmologist should assist other specialists in determining the priority for repair of the patient's injuries.

- Examine and treat the patient for *all* injuries

HISTORY

Mechanism of Injury

Even before seeing the patient, the ophthalmologist can anticipate the types of injuries that are most likely to be encountered from a knowledge of the mechanism of injury. An accurate history is essential, but in many instances, the history may be inaccurate, e.g., self-inflicted trauma, a child whose injury was not witnessed.

> **KEY POINT**
>
> Apparently trivial eyelid trauma may be associated with serious sight-threatening or even life-threatening injury which will go undetected unless a high index of suspicion is maintained during the patient's evaluation.

The examination of patients who have sustained eyelid and/or orbital trauma should be performed very delicately and meticulously to exclude associated trauma to the globe (Fig. 24.1).

> **KEY POINT**
>
> Lacerations of the eyelid have an underlying perforating injury of the globe, or even a penetrating injury of the brain, until proven otherwise (Fig. 24.2).

> **KEY POINT**
>
> Lacerations of the medial canthal area involve the lacrimal drainage apparatus until proven otherwise (Fig. 24.3).

- Maintain a high index of suspicion for undetected injury

Eyelid and orbital injuries occur after contact with sharp or blunt objects, toxic substances, or sources of thermal or electromagnetic energy. Combination injuries may be present, such as those seen in road traffic accidents.

Sharp Trauma

Sharp trauma tends to produce a clean wound to the eyelids without actual tissue loss. Sharp trauma can be associated with ocular injury, injury to extraocular muscles or other orbital structures, or through penetration of the orbital walls, craniocerebral or upper respiratory tract injuries.

> **KEY POINT**
>
> The ophthalmologist must maintain a high index of suspicion for undetected injury and for retained foreign bodies, e.g., in young children whose injury has not been witnessed (Fig. 24.4).

Blunt Trauma

Abrasions, irregular lacerations and partial avulsions are more common with blunt trauma than with sharp trauma. Associated neurological injury (intracranial or cervical), facial fractures, orbital wall blowout fractures, concussive ocular injury, or globe rupture must be ruled out.

> **KEY POINT**
>
> A computed tomography (CT) scan examination should be performed whenever there is clinical evidence of orbital trauma or the suspicion of an intraorbital foreign body.

Bites

Eyelid injuries caused by bites pose unique problems. The injuries themselves can be a combination of sharp and blunt trauma, causing lacerations and tearing-type injuries and, rarely, actual tissue loss. Most periorbital bites are caused by domestic dogs (Fig. 24.5). Facial and eyelid bites from other animals are extremely rare. Periorbital human bites are also rare but potentially serious.

> **KEY POINT**
>
> All bite wounds should be considered contaminated, and preventive measures must be taken against possible infection.

PATIENT EVALUATION

Eyelid trauma is highly visible and, in most cases, alarming in appearance to the patient. Anxiety about the possibility of loss of vision and disfigurement is high and must be managed tactfully. Patients who are under the influence of drugs or alcohol are often particularly difficult to evaluate satisfactorily. Steps should be taken to prevent further inadvertent injury.

> **KEY POINT**
>
> It should be borne in mind that legal actions often result from the injury, and possibly from the treatment, if the results are unsatisfactory.

Systemic Considerations

The ophthalmologist may be working alone in the case of a patient who has sustained an eyelid laceration and a penetrating eye injury, or he/she may be part of a multidisciplinary team managing a severely traumatized patient, e.g., following a road traffic accident. After life-threatening associated injuries have been ruled out, acute sight-threatening conditions must be assessed. The patient's injuries must be dealt with in their order of importance and severity. It is obvious to an ophthalmologist that the repair of a penetrating injury takes precedence over the repair of eyelid lacerations. It may not be obvious to another team, however, that the immediate management of a sight-threatening orbital hematoma takes precedence over visually dramatic facial lacerations once hemostasis has been obtained (Fig. 24.6). The evaluation of

---

Table 24.1 Cardinal Principles

- Examine and treat the patient for all injuries
- Maintain a high index of suspicion for undetected injury
- Determine the priority for repair
- The results of primary repair are superior to secondary repair
- Delay major reconstruction if the necessary expertise is not available
- Delay the repair until operating conditions are optimal
- Document all injuries very carefully
- Remove dirt and debris
- Reposition tissues to their correct anatomical alignment
- Do not discard or excise tissue unnecessarily

---

the unconscious patient is particularly difficult. The ophthalmologist plays a very important role in such a situation where the proper evaluation of a relatively afferent pupil defect cannot be delegated to other clinicians.

- Determine the priority for repair

Resuscitation, if needed, and stabilization of vital signs are the initial goals for the treatment of any trauma patient. It must be borne in mind that any patient who has sustained trauma has the potential to develop shock during the evaluation process as a result of occult serious or life-threatening injury (see Fig. 24.2). Periodic monitoring of vital signs during the examination process is therefore mandatory. Once the patient has been stabilized, the presence of life-threatening associated injury must be ruled out. Understanding the mechanism of injury is most helpful in this regard, e.g., an eyelid injury from a screwdriver in a child may be associated with a serious central nervous system (CNS) injury.

All patients with significant eyelid trauma should receive a complete ophthalmic examination, but the order and venue for the examination (in the emergency department or the operating room) are dictated by the severity of associated ocular injury. It is important to ensure that all steps have been taken to exclude possible associated trauma (e.g., CNS injury in a patient with an upper lid puncture wound) by CT scanning, before the patient is anesthetized. It is highly unsatisfactory to discover other injuries, which require the expertise of other specialists/operating facilities that are located elsewhere, once the patient has been anesthetized.

In patients with animal bites it is important to establish whether or not the patient is immuno-compromised and, in particular, whether or not a prior splenectomy has been performed, so that the increased risk of possible post-traumatic infection with unusual organisms can be assessed. The management of any secondary infection in this situation should be undertaken with the assistance of a microbiologist. The patient's tetanus immunization status should be investigated and tetanus toxoid given where appropriate. The risk of contracting rabies in the United Kingdom is extremely low, but must be borne in mind when managing such injuries in other countries.

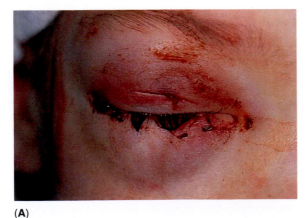

(A)

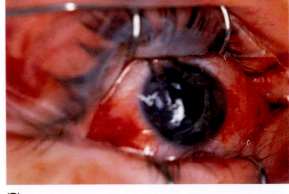

(B)

Figure 24.1 (**A**) A patient presenting with an apparently trivial upper eyelid laceration. (**B**) Careful examination of the globe revealed a penetrating eye injury with an iris prolapse.

Evaluation of Eyelid Injuries

It is convenient to divide eyelid injuries into the following categories:

- Marginal injuries
- Extra marginal injuries
- Avulsion injuries
- Injuries involving tissue loss

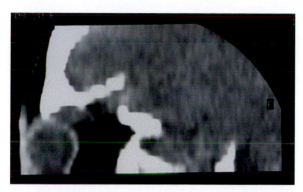

Figure 24.2 A sagittal computed tomography (CT) scan of a patient with apparently trivial upper eyelid injury but who developed a frontal lobe abscess 3 days following her fall onto a rose bush. She had sustained a fracture of the roof of her orbit and a penetrating injury of her brain. She had no other symptoms of presentation.

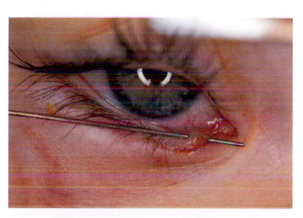

Figure 24.3 A right lower eyelid laceration involving the inferior canaliculus.

Marginal Injuries

Most full-thickness marginal lid lacerations are easily identified. It is easy, however, to overlook medial canthal injuries, particularly when dried coagulum obscures the area in a child. Relatively minor trauma, even to the lateral aspect of the eyelids, can result in rupture of the attachment of the medial can-

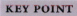

> **KEY POINT**
>
> All marginal trauma to the medial canthal region should be assumed to have damaged the canalicular system, unless proved otherwise (see Fig. 24.3).

thal tendon to the tarsus, an area of anatomical weakness, with resulting disruption of the canalicular system. This is particularly true of dog bites, injuries from hooks, and even finger-poking injuries.

Assessing the lacrimal system may be difficult in a child with an injury to the medial canthus and, in some situations, the patient must be anesthetized for the examination. Failure to identify and repair a canalicular laceration primarily will have long-term consequences for the patient (Fig. 24.7).

- The results of primary repair are superior to secondary repair

Extra Marginal Injuries

In most instances, extra marginal lid lacerations tend to follow the relaxed skin tension lines (RSTLs) and are oriented parallel to the free margin of the eyelid (see Fig. 24.1). All such lacerations should be considered to be associated with a possible underlying injury to the eye, the orbit, or contiguous structures such as the cranial cavity. Depending on the mechanism of injury and the clinical findings, appropriate imaging studies should be undertaken to evaluate the extent of associated orbital trauma and to rule out the presence of retained foreign bodies. The wound should be gently explored to measure its depth. The presence of fat in the wound indicates that the wound has at least breached the orbital septum (Fig. 24.8).

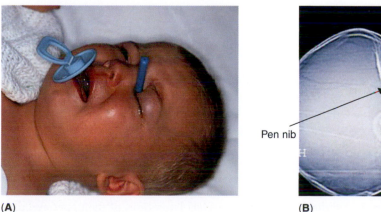
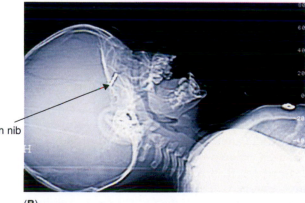

Pen nib

(A)   **(B)**

Figure 24.4 This infant was unsupervised playing with a pen when he fell. The pen nib was embedded in the body of the sphenoid with no other intracranial or ophthalmic injury. It was removed and the infant made a full recovery. Had the infant pulled the pen out the only visible sign of injury would have been a minor medial canthal wound.

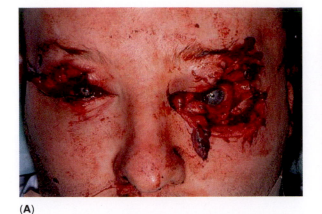
(A)

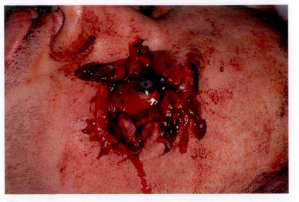
(B)

Figure 24.5 A severe dog bite injury with tissue loss.

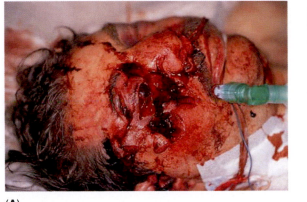
(A)

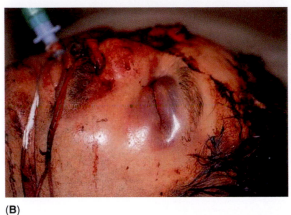
(B)

Figure 24.6 A patient who has sustained severe blunt facial trauma. (**A**) The right globe has been damaged beyond repair. (**B**) The left orbit has an expanding orbital haematoma whose management takes precedence over his other facial injuries once haemostasis has been obtained and his airway protected.

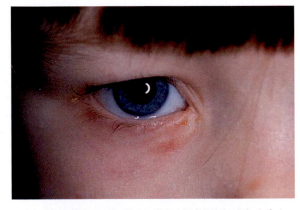

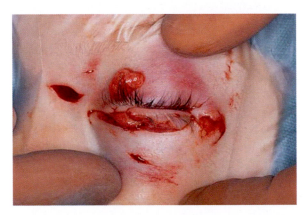

Figure 24.7 A lower lid marginal laceration, which involved the inferior cana-liculus. The canalicular injury was not recognized. The small laceration was managed with Steri-strips. The patient now has constant epiphora and will require a conjunctivodacryorhinostomy (CDCR) with a Leseter Jones tube.

Figure 24.8 A dog bite injury with several eyelid puncture wounds with orbital fat prolapse and a lower lid marginal laceration.

In the upper lid it is important not to confuse fat with the lacrimal gland. The fat may be cleaned and gently reposited. It is not necessary to attempt a repair of the orbital septum. If the fat has been exposed for a long period of time, it may be difficult to reposit it. If it is removed, it should be very carefully cross-clamped with a curved artery clip, first taking care not to apply any traction to the fat. The fat should then be removed with Westcott scissors and the stump cauterized carefully and the artery clip gently released but immediately reclamped in the event of any bleeding. In general, the fat

should be left alone to prevent postoperative eyelid asymmetry.

Tissue loss is sometimes seen with extra marginal lacerations, particularly in lacerations from a broken windshield, which produce a characteristic series of partial and some-times full-thickness linear gouges together with irregular lac-erations and abrasions. It may also be seen with some animal bites (see Fig. 24.5).

Extra marginal lacerations of the upper eyelid may involve the levator aponeurosis or levator muscle. Any laceration of these structures should be explored and repaired as soon as possible. In an adult it is helpful if the repair can be undertaken

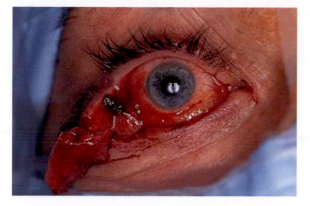

Figure 24.9 A lower eyelid avulsion injury with typical tangential extension of the laceration at the level of the eyelid crease.

under local anesthesia so that the height and contour of the lid can be adjusted appropriately.

Avulsion Injuries
Full-thickness marginal lacerations of the eyelids in the medial canthal area can also be associated with tangential extensions of the lacerations at the level of the eyelid creases and distal borders of the tarsi (Fig. 24.9). Disruption of the orbicularis muscle allows retraction of the cut edges, and gives the appearance of tissue loss. This is, however, very rarely the case.

Injuries Involving Tissue Loss
Although tissue loss in the periocular region is rare, it is important to recognize, as a formal reconstruction may be required. This requires particular oculoplastic expertise (see Fig. 24.5). Attempts to undertake such work in inexperienced hands may seriously compromise the result.

- Delay major reconstruction if the necessary expertise is not available

MANAGEMENT DECISIONS

After the nature and extent of the injuries have been appropriately evaluated, management decisions can be made. The repair of eyelid injuries may be delayed for up to 72 hours if the operating conditions are not optimal. It is preferable, however, to repair such injuries as soon as possible after trauma for the following reasons:

1. Decontamination of the wounds is far more effective the earlier it is performed
2. Post-traumatic tissue edema increases during the first 24 hours after injury
3. The surgical repair becomes more difficult to perform after the first 24 hours

If the ophthalmologist has doubts about the suitability of the facilities in the Accident and Emergency Department or about the patient's cooperation, the surgical repair should be undertaken in the operating room. If a formal repair of a lacrimal drainage system injury is contemplated, it is preferable to undertake such surgery under general anesthesia. If the surgical repair must be delayed, e.g., because of potential anesthetic problems, decontamination of the wounds should be carried out, and a suitable

protective dressing should be applied until surgery can be performed. This is particularly important with respect to bite wounds.

- Delay the repair until operating conditions are optimal

Medicolegal Considerations

> **KEY POINT**
>
> Accurate and detailed documentation is essential. Many injuries will result in civil or criminal legal proceedings.

An accurate detailed legible history must be recorded and signed. It is particularly important to record any eye-witness statements and to record the names of anyone who administered any first aid. In the case of road traffic accidents it is important to record who was driving the vehicle. A record of the patient's vision is mandatory, unless this cannot be measured. A detailed description of the ocular and systemic examination findings with drawings should be recorded.

Photographic documentation of the nature and extent of the injuries is particularly helpful and should always be considered (Fig. 24.10). Photographic documentation offers significant advantages over drawings:

- Photographs provide objective documentation of the patient's preoperative appearance
- Objective documentation may be useful in supporting claims filed with solicitors, insurance companies, or the Criminal Injury Compensation Board
- The photographs can illustrate the ophthalmologist's testimony should it be required in the future
- Document all injuries very carefully

SURGICAL MANAGEMENT
Wound Decontamination

In is essential that all wounds are thoroughly cleaned and all foreign bodies removed before any surgical repair is undertaken. Wounds should be carefully explored and a high degree of suspicion maintained that retained foreign material is present, depending on the circumstances of the injury (see Fig. 24.2). Failure to remove particulate matter, as seen following explosions or contact from road surfaces in road traffic accidents, will lead to a traumatic tattoo that will prove extremely difficult to remove at a secondary procedure.

The role of prophylactic antibiotic administration in the treatment of traumatic eyelid and facial wounds remains controversial and is no substitute for meticulous wound decontamination. Grossly contaminated wounds, wounds associated with significant tissue devitalization, wounds involving the orbit, and animal/human bites certainly warrant antibiotic therapy, which should be commenced as soon as possible in consultation with a microbiologist (Fig. 24.11).

- Remove dirt and debris

Tetanus prophylaxis must be considered in all patients. Patients with clean wounds who have been immunized within the last 10 years do not require tetanus toxoid injections. This

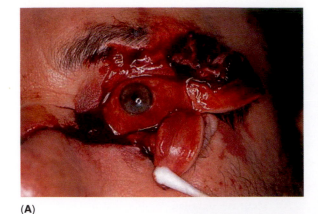
(A)

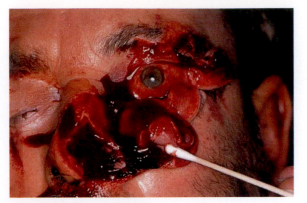
(B)

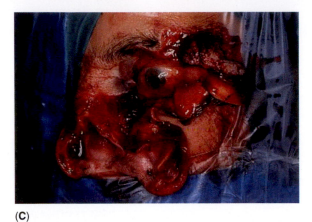
(C)

Figure 24.10 (**A–C**) Severe facial trauma caused by a relative of the patient. The photographs were used in legal proceedings.

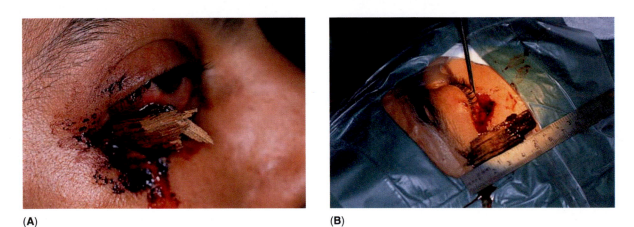
(A)   (B)

Figure 24.11 (**A**) A wooden foreign body removed under general anaesthesia. (**B**) Careful orbital wound exploration was essential to ensure no residual foreign bodies were left in situ.

criterion is reduced to 5 years for wounds with devitalized tissue or for contaminated wounds. Patients with clean wounds who have not been immunized should be treated with tetanus toxoid. Patients with contaminated wounds or devitalized tissue should also receive tetanus immunoglobulin.

Sequence of Periocular Laceration Repair

It is important to approach the repair of periocular wounds in a systematic fashion. Many periocular wounds are simple and straightforward to repair but some are complex lacerations with associated damage to the lacrimal drainage system, the globe, and the bony orbital walls (Fig. 24.12).

Lacrimal Drainage System Wounds

After the wound has been decontaminated, it should be repaired in a methodical fashion. Canalicular lacerations should be repaired meticulously. In the past, many surgeons have advocated a very conservative approach to the management of canalicular lacerations for fear of causing iatrogenic damage not only to the affected canaliculus but also to the uninvolved canaliculus or to the common canaliculus. It is mandatory to avoid such iatrogenic trauma, which was particularly seen with the use of the pigtail probe, for which reason it has fallen into disrepute. The technique of passing bi-canalicular silicone stents is much simpler than using a pigtail probe. In the hands of a

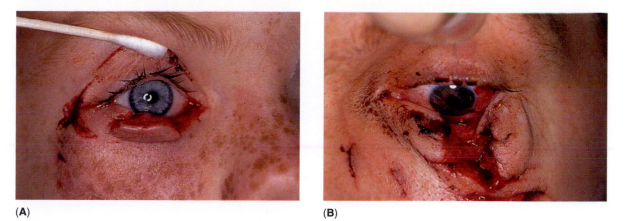

(A)   (B)

Figure 24.12 (**A**) This patient has sustained a lower lid avulsion injury in addition to a lateral marginal laceration. It is preferable to repair the avulsion injury and the inferior canalicular laceration before proceeding with a repair of the lateral marginal laceration. (**B**) This patient has a severe lower lid marginal laceration and a penetrating eye injury with iris prolapse. The globe must be repaired first followed by a meticulous eyelid repair, taking care to avoid undue pressure on the globe.

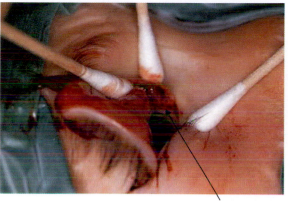

Lacerated superior
canaliculus

Figure 24.13 A patient with an upper eyelid avulsion injury. The lighter colour of the lacerated superior canaliculus is contrasted with the surrounding orbicularis muscle.

skilled and experienced surgeon bi-canalicular silicone intubation causes little if any iatrogenic trauma and offers significant advantages over mono-canalicular intubation:

- When tightened, the silicone loop aids in the ana-tomical realignment of the eyelid, although the loop must be loosened once the sutures are in place to avoid any cheese wiring of the puncta and canaliculi.
- Patients more readily tolerate the loop of silicone at the medial canthus for long periods than mono-canalicular stents, which occlude the puncta and cause secondary epiphora.

It is therefore reasonable for the skilled and experienced surgeon to attempt a repair of a lacerated superior canaliculus when the inferior canaliculus is intact. If the surgeon is inexperienced, however, the priorities are to avoid iatrogenic trauma and to achieve a good anatomical alignment of the eyelid. Under these circumstances, the use of a mono-canalicular stent is preferable. A Crawford style, mono-canalicular stent is preferred. When both canaliculi have been severed, it is mandatory to attempt a repair of these.

Numerous methods have been described to assist in the identification of the proximal end of a lacerated canaliculus. These are very rarely required, as the proximal end of the

lacerated canaliculus can almost always be readily identified using the operating microscope. It is more difficult to locate following an avulsion injury when good retraction of the surrounding edematous tissues is essential using cotton-tipped applicators. The lighter color of the canaliculus is contrasted with the surrounding orbicularis muscle (Fig. 24.13).

At induction of anesthesia the nose should be packed with small neurosurgical patties moistened with a vasoconstrictor, e.g., 5% cocaine solution. These should be placed under and around the inferior turbinate. Shrinkage of the mucosa of the inferior turbinate will permit much easier retrieval of the silicone stent from the nose without bleeding. The mucosa of the inferior turbinate can also be injected with 2% Lidocaine with 1:80,000 units of adrenaline.

It is essential to insert good-quality silicone stents atraumatically. The author's first choice is the Crawford silicone stent. This is reinforced with a white thread within the silicone and has a fine flexible wire introducer with a small olive tip (Fig. 24.14). It is essential to check the attachment of the silicone to the introducer. This should be rounded and smooth, permitting easy passage through the canaliculi. Some stents have a flattened attachment that causes trauma to the canaliculi. Such stents should be avoided.

The flexible wire introducer is easily retrieved from beneath the inferior turbinate, either with the use of a nasal endoscope and a hook retriever or with a Tse–Anderson grooved director placed under the inferior turbinate and used by "feel." This is a modified Quickert grooved director with a tip designed to catch the olive tip of the wire introducer (Fig. 24.15). A similar device, the Anderson Hwang grooved director, is now available from Altomed Limited. The wire introducers are then removed. If a mono-canalicular stent has been placed, the stent is shortened with scissors so that the stent retracts beneath the inferior turbinate. If a bi-canalicular stent has been placed, the ends of the stent are pulled down and a Castroviejo needle holder placed across the tubing. Another needle holder is used to tie a simple knot, which is tightened. The stent is cut 4 to 5 mm below the knot and the stent allowed to retract under the inferior turbinate. The stent is then loosened at the medial canthus so that this is under no tension.

It is essential that an attempt be made to pass the stent via the lacerated canaliculus first. Only if this maneuver is successful should the stent then be passed via the uninvolved

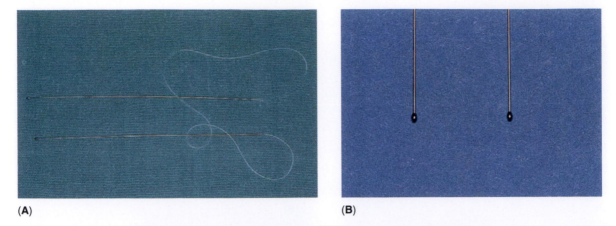

(A)   (B)

Figure 24.14 (**A**) A Crawford silicone stent. (**B**) The olive tip of the stent introducer.

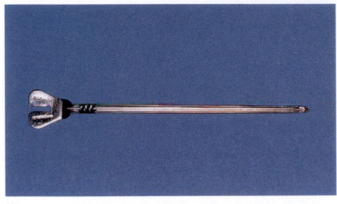

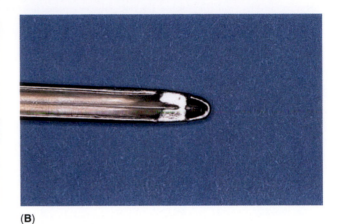

(A)   (B)

Figure 24.15 (**A**) A Tse-Anderson grooved director. (**B**) The modified tip of the grooved director.

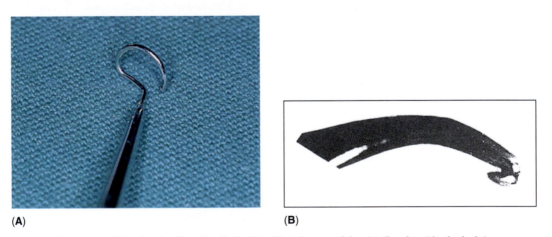

(A)   (B)

Figure 24.16 (**A**) A pigtail probe with a barbed tip. (**B**) A diagram of the pigtail probe with a barbed tip.

canaliculus. The stent is left in place and removed after 9 to 12 months in the absence of any problems.

If the stents cannot be passed into the nose successfully, e.g., there is an associated nasal fracture, the pigtail probe can be used. This requires more skill and care and does not offer the advantage of assisting the anatomical realignment of the eyelid in contrast to bi-canalicular intubation. The pigtail probe is passed via the uninvolved canaliculus. A single attempt should be made to gently rotate the probe into position. If this is difficult, or any resistance is encountered, the attempt should be abandoned.

It is important to select a pigtail probe of appropriate size. A common error is to assume that one size fits all because only a single size is available. The probe should be smooth, with a small eye at the tip through which a 6/0 nylon suture is passed. No probe should be used which has a barb at the tip. This causes severe trauma to the canaliculi and its use is largely responsible for the pigtail probe falling into disrepute (Fig. 24.16).

Once the nylon has been retrieved and the probe removed, a fine silicone tube is passed over the suture. A Crawford stent is ideal. This is cut and the central thread removed, leaving a hollow tube. The tubing is then trimmed to size, taking great care not to cut the suture. The suture is then tied and cut and the knot rotated into the lacrimal sac (Fig. 24.17).

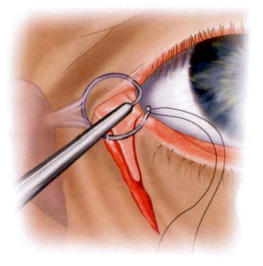

(A)

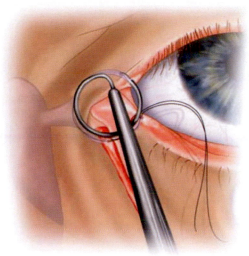

(B)

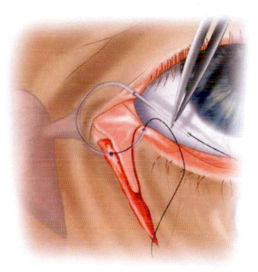

(C)

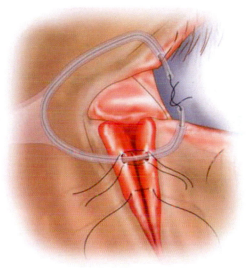

(D)

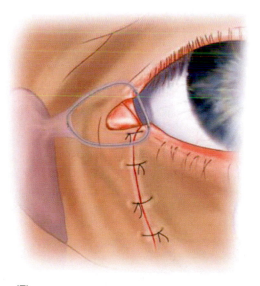

(E)

Figure 24.17 (**A**) A pigtail probe has been passed via the superior canaliculus and a 6/0 nylon suture threaded through the eye of the probe. (**B**) The probe is rotated back and the suture withdrawn through the superior canaliculus. (**C**) Silicone tubing is threaded over the suture. (**D**) 8/0 Vicryl sutures are placed through the substantia propria of the canaliculus. (**E**) The tubing is cut to size and the central nylon suture tied and the knot rotated into the lacrimal sac.

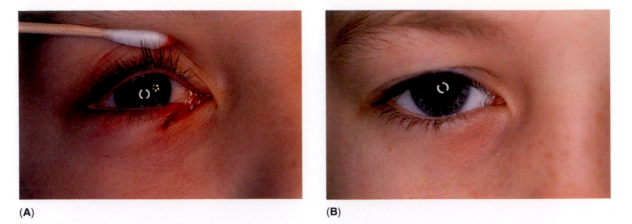

(A)   (B)

Figure 24.18 **(A)** A minor lower lid marginal laceration involving the inferior canaliculus. **(B)** The canalicular laceration has been repaired using a pigtail probe. The nylon suture is visible in the silicone stent.

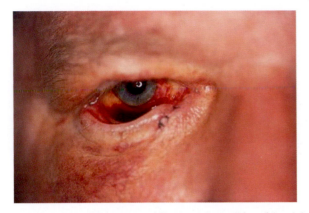

Figure 24.19 A lower lid ectropion following a lower lid avulsion injury. No attempt has been made to repair the medial canthal tendon.

This procedure is ideally suited to minor lacerations (Fig. 24.18).

With more major lacerations or avulsion injuries of the lower eyelid, the medial canthal ligament should be reconstructed with a permanent suture (e.g., 5/0 Ethibond on a half circle needle) after the silicone tubing has been placed but not yet tied. It is essential to ensure that the suture is initially placed through the posterior lacrimal crest. This requires good assistance and retraction of the tissues. The posterior lacrimal crest is approached by dissection between the caruncle and the plica semilunaris. The crest can be felt with a Freer periosteal elevator. The use of a 1/2–circle needle is essential to facilitate good fixation to the posterior lacrimal crest and easier retrieval of the needle. Failure to attach the avulsed lid to this position will lead to antero-positioning of the lower lid, poor cosmesis, and epiphora (Fig. 24.19).

The Ethibond suture is passed through the tarsus, taking care not to damage the canaliculus further, and is then tied with a slipknot to ensure correct anatomical placement of the eyelid, but then loosened so that a microsurgical repair of the canaliculus itself can proceed. When possible, the canaliculus should be repaired with three equally spaced 8/0 Vicryl sutures placed through the substantia propria of the canaliculus. These sutures should be left untied until all three have been placed.

The silicone tubing can then be gently tightened and the Ethibond posterior fixation suture tied. This action takes all tension off of the 8/0 sutures, which can then be tied blindly and cut. The orbicularis muscle is repaired with the remaining Vicryl suture. The lid margin is sutured with two interrupted 6/0 Vicryl sutures placed in a vertical mattress fashion, again taking care not to damage the canaliculus or the stent. Finally, the stent is tied in the nose and loosened so that there is no tension on it (Fig. 24.20).

Marginal Injuries

Marginal injuries can be difficult to repair because of secondary eyelid bruising and swelling as well as irregularity of the wound (Fig. 24.21). Although it is reasonable to debride shredded devitalized tissue, this should be kept to a minimum. The blood supply to the periorbital area is excellent and the tissue, which may appear non-viable, will usually survive even if replaced as a free graft.

• Reposition tissues to their correct anatomical alignment

The goals in the repair of marginal lacerations are:

• Meticulous anatomical alignment of the eyelid margin
• Avoidance of secondary trichiasis and eyelid notching
• Restoration of the structural integrity of the tarsus
• Avoidance of any eyelid retraction or lagophthalmos
• A limitation of cutaneous and deep scar formation

Failure to observe the basic principles of eyelid repair and postoperative wound management will result in failure to achieve these goals and poor results (Figs. 24.22 and 24.23). Secondary surgery will not achieve as good a result.

Figure 24.23 illustrates the reconstructive problems caused by a poor attempt at a primary repair.

• The results of primary repair are superior to secondary repair

The principles involved in the repair of eyelid marginal lacerations are very similar to those involved in the closure of wedge resection defects of the eyelid. It is rarely the case that tissue is missing from the eyelid. Depending on the age of the patient, it may be possible to convert a wound to a standard wedge excision by segmental excision of the involved area.

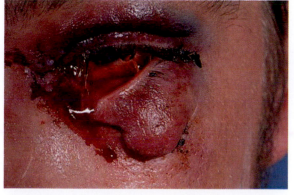

(A)

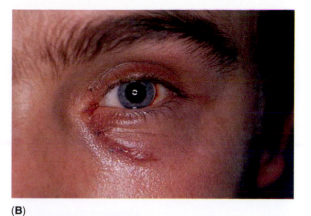

(B)

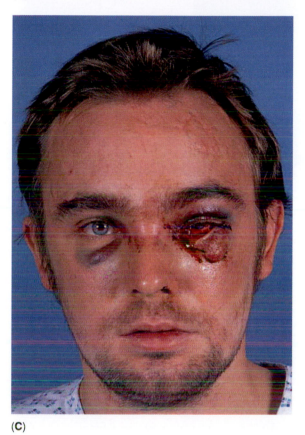

(C)

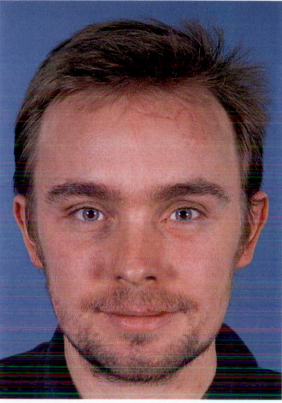

(D)

Figure 24.20 (**A**) A severe left lower eyelid avulsion injury with secondary eyelid oedema and bruising. (**B**) One week following the repair with a bicanalicular silicone intubation. (**C**) A full face photograph of the same patient with a left lower eyelid avulsion injury. (**D**) The same patient eight weeks following the repair with a bicanalicular silicone intubation.

If, however, the extent of the tissue loss is too great, a formal reconstruction will be required.

After the eyelid margin and tarsus have been repaired, any horizontal defects of the upper eyelid retractors should be repaired before the orbicularis and skin are closed as separate layers (Fig. 24.24). Failure to repair defects of the upper eyelid retractors may result in a severe ptosis that is much more difficult to correct secondarily (Fig. 24.25). Following windscreen injuries, multiple flaps and puncture wounds may be present and it may be a very difficult task to ascertain the correct anatomical location for the tissues. This task is made even more difficult by the possibility of tissue loss.

Extra Marginal Injuries

It is to be re-emphasized that extra marginal lacerations are associated with more serious underlying injuries until proved otherwise.

The goals in the repair of extra marginal lacerations are:

- Meticulous anatomical alignment of the eyelid tissues
- Avoidance of any eyelid retraction or lagophthalmos (Fig. 24.26)
- A limitation of cutaneous and deep scar formation

In the upper lid, if the lacerations extend to the eyebrow, it is preferable to realign the eyebrow first. Suturing of the

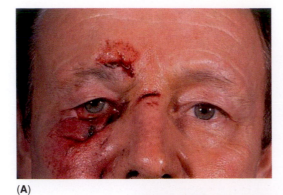

(A)

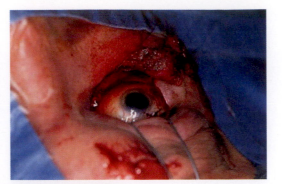

(B)

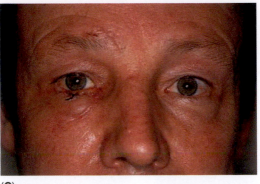

(C)

Figure 24.21 (**A**) A severe right lower eyelid avulsion injury combined with a marginal laceration. (**B**) A small pedicle of attachment with a dusky appearance to the avulsed eyelid tissue. (**C**) The result of a good anatomical realignment 2 weeks later prior to lid margin suture removal.

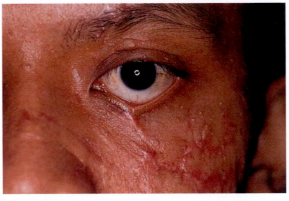

(A)

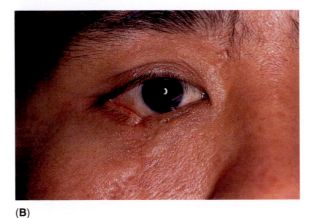

(B)

Figure 24.22 (**A**) Lower eyelid retraction with severe cutaneous and deep scar formation. (**B**) A central lower eyelid notch with retraction.

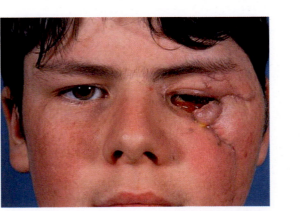

Figure 24.23 Severe periocular scarring and a dehiscence of a left lower lid wound repair.

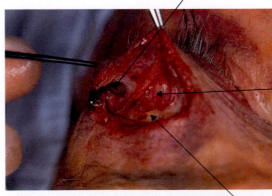

Full-thickness wound

Müller's muscle

Levator aponeurosis

Figure 24.24 An upper eyelid extramarginal laceration with a full-thickness hole laterally and a lacerated levator aponeurosis. The skin wound was extended to effect a repair of the levator aponeurosis.

orbicularis muscle with 5/0 Vicryl aids in the alignment of irregular skin flaps and removes the tension from the skin sutures. The minimal number of sutures should be placed in order to limit deep scarring. The sutures should not strangulate tissue. As in all repairs, slight eversion of the skin edges minimizes the chances of depressed scars. The skin wounds are closed with interrupted 7/0 Vicryl sutures.

- Do not discard or excise tissue unnecessarily

Eyelid Injuries with Associated Severe Penetrating Globe Injury

KEY POINT

The decision to repair a severely traumatized eye with no prospect of useful vision may compromise the patient's outcome if this decision prevents the adequate primary repair of associated complex eyelid lacerations and orbital fractures (Fig. 24.27).

This may save the patient from numerous further operative procedures. This can be extremely difficult and any decision to proceed with a primary enucleation must be made at the most senior level. It is particularly important when the ophthalmic surgeon is operating as part of a multidisciplinary team. Good communication with other members of the team is vital. Detailed pre and postoperative documentation is also imperative.

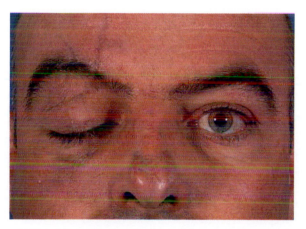

Figure 24.25 A right traumatic ptosis due to failure to explore and primarily repair the transected levator muscle.

Postoperative Care

Measures should be taken to prevent excessive postoperative eyelid edema, which can adversely affect the outcome. These are:

- Elevation of the patient's head
- Application of a pressure dressing
- Ice packs

For most injuries the pressure dressing can be removed the following day. The prolonged application of a pressure dressing should be avoided in young children, in order to avoid occlusion amblyopia. The eyelid can instead be protected with a clear Cartella shield.

In the case of severe eyelid avulsion injures where the wound is under tension (see Fig. 24.20), the tarsal fixation suture should be supported by a pressure dressing, which is applied with the use of Micropore tape fixated to the cheek area and then drawn up to the forehead. The prior application of Tincture of Benzoin to the skin of the cheek and the forehead assists this process. This dressing holds tension off the wound until the wound has had a chance to heal and also reduces the chances of further postoperative edema developing, which can cause the sutures to "cheese wire" and the wound to dehisce (see Fig. 24.23). Such a dressing should be further supported with the use of a head bandage and can be maintained in place for up to 1 week postoperatively.

Eyelid margin sutures should be removed 2 weeks postoperatively along with the skin sutures.

The patient should be advised to undertake regular and frequent postoperative wound massage using Lacrilube ointment. The application of a silicone gel preparation e.g., Kelocote or Dermatix, can also help to prevent wound contracture and to soften the resultant scar.

Secondary Repair

Although the aim of a good primary repair of eyelid injuries is to avoid the necessity for any secondary reconstructive surgery, such secondary intervention is occasionally necessary for a variety of reasons:

- A severe aesthetic deformity (see Fig. 24.23)
- Lagophthalmos with exposure keratopathy (see Fig. 24.26)

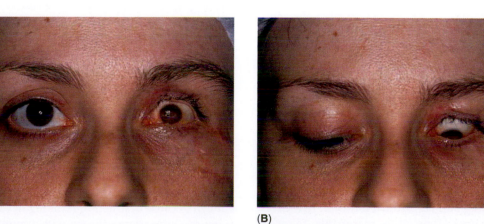

(A)   **(B)**

Figure 24.26 (A) A left upper eyelid retraction, phthisis bulbi and periorbital severe cutaneous and deep scar formation following a road traffic accident. (B) Severe lag on downgaze due to overzealous debridement of the upper lid tissues which appeared to be devitalized.

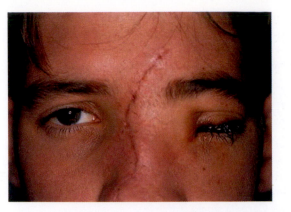

Figure 24.27 This patient suffered a severe left globe rupture and a comminuted nasoethmoidal fracture. A maxillofacial surgeon undertook the repair of the nasoethmoidal fracture after the severe globe rupture had been repaired. The maxillofacial surgeon was unable to effect a satisfactory repair of the fractures for fear of damaging the globe. The globe had no visual prospects and was enucleated the next day.

- Mechanical keratitis from eyelid malposition/ trichiasis
- Lower lid retraction/ectropion (see Fig. 24.22)
- An overlooked foreign body
- Tattooing of the wound
- An overlooked injury to the canalicular system (see Fig. 24.7)
- A deformity of the medial or lateral canthi (see Fig. 24.23)
- Ptosis (see Fig. 24.25)
- Conjunctival scarring with restriction of ocular motility

The timing of the secondary intervention depends on the degree of urgency of the problem and can be categorized as early, intermediate, or late, e.g., lagophthalmos with exposure keratopathy, which cannot be managed conservatively, requires an early secondary intervention.

If the opportunity arises to reintervene early where there has been a failure to apply the basic principles discussed earlier, the wound can be simply recreated and repaired more appropriately. An alternative strategy may need to be employed, however, for an eyelid that is shortened by loss of tissue or scar formation. A superior result may be achieved by a reconstruction with a full-thickness skin graft combined with an orbicularis muscle advancement undertaken as an aesthetic procedure (Fig. 24.28A and B), or with the additional use of fat grafting to prevent re-adhesion to deeper structure (Fig. 24.28C–F).

The management of a ptosis following trauma can be a challenge. It can be very difficult to differentiate a mechanical ptosis due to eyelid swelling and hematoma from a neurogenic ptosis or from a myogenic/aponeurotic ptosis following a direct laceration to the levator muscle or its aponeurosis. The ptosis may in fact have a mixed etiology. If it is known that the levator muscle or its aponeurosis has been transected, it is preferable to reintervene early and repair the laceration with the patient under local anesthesia. The presence of eyelid swelling and hematoma, however, may make this impractical. Alternatively, it is reasonable to delay reintervention for some months unless there is a risk of

amblyopia in an infant. The ptosis and levator function may improve spontaneously. The ptosis can then be re-evaluated and the ptosis managed according to basic principles (see chap. 7).

If the opportunity for an early reintervention for canalicular lacerations has been missed the secondary reconstruction can be particularly difficult and may fail to achieve freedom from epiphora without a conjunctivo-dacryocystorhinostomy (CDCR) and placement of a Lester Jones tube.

Late reintervention for the revision of scars is indicated once the scars have matured and the wounds have been extensively massaged.

BURNS
Burns can be classified as:

- Thermal
- Chemical
- Electrical
- Radiational

This section will deal only with thermal burns.

Patients who have sustained thermal burns to the eyelids are often critically ill. The majority of such patients are managed in a specialist burns unit. Severe burns are rarely confined to the eyelids and periocular region (Fig. 24.29).

Fortunately, the eye is rarely affected acutely by facial burns because of the protective mechanisms afforded by reflex eyelid closure and the Bell's phenomenon.

Burns are further classified as:

- First degree
- Second degree
- Third degree

A first-degree burn only involves the epidermis and is characterized by erythema typically seen in a mild sunburn. A second-degree (partial thickness) burn involves the epidermis and superficial layers of the adjacent dermis. Regeneration of the skin occurs from remaining epithelial elements. This degree of burn is characterized by pain, erythema, blistering, and weeping, as typically seen following CO_2 laser resurfacing (Fig. 24.30). A third-degree burn (full thickness) involves total and irreversible destruction of both the epidermis and dermis. Such a burn is painless and is characterized by the absence of edema, with the area affected by the burn appearing hard and inelastic (see Fig. 24.29).

Management
The immediate management of thermal burns of the eyelids is conservative. The goals are:

- To prevent infection
- To prevent secondary corneal complication

First-degree burns usually require no further treatment. Second and third-degree burns should be cleaned and any foreign material removed. If the burned tissue is extensive enough to cause destruction resulting in corneal exposure, it is imperative to protect the eye with a combination of topical lubricants and antibiotics. If corneal protection cannot be

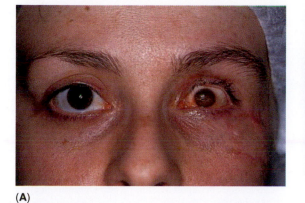
(A)

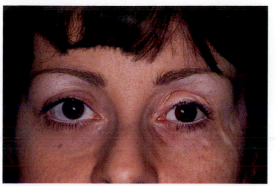
(B)

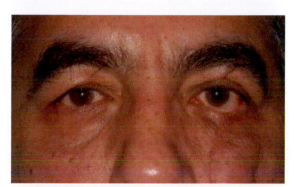
(C)

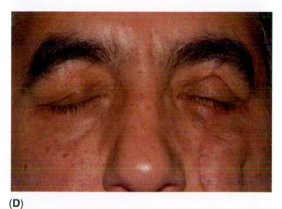
(D)

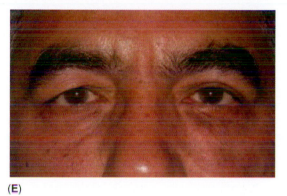
(E)

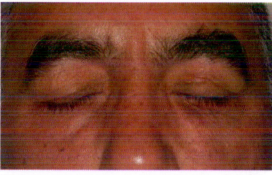
(F)

Figure 24.28 (**A**) Left upper eyelid retraction, phthisis bulbi, and periorbital severe cutaneous and deep scar formation following a road traffic accident. (**B**) The result after a full-thickness postauricular skin graft combined with an orbicularis muscle advancement and fitting of a cosmetic shell. (**C**) A patient with a left lower lid retraction and a facial depression with a long, deep, vertical lower lid and facial scar following a facial knife wound. (**D**) The same patient demonstrating lagophthalmos, an upper lid sulcus defect, and lid lag on down gaze from a deep upper lid scar. (**E**) The same patient 6 months following upper and lower lid skin grafts with the placement of a dermis fat graft in the mid-face. (**F**) The patient showing improvement in his lagophthalmos.

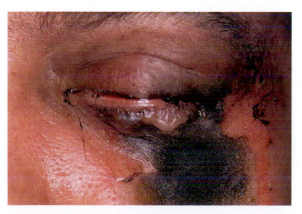

Figure 24.29 A self-inflicted third-degree burn of lower eyelid, lateral aspect of upper eyelid and cheek in a schizophrenic patient caused by direct contact with a cigarette lighter flame.

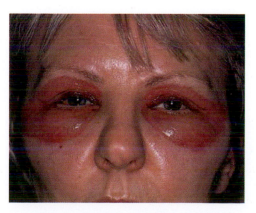

Figure 24.30 CO_2 laser resurfacing burns.

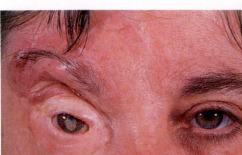

Figure 24.31 Corneal scarring in spite of extensive periocular skin grafting combined with a lateral tarsorrhaphay and a medial canthoplasty.

achieved satisfactorily a temporary suture tarsorrhaphy may be necessary.

Once cicatricial changes begin in the eyelids with ectropion and lagophthalmos, there is often a rapid deterioration of the ocular surface. More aggressive treatment may be necessary to prevent irreversible ocular morbidity (Fig. 24.31). Although skin grafting is usually delayed until cicatricial changes stabilize, the use of early full-thickness skin grafts may be necessary to reduce ocular morbidity.

The late management of thermal eyelid burns involves excision of the scar with the use of full-thickness skin grafts. The recipient lid should be placed on maximum stretch with the use of eyelid margin silk sutures in order to increase the area to be grafted. This allows for postoperative skin graft contraction, which should be minimized by a strict protocol of postoperative massage using Lacrilube ointment and the application of a silicone gel preparation, e.g., Kelocote or Dermatix.

FURTHER READING

1. American Academy of Ophthalmology. Basic and Clinical Science Course: Orbit, Eyelids and Lacrimal System, section 7. San Francisco, CA: American Academy of Ophthalmology, 1998–1999: 101–9, 138–41.
2. Gonnering RS. Eyelid trauma. In: Bosniak S, ed. Principles and Practice of Ophthalmic Plastic and Reconstructive Surgery, vol. 1. Philadelphia, PA: WB Saunders, 1996: 452–64.
3. Green J, Charonis GC, Goldberg RA. Eyelid trauma and reconstructive techniques. In: Yanoff M, Duker J, eds., Ophthalmology Philadelphia, PA: Mosby, 2004: 720–7.
4. Grossman MD, Berlin AJ. Management of acute adnexal trauma. In: Stewart WB, ed., Surgery of the Eyelids, Orbit and Lacrimal System, vol. 1. Ophthalmology Monographs 8. San Francisco, CA: American Academy of Ophthalmology, 1993: 170–85.
5. Jordan DR, Nerad JA, Tse DT. The pigtail probe revisited. Ophthalmology 1990; 97: 512–9.
6. Kulwin DR. Thermal, chemical and radiation burns. In: Stewart WB, ed., Surgery of the Eyelids, Orbit and Lacrimal System, vol. 1, Ophthalmology Monographs 8. San Francisco, CA: American Academy of Ophthalmology, 1993: 186–97.
7. Mustarde JC. Repair and Reconstruction in the Orbital Region. Edinburgh: Livingstone, 1966.
8. Nerad JA, Carter KD, Alford MA. Disorders of the eyelid: eyelid trauma. In: Rapid Diagnosis in Ophthalmology-Oculoplastic & Reconstructive Surgery. Philadelphia, PA: Mosby Elsevier, 2008: 62–5.
9. Nerad JA, Carter KD, Alford MA. Disorders of the orbit: trauma. In: Rapid Diagnosis in Ophthalmology-Oculoplastic & Reconstructive Surgery. Philadelphia, PA: Mosby Elsevier, 2008: 242–57.
10. Shore JW, Rubin PA, Bilyk JR. Repair of telecanthus by anterior fixation of cantilevered miniplates. Ophthalmology 1992; 99: 1133–8.

25 Orbital wall blowout fractures

INTRODUCTION

The term "pure orbital blowout fracture" is used to describe a fracture of the orbital floor, the medial orbital wall, or both, with an intact bony orbital margin. The term "impure orbital blowout fracture" is used when such fractures occur in conjunction with a fracture of the orbital rim, e.g., as part of a zygomatic complex fracture. The most common site for a blowout fracture to occur is the postero-medial aspect of the orbital floor medial to the infraorbital neurovascular bundle where the maxillary bone is very thin. As the lamina papyracea is also very thin, the medial orbital wall is also prone to fracture, either in isolation or in association with a fracture of the orbital floor or other facial bones.

ETIOLOGY

There are two mechanisms thought to be responsible for pure orbital wall blowout fractures:

1. The backward displacement of the globe caused by a blunt non-penetrating object, e.g., a tennis ball, which raises the intraorbital pressure sufficiently to fracture the postero-medial orbital floor and/or the lamina papyracea of the ethmoid
2. A transient deformation of the orbital rim transmits the force of injury directly to the orbital wall

These fractures may occur following any blunt trauma to the periorbital region, e.g., following a blow with a fist (Fig. 25.1). The weak areas of the orbital walls provide some means of protection to the globe and orbital tissues, permitting these to expand into the maxillary antrum and/or ethmoid sinus rather than being compressed against the other more rigid areas of the orbit. The periorbita overlying the fracture is usually ruptured allowing the adjacent orbital fat to prolapse into the fracture site. Occasionally part of an adjacent extraocular muscle will also prolapse into the fracture site.

Although a rupture of the globe can complicate such fractures, this occurrence is rare. Conversely, any patient who has suffered blunt trauma sufficiently severe to cause a ruptured globe has an orbital wall blowout fracture until proven otherwise.

DIAGNOSIS

A high index of suspicion should be maintained for the presence of a blowout fracture in any patient who has sustained blunt periorbital trauma. The patient's clinical signs will depend on the timing of the examination in relation to the traumatic episode. A patient presenting some months after the traumatic event may have enophthalmos as the only physical sign.

Clinical Signs and Symptoms
1. Eyelid ecchymosis/hematoma
2. Subcutaneous emphysema
3. A neurosensory loss in the distribution of the infraorbital nerve
4. A limitation of ocular motility with diplopia
5. Enophthalmos/proptosis/hypoglobus
6. An upper eyelid sulcus deformity
7. Pseudoptosis
8. Headache
9. Nausea/vomiting
10. Bradycardia

Eyelid Ecchymosis/Hematoma
Although eyelid ecchymosis, hematoma, or edema are usually present when the patient is seen soon after trauma has occurred, these signs may be absent as seen in the so-called "white eyed blowout fracture" in pediatric patients. In these patients, the flexible bone of the orbital floor is fractured and forced inferiorly. The periorbita is ruptured resulting in a prolapse of inferior orbital fat. Part of the inferior rectus muscle may also be forced into the fracture. The flexible bone of the orbital floor then springs back into position causing a severe entrapment of the prolapsed tissues.

Subcutaneous Emphysema
A blowout fracture communicates with an air-filled sinus. Air may be forced into the orbit and/or eyelids, particularly in medial orbital wall blowout fractures, when the patient blows the nose or sneezes. Subcutaneous emphysema may result in palpable crepitus. Patients should be urged not to blow their nose or to hold the nose when sneezing, or the subcutaneous emphysema may be greatly exacerbated. Very rarely, air forced into the orbit can cause a severe proptosis, and an orbital compartment syndrome with a compromise of the blood supply to the optic nerve or globe (Fig. 25.2).

Neurosensory Loss in the Distribution of the Infraorbital Nerve
Dysfunction of the infraorbital nerve is almost pathognomonic of an orbital floor blowout fracture. The patient is usually aware of altered sensation in the ipsilateral cheek, upper teeth and upper lip. This occurs because the fracture extends along the infraorbital groove or canal, injuring the infraorbital nerve. Not all patients with an orbital floor blowout fracture, however, experience such sensory deficits. These annoying sensory deficits tend to resolve spontaneously with time but may be exacerbated by surgical intervention for the fracture. Very rarely, persistent pain in the distribution of the infraorbital nerve may be an indication for surgical decompression of the nerve, which may be compressed by bone fragments.

Limitation of Ocular Motility
The patient with an orbital floor blowout fracture may have vertical diplopia due to a variety of different mechanisms. Horizontal diplopia in the presence of a medial orbital wall

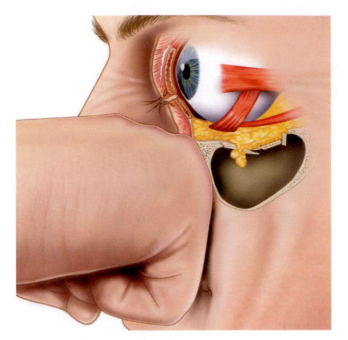

Figure 25.1 Production of an orbital floor blowout fracture with a prolapse of orbital fat into the maxillary antrum.

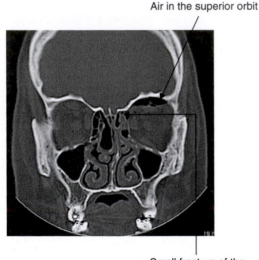

Air in the superior orbit

Small fracture of the lamina papyracea

Figure 25.2 This patient sustained a small medial orbital wall blowout fracture complicated by air forced into the orbit under pressure when the patient sneezed.

blowout fracture is less commonly seen. The mechanisms which may be responsible for limitation of ocular motility are:

1. Entrapment of connective tissue septa or of an extraocular muscle within the fracture
2. Hematoma and/or edema in the orbital fat adjacent to the fracture
3. Hematoma or contusion of an extraocular muscle(s)
4. Palsy of an extraocular muscle(s) due to neuronal damage
5. Volkmann's ischemic contracture of an entrapped extraocular muscle

Enophthalmos/Proptosis/Hypoglobus
Enophthalmos is produced by an enlarged orbital volume and varies from insignificant to cosmetically disfiguring depending on the degree of orbital bony expansion. Fat atrophy usually contributes little if anything to the enophthalmos. Enophthalmos may be masked by orbital hematoma, edema, or air, which may even cause proptosis in the first few days following trauma. Proptosis, however, may be associated with a "blow-in" fracture where the fragmented bones of the orbital floor are displaced into the orbit. This is more often seen in the context of fractures involving the roof of the orbit. Enophthalmos is always significant in the presence of combined fractures of the orbital floor and medial orbital wall. Hypoglobus is seen in the presence of extensive orbital floor blowout fractures. In some patients, the maxillary antrum extends laterally for some distance beyond the infraorbital neurovascular bundle, with the ensuing orbital floor defect occupying almost the whole of the orbital floor. Very rarely, the globe may come to lie within the maxillary antrum or even within the ethmoid sinus (Figs. 25.3 and 25.4).

Upper Eyelid Sulcus Deformity/Pseudoptosis
Enophthalmos results in a decreased support of the upper eyelid, which in turn leads to a secondary pseudoptosis and an upper eyelid sulcus deformity (Fig. 25.5).

Headache/Nausea/Vomiting/Bradycardia
In pediatric patients with a "white-eyed blowout fracture", the symptoms of headache with nausea and vomiting associated with a bradycardia, may be misinterpreted as signs of blunt head trauma requiring admission to hospital for head injury observations. These symptoms and signs in the presence of such a fracture are produced by the oculocardiac reflex.

Clinical Evaluation
Any patient who has sustained blunt orbital trauma should undergo a complete ophthalmic examination to exclude associated ocular injuries (Table 25.1 and Fig. 25.6). The incidence of ocular injuries has been reported as 14% to 30%. The possibility of a globe rupture must always be considered and excluded before a forced duction test is performed.

Any proptosis or enophthalmos should be measured using a Hertel exophthalmometer. Any vertical displacement of the globe should also be measured and recorded. The eyelids and periorbital tissues should be palpated for subcutaneous emphysema and for any orbital rim fractures. The malar eminences should be palpated and any depression or displacement noted (Fig. 25.7).

The patient should be asked to open and close his/her mouth to ensure there is no associated pain or trismus. Such signs and symptoms are suggestive of a zygomatic complex fracture. A record of the extent of any infraorbital sensory loss should be made.

A full orthoptic assessment should be performed with prism measurements in nine positions of gaze, a Hess chart, and a monocular and binocular visual field assessment. A forced duction test and an active force-generation test should be performed. Prior to the performance of a forced duction test, a cotton-tipped applicator is soaked with topical anesthetic drops and held against the limbus for a few minutes. The patient should be recumbent. Fine-toothed forceps are then used to grasp the conjunctiva and Tenon's capsule just posterior to the limbus. The patient is then asked to look in the direction of restriction of movement of the eye

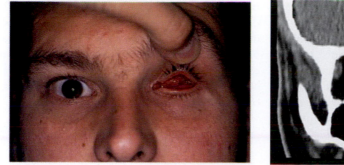

(A)

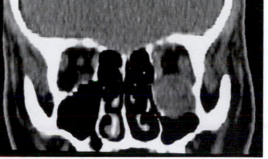

(B)

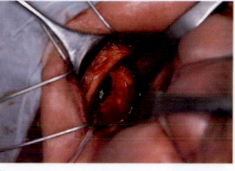

(C)

Figure 25.3 (**A**) This patient was referred for the management of an apparent anophthalmic socket. (**B**) A coronal CT scan of the patient demonstrating an extensive orbital floor blowout fracture with the globe prolapsed into the maxillary antrum. (**C**) The position of the globe below the inferior orbital margin seen intraoperatively.

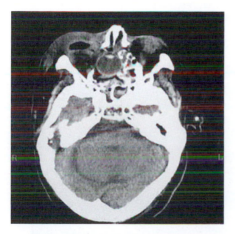

Figure 25.4 An extensive medial orbital wall and orbital floor blowout fracture with the globe prolapsed into the ethmoid sinus and nasal cavity.

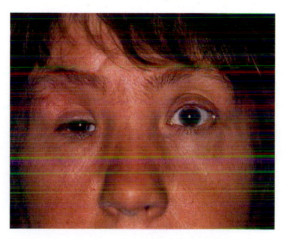

Figure 25.5 A patient demonstrating enophthalmos, ptosis and an upper lid sulcus deformity following extensive orbital floor and medial wall blowout fractures.

while the examiner attempts to move the globe in the same direction (Fig. 25.8). A patient with tissue entrapment will usually experience pain on attempted globe movement in the direction of restriction. The results of this test need to be interpreted with caution. If the examiner is unable to move the globe normally, this implies entrapment of the inferior orbital septa, but a positive forced duction test can also be caused by extraocular muscle/orbital hematoma and edema. A strongly positive forced duction test, in a patient with evidence of a blowout fracture on a computed tomography (CT) scan, does suggest tissue entrapment as the cause of ocular restriction.

In an active force-generation test, the globe is again grasped with fine-toothed forceps and the patient asked to

try as hard as possible to move the eye in the direction of action of the muscle under investigation. The examiner can feel muscle contraction from a tug on the forceps. An active

Table 25.1 Ocular Injuries Complicating Blowout Fractures

Globe rupture	Lens subluxation
Retinal tears	Traumatic cataract
Retinal dialysis	Choroidal rupture
Vitreous hemorrhage	Commotio retinae
Angle recession	Macular scarring
Hyphema	Traumatic mydriasis

force-generation test is useful in differentiating extraocular muscle paralysis from tissue entrapment.

If a patient has symptoms and signs suggestive of an orbital wall blowout fracture, a CT scan should be performed in an axial plane with coronal and sagittal reconstructions (Fig. 25.9). With modern CT scanners, this investigation can be performed very quickly. Images available in three planes are extremely valuable in assessing the full extent of the injury. A plain skull X-ray is of little use in the evaluation of a blowout

fracture. A CT scan demonstrates the relationship of the soft tissues to the fracture sites, permits an evaluation of any secondary effects of trauma, e.g., retrobulbar hemorrhage, intra-optic nerve sheath hematoma, subperiosteal hematoma, and can help to demonstrate any complications of trauma, e.g., orbital cellulitis, orbital or subperiosteal abscess, and retained orbital foreign bodies.

> **KEY POINT**
>
> In a pediatric patient with a "white eyed blowout fracture", there may be very little evidence of a fracture on a CT scan and the scan may be reported by a radiologist as showing no fracture.

Management

Patients should be urged not to blow their nose or to hold the nose when sneezing. The role of antibiotic prophylaxis is controversial. If the CT scan shows evidence of chronic sinusitis, antibiotics should be prescribed to prevent a secondary orbital cellulitis (Fig. 25.10).

A number of different surgical specialties may be involved in the management of patients with an orbital wall blowout fracture(s), and opinions differ concerning the indications for surgery, the timing of surgery, the surgical approach, and the use of orbital implant materials. Although there are guidelines, which can be used to advise the patient about surgical intervention, each

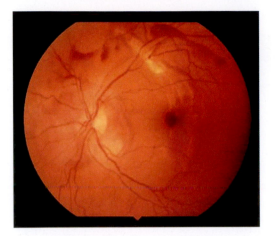

Figure 25.6 A choroidal rupture, macular haemorrhage and widespread retinal haemorrhages following blung ocular trauma.

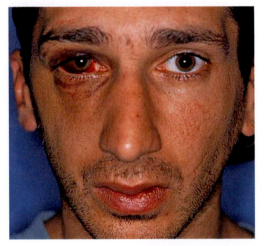

(A)

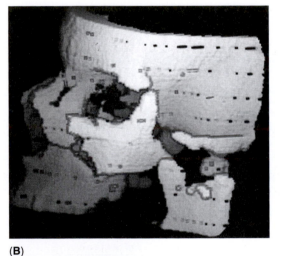

(B)

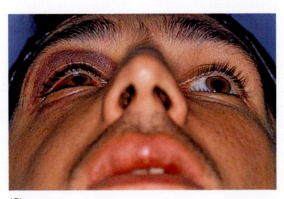

(C)

Figure 25.7 (**A**) Patient with a right zygomatic complex fracture showing a depression over the right malar eminence. (**B**) The abnormality is better appreciated from below. (**C**) This three-dimensional CT scan reconstruction demonstrates why the patient is experiencing trismus.

patient should be managed on an individual basis, after a careful consideration of the pros, cons, risks, and potential complications of such surgical intervention. In general, the indications for the surgical repair of a blowout fracture are:

- Unresolving soft tissue entrapment with disabling diplopia
- Enophthalmos greater than 2 mm
- CT scan evidence of a large fracture

Patients with diplopia are observed for a period of approximately 2 to 3 weeks. If the diplopia resolves with a small fracture evident on CT, no surgical intervention is required.

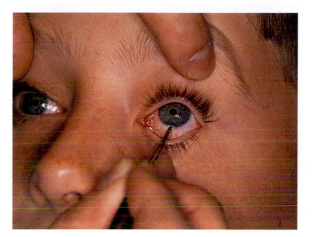

Figure 25.8 A forced duction test.

There is an important exception to this. Pediatric patients with marked tissue entrapment and a linear fracture on a CT scan (a "trapdoor" fracture) are at risk of developing an ischemic contracture unless the tissue entrapment is released very early (Figs. 25.11–25.14). This is an indication for very early surgery.

KEY POINT

An orbital wall blowout fracture in a pediatric patient should be evaluated urgently and in the presence of restriction of ocular motility may require surgical intervention without delay.

It is reasonable to defer operative decisions on the basis of the degree of enophthalmos for 2 to 3 weeks to determine with the patient whether or not the enophthalmos is cosmetically significant. This allows orbital edema and any hematoma to resolve, which in turn makes the surgery somewhat easier to perform. Extensive defects, particularly involving both the orbital floor and medial wall, suggest a high chance of progressive unsightly enophthalmos and support the decision for surgical intervention. The patient must be fully informed of the risks and potential complications of such surgery, *including the risk of blindness* (see below).

Surgical Management

The surgical approach is the same whether the surgery is performed early (within 2 to 3 weeks of the trauma) or is delayed. It is essential to use an operating headlight and magnifying surgical loupes. The surgery is performed under general anesthesia.

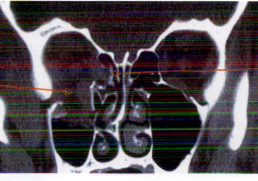

Orbital floor blowout fracture

Medial orbital wall blowout fracture

(A)

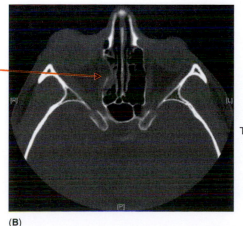

Medial orbital wall blowout fracture

(B)

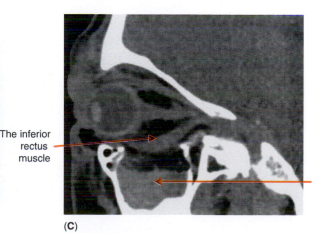

The inferior rectus muscle

Blood in the maxillary sinus

(C)

Figure 25.9 (**A**) A coronal CT scan demonstrating orbital floor and medial orbital wall blowout fractures. (**B**) An axial CT scan demonstrating a medial orbital wall blowout fracture. (**C**) A sagittal CT scan demonstrating an extensive orbital floor blowout fracture extending to the posterior limit of the maxillary sinus.

An orbital floor blowout fracture is usually approached via a lower eyelid incision. There is very rarely an indication for a Caldwell–Luc approach in which an opening is made into the maxillary sinus in the area of the superior gingiva. A medial wall fracture can also be repaired via the same lower eyelid incision. Alternatively, a transcaruncular approach can be used. If a patient already has a significant eyelid laceration in association with the fracture, this can be utilized for access to the fracture.

The lower eyelid incision can be made through the skin or through the conjunctiva (Fig. 25.15). The preferred incision is transconjunctival via a "swinging lower eyelid" flap approach (Fig. 25.16). This provides excellent access to the whole of the orbital floor and to the medial orbital wall. For the management of small "trapdoor" orbital floor fractures, the transconjunctival approach without a lateral canthotomy and inferior cantholysis is adequate. If preferred, a transcutaneous approach is adequate for relatively small fractures, and the lateral canthus is not disturbed. The resultant subciliary scar, if the wound is properly constructed, closed, and cared for postoperatively with massage, is barely visible (see Fig. 25.14).

The majority of orbital floor fractures involve the postero-medial aspect of the orbital floor, which is adjacent to the inferior orbital groove and the infraorbital canal. The infraorbital nerve is at risk from injury during the dissection as are the infraorbital artery and vein. Great care must

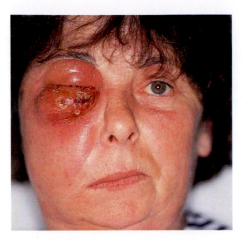

Figure 25.10 This patient sustained an orbital floor blowout fracture following accidental blunt trauma. She represented to the A&E Department 2 days later with a severe orbital cellulitis and a blind eye.

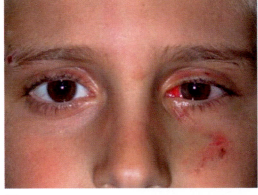

(A)

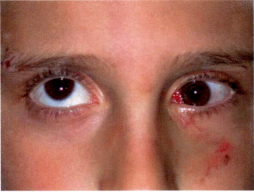

(B)

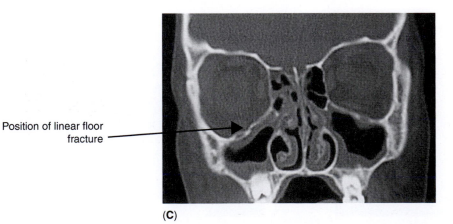

Position of linear floor fracture

(C)

Figure 25.11 (**A**) A boy presenting with diplopia on upgaze 2 days following blunt trauma to the left orbit. (**B**) Marked limitation of upgaze. A forced duction test was markedly positive. Early surgical release of the entrapped tissue is indicated. (**C**) A coronal CT scan of same patient. The radiographic images may be misleading in the absence of any obvious bony displacement.

be taken with the dissection to avoid damage to these vascular structures. Thermocautery should be used sparingly to avoid damage to the infraorbital nerve. All margins of the fracture should be exposed and prolapsing structures

Linear 'trapdoor' fracture of the orbital floor
after release of entrapped orbital contents

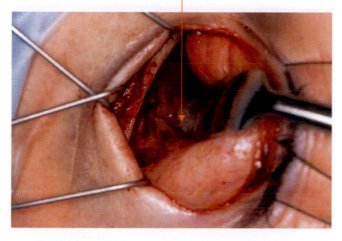

Figure 25.12 The same patient as in Figure 25.12 demonstrating a linear fracture of the orbital floor in which orbital tissue was entrapped. The tissue was released with full recovery of ocular motility. No orbital floor implant was required.

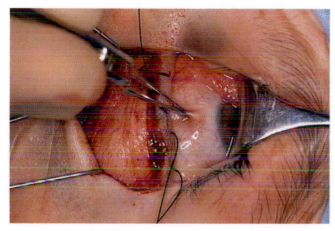

Figure 25.13 The forced duction test is repeated after release of the entrapped orbital tissue.

repositioned in the orbit. Overly aggressive dissection posteriorly risks damage to the optic nerve and other orbital apical structures.

KEY POINT

It is useful to use a piece of Supramid with a Sewell retractor to help to keep prolapsing orbital fat from the surgical field during the orbital dissection.

TRANSCONJUNCTIVAL APPROACH

This approach utilizes an incision through the conjunctiva of the lower eyelid, usually combined with a lateral canthotomy and an inferior cantholysis. The eyelid is thereby detached from the lateral orbital rim and swung inferiorly (a "swinging eyelid flap" approach).

Surgical Approach

1. A forced duction test is performed and the findings recorded.
2. A lateral canthal incision 5 to 8 mm in length is marked along a skin crease with gentian violet.
3. 1.5 to 2 ml of 0.5% Bupivacaine with 1:200,000 units of adrenaline mixed 50:50 with 2% lidocaine with 1:80,000 units of adrenaline are injected subcutaneously into the lower eyelid and lateral canthus. It is important to avoid any subconjunctival injections as these will affect the pupil.
4. The patient is prepped and draped leaving the fellow eye uncovered so that the symmetry of the globe positions can be compared and, if necessary, pupillary reactions to light assessed. The fellow eye should be protected with the instillation of Lacrilube ointment.
5. A 4/0 silk traction suture is passed through the gray line of the lower eyelid.
6. A lateral canthal skin incision is made along the previously marked crease using a Colorado needle. The incision is deepened to expose the periosteum of the lateral orbital margin.
7. Next, a lateral canthotomy is performed using the Colorado needle or using blunt-tipped Westcott scissors.

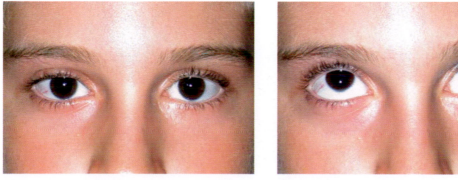

(A)   (B)

Figure 25.14 (**A**) The same patient as in Figures 25.11–25.13 12 months following release of the entrapped orbital tissue. (**B**) The limitation of upgaze has completely resolved.

8. The lower eyelid is then everted over a small Desmarres retractor. The silk suture is fixated to the face drapes using a small curved artery clip.

9. A conjunctival incision is made just below the inferior border of the tarsus extending from just below the inferior punctum to the lateral canthus using the Colorado needle.

10. Hemostasis is achieved using bipolar cautery when required.

11. A plane of dissection is created anterior to the orbital septum (Fig. 25.15). The orbicularis muscle is clearly seen using the bloodless approach with a Colorado needle and the dissection is continued keeping immediately posterior to this muscle.

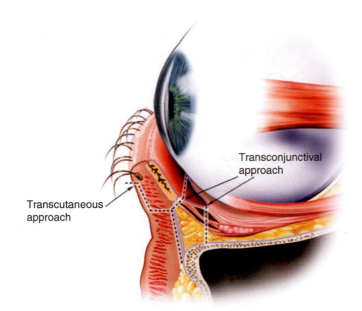

Figure 25.15 A diagram showing the planes of dissection when exposing the inferior orbital margin using a transcutaneous or a transconjunctival approach.

12. This plane is dissected all the way to the inferior orbital margin.

13. 4/0 silk traction sutures are placed through the medial and lateral aspects of the conjunctival/ lower eyelid retractor complex. The sutures are then fixated to the forehead drapes using curved artery clips to protect the cornea during the rest of the surgery. Care is taken to ensure that the sutures are pulled up on either side of the globe and do not abrade the cornea.

14. Jaffe lid retractors are inserted into the wound and fixated to the face drapes using curved artery clips.

15. Using the Colorado needle the periosteum is incised 2 mm below the rim commencing medially and carrying this incision to a slightly lower position laterally (Fig. 25.16).

16. The periosteum is elevated from the underlying bone using the sharp end of a Freer periosteal elevator.

17. The periorbita is then elevated from the orbital floor medially using the Freer periosteal elevator.

18. The blade of a Sewall retractor is placed carefully into the subperiosteal space and the orbital contents are retracted (Fig. 25.17).

19. A constant vessel is encountered along the center of the orbital floor passing from the infraorbital neurovascular bundle to the orbit. This should be cauterized as it enters the periorbita and cut with Westcott scissors.

20. The margins of the fracture are carefully exposed using the Freer periosteal elevator taking care to release the pressure on the retractors at regular intervals. The patient's pupil is also checked at regular intervals.

21. Once the prolapsing orbital contents have been lifted out of the fracture site, a forced duction test is repeated. This should now demonstrate unrestricted movement of the globe.

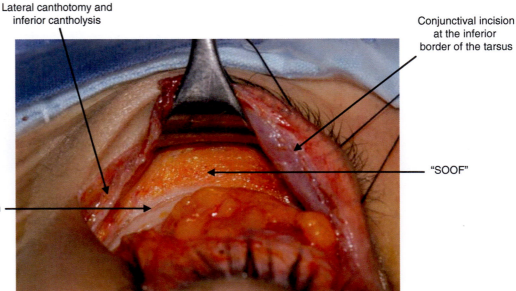

Figure 25.16 A "swinging eyelid" flap approach to the inferior orbital margin.

22. A Supramid sheet is cut to the appropriate size and shape.
23. The implant is placed over the fracture site ensuring that all margins are covered and that no tissue is allowed to herniate from the orbit again. The implant should be of an adequate size and shape to fulfill this objective. The posterior margin of the fracture should be adequately exposed; this helps to support the implant, preventing it from prolapsing into the maxillary antrum or into the ethmoid sinus (Fig. 25.18).
24. The Supramid sheet is removed and used as a template against which the definitive orbital implant to be used is cut to size.

KEY POINT

It is very important to avoid the use of an unnecessarily large implant, to avoid compression of orbital apical structures. Likewise, it is important not to place the implant too far posteriorly in the orbit. The forced duction test should be repeated to ensure that the movement of the globe remains unrestricted. The globe position should also be compared with that of the fellow eye to ensure that a hyperglobus has not been created.

---

25. Fixation of an implant is usually unnecessary. To prevent migration of the implant anteriorly, two small relieving incisions can be made into the anterior margin of the implant and part of the implant folded inferiorly to lie within the anterior aspect of the fracture.
26. If the fracture is so large that there is no posterior support for the implant, the implant should then be cantilevered over the fracture with microplates, which are fixated below the inferior orbital margin with screws (Fig. 25.19).
27. The edges of the periosteum are identified over the inferior orbital margin and closed with interrupted 5/0 Vicryl sutures, taking care to ensure that

the orbital septum is not inadvertently included in the closure as this will cause retraction of the lower eyelid.
28. The conjunctiva and inferior retractors are reapproximated to the inferior border of the tarsus with interrupted 7/0 Vicryl sutures ensuring that the knots are buried.
29. The lateral aspect of the tarsus is attached to the periosteum of the lateral orbital margin using a single 5/0 Vicryl suture.
30. The 4/0 silk traction suture is removed and antibiotic ointment instilled into the eye.
31. A compressive dressing is applied.

Postoperative Care

The compressive dressing is removed in the recovery room as soon as the patient is awake and co-operative. The patient's visual acuity and pupil reactions are checked. These are checked hourly for the first 12 hours postoperatively to ensure that the visual acuity does not diminish in the event of a sudden retrobulbar hemorrhage. The patient should also be monitored regularly for the development of orbital pain or proptosis. Ice packs are applied intermittently and the patient's head is kept elevated. Postoperative lower eyelid massage is commenced in a vertical direction 5 days after surgery to prevent wound contracture and any eyelid retraction. This is undertaken for approximately 3 min three times a day after the application of Lacrilube ointment to the eyelid skin for a period of 6 weeks. Prophylactic broad-spectrum antibiotics are prescribed for 7 days postoperatively. The patient must be instructed not to blow the nose or hold the nose when sneezing for 6 weeks postoperatively.

TRANSCUTANEOUS APPROACH

The subciliary skin incision is the preferred transcutaneous approach although in some patients a lower lid skin crease incision provides a quick exposure with a good postoperative scar. An incision placed directly over the inferior orbital margin should be avoided as this is cosmetically unsatisfactory and is associated with prolonged postoperative eyelid lymphedema.

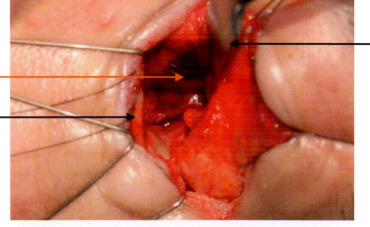

Orbital floor fracture —

The inferior orbital margin —

Sewall retractor —

Figure 25.17 The orbital floor fracture is being exposed via a "swinging lower eyelid" flap approach.

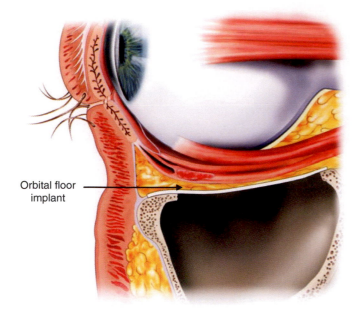

Orbital floor implant

Figure 25.18 An orbital implant placed over margins of orbital floor blowout fracture. No fixation of the implant should normally be required.

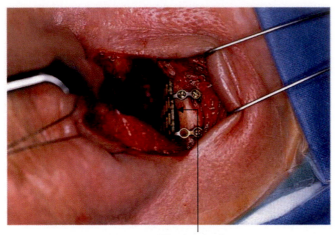

Titanium implant

Figure 25.19 A titanium orbital implant fixated with screws to the inferior orbital margin and cantilevered back to the posterior margin of the fracture.

Surgical Approach

1. 1.5 to 2 ml of 0.5% Bupivacaine with 1:200,000 units of adrenaline mixed 50:50 with 2% lidocaine with 1:80,000 units of adrenaline are injected subcutaneously into the lower eyelid.
2. A 4/0 silk traction suture is passed through the gray line of the lower eyelid and fixated to the head drapes with a curved artery clip. This places the lower eyelid tissues under tension to assist with the dissection through the tissue planes but it also permits the complete protection of the eye from the surgical instruments.
3. A subciliary skin incision is made with a Colorado needle.
4. The skin is separated from the pretarsal orbicularis muscle with blunt-tipped Westcott scissors.
5. The orbicularis muscle is then opened below the tarsus using the Colorado needle, exposing the underlying orbital septum.

6. The rest of the procedure is undertaken as described above.
7. The skin is closed with interrupted 7/0 Vicryl sutures.

Postoperative Care
This is as described above.

ORBITAL IMPLANT MATERIALS
A variety of autogenous and synthetic materials have been used to cover an orbital wall blowout fracture, including silicone, Teflon, supramid, gelfilm, hydroxyapatite, methylmethacrylate, titanium, autogenous cartilage, and autogenous bone. Autogenous bone can be harvested from the iliac crest or from the outer table of the skull. This entails a lengthier operation, a longer in-patient stay and risks donor site morbidity and complications. The author's preference is porous polyethylene (Medpor), which is easy to cut and shape to the precise dimensions required. It lends good support for the majority of fractures and becomes ingrown by fibrovascular tissue. For larger fractures, channeled Medpor or a Medpor Titan are preferred to lend greater support for the orbital contents, particularly when there is a large orbital floor fracture combined with a large medial wall fracture (see Figs. 25.20 and 25.21).

Delayed Treatment of Diplopia
Long-term motility problems are quite rare in all types of orbital wall blowout fracture, with the exception of the linear "trapdoor" fracture in the young. Spontaneous improvement in motility with resolution of diplopia is more common over a period of weeks to months whether a surgical repair of the fracture has been undertaken or not. There may be residual diplopia even after a successful repair of the fracture if there has been extraocular muscle or neuronal damage. Diplopia can, however, occur in the presence of normal extraocular muscles but with a large fracture and a markedly displaced globe. This is due to a change in the line of muscle pull. Such patients have clinically significant enophthalmos and the decision to proceed with a surgical repair of the fracture is made on this basis.

A period of 4 to 6 months should be permitted to allow the diplopia to resolve or stabilize. Temporary relief can be provided with Fresnel prisms, which can be easily changed as alterations in the pattern of motility defect occur. Diplopia that does not resolve may not require any treatment if the patient is not disadvantaged by it, e.g., diplopia which occurs only in an extreme gaze position. Alternatively, a permanent spectacle prism may be considered or strabismus surgery may be required.

In general, the goals of strabismus surgery following an orbital wall blowout fracture are to either enhance the action of the underacting muscles or weaken the action of the secondarily overacting muscles. The inverse Knapp procedure involves the transposition of the medial and lateral recti to the inferior rectus insertion to enhance the degree of depression of the affected eye. This can be combined with a recession of the inferior rectus, where this muscle shows contracture. A forced duction test must be performed before making a decision to recess this muscle. The risk of the development of anterior segment ischemia must also be taken into consideration. Surgery on

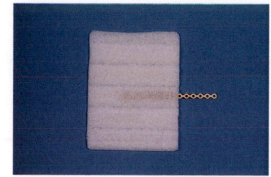

(A)

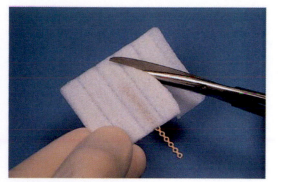

(B)

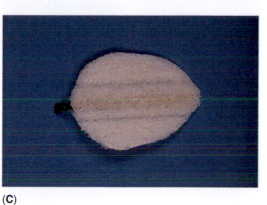

(C)

Figure 25.20 (**A**) A channeled Medpor implant. (**B**) The implant is cut to the appropriate size and shape using a template (usually a sheet of Supramid). (**C**) The implant ready for insertion to cover a large orbital floor fracture.

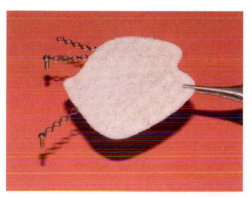

(A)

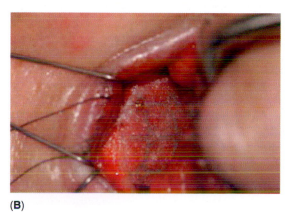

(B)

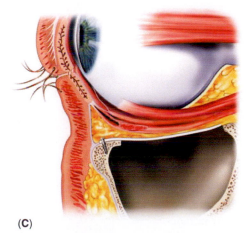

(C)

Figure 25.21 (**A**) A Medpor Titan orbital floor implant shown with titanium screws. (**B**) A Medpor Titan orbital floor implant has been placed over the orbital floor blowout fracture and the implant has been fixated to the inferior orbital margin using a titanium screw. The protruding titanium plates were redundant in this case and have been removed. (**C**) A drawing showing the orbital floor implant screwed to the inferior orbital margin in a case where the implant could not be fixated to a posterior bony lip. The implant has instead been cantilevered in this position.

other extraocular muscles may also be required to improve the field of binocular single vision. Patients must be counseled carefully prior to this surgery to ensure that they have realistic expectations. Such surgery should be undertaken by a surgeon expert in the management of ocular motility disorders.

COMPLICATIONS OF ORBITAL WALL BLOWOUT FRACTURE SURGERY
Blindness
Postoperative blindness is a rare complication. Nevertheless, the risk of this complication should be discussed with patients preoperatively and the risk weighed against the potential benefits of a surgical repair. It may be caused by:

- Intraoperative damage to the globe and/or optic nerve
- Postoperative orbital hemorrhage
- Compression of the optic nerve by misplacement of the orbital implant

Every precaution should be taken to prevent the occurrence of blindness. The development of any intraoperative enlargement of the pupil should be a cause for concern and should be investigated. A swinging flashlight test can be undertaken to exclude the presence of a relative afferent pupil defect and the fundus should be examined.

KEY POINTS

A ruptured globe must be excluded before a patient undergoes an orbital wall blowout fracture repair

Pressure applied to retractors in the orbit must be released at regular intervals

The patient's pupil should be monitored intraoperatively at regular intervals

Meticulous hemostasis must be obtained before closure of the wounds is undertaken

The patient's vision must be monitored on recovery from general anesthesia and at regular intervals thereafter for at least 12 hours

Great care must be taken to ensure that the orbital implant is of the correct size and shape and is not forced into the orbit beyond the posterior limit of the fracture

---

Diplopia
It is important to warn patients that it is not uncommon for diplopia to be worse in the first few weeks following surgery as a consequence of iatrogenic trauma from the surgical dissection to free entrapped orbital contents. It is important, however, to ensure that further inadvertent tissue entrapment has not been caused by misplacement of the orbital implant. For this reason, the forced duction test must be repeated after placement of the orbital implant.

Lower Lid Retraction
Lower eyelid retraction may be caused by:

- Incorrect closure of the periosteum over the infraorbital margin with inadvertent incorporation of the orbital septum in the sutures
- Adhesions of the orbital septum to the infraorbital margin (Fig. 25.22)

Careful identification of the periosteal edges will avoid incorrect wound closure. Adhesions can be avoided by ensuring a meticulous dissection between the orbicularis oculi and the orbital septum, preventing any hematoma, and by early and prolonged postoperative eyelid massage.

The surgical correction of postoperative lower lid retraction is difficult. This is managed via a conjunctival incision at the lower border of the tarsus, with a recession of the conjunctiva and the lower lid retractors, and a dissection of all adhesions to the inferior orbital margin. A spacer, e.g., a hard palate graft or dermal graft, is then interposed between the lower lid retractors and the lower border of the tarsus. In cases where there are extensive adhesions to the inferior orbital margin with a loss of preaponeurotic fat, a dermis fat graft is placed over the rim to prevent further adhesions.

Lower Lid Entropion
A lower lid entropion may very rarely occur after contracture of the wound following a transconjunctival approach to an orbital floor fracture (Fig. 25.23). It is managed in a similar manner to lower lid retraction.

Implant Extrusion
Extrusion of an orbital implant may occur early or late after surgery for a blowout fracture. It may be seen many years after surgery (Figs. 25.24 and 25.25). It may occur for a number of following reasons:

- Infection
- The use of an oversized implant
- Inadequate closure of the periosteum along the inferior orbital margin

In the presence of an infection, the implant has to be removed. Further surgery can be undertaken later when the infection has resolved. An over-sized implant can be removed and exchanged for an appropriate size. Late extrusion requires the removal of the implant but usually no replacement is required as the fracture site will have healed and the risk of the subsequent development of significant enophthalmos is small.

Infection
Although an infection must be treated with systemic antibiotics, the implant will usually require removal.

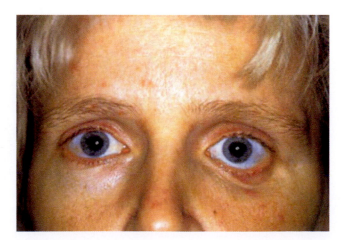

Figure 25.22 Left lower eyelid retraction following an orbital floor blowout fracture repair performed via a subciliary transcutaneous approach.

Infraorbital Sensory Loss

Patients should be warned about the potential for sensory loss in the distribution of the infraorbital nerve. Great care should be taken not to cause unnecessary intraoperative trauma to the nerve and to remove any bone fragments which impinge on the nerve. Identification of the nerve may be difficult in the late management of large orbital floor fractures.

UNDERCORRECTION OF ENOPHTHALMOS

Residual enophthalmos is usually the result of:

- Failure to reposition all prolapsed orbital tissues

- Failure to place the orbital implant over the whole of the fracture (Fig. 25.26)
- Failure to treat any additional medial wall fracture

Although post-traumatic orbital fat atrophy can occur, this is usually overstated and the real cause of residual enophthalmos overlooked.

PROPTOSIS/HYPERGLOBUS

Proptosis or hyperglobus may occur from the use of oversized orbital implants, e.g., autogenous bone grafts (Fig. 25.27). Care should be taken during surgery to avoid this complication by

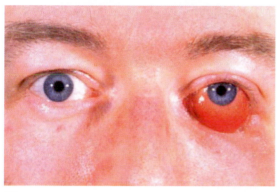

(A)

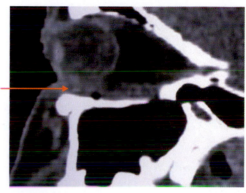

The lower lid is lying along the anterior aspect of the orbital floor

(B)

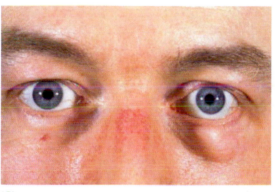

(C)

Figure 25.23 (**A**) Severe lower eyelid contracture and chemosis following infection of an orbital floor silastic implant. (**B**) A CT scan demonstrating the position of the lower eyelid. (**C**) The result following removal of the implant and insertion of a dermis fat graft to prevent adhesion of the lower eyelid to the inferior orbital margin.

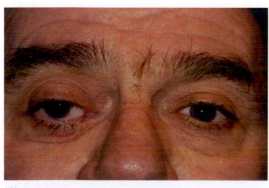

(A)

Inferior fornix foreign body granuloma overlying an extruding silicone implant

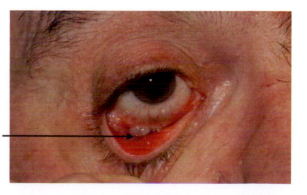

(B)

Figure 25.24 (**A**) A patient complaining of a sore discharging eye. He had undergone an orbital floor blowout fracture repair 15 years earlier. (**B**) An examination of his inferior fornix revealed a foreign body granuloma and an extruding silicone orbital floor implant.

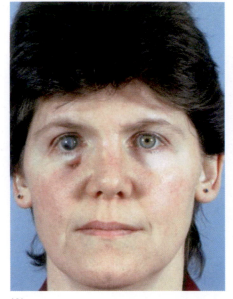
(A)

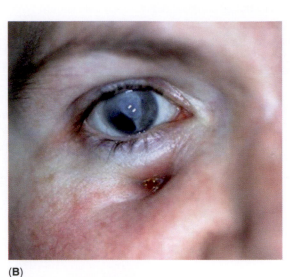
(B)

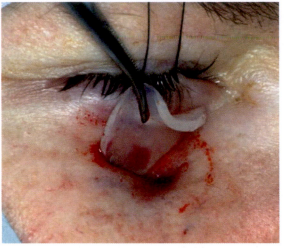

(C)

Figure 25.25 (**A**) A patient who presented with a discharging sinus in the lower eyelid. She had undergone the repair of an orbital floor blowout fracture 15 years earlier. (**B**) A close-up photograph of her lower eyelid sinus. She had also suffered a penetrating eye injury previously. (**C**) A silicone orbital floor implant was removed on exploring the lower eyelid sinus.

comparing the intraoperative position of the globe with that of the fellow globe in unilateral cases.

Cyst Formation
Synthetic implants can be associated with the development of cysts which can result in a displacement of the globe and diplopia (Fig. 25.28). Rarely such cysts can be associated with a spontaneous orbital hemorrhage which can be sight-threatening.

Lower Lid Lymphedema
Lower lid lymphedema is usually seen following the use of a skin incision directly over the inferior orbital margin. Such an incision leaves an unsightly scar, predisposes the patient to implant extrusion and should be avoided unless there is already a laceration in this location.

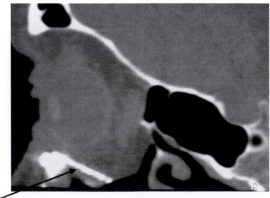
Orbital floor implant

Figure 25.26 A malpositioned and inadequately sized orbital floor implant.

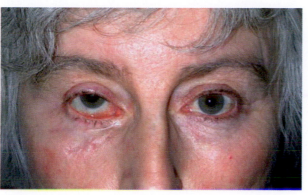

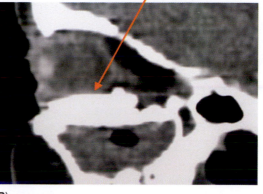

A very bulky calvarial
bone graft lying along the
orbital floor

(A)   (B)

Figure 25.27 (**A**) A patient seen 6 weeks following the repair of an orbital floor blowout fracture undertaken by a maxillo-facial surgeon using a calvarial bone graft. She has a right hyperglobus and lower eyelid retraction. (**B**) A sagittal CT scan of the same patient demonstrating that an inappropriately sized bone graft is the cause of the hyperglobus.

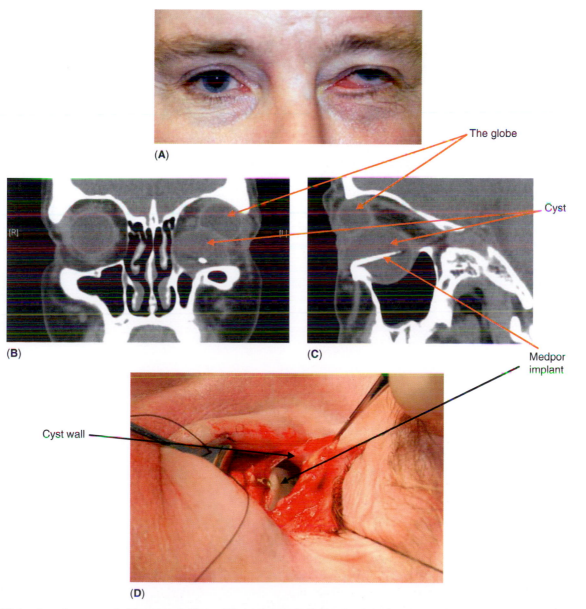

Figure 25.28 (**A**) A patient who presented with an acute left hyperglobus and diplopia after previously undergoing an orbital floor fracture repair using a channeled Medpor implant. (**B**) A coronal CT scan demonstrating a large intraorbital cyst. (**C**) A sagittal CT scan demonstrating the size and posterior extension of the cyst. (**D**) An intraoperative photograph of the cyst being opened and the channeled Medpor implant being exposed prior to its removal.

Chemosis

Postoperative chemosis is more commonly seen following a transconjunctival approach to the repair of an orbital wall blowout fracture. It is rarely severe and usually resolves with the use of topical lubricants.

FURTHER READING

1. Albert DM, Lucarelli MJ. Orbital fractures: diagnosis and management. In: Clinical Atlas of Procedures in Ophthalmic Surgery. Chicago, IL: AMA Press, 2004: 347–59.
2. American Academy of Ophthalmology. Basic and clinical science course: orbit, eyelids, and lacrimal system, section 7. San Francisco, CA: The American Academy of Ophthalmology, 2006/7: 97–108, 184–7.
3. Belli E, Matteini C, Mazzone N. Evolution in diagnosis and repairing of orbital medial wall fractures. J Craniofac Surg 2009; 20: 191–3.
4. Berkowitz RA, Putterman AM, Patel DB. Prolapse of the globe into the maxillary sinus after orbital floor fracture. Am J Ophthalmol 1981; 91: 253–7.
5. Cole P, Kaufman Y, Hollier L. Principles of facial trauma: orbital fracture management. J Craniofac Surg 2009; 20: 101–4.
6. Dutton GN, Al-Qurainy I, Stassen LFA, et al. Ophthalmic consequences of mid-facial trauma. Eye 1992; 6: 86–9.
7. Dutton JJ. Atlas of Clinical and Surgical Orbital Anatomy. Philadelphia, PA: WB Saunders, 1994.
8. Holck DE, Ng JD. Evaluation and Treatment of Orbital Fractures. Philadelphia, PA: Saunders, 2005.
9. Jordan DR, Allen LH, White J, Harvery J, Pashby R, Esmaeli B. Intervention within days for some orbital floor fractures: the white-eyed blowout. Ophthal Plast Reconstr Surg 1998; 14: 379–90.
10. Jordan DR, St Onge P, Anderson RL, Patrinely JR, Nerad JA. Complications associated with alloplastic implants used in orbital fracture repair. Ophthalmology 1992; 99(10): 1600-8.
11. Jordan DR, White GL, Anderson RL, Thiese SM. Orbital emphysema: a potentially blinding complication following orbital fractures. Ann Emerg Med 1988; 17: 853–5.
12. Koornneef L. Orbital septa: anatomy and functions. Ophthalmology 1979; 86: 876–80.
13. Lyon DB, Newman SA. Evidence of direct damage to extraocular muscles as a cause of diplopia following orbital trauma. Ophthal Plast Reconstr Surg 1989; 5: 81–91.
14. McGurk M, Whitehouse RW, Taylor PM, Swinson B. Orbital volume measured by a low-dose CT scanning technique. Dentomaxillofac Radiol 1992; 21: 70–2.
15. Putterman AM, Stevens T, Urist MJ. Nonsurgical management of blowout fractures of the orbital floor. Am J Ophthalmol 1974; 77: 232–9.
16. Putterman AM. Management of orbital fractures: the conservative approach. Surv Ophthalmol 1991; 92: 523–8.
17. Rubin PA, Bilyk JR, Shore JW. Orbital reconstruction using porous polyethylene sheets. Ophthalmology 1994; 101: 1697–708.
18. Smith B, Lisman RD, Simonton J, Della Rocca R. Volkmann's contracture of the extraocular muscles following blowout fracture. Plast Reconstr Surg 1984; 74: 200–9.
19. Smith B, Regan WF. Blow-out fractures of the orbit. Mechanism and correction of internal orbital fracture. Am J Ophthalmol 1957; 11: 733–9.
20. Nerad JA. Techniques in Ophthalmic Plastic Surgery—A Personal Tutorial(ISBN: 978-1-4377-0008-4) Philadelphia, PA: Elsevier Inc., 2010: 113–26, 355–87.
21. Westfall CT, Shore JW. Isolated fractures of the orbital floor: risk of infection and the role of antibiotic prophylaxis. Ophthalmic Surg 1991; 22: 409–11.

26 Zygomatic complex fractures

INTRODUCTION

A zygomatic complex fracture refers to a traumatic displacement of the zygoma and is often referred to as a tripod or tripartite fracture. This usually involves three areas of dislocation: the area of the fronto-zygomatic suture, the zygomatico-maxillary suture, and the zygomatic arch (Figs. 26.1 and 26.2).

ETIOLOGY

Zygomatic fractures usually occur following direct blunt trauma to the cheek.

DIAGNOSIS

The presence of a zygomatic complex fracture should be suspected in any patient who has sustained blunt trauma to the cheek. The patient should be observed from below, looking for malar flattening. This may, however, be masked by edema. The patient should be asked to open the mouth, looking for trismus (Fig. 26.3). The orbital margin should be carefully palpated for gaps, steps, and areas of tenderness. A neurosensory examination of the area should be performed, as hypoesthesia or anesthesia of the lower eyelid and cheek may be present. Imaging should be performed if there is a clinical suspicion of such a fracture.

CLINICAL SIGNS

Flattening of the cheek is usually noted (Fig. 26.4).

Palpation of the inferior orbital margin may reveal gaps or steps. *The signs and symptoms of such a fracture depend on the degree of displacement of the zygoma and the direction of the displacement*. The lower eyelid may be dragged inferiorly, the lateral canthus may be displaced inferiorly, or there may be a bulge in the lateral cheek area (Fig. 26.5).

There is usually an associated orbital floor fracture with enophthalmos but rarely signs of soft tissue entrapment. The fracture may be associated with other fractures, e.g., inferior orbital rim fractures.

MANAGEMENT

If the fracture is very minor, with no significant displacement of the zygoma, the patient should be managed conservatively. No surgery is indicated.

There are two basic surgical approaches for the management of a zygomatic complex fracture:

1. Gillies temporal approach
2. Direct approach

Gillies Temporal Approach

This approach is used where the fractures are regular, recent, and the displaced bone fragment is impacted on adjacent bone. A 5-cm incision is made approximately 2 to 3 cm behind the hairline over the temporal fossa, avoiding the superficial temporal vessels. The deep temporalis fascia is located and incised, exposing the underlying temporalis muscle (Fig. 26.6).

Blunt dissection is performed in the plane between the temporalis fascia and the temporalis muscle. A Kilner elevator is then inserted and the blade manipulated under the zygoma (Fig. 26.7). The instrument is then used to disimpact the bone fragment. This approach has the advantage of being relatively simple and fast but it does not permit an inspection of any associated orbital floor fracture.

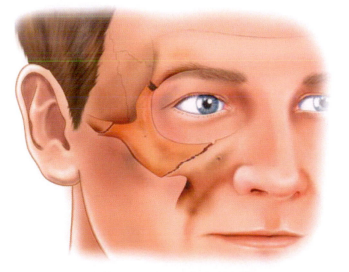

Figure 26.1 A right zygomatic complex fracture demonstrating the areas of dislocation of the zygomatic bone.

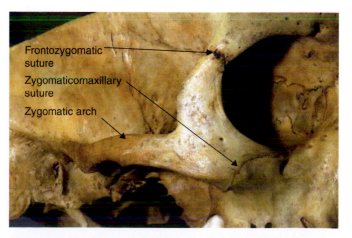

Frontozygomatic suture

Zygomaticomaxillary suture

Zygomatic arch

Figure 26.2 A lateral view of a skull demonstrating the potentially weak areas of the zygoma.

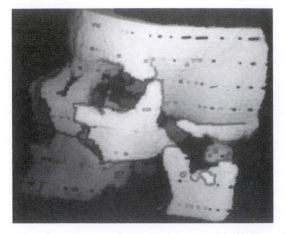

Figure 26.3 A three-dimensional CT scan reconstruction demonstrating a depressed zygomatic arch. This impinges on the coronoid process of the mandible and the adjacent temporalis muscle, causing both limitation of mouth opening and pain.

Direct Approach

This approach is used if there is a marked degree of displacement of the zygoma or if the bone fragments are comminuted. Titanium compression plates are used to gain stability at two fracture sites, usually the fronto-zygomatic and zygomatico-maxillary suture line areas. The fronto-zygomatic area is exposed by a direct incision in the lateral brow area (Fig. 26.8). The zygomatico-maxillary area is exposed either by a subciliary transcutaneous approach or by a "swinging lower eyelid flap" transconjunctival approach (Fig. 26.9).

Three examples of the outcome following these surgical approaches are shown in Figures 26.8 and 26.9.

The bone fragments are manipulated into the correct position using an elevator inserted via the brow incision. The orbital floor can be inspected at the same time, any herniated orbital contents replaced, and an orbital floor implant placed.

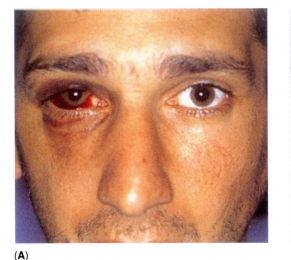
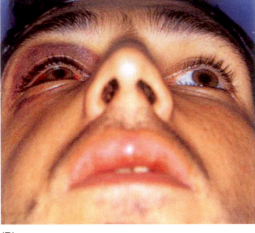

(A)   **(B)**

Figure 26.4 (**A**) A patient with a right zygomatic complex fracture demonstrating flattening of the right malar eminence. (**B**) This is best seen from below.

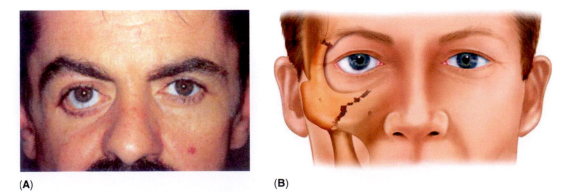

(A)   **(B)**

Figure 26.5 (**A**) A patient with a right zygomatic complex fracture with lower eyelid retraction, malar flattening and inferior displacement of the lateral canthus. (**B**) A diagram demonstrating the zygomatic bone hinged at the fronto-zygomatic suture line. The attachment of the orbital margin causes lower eyelid retraction.

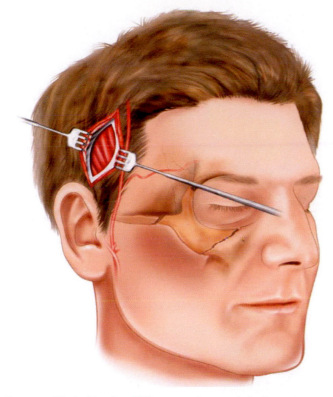

Figure 26.6 The incision for a Gillies temporal approach for the management of a zygomatic complex fracture.

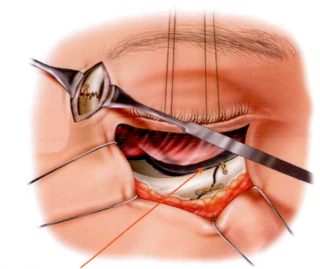

Medpor Titan implant

Figure 26.8 The incisions for the direct approach to the management of a zygomatic complex fracture.

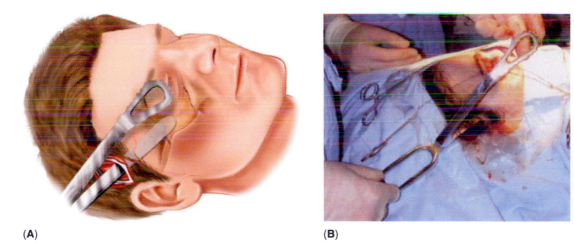

(A)   (B)

Figure 26.7 (A) A diagram demonstrating a Kilner elevator blade inserted under the zygoma. (B) An intraoperative photograph of a patient undergoing a Gillies approach repair of a zygomatic complex fracture.

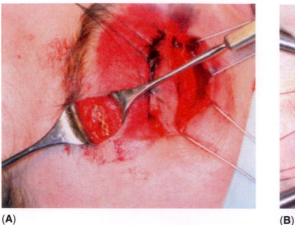 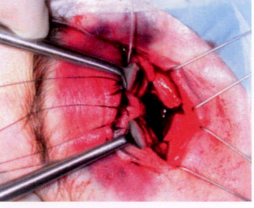

(A)   **(B)**

Figure 26.9 (**A**) The frontozygomatic fracture has been stabilized with a microplate. A transcutaneous approach to the inferior orbital margin has been used, as there was a large inferior eyelid laceration. A lateral canthotomy and inferior cantholysis had been performed for the urgent management of an orbital haematoma with compressive optic neuropathy. (**B**) The inferior orbital margin has comminuted fractures. These were reduced and fixated with microplates. A large orbital floor fracture is also visible. This was repaired with a channeled Medpor implant.

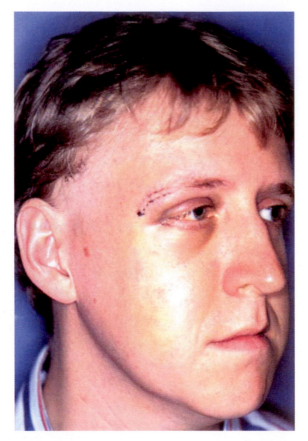

Figure 26.10 A patient who has undergone both a direct approach and a Gillies temporal approach to the repair of a right zygomatic complex fracture with a large orbital floor fracture. Incisions are seen in the temporal area, over the lateral aspect of the brow and in the lower eyelid.

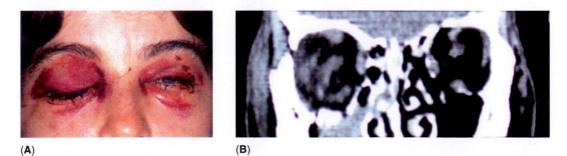

(A)   **(B)**

Figure 26.11 (**A**) A female patient following an assault with a hammer. (**B**) A coronal CT scan demonstrating a right zygomatic complex fracture and comminuted inferior orbital rim fractures. This patient's bony repairs are demonstrated in Figures 26.7 and 26.9.

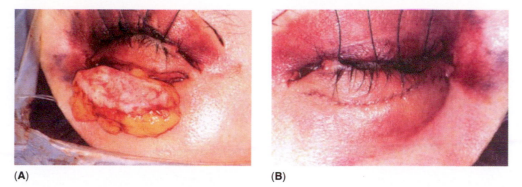

(A) (B)

Figure 26.12 (**A**) A dermis fat graft was placed over the orbital rim to prevent adhesions and eyelid retraction or hollowing. (**B**) The appearance at the completion of surgery.

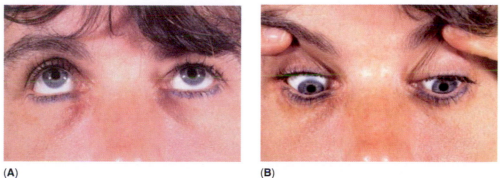

(A) (B)

Figure 26.13 The appearance of the patient shown in Figure 26.11 at 3 months postoperatively.

A titanium miniplate

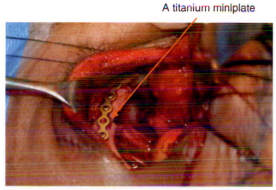

A large orbital floor blowout fracture

The margins of the orbital floor blowout fracture

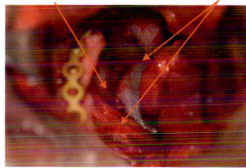

(A) (B)

A Medpor implant covering all margins of the fracture

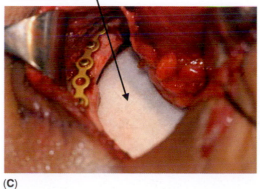

A dermis fat graft placed over the titanium miniplate and inferior orbital margin to prevent adhesions

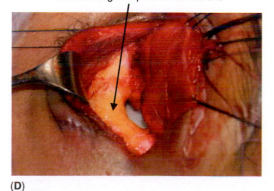

(C) (D)

Figure 26.14 (**A**) An intraoperative photograph of an old orbital floor blowout fracture and a previous titanium miniplate fixation of a fractured inferior orbital margin as part of the repair of a zygomatic complex fracture. The orbital floor blowout fracture had not been repaired. (**B**) A close-up photograph demonstrating the horizontal extent of the fracture and its medial and lateral margins. (**C**) A Medpor orbital implant has been placed over all the margins of the fracture. No fixation of the implant was required. (**D**) An abdominal dermis fat graft has been placed over the titanium miniplate and the exposed inferior orbital margin to prevent adhesions. The dermis is placed against the bone and periosteum. No suture fixation of the graft is usually necessary.

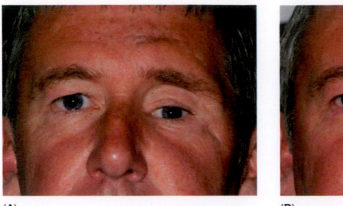

(A)   (B)

Figure 26.15 (**A**) The same patient with an extensive old orbital floor blowout fracture which had not been treated. (**B**) The same patient 6 months following the repair of his orbital floor blowout fracture with placement of a Medpor sheet implant and a lower lid dermis fat graft.

Two examples of the outcome following the use of these surgical approaches are given in Figures 26.10–26.13.

Figures 26.14 and 26.15 show a patient whose zygomatic complex fracture had been repaired directly by a maxillo-facial surgeon but whose orbital floor fracture repair had been left untreated because of concerns about the patient's associated globe injury.

FURTHER READING

1. Aguilar EA. The reevaluation of the indications for orbital rim fixation and orbital floor exploration in zygomatic complex fractures. Arch Otolaryngol Head Neck Surg 1989; 115: 1025.
2. Holck DE, Ng JD. Evaluation and Treatment of Orbital Fractures. Philadelphia, PA: Saunders, 2005.
3. Manson PN. Analysis of treatment for isolated zygomaticomaxillary complex fractures. Discussion. J Oral Maxillofac Surg 1996; 54: 400–1.
4. Murphy ML, Nerad JA. Complex orbital fractures. Ophthalmol Clin North Am 1996, 9(4). 607–27.

27 Other orbital fractures

INTRODUCTION
Midfacial Fractures
The site and extent of midfacial fractures depends on the type of impact and its direction and degree of severity. It is useful to have an understanding of the Le Fort classification of these fractures although pure Le Fort fractures are rarely encountered in clinical practice: they are often quite asymmetric.

Le Fort Classification
1. A Le Fort I fracture is a transverse fracture through the lower part of the maxilla above the teeth. The orbit is not involved (Fig. 27.1).
2. A Le Fort II fracture has a pyramidal configuration involving the nasal, lacrimal, and maxillary bones. The fracture lines extend through the frontal processes of the maxilla, through the lacrimal bones, the floor of the orbits, the area of the zygomatico-maxillary suture lines, and involve the pterygoid plates (Fig. 27.2). Orbital wall blowout fractures may be present and the lacrimal drainage system may also be involved.
3. A Le Fort III fracture represents a true craniofacial dysjunction in which the entire facial skeleton is detached from the skull base and suspended only by soft tissues. This fracture involves the medial and lateral orbital walls and orbital floor. The fracture lines extend through the superior aspect of the nasal bones, the fronto-maxillary suture area, through the ethmoid sinuses and medial orbital walls, below the optic canal to the inferior orbital fissures, and through the fronto-zygomatic suture areas (Fig. 27.3).

NASO-ORBITAL FRACTURES
Naso-orbital fractures comprise one of the most common patterns of fracture affecting the facial skeleton. They are most commonly the result of a severe impact across the bridge of the nose, e.g., in a motor vehicle accident in which an unrestrained passenger's face strikes the dashboard. The nasal bones are fractured and depressed. The medial canthal tendons are displaced laterally, leading to telecanthus. There are usually medial orbital wall blowout fractures. Damage to the cribriform plate may result in cerebrospinal fluid (CSF) rhinorrhoea. A severe epistaxis may result from a laceration or an avulsion of the anterior ethmoid arteries. Clinically, the patient usually presents with a flattened bridge of the nose and swollen medial canthal areas (Fig. 27.4). Dacryostenosis is a common complication, requiring a dacryocystorhinostomy (DCR). Management of these injuries involves early surgical reduction of the fractures with the use of mini- and microplates. These fractures, along with mid facial fractures, are best managed by a multidisciplinary team of surgeons.

ORBITAL ROOF FRACTURES
Orbital roof fractures (Fig. 27.5) may also involve the brain, cribriform plate, and the frontal sinuses. They are usually caused by severe blunt trauma or occasionally by penetrating injuries. It is important to bear in mind the possibility of such an injury in children who may present with only a minor periocular laceration after falling on a pointed object. These fractures can lead to serious complications, e.g., intracranial haemorrhage, brain contusion or laceration, infection, CSF rhinorrhea, caroticocavernous fistula, pneumocephalus (Fig. 27.6), and traumatic optic neuropathy.

Damage to the trochlea may result in diplopia. The patients may also experience painful limitation of up gaze due to inferior displacement of bone fragments. Ptosis may result from direct trauma to the levator muscle or to the oculomotor nerve.

The brain often sustains a concussion injury and may even be lacerated if there is a comminuted fracture. The supraorbital margin may be depressed with a palpable step-like deformity. Occasionally the roof of the orbit is displaced inferiorly and constitutes a "blow-in" fracture with a resultant hypoglobus (Fig. 27.6). The management of these fractures should be undertaken in close cooperation with a neurosurgeon.

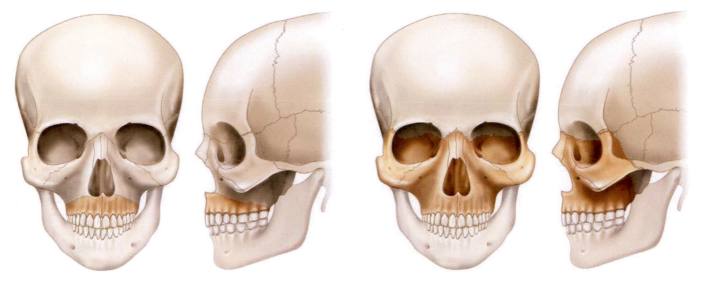

Figure 27.1 Le Fort I fracture.

Figure 27.3 Le Fort III fracture.

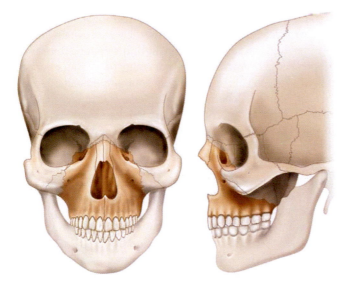

Figure 27.2 Le Fort II fracture.

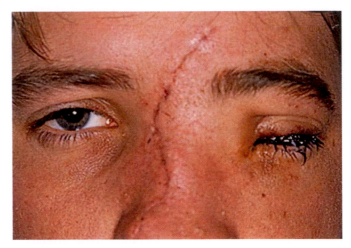

Figure 27.4 This patient suffered a severe comminuted nasoethmoidal fracture. A severe globe rupture necessitated enucleation. The failure to reduce the fractures adequately at the initial surgical repair will inevitably result in a severe secondary facial deformity.

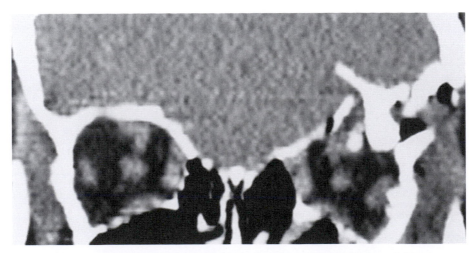

Figure 27.5 A severe left orbital roof fracture in a patient who fell 15 feet from a ladder.

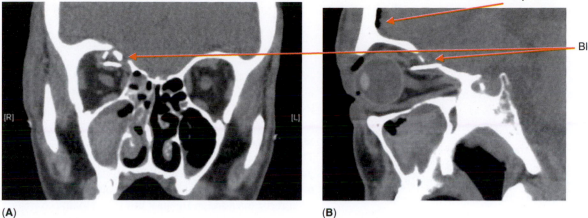

Figure 27.6 (**A**) A coronal CT scan demonstrating an orbital roof "blow in" fracture. The patient had marked restriction of elevation of his eye. (**B**) A sagittal CT scan demonstrating the impingement of the displaced orbital roof fracture on the superior rectus muscle.

FURTHER READING

1. Albert DM, Lucarelli MJ. Orbital fractures: diagnosis and management. In: Clinical Atlas of Procedures in Ophthalmic Surgery. Chicago, IL: AMA Press, 2004: 347–59.
2. American Academy of Ophthalmology. Orbit, eyelids, and lacrimal system (Section 7). In: Basic and Clinical Science Course. San Francisco: The American Academy of Ophthalmology, 2006/7: 97–108, 184–7.
3. Fulcher TP, Sullivan TJ. Orbital roof fractures: management of ophthalmic complications. Ophthal Plast Reconstr Surg 2003; 19(5): 359–63.
4. Greenwald MJ, Boston D, Pensler JM, Radkowski MA. Orbital roof fractures in childhood. Ophthalmology 1989; 96: 491–7.
5. Holck DE, Ng JD. Evaluation and Treatment of Orbital Fractures. Philadelphia, PA: Saunders, 2005.
6. Markowitz BL, Manson PN. Panfacial fractures: organization and treatment. Clin Plast Surg 1989; 16: 105–14.
7. Markowitz BL, Manson PN, Sargent L, et al. Management of the medial canthal tendon in nasoethmoid orbital fractures: the importance of the central fragment in classification and treatment. Plast Reconstr Surg 1991; 87: 843–53.
8. Nerad JA. Techniques in Ophthalmic Plastic Surgery: A Personal Tutorial. Philadelphia, PA: Elsevier Inc., 2010: 113–26, 355–87 (ISBN: 978-1-4377-0008-4).

28 Traumatic optic neuropathy

INTRODUCTION

Injuries to the optic nerve are rare and may result from a variety of mechanisms:

- Direct injury to the optic nerve
  - penetrating orbital trauma (Fig. 28.1)
  - partial or complete avulsion (Fig. 28.2)
  - intraoptic nerve sheath hematoma (Fig. 28.3)
- Indirect injury to the optic nerve
  - optic canal fracture with contusion of the optic nerve/edema within the optic canal following a blow to the supraorbital area
  - expanding intraorbital hematoma (Fig. 28.4)

APPLIED ANATOMY

See chapter 2.

PATIENT EVALUATION

Evaluation of the patient may be difficult, especially if the patient is unconscious. It is essential to monitor optic nerve function and pupillary reactions. It is important to establish the time of onset of visual loss. Immediate visual loss following trauma is associated with a very poor prognosis. This is usually due to severe direct penetrating trauma, severe intracanalicular contusion, or optic nerve avulsion. A secondary visual loss is usually due to a circulatory disturbance subsequent to the initial trauma. This can occur from continued bleeding into the intraconal, extraconal, or subperiosteal spaces.

It is extremely important to exclude other causes of visual loss, e.g., a posterior globe rupture. High-resolution CT scanning examination of the orbits, paranasal sinuses, optic canals, and brain should be performed. Plain skull X-rays have no role in the evaluation of the patient with traumatic optic neuropathy. It is imperative, however, that an urgent orbital decompression, if indicated, is not delayed by any imaging studies.

MANAGEMENT

The treatment for posterior indirect traumatic optic neuropathy is determined on an individual basis. Immediate treatment with high-dose intravenous methylprednisolone has been recommended in the past but this remains controversial with no firm evidence to support its use. Endoscopic optic canal decompression may be considered on an individual basis, but the overall results are poor, and again there is no firm evidence available to support its use.

Hemorrhage and edema in the orbit following trauma can result in an increased pressure within the orbit causing an orbital compartment syndrome, with the risk of vascular compromise. An acute rise in intraorbital pressure can compress the optic nerve at the orbital apex or can result in a closure of the central retinal artery. Under these circumstances an immediate lateral canthotomy and inferior cantholysis should be performed for decompression of the anterior orbit and for the relief of secondarily elevated intraocular pressure (Fig. 28.5). Intravenous acetazolamide should be given in addition to topical therapy to lower intraocular pressure.

A formal orbital decompression may have to be performed in selected cases. An orbital hemorrhage cannot be drained through a needle, and blind stabs into the orbit in the vain hope of draining blood should *never* be considered. In contrast, a needle aspiration of entrapped air within the orbit may be undertaken with extreme care and under radiological guidance if visual function is compromised.

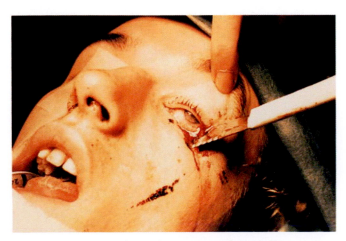

Figure 28.1 Direct optic nerve trauma from a knife.

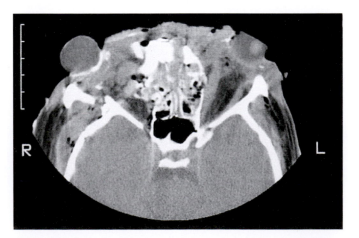

Figure 28.2 Severe orbital trauma following a motor vehicle accident with complete avulsion of both optic nerves.

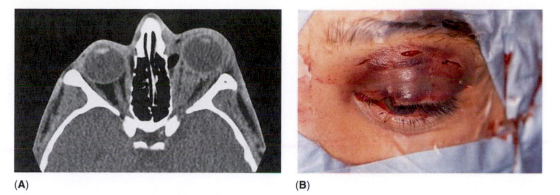

(A)   **(B)**

Figure 28.3 (**A**) A left intraoptic nerve sheath hematoma. (**B**) The same patient referred after inappropriate blind stabs had been made in the upper eyelid in a vain attempt to drain an orbital hematoma.

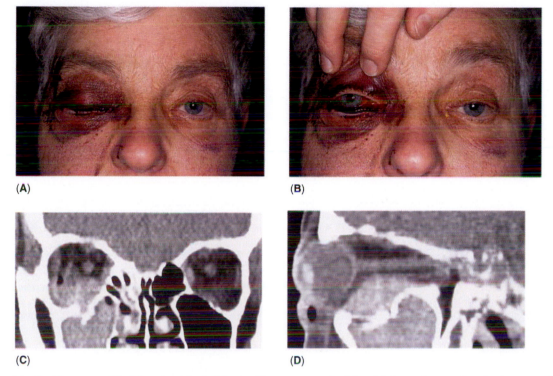

(A)   **(B)**

(C)   **(D)**

Figure 28.4 Complete visual loss occurred in this patient 30 min following blunt trauma to the right orbit due to the secondary development of a large subperiosteal hematoma. (**A**) A periorbital hematoma. (**B**) Proptosis and hyperglobus. (**C**) A coronal CT scan demonstrating an orbital floor fracture and an inferior orbital hematoma. (**D**) A sagittal CT scan demonstrating proptosis, an orbital floor fracture and a subperiosteal hematoma extending to the orbital apex.

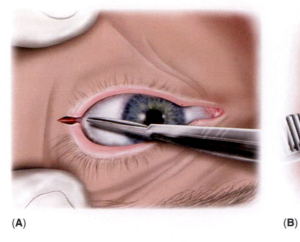

(A)

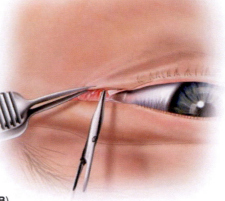

(B)

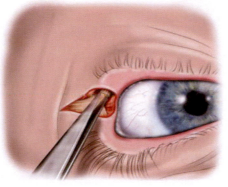

(C)

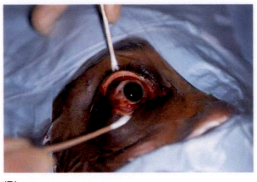

(D)

Figure 28.5 (**A**) A lateral canthotomy is performed. (**B**) The eyelid is grasped with a pair of Paufique forceps and drawn supero-laterally while all eyelid attachments to the lateral orbital margin between the skin and the conjunctiva are divided with scissors. (**C**) This drawing demonstrates an inferior cantholysis being performed. (**D**) A lateral canthotomy and inferior cantholysis have been performed on this patient by the bedside prior to a formal exploration and repair of a displaced lateral orbital wall fracture.

FURTHER READING

1. Alford MA, Nerad JA, Carter KD. Predictive value of the initial quantified relative afferent pupillary defect in 19 consecutive patients with traumatic optic neuropathy. Ophthal Plast Reconstr Surg 2001; 17: 323.
2. Bilyk JR, Joseph MP. Traumatic optic neuropathy. Semin Ophthalmol 1994; 9: 200–11.
3. Goodall KL, Brahma A, Bates A, Leatherbarrow B. Lateral canthotomy and inferior cantholysis: an effective method of urgent orbital decompression for sight-threatening acute retrobulbar haemorrhage. Injury 1999, 30: 485–90.
4. Levin LA, Beck RW, Joseph MP, Seiff S, Kraker R. The Treatment of Traumatic Optic Neuropathy. Ophthalmology 1999; 106: 1268–77.
5. Lima V, Burt B, Leibovitch I, et al. Orbital compartment syndrome: the ophthalmic surgical emergency. Surv Ophthalmol 2009; 54(4): 441–9.
6. Miller NR. The management of traumatic optic neuropathy. Editorial. Arch Ophthalmol 1990; 108: 1086–7.
7. Newton TH, Bilaniuk LT. Radiology of the Eye and Orbit. New York, NY: Raven Press, 1990.
8. Steinsapir KD, Goldberg RA. Traumatic optic neuropathy. Surv Ophthalmol 1994; 38: 487–518.

Index

Page numbers in italics refer to figures and tables

abducens nerve, 60
aberrant reinnervation, 136, 204
absorbable sutures, 16
achrochordon (papilloma), 205
acquired upper eyelid entropion, 94, *95*
acute spastic entropion, 75
acute thyroid orbitopathy, 375
adenoid cystic carcinoma, 385
advancement flap, 21
afrazine, 453
allergy, 6
Allevyn Cavity®, 525
Allevyn Thin®, 283
alopecia, 361
analgesia, postoperative, 22
anesthesia
    enucleation, 485
    general, 4
    local, 3
    orbital exenteration, 522
    regional, 4
    topical, 3
angiosarcoma, 231
anterior face of maxilla, 297
anterior orbitotomy
    lower eyelid transconjunctival, 403–5
    transcutaneous, 403
    upper eyelid vertical split, 405–6
apocrine hidrocystoma, 212
aponeurotic ptosis, 146
Aquacel®, 525
argon laser ablation, 106
arteriography, 373
arteriovenous shunts, 390–1
artery clips, 6
auricular cartilage graft, 105, *263*
    indications, 287
    postoperative care, 288
    surgical procedure, 288
autogenous grafts, 279
    see also auricular cartilage graft; dermis
        fat graft; fascia lata graft; hard palate
        graft; mucous membrane graft; skin
        graft; temporalis fascia graft
autogenous implant, 483–4
avulsion injuries, 535

bandage contact lens, 106
basal cell carcinoma (BCC)
    malignant eyelid tumors, 217–8
    periocular tumors
        cryotherapy, 229
        irradiation, 228–9
        Mohs' micrographic surgery, 229–30
        photodynamic therapy, 230

surgical management of, 227–8
        topical chemotherapeutic
            agents, 230
basal cell nevus syndrome, 218–9
baseball implant, 483
Bell's palsy *see* facial palsy
benign eyelid tumors *see* eyelid tumors
    lesions of adnexa, 211–2
    lesions of dermis, 207–11
    lesions of epidermis, 205–7
    pigmentary lesions, 214–7
    tumors of hair follicle origin, 212–4
    tumors of sweat gland origin, 212
Berke–Reese lateral orbitotomy, 412
bi-coronal flap incision, *9*
bilateral proptosis, causes of, 366
bilobed flap, 21, *23*, 272
biomicroscopy, 447
bites, 531
blepharochalasis, 320
blepharoplasty
    vs. dermatochalasis, 319–20
    applied anatomy
        lower eyelids, 314–8
        mid-face, 318–9
        upper eyelids, 310–3
    cheek implant, 333–4
    complications for surgery, *340*
    lower eyelid
        goals, 326
        preoperative patient evaluation,
            326–7
        surgical approaches, 327–8
        surgical technique, 328
    medicolegal pitfalls, 342–3
    mid-face lift, 331, 333
    SOOF lift, 331
    structural fat grafting, 331
    in thyroid eye disease, 190–1
    transconjunctival
        postoperative care, 338–40
        surgical procedure, 335–8
    transcutaneous
        with fat debulking, 334–5
        postoperative care, 331
        surgical procedure, 328–31
    upper eyelid
        anesthesia, 325
        goals of, 320
        informed consent, 323–4
        postoperative care, 326
        preoperative patient evaluation,
            320–3
        surgical procedure, 325–6
        surgical technique, 324

blepharoptosis
    complications of surgery, 169–75
    patient assessment, 147–50
    ptosis classification, 136–47
    surgical procedures, 151–68
blindness, 442
    orbital wall blowout fractures, 558
blunt trauma, 531
bone graft, 297
bone wax, 13
bony orbit, 45–6
bony orbital decompression
    bicoronal flap approach, 436
    lateral canthal, 436
    lateral orbitotomy, 436
    lower eyelid approach, 435–6
    medial canthal skin incision, 436
    nasal endoscopic approach, 434–5
    transantral approach, 436
    transcaruncular approach, 436
    upper eyelid incision, 436
botulinum toxin injections
    chin, 303
    contraindications, 303
    forehead, 302–3
    glabella, 302
    lateral canthus, 302
    lower eyelid, 303
    neck, 303
    procedure, 301–2
    side effects, 304
    upper lip, 303
botulism, 143–4
bradycardia, 548
brow depressor muscle, *31*
brow lift, 359
brow ptosis, 137
    applied anatomy, 346
    complications of brow lift surgery
        alopecia, 361
        facial nerve trauma, 360
        hematoma, 360–1
        scarring, 361
        sensory nerve trauma, 360
    direct brow lift, 203
    endoscopic brow lift, 203–4
    preoperative patient evaluation
        anesthesia, 348
        examination, 346–7
        history, 346
        surgical planning, 347–8
    surgical procedures
        coronal forehead and brow lift, 359
        direct brow lift, 348–9
        endoscopic brow lift, 355–9

brow ptosis (*Continued*)
    gull-wing direct brow lift, 350
    mid-forehead brow lift, 350–1
    pretrichial forehead and brow lift,
        359–60
    temporal eyebrow lift, 351–2
    transblepharoplasty browpexy, 352–3
    transblepharoplasty endotine brow
        lift, 353–5
buccomaxillary ligaments, 73
buried integrated implants, 480–1
burns
    management, 544, 546
    thermal, 544

canaliculi, 62
canaliculo-dacryocystorhinostomy
    indications, 470
    surgical procedure, 470–1
canaliculotomy, 456
canthal tendon, lateral
    granuloma, 89
    laxity, 122
    reconstruction, 278
canthal tendon, medial
    laxity, 119
    reconstruction
        bilobed flap, 272
        full-thickness skin grafting, 269
        glabellar flap, 271, *272*
        laissez-faire, 269, *271*
        local flap, 271
        median forehead flap, 272
        rhomboid flap, 271–2, *273*
cantholysis, 257
canthotomy, 257
capillary hemangioma, 207–8, 382–4
cartilage graft, 263
Castroviejo implant, 483
Castroviejo needle holders, 6
cavernous hemangioma, 208, 381–2
cellulitis, orbital, 375
    clinical features, 376
    complications, 379
    diagnosis of, 377
    etiology, 376
    management of, 377–9
central retinal vein, 61
cerebral ptosis, 143
cerebrospinal fluid (CSF) leak, 442
chalazion, 211–2
cheek flaps, 243
chemical peels, 307
chemosis, 342, 562
chemotherapy, 388
chronic progressive external
        ophthalmoplegia (CPEO), 145–6
cicatricial ectropion, 75
    causes of, 129
    complications, 91
    lateral tarsal strip procedure, 130–2
    lateral wedge resection, 130–2
    skin graft, 130
    surgical procedures
        posterior lamellar graft, 90–1

retractor advancement, 89
    tarsal fracture, 89–90
coated Vicryl Plus antibacterial, 16
Colorado needle, *5*
combined orbitotomies, 416
computed tomography, 369, 371
    imaging in epiphora, 451
    thyroid eye disease, 428–9
congenital dystrophy, 144
    chronic progressive external
        ophthalmoplegia, 145–6
    motonic dystrophy, 144
    muscle trauma, 146
congenital epiblepharon, 92
    postoperative management, 92–3
    surgical procedure, 93
congenital lower eyelid ectropion, 135
congenital lower eyelid entropion, 75
    postoperative care, 92
    surgical procedure, 91–2
congenital nasolacrimal duct obstruction,
        453
congenital upper eyelid entropion, 94, *95*
conjunctiva, 39
conjunctival lymphoma, 388
conjunctival prolapse, 173, 491
conjunctivo-dacryocystorhinostomy
        (CDCR)
    endoscopic, 474–5
    external, 472–4
    indications, 471
    patient evaluation, 472
contralateral upper eyelid
        retraction, 136
corneal exposure management
    gold weight insertion, 200–2
    lateral tarsorrhaphy, 196–8
    levator aponeurosis recession,
        199–200
    medial canthoplasty, 198–9
    müllerectomy, 199–200
    punctal occlusion, 196
    temporary suture tarsorrhaphy, 196
corneal irritation, 341
corneal neurotization, 204
coronal forehead, 359
corrugator supercilii muscle, 43
cosmetic blepharoplasty, 310
cosmetic patient
    non-surgical treatment
        botulinum toxin injections, 301–4
        chemical peels, 307
        cutaneous laser resurfacing, 307
        dermal filler injections, 304–5
        intense pulsed light treatment, 307
    patient consultation
        consultation facility, 300
        patient selection for surgery, 301
        pre-consultation, 300
        surgeon consultation, 300–1
    surgical treatment options, 307–9
cribriform plate, 48
Cryojet cryotherapy device, *108*
cryotherapy, 106–7, 229
current orbital implants, 482

cutaneous horn, 205–6
Cutler–Beard reconstruction
    complications, 264
    first and second stages of, 261–4
    full-thickness eyelid composite graft,
        264, 266
    lower lid rotation, 266–9
cyanoacrylate adhesive, 18
cyclic oculomotor nerve palsy, 137

dacryocystectomy, 476–7
dacryocystocoele
    lacrimal sac fistula, 455
    punctal atresia, 455–6
dacryocystography (DCG), 450
dacryocystorhinostomy (DCR)
    contraindications, 457
    endonasal laser-assisted, 469–70
    endoscopic non-laser assisted,
        466–9
    goals and risks of operation, 458
    indications, 457
    redo external, 464
dacryocystorhinostomy (DCR), external
    patient preparation, 458–9
    postoperative care, 464
    surgical procedure
        exposure, 459–60
        flaps, 461–3
        incision, 459–60
        osteotomy, 460–1
        retraction, 459–60
        wound closure, 463
dacryocystostomy, 456–7
dacryoscintigraphy, 451
deep perioral muscles, 73
depressor supercilii muscle, 44
Dermabond® Ethicon, 18
dermal filler injections, 304–5
Dermatix, 281
dermatochalasis, 137, 319–20
dermis fat graft, 483
    enucleation
        postoperative care, 495
        surgical procedure, 493–4
    indications, 290
    postoperative care, 291
    socket reconstruction, 505, 507
    surgical procedure, 290–1
dermoid cyst, 206, 395
dietary restriction, 26
diplopia, 342, 442
    botulinum toxin injections, 304
    delayed treatment of, 556, 558
    orbital wall blowout fractures, 558
    in ptosis, 175
direct brow lift, 203, 348–9
direct injury, 572
dog-ear deformity, 21–2, *25*
double elevator palsy, 136–7
Down syndrome, *135*
drains, 26
dressings, 26
dry eye syndrome, 341
Duane's retraction syndrome, 137

eccrine spiradenoma, 212
ectropion, lower eyelid
  cicatricial
    causes of, 129
    lateral tarsal strip procedure, 130–2
    lateral wedge resection, 130–2
    skin graft, 130
  classification, 110
  congenital, 135
  correction of, 202–3
  involutional
    medial ectropion, 113–22
    punctal ectropion, 113
    tarsal ectropion, 126, 128–9
    of whole length of lower eyelid, 122
  mechanical, 132
  medical management and factors, 111–2
  paralytic, 132–3, 135
  patient evaluation, 110
elasticity, 16
electrolysis, 106
Ellman–Surgitron radiofrequency device,
    106, 108
endonasal laser-assisted DCR, 469–70
endoscopic brow lift, 203–4, 355–9
endoscopic brow lift instrument, 5
endoscopic conjunctivo-
    dacryocystorhinostomy, 474–5
endoscopic nasal examination, 448–9
endoscopic nasal septoplasty, 475–6
endoscopic non-laser assisted DCR
  patient preparation, 466
  postoperative care, 468–9
  surgical procedure
    flaps creation, 468
    nasal mucosal flap, 467
    osteotomy, 467
endoscopic orbitotomy, 415–6
enophthalmos, 366, 443, 548
  undercorrection of, 559
entropion, lower eyelid
  acute spastic, 75
  cicatricial, 75
    complications, 91
    posterior lamellar graft, 90–1
    retractor advancement, 89
    tarsal fracture, 89–90
  congenital, 75
    postoperative care, 92
    surgical procedure, 91–2
  involutional, 75
    complications, 89
    everting sutures, 79–80, 81
    lateral tarsal strip procedure, 83–5
    retractor advancement, 80–3
    wedge resection, 85–9
  medical management, 78
  orbital wall blowout fractures, 558
  patient assessment
    examination, 78
    history, 77–8
  surgical anatomy, 75–7
entropion, upper eyelid
  acquired, 94, 95
  classification, 94, 95

congenital, 94, 95
  patient assessment, 94
  surgical management
    anterior lamellar reposition with gray
      line split, 95–6
    auricular cartilage graft, 105
    factors influencing, 95
    lamellar split and posterior lamellar
      advancement, 99
    posterior lamellar mucous membrane
      graft, 101–3
    tarsal wedge excision, 96, 98
    terminal tarsal rotation, 99–101
    upper lid auricular cartilage graft,
      94, 98
enucleation
  vs evisceration, 495–8
  anesthesia, 485
  complications
    conjunctival prolapse, 491
    implant exposure, 490–1
    orbital hematoma, 491
    over-sized implant, 491
  dermis fat graft
    postoperative care, 495
    surgical procedure, 493–4
  goals of, 479
  hydroxyapatite implant
    complications, 492–3
    postoperative care, 492
    surgical procedure, 491–2
  indications, 479
  orbital implants, 479–85
  postoperative care, 489–90
  preoperative preparation, 479
  surgical procedure, 485–9
enucleation scissors, 6
epiblepharon, 92
epidermoid cyst, 206
epilation, 106
epiphora, 341, 443
  adults
    eyelid surgery, 456
    Kelly punch punctoplasty, 456
    punctoplasty, 456
    three-snip punctoplasty, 456
  applied anatomy, 445
  children
    congenital nasolacrimal duct
      obstruction, 453
    nasolacrimal duct probing, 453–5
  external examination, 445, 447
  history, 445
  imaging
    computed tomography, 451
    dacryocystography, 450
    dacryoscintigraphy, 451
  infants
    congenital nasolacrimal duct
      obstruction, 453
    nasolacrimal duct probing, 453–5
  slit lamp examination, 447
Ethibond sutures, 17
Ethilon sutures, 17
ethmoidal arteries, 61

ethmoidal sinuses, 67–8
everting sutures, 79–80, 81
evisceration, 495–6
  vs enucleation, 485–8
  postoperative care, 498
  surgical procedure, 496–8
exenteration, 228
  classification, 520
  extended, 526
  orbital reconstruction, 526
  subtotal, 526
  surgical technique, 522
  total, 522, 524–6
exposed integrated implants, 481–2
exposure keratopathy, 171, 194–5
extended exenteration, 526
external carotid artery, 60
external conjunctivo-
    dacryocystorhinostomy, 472–4
extra marginal injuries, 533–5, 541, 543
extraconal orbital space, 54
eyebrow
  applied anatomy, 346
  corrugator supercilii muscle, 43
  depressor supercilii muscle, 44
  frontalis muscle, 40, 42–3, 45
  orbicularis oculi muscle, 44
  procerus muscle, 44
eyelash
  argon laser ablation, 106
  bandage contact lens, 106
  cryotherapy, 106–7
  electrolysis, 106
  epilation, 106
  loss of, 174
  ptosis, 173
  surgical excision, 107–9
  see also Trichiasis
eyelid
  canthal tendon, 33, 34
  conjunctiva, 39
  contour defects, 171
  eyelid retractor, 35–9
  hollowing of, 341
  lateral canthal reconstruction, 278
  lymphatic drainage of, 42
  medial canthal reconstruction
    bilobed flap, 272
    full-thickness skin grafting, 269
    glabellar flap, 271, 272
    laissez-faire, 269, 271
    local flap, 271
    median forehead flap, 272
    rhomboid flap, 271–2, 273
  orbicularis oculi muscle,
      28–9
  orbital septum, 29–32
  pre-aponeurotic fat pads, 33–5
  sensory nerve supply of, 39
  skin, 28
  surgery in adults, 456
  tarsal plates, 32–3
  vascular supply to, 39–40, 41
eyelid composite graft, 297
eyelid ecchymosis, 547

eyelid injuries
  avulsion injuries, 535
  extra marginal injuries, 533–5
  marginal injuries, 533
  tissue loss, 535
eyelid, lower
  blepharoplasty, 310
    goals, 326
    preoperative patient evaluation, 326–7
    surgical approaches, 327–8
    surgical technique, 328
  fascial sling, 510–12
  full-thickness loss of, 269
  laxity, 510
  reconstruction
    free tarsoconjunctival graft, 241–3
    large defects, 235–40
    lateral periosteal flap, 240
    lower eyelid island flap, 249
    medial periosteal flap, 240–1
    moderate defects, 234–5
    Mustardé cheek rotation flap, 243, 245–6, *248*, 249
    periosteal flaps, 240
    semicircular rotation flap, 235
    small defects, 233–4
  retraction, orbital wall blowout fractures, 558
  thyroid-related eyelid retraction
    free tarsal graft spacer, 189
    hard palate graft spacer, 186–9
  see also ectropion, lower eyelid; entropion, lower eyelid
eyelid repositioning surgery, 443
eyelid tumors
  benign lesions of adnexa, 211–2
  benign lesions of dermis
    capillary hemangioma, 207–8
    cavernous hemangioma, 208
    plexiform neurofibroma, 208–9
    pyoderma gangrenosum, 210
    pyogenic granuloma, 209–10
    varix, 211
    xanthelasma, 210
    xanthoma, 210
  benign lesions of epidermis
    achrochordon (papilloma), 205
    cutaneous horn, 205–6
    dermoid cyst, 206
    epidermoid cyst, 206
    inverted follicular keratosis, 205
    milia, 207
    molluscum contagiosum, 207
    phakomatous choristoma, 207
    seborrhoeic keratosis, 205
    verruca vulgaris, 207
  benign pigmentary lesions
    lentigines, 216–7
    melanocytic nevus, 214–6
    nevus of ota, 216
  benign tumors of hair follicle origin
    pilomatrixoma, 212
    sebaceous adenoma, 212–3
    sebaceous cyst, 212

    trichoepithelioma, 213–4
    tricholemmoma, 213
  benign tumors of sweat gland origin
    apocrine hidrocystoma, 212
    eccrine spiradenoma, 212
    syringoma, 212
  biopsy of eyelid and periocular lesions, 217
  biopsy technique, 217
  malignant eyelid tumors
    basal cell carcinoma, 217–8
    basal cell nevus syndrome, 218–9
    Kaposi's sarcoma, 224, *226*
    keratoacanthoma, 219–220
    melanoma, 221, 223–4
    Merkel cell tumor, 221
    metastatic tumors, 224
    mycosis fungoides, 224, *226*
    sebaceous gland carcinoma (SGC), 220–1
    squamous cell carcinoma (SCC), 219
eyelid, upper
  blepharoplasty, 310
    anesthesia, 325
    goals of, 320
    informed consent, 323–4
    postoperative care, 326
    preoperative patient evaluation, 320–3
    surgical procedure, 325–6
    surgical technique, 324
  Cutler–Beard reconstruction
    complications, 264
    first and second stages of, 261–4
    full-thickness eyelid composite graft, 264, 266
    lower lid rotation, 266–9
  eyelid defects not involving the eyelid margin, 269
  full-thickness loss of, 269
  reconstruction
    canthotomy and cantholysis, 257
    free tarsoconjunctival graft, 259–61
    semicircular rotation flap, 259
    sliding tarsoconjunctival flap, 257–9
    small defects, 256–7
  skin creases, 341–2
  thyroid-related eyelid retraction
    anterior approach levator recession, 183–5
    anterior approach Z-myotomy, 185–6
    graded full-thickness anterior blepharotomy, 186
    müllerectomy, 180–1
    posterior approach levator recession, 181–2
  see also entropion, upper eyelid

face
  muscles in, 73
  retaining ligaments, 70, *72*, 73
  scalp, 69
  superficial musculoaponeurotic system, 70
  temple, 69–70
facial incision, *8*

facial nerve
  aberrant reinnervation of, 136, 204
  cervical branch, 45
  marginal mandibular nerve, 45
  temporal branch, 44
  zygomatic and buccal branches, 44
  trauma, 360
facial palsy
  causes of, *193*
  examination of, 192–4
  general treatment, 194
  history, 192
  medical treatment, 194–5
  surgical treatment
    aberrant reinnervation, 204
    brow ptosis, 203–4
    corneal exposure, 196–202
    corneal neurotization, 204
    correction of lower eyelid ectropion, 202–3
false retaining ligaments, 318
Fasanella–Servat procedure, 151–2
fascia lata graft
  indications, 295
  surgical technique, 295–6
fat herniation, 328
fat necrosis, 342
fat pearl graft, 295
fibrin sealant, 13–14
fine-needle aspiration biopsy, 374
first-degree burn, 544
flap techniques, 19–21
fluorescein dye disappearance test, 447
forced duction test, 552
fornix-deepening sutures, 517–9
free flaps, 21, 529
free tarsoconjunctival graft, 241–3, 259–61
fricke flap, 249–53
frontal sinuses, 67
frontal transcranial craniotomy, 416–7
frontalis muscle, 40, 42–3, 45
frontalis suspension procedure, 163–8
Frost suture, 26
full-thickness eyelid composite graft, 264, 266
full-thickness skin graft
  donor sites of, 279
  medial canthal reconstruction, 269
  periocular flaps, 255, 274–7
  postoperative care, 281
  surgical procedure, 279–81

galea aponeurotica, 69
Gamgee®, 283
general anesthesia, 4
glabellar flap, 271, *272*
gold weight implantation, 200–2
Gorlin's syndrome, 218–9
granulomatous disorders, 380
Guillain–Barré syndrome, 143
gull-wing direct brow lift, 350

hard palate, 186
hard palate graft, 285
  indications, 286

postoperative care, 286
surgical procedure, 286
headache, 548
hematoma, 89, 360–1, 547
hemifacial spasm, 136
hemophilus influenza, 376
hemorrhage, 175, 442–3
hemostasis
cautery, 13
instrumentation, 13
nasal packing, 11
postoperative, 14
preoperative evaluation, 11
preoperative injection, 11
suction, 11–13
topical hemostatic agents, 13–14
high-flow shunts, 391
Horner's muscle, 31
Horner's syndrome, 138–40
House–Brackmann score, 194
hyaluronic acid filler injections, 327
hydroxyapatite implant
complications, 492–3
postoperative care, 492
surgical procedure, 491–2
5-hydroxytryptamine (5-HT), 388
hyperglobus, 559
hypoglobus, 443, 548

idiopathic sclerosing inflammation, 380
implant malposition, 515
indirect injury, 572
inferior ophthalmic vein, 61
inflammatory lesions, 384
infraorbital anesthesia, 443
infraorbital nerve, 547
infraorbital sensory loss, 559
infratrochlear artery, 60
injuries
marginal, 533, 540–41
optic nerve, 572
injuries, eyelid
avulsion injuries, 535
extra marginal injuries, 533–5
globe injury, 543
marginal injuries, 533
mechanism, 531
secondary repair, 543–4
tissue loss, 535
integrated implants, 480
intense pulsed light treatment, 307
internal carotid artery, 60
intraconal orbital space, 53–4
intralesional corticosteroid injections, 382
inverted follicular keratosis, 205
involutional ectropion
medial ectropion
with horizontal eyelid laxity, 116, 119
with medial canthal tendon laxity, 119–20, 122
without horizontal eyelid laxity, 113, 115–6
punctal ectropion, 113
tarsal ectropion, 126, 128–9
of whole length of lower eyelid, 122

involutional entropion, 75
complications, 89
everting sutures, 79–80
lateral tarsal strip procedure, 83–5
lower eyelid
retractor advancement, 80–3
wedge resection, 85–9
irradiation, 228–9

Jaffe retractors, 10

Kaposi's sarcoma, 224, 226, 231
Kearns–Sayre syndrome (KSS), 146
Kelly punch punctoplasty, 456
Kelocote, 281
Keloid scarring, 8
keratoacanthoma, 219–220
keratoconjunctivitis sicca, 341

Lacrilube (liquid paraffin) ointment, 281
lacrilube ointment, 359
lacrimal artery, 60
lacrimal drainage system, 62
endoscopic nasal
examination, 448–9
fluorescein dye
disappearance test, 447
probing of canaliculi, 448
syringing of, 447–8
lacrimal gland, 62
lacrimal gland tumors, 384–5
lacrimal nerve, 59
lacrimal sac, 63–64
lacrimal sac fistula, 455
lacrimal system
canaliculi, 62
lacrimal drainage system, 62
lacrimal gland, 62
lacrimal sac, 63–64
nasolacrimal duct, 64
puncta, 62
tear film, 62
lagophthalmos, 171, 341
botulinum toxin injections, 304
laissez faire, 269, 271
advantages, 526, 528
disadvantages, 528
lamellar split and posterior lamellar
advancement, 99
laser resurfacing, 307
late implant exposure, 515
lateral canthal reconstruction, 278
lateral canthotomy, 574
lateral orbital wall, 51–2
lateral orbitotomy, 412–5
lateral periosteal flap, 240
lateral tarsorrhaphy, 189–90, 196–8
Le Fort fractures, 569, 570
Lemagne procedure, 168
lentigines, 216–7
levator aponeurosis advancement
procedure, 155–9
levator aponeurosis recession, 199–200

levator muscle resection, 159–162
Limberg rhomboid flap, 21
LJ tube, 474–5
local anesthesia, 3
local flaps, 271, 528–9
advancement flap, 21
rotation flap, 21
transposition flap, 21
lower eyelid island flap, 249
lower eyelid transconjunctival anterior
orbitotomy, 403–5
lower face muscles, 73
lower lid lymphedema, 560
lymphoma, 231
Lynch skin incision medial orbitotomy, 406–9

magnetic resonance angiography
(MRA), 373
magnetic resonance imaging (MRI), 371–2, 429
Malar mounds, 319
malignant disorders, 520
malignant eyelid tumors
basal cell carcinoma, 217–8
basal cell nevus syndrome, 218–9
goals in surgical management, 227
Kaposi's sarcoma, 224, 226
keratoacanthoma, 219–220
management of, 227
melanoma, 221, 223–4
Merkel cell tumor, 221
metastatic tumors, 224
mycosis fungoides, 224, 226
sebaceous gland carcinoma (SGC), 220–1
squamous cell carcinoma (SCC), 219
malleable retractor, 9
marginal injuries, 533, 540–41
marginal mandibular nerve, 45
marginal reflex distance-1 (MRD-1), 321
marginal reflex distance-2 (MRD-2), 321
maxillary sinuses, 69
mechanical ectropion, 132
mechanical ptosis, 147
medial canthal reconstruction
bilobed flap, 272
full-thickness skin grafting, 269
glabellar flap, 271, 272
laissez-faire, 269, 271
local flap, 271
median forehead flap, 272
rhomboid flap, 271–2, 273
medial canthoplasty, 133, 135, 198–9
medial orbital wall, 48–9
medial orbitotomy
Lynch skin incision, 406–9
transcaruncular, 411–2
transconjunctival, 409–11
medial palpebral arteries, 60
medial periosteal flap, 240–1
median forehead flap, 272
Medihoney®, 526
Medpor Titan, 556
melanocytic nevus, 214–6

melanoma
  classification, 221
  clinical features, 221, 223–4
  radiation, 231
  surgery, 230–1
  topical chemotherapeutic agents, 231
memory, 16
meningitis, 442
Merkel cell tumor, 221, 231
metastatic eyelid tumor, 231
metastatic tumors, 224
microcystic adnexal carcinoma, 231
middle turbinate, anatomical variations of,
    449–50
mid-face lift, 132
mid-face muscles, 73
midfacial fractures, 569
mid-forehead brow lift, 350–1
mild lower eyelid retraction, 341
milia, 207
Mohs' micrographic surgery, 227, 229–30
molluscum contagiosum, 207
monofilament sutures, 16
motor nerves
  abducens nerve, 60
  oculomotor nerve, 59
  trochlear nerve, 59–60
mucosa associated lymphoid tissue (MALT
    lymphoma), 388
mucous membrane graft, 517–9
  indications, 283
  postoperative care, 285
  surgical procedure, 283–5
müllerectomy
  anterior approach levator recession,
    183–5
  anterior approach Z-myotomy, 185–6
  corneal exposure management,
    199–200
  graded full-thickness anterior
    blepharotomy, 186
  posterior approach levator recession,
    181–2
  postoperative care, 181
  surgical procedure, 180–1
Müller's muscle, 38–9, 40
Müller's muscle resection, 152–4
multifilament sutures, 16
muscle
  lower face, 73
  mid-face, 73
  recession, 443
  trauma, 146
Mustardé cheek rotation flap, 243, 245–6,
    248, 249
myasthenia gravis, 140–1
mycosis fungoides, 224, 226
myogenic ptosis, 144
myotonic dystrophy, 144

nasal packing, 11
nasal septal cartilage graft
  postoperative care, 290
  surgical procedure, 289
nasociliary nerve, 56, 58

nasojugal flap, 253–4, 255
nasolacrimal duct ostium, 64
nasolacrimal duct probing, 453–5
naso-orbital fractures, 569
nausea, 548
negative vector, 327
nerve
  abducens, 60
  lacrimal, 59
  marginal mandibular, 45
  nasociliary, 56, 58
  oculomotor, 59
  ophthalmic, 55
  supraorbital, 55
  supratrochlear, 55
  trigeminal, 55–9
  trochlear, 59–60
  zygomatic, 59
neurogenic ptosis
  botulism, 143–4
  cerebral ptosis, 143
  Guillain–Barré syndrome, 143
  Horner's syndrome, 138–140
  myasthenia gravis, 140–1
  oculomotor nerve palsy, 137–8
  synkinetic ptosis, 142–3
neurosensory loss, 547
nevocellular nevus, 214–6
nevus of ota, 216
nodular melanoma, 223, 226
nonabsorbable sutures, 16
non-integrated implants, 480
non-malignant disorders, 520
non-specific orbital inflammatory disease,
    379–80
non-steroidal anti-inflammatory drug
    (NSAID) therapy, 489–90
nose
  nasal septum, 64–5
  paranasal sinuses
    ethmoidal sinuses, 67–8
    frontal sinuses, 67
    maxillary sinuses, 69
    sphenoidal sinuses, 68
  turbinates, 65, 67
Novafil, 17
Nylon, 17

ocular adnexa, 499
ocular motility, 547
ocular muscle surgery, 443
oculocardiac reflex, 341
oculodermal melanocytosis, 216
oculomotor nerve, 59
oculomotor nerve palsy, 137–8
oculopharyngeal muscular dystrophy, 146
oculosympathetic paresis, 138–140
ophthalmic artery, 60
ophthalmic nerve, 55
ophthalmologist, 192
ophthalmoplegia plus, 146
Opsite Flexifix® (Smith and Nephew), 283
optic canal, 53
optic nerve, 54–5
  glioma, 384

injuries, 572
oral propranolol, 383
orbicularis oculi muscle, 28–9, 44
orbit
  applied anatomy, 398
  extraconal space, 398
  intraconal space, 398
  subperiosteal space, 398
  sub-Tenon's space, 398
  surgery
    approaches, 397–8
    biopsy specimen, 402
    dissection, 401–2
    exposure, 401
    goal, 398
    hemostasis, 402–3
    illumination, 400–1
    imaging techniques, 400
    instrumentation, 400
    magnification, 400–1
    postoperative management, 417–8
    principles, 398–403
  surgical spaces, 398
  suspected pathology, 397–8
orbital and periocular arterial system, 60
  ethmoidal arteries, 61
  external carotid artery, 60
  infratrochlear artery, 60
  internal carotid artery, 60
  lacrimal artery, 60
  medial palpebral arteries, 60
  ophthalmic artery, 60
  supraorbital artery, 60
  supratrochlear artery, 60
orbital apex, 51
orbital cellulitis, 375, 443
  clinical features, 376
  complications, 379
  diagnosis of, 377
  etiology, 376
  management of, 377–9
orbital disorder
  degenerations and depositions, 395
  evaluation of, 362
  examination
    general physical examination, 366–7
    specific orbital examination,
      363–4, 366
  history of, 363
  laboratory investigations, 367
  orbital biopsy, 373–4
  orbital imaging, 367–73
  orbital inflammation, 375–80
  orbital tumors, 381–90
  pathophysiological orbital process, 362
  specific orbital inflammatory disease, 380
  structural disorders, 394–5
  vascular disorders, 390–4
orbital exenteration
  anesthesia, 522
  applied surgical anatomy, 522
  free flaps, 529
  local flaps, 528–9
  osseointegrated titanium implants, 529
  preoperative evaluation, 520

preoperative patient preparation, 520
prosthetic options, 529
split-thickness skin graft, 528
orbital floor, 49–51
orbital fractures
Le Fort fractures, 569, *570*
midfacial fractures, 569
naso-orbital fractures, 569
orbital roof fractures, 569, *570*
orbital hematoma, 491
orbital imaging, 367
arteriography, 373
computed tomography (CT), 369, 371
magnetic resonance angiography (MRA), 373
magnetic resonance imaging (MRI), 371–2
review of images, 373
ultrasonography (USG), 369
orbital implant
advantages, 479–80, 482
alternative implants, 483–5
buried integrated implants, 480–1
current orbital implants, 482
disadvantages, 482–3
exposed integrated implants, 481–2
extrusion of, 558
factors, 499
integrated implants, 480
non-integrated implants, 480
orbital wall blowout fractures, 556, 558
primary orbital implant, 480
rationale for implant use, 483
secondary orbital implant, 480
see also enucleation; evisceration
orbital inflammation
acute thyroid orbitopathy, 375
non-specific orbital inflammatory disease, 379–80
orbital cellulitis, 375–9
specific orbital inflammatory disease, 380
orbital ligaments, 73
orbital lymphoma, 385, 388
orbital margin, 46–8
orbital metastases, 388–9
orbital roof, 52–3
orbital roof fractures, 569, *570*
orbital septum, 29–32
orbital spaces
extraconal space, 54
intraconal space, 53–4
subperiosteal space, 54
sub-Tenon's space, 53
orbital structural disorders, 394–5
orbital tumors
capillary hemangioma, 382–4
cavernous hemangioma, 381–2
lacrimal gland tumors, 384–5
optic nerve glioma, 384
orbital lymphoma, 385, 388
orbital metastases, 388–9
rhabdomyosarcoma, 389
secondary orbital tumors, 389–90
sphenoid wing meningioma, 384
orbital vascular disorders

arteriovenous shunts, 390–1
lymphangiomas, 392, 394
orbital varices, 391–2
orbital vascular lesions, 390
orbital venous system
central retinal vein, 61
inferior ophthalmic vein, 61
superior ophthalmic vein, 61
supraorbital vein, 61
orbital wall blowout fractures
clinical evaluation, 548–550
clinical signs and symptoms, 547–8
complications, 558–9
diagnosis, 547
etiology, 547
management, 550–1
orbital implant materials, 556, 558
surgical management, 551–3
transconjunctival approach, 553–5
transcutaneous approach, 555–6
orbito-malar ligament, 318–9
orbitotomy
anterior
lower eyelid transconjunctival, 403–5
transcutaneous, 403
upper eyelid vertical split, 405–6
combined, 416
endoscopic, 415–6
lateral, 412–5
medial
Lynch skin incision, 406–9
transcaruncular, 411–2
transconjunctival, 409–11
transcranial
frontal craniotomy, 416–7
pterional craniotomy, 417
osseointegrated titanium implants, 529
over-sized implant, 491
oversized orbital implant, 515
oxymetazoline, 453

palpebral spring implantation, 202
Pang sutures, 172
paralytic ectropion, 132–3, 135
paranasal sinuses
ethmoidal sinuses, 67–8
frontal sinuses, 67
maxillary sinuses, 69
sphenoidal sinuses, 68
patient consultation
consultation facility, 300
patient selection for surgery, 301
pre-consultation, 300
surgeon consultation, 300–1
pericranium, 69
periocular flaps
eyelid defects not involving the eyelid margin, 254–5
fricke flap, 249–53
full thickness skin graft, 255, 274–7
nasojugal flap, 253–4, *255*
periocular incisions, *8*
periocular squamous cell carcinoma, 230
periocular tumors
basal cell carcinoma

cryotherapy, 229
irradiation, 228–9
Mohs' micrographic surgery, 229–30
photodynamic therapy, 230
surgical management of, 227–8
topical chemotherapeutic agents, 230
melanoma
radiation, 231
surgery, 230–1
topical chemotherapeutic agents, 231
periorbita, 53
periorbital sensory innervation, 55–9
periosteal flaps, 240
Perlane, 305
phakomatous choristoma, 207
photodynamic therapy (PDT), 230
pilomatrixoma, 212
pin cushion effect, 279
plasticity, 16
pleomorphic adenoma, 385
plexiform neurofibroma, 208–9
pliability, 16
polybutester, 17
polyester, 17
Polyglactin 910, 16
polypropylene, 17
postauricular skin, 279
post-enucleation socket syndrome (PESS), 136, 480, 499
posterior lamellar graft, 90–1
posterior lamellar granuloma, 174
posterior lamellar mucous membrane graft, 101–3
postoperative analgesia, 489
postoperative nausea and vomiting (PONV), 490
pre-aponeurotic fat pads, 33–5
preauricular skin, 279
pre-consultation, 300
preseptal cellulitis, 377
pretrichial forehead and brow lift, 359–60
primary chemotherapy, 388
primary mucinous carcinoma, 231
primary orbital implant, 480
probing of canaliculi, 448
procerus muscle, 44
Prolene, 17
proptosis, 548, 559
proxymethocaine, 3
pseudoptosis, 548
pterional transcranial craniotomy, 417
ptosis
botulinum toxin injections, 304
classification
pseudoptosis, 136–7
true ptosis, 137–147
complications of surgery
conjunctival prolapse, 173
diplopia, 175
exposure keratopathy, 171
extrusion/infection of frontalis suspension material, 174–5
eyelash ptosis, 173
eyelid contour defects, 171
hemorrhage, 175

ptosis (*Continued*)
  lagophthalmos, 171
  loss of eyelashes, 174
  over-correction, 170–1
  posterior lamellar granuloma, 174
  skin crease defects, 172
  suture exposure, 174
  under-correction, 169–170
  upper lid entropion/ectropion, 173
  patient assessment
    applied anatomy, 150
    examination, 147–150
    history, 147, *150*
  socket reconstruction, 512
  surgical procedures
    Fasanella–Servat procedure, 151–2
    frontalis suspension procedure, 163–8
    Lemagne procedure, 168
    levator aponeurosis advancement procedure, 155–9
    levator muscle resection, 159–162
    Müller's muscle resection, 152–4
    Whitnall's sling procedure, 162
puncta, 62
punctal atresia, 455–6
punctal ectropion, 113
punctal occlusion, 196
punctoplasty, 456
pure orbital blowout fracture, 547
pyoderma gangrenosum, 210
pyogenic granuloma, 209–10

radiation, 231
radiotherapy, 388
rare eyelid tumors, 224
rarer malignant eyelid tumors
  angiosarcoma, 231
  Kaposi's sarcoma, 231
  lymphoma, 231
  Merkel cell tumor, 231
  metastatic eyelid tumor, 231
  microcystic adnexal carcinoma, 231
  primary mucinous carcinoma, 231
redo external dacryocystorhinostomy, 464
regional anesthesia, 4
Restylan® fillers, 304
retaining ligaments, 70, *72*, 73
retraction, lower eyelid
  free tarsal graft spacer, 189
  hard palate graft spacer, 186–9
retractor advancement, lower eyelid
  lateral tarsal strip procedure, 83–5
  postoperative care, 84–5
  surgical procedure, 80–3
  wedge resection
    postoperative care, 89
    surgical procedure, 85–9
retractor, eyelid, 35–9
reverse cutting needles, 15
rhabdomyosarcoma, 389
rhomboid flap, 271–2, *273*
rib grafts, 297
ring handle needle holders, 6

Ritleng stent, 453
rotation flap, 21

scarring, 361
sclerosing agents, 394
sebaceous adenoma, 212–3
sebaceous cyst, 212
sebaceous gland carcinoma (SGC), 230
  clinical features, 220
  diagnosis of, 220–1
  prognostic factors, 220
seborrhoeic keratosis, 205
secondary orbital implant, 480
  orbital implants of, 499–500
  procedure, 502
secondary orbital tumors, 389–90
second-degree burn, 544
sedation, 3
semicircular rotation flap, 235, 259
sensory loss, 342
sensory nerve trauma, 360
Sewall retractor, 9
sharp trauma, 531
silicone rod cerclage, 202
silk, 17
simple acrylic sphere implant, 483
simple silicone sphere implant, 483
skin crease
  defects, 172
  upper eyelid, 341–2
skin graft, 130, 279, *282*
  cicatricial ectropion, 130
  full-thickness
    vs split-thickness, 279
    donor sites of, 279
    postoperative care, 281
    surgical procedure, 279–81
  split-thickness
    vs full-thickness, 279
    postoperative care, 283
    surgical procedure, 281–3
skin incisions, 7
skin suturing techniques, 18–19
skin–muscle flap, *265*
sliding tarsoconjunctival flap, 257–9
socket
  contracture
    fornix-deepening sutures, 517–9
    management of, 515–7
    mild, 517
    moderate, 517
    mucous membrane graft, 517–9
    severe, 519
  ocular adnexa, 499
  patient evaluation, 499
  preoperative preparation, 501–2
  reconstruction
    dermis fat graft, 505, 507
    fornix deepening sutures, 513
    inferior fornix shallowing, 512–3
    lower eyelid fascial sling, 510–12
    lower eyelid laxity, 510
    orbital implant complications, 513–5
    ptosis, 512

residual orbital volume deficiency correction, 507–8
  spherical implant, 502–5
  structural fat grafting, 509–10
  subperiosteal orbital implant, 508–9
soft tissue expander, *253*
soft tissue expansion, 132
specific orbital inflammatory disease
  granulomatous disorders, 380
  idiopathic sclerosing inflammation, 380
  vasculitides, 380
sphenoid wing meningioma, 384
sphenoidal sinuses, 68
spherical implant, 502–5
split-thickness skin graft, 528
  vs full-thickness skin graft, 279
  postoperative care, 283
  surgical procedure, 281–3
spring handle needle holders, 6
squamous cell carcinoma (SCC), 219, 230
Stallard–Wright lateral orbitotomy, 412–5
staples, 17–18
structural fat grafting, 291–2
  blepharoplasty, 331
  complications, 309
  donor site selection, 309
  indications, 292, 309
  postoperative care, 294–5
  socket reconstruction, 509–10
  surgical procedure, 292–4
structural lesions, 384
subcutaneous emphysema, 547
sub-orbicularis oculi muscle fat (SOOF) lift, 331
subperiosteal orbital implant, 508–9
subperiosteal orbital space, 54
sub-Tenon's orbital space, 53
subtotal exenteration, 526
sump syndrome, 464
superficial muscles, 73
superficial musculoaponeurotic system (SMAS), 70
superficial spreading melanoma, 223
superior ophthalmic vein, 61
supraclavicular fossa skin, 130
supraorbital artery, 60
supraorbital nerve, 55
supraorbital vein, 61
supratrochlear artery, 60
supratrochlear nerve, 55
surgeon consultation, 300–1
surgical excision, 107–9
surgical instruments
  artery clips, 6
  Colorado needle, 5
  endoscopic brow lift instrument, *5*
  enucleation scissors, 6
  external DCR, *4*
  spring handle needle holders, 6
  Valley Lab diathermy machine, *5*
surgical principles
  anesthesia selection, 2–4
  correct surgical site marking and allergy check, 6

documentation, 1–2
hemostasis
  cautery, 13
  instrumentation, 13
  nasal packing, 11
  postoperative, 14
  preoperative evaluation, 11
  preoperative injection, 11
  suction, 11–13
  topical hemostatic agents, 13–14
postoperative care, 23–27
postoperative pain management, 22
preoperative patient evaluation, 1
preparation and draping of patient, 6
selection of surgical procedure, 2
surgical incision and exposure, 6–10
surgical instrumentation, 4–6
surgical planning and communication, 2
wound closure
  dog-ear deformity, 21–22
  flap techniques, 19–21
  skin suturing techniques, 18–19
  suture materials, 16–18
  suture needles, 14–15
surgical tapes, 18
Surgicel, 13
sutures
  absorbable, 16
  everting, 79–80, *81*
  exposure, 174
  Frost, 26
  materials, 16–18
  monofilament, 16
  multifilament, 16
  needles, 14–15
  nonabsorbable, 16
  Pang, 172
  percutaneous, *19*
  running subcuticular, 18–19
  vertical mattress, 19, *20*
switch flap, 266–9
synkinetic ptosis, 142–3
synthetic implants, 560
synthetic multifilamentous
  materials, 16
syringoma, 212

Taper needles, 15
tarsal ectropion, 126, 128–9
tarsal plates, 32–3
tarsal wedge excision, 96, 98
tear film, 62
tear trough injections
  complications, 306–7
  contraindications, 305
  procedure, 306
temporal eyebrow lift, 351–2
temporalis fascia graft
  indications, 296
  surgical technique, 296–7
temporalis fascia transfer, 202
temporary lower eyelid ectropion, 341
temporary suture tarsorrhaphy, 196
tenzel flap, 235
terminal tarsal rotation, 99–101

thermal burn, 544
third nerve palsy, 137–8
third-degree burn, 544
three-snip punctoplasty, 456
thrombin, 13
thyroid eye disease
  bony orbital decompression
    bicoronal flap approach, 436
    lateral canthal, 436
    lateral orbitotomy, 436
    lower eyelid approach, 435–6
    medial canthal skin incision, 436
    nasal endoscopic approach, 434–5
    transantral approach, 436
    transcaruncular approach, 436
    upper eyelid incision, 436
  classification of severity of, 428
  clinical presentation, 421–2
  clinical signs, 422–6
  clinical symptoms, 422
  differential diagnosis, 429–30
    increasing orbital volume, 434
    medical management, 432
    orbital fat removal, 433–4
    surgical management, 432–3
    surgical orbital decompression, 433
  epidemiology, 420–1
  orbital imaging
    computerized tomography, 428–9
    magnetic resonance imaging, 429
    ultrasound, 429
  pathogenesis, 419
  pathology, 419
  pathophysiology, 419–20
  patient evaluation, 426–8
  surgical approach
    postoperative management, 441
    potential complications, 441–2
    preoperative preparation, 436
    surgical technique, 436–41
thyroid-related eyelid retraction
  blepharoplasty, 190–1
  lateral tarsorrhaphy, 189–190
  lower eyelid retraction
    free tarsal graft spacer, 189
    hard palate graft spacer, 186–9
  orbital decompression *vs.* eyelid surgery,
    178–9
  patient evaluation, 177
  surgical intervention, 177
  upper eyelid retraction
    anterior approach levator recession,
     183–5
    anterior approach Z-myotomy, 185–6
    graded full-thickness anterior
     blepharotomy, 186
    müllerectomy, 180–1
    posterior approach levator recession,
     181–2
thyroid-related orbitopathy, 362, 375
time-resolved imaging of contrast kinetics
  (TRICKS), 373
Tisseel®, 13, 394
tissue adhesives, 18
topical anesthesia, 3

topical antibiotic ointment, 26
topical chemotherapeutic agents, 230–1
topical cocaine, 3
topical hemostatic agents, 13–14
total exenteration, 522, 524–6
transblepharoplasty browpexy, 352–3
transblepharoplasty endotine brow lift,
  353–5
transcaruncular medial orbitotomy,
  411–2
transconjunctival blepharoplasty
  postoperative care, 338–40
  surgical procedure, 335–8
transconjunctival medial orbitotomy,
  409–11
transcranial orbitotomy
  frontal craniotomy, 416–7
  pterional craniotomy, 417
transcutaneous anterior orbitotomy, 403
transcutaneous blepharoplasty
  with fat debulking, 334–5
  postoperative care, 331
  surgical procedure, 328–31
transposition flap, 21
trauma, eyelid
  bites, 531
  blunt trauma, 531
  injury mechanism, 531
  management decisions, 535
  patient evaluation, 532–5
  sharp trauma, 531
  surgical management
    extra marginal injuries, 541, 543
    lacrimal drainage system wounds,
     536–8, 540
    marginal injuries, 540–41
    periocular laceration repair
     sequence, 536
    wound decontamination, 535–6
traumatic optic neuropathy, 572
trichiasis, 106, *107*
trichoepithelioma, 213–4
tricholemmal cyst, 212
tricholemmoma, 213
trigeminal nerve
  maxillary divisions of, 59
  ophthalmic division of, 55–9
trochlear nerve, 59–60
true ptosis
  aponeurotic, 146
  mechanical, 147
  myogenic, 144–6
  neurogenic, 137–144
true retaining ligaments, 318
turbinates, 65, 67

ultrasonography (USG), 369
ultrasound, 429
universal implant, 483
upper eyelid skin, 130
upper eyelid sulcus deformity, 548
upper eyelid tarsal graft
  indications, 286
  postoperative care, 287
  surgical procedure, 286–7

upper eyelid vertical split anterior
    orbitotomy, 405–6
upper inner arm skin, 130
upper lid auricular cartilage graft, 94
upper lid tarsoconjunctival pedicle flap,
    235–40

Valley Lab diathermy machine, *5*
valve of Hasner, 64
valve of Rosenmüller, 64
varix, 211
vasculitides, 380
verruca vulgaris, 207
Vicryl Rapide, 16
vomiting, 548
V–Y flap, 271

wedge resection, lower eyelid
    postoperative care, 89
    surgical procedure, 85–9
Wegener's granulomatosis, 380
Whitnall's ligament, 36, *37*
Whitnall's sling procedure, 162
World Health Organization (WHO), 388
wound care, postoperative, 26
wound closure
    dog-ear deformity, 21–22
    flap techniques, 19–21
    skin suturing techniques, 18–19
    suture materials, 16–18
    suture needles, 14–15
wound decontamination, 535–6
Wright's retractor, 9, *401*

xanthelasma, 210
xanthoma, 210

Z-plasty, 21, *24*
zygomatic complex fracture
    clinical signs, 563
    diagnosis, 563
    direct approach, 564
    etiology, 563
    Gillies temporal approach,
        563, 565
zygomatic facial nerve, 44
zygomatic ligaments, 73
zygomatic nerve, 59
zygomatic retaining ligament,
    318